PROTECTIVE STRATEGIES FOR NEURODEGENERATIVE DISEASES

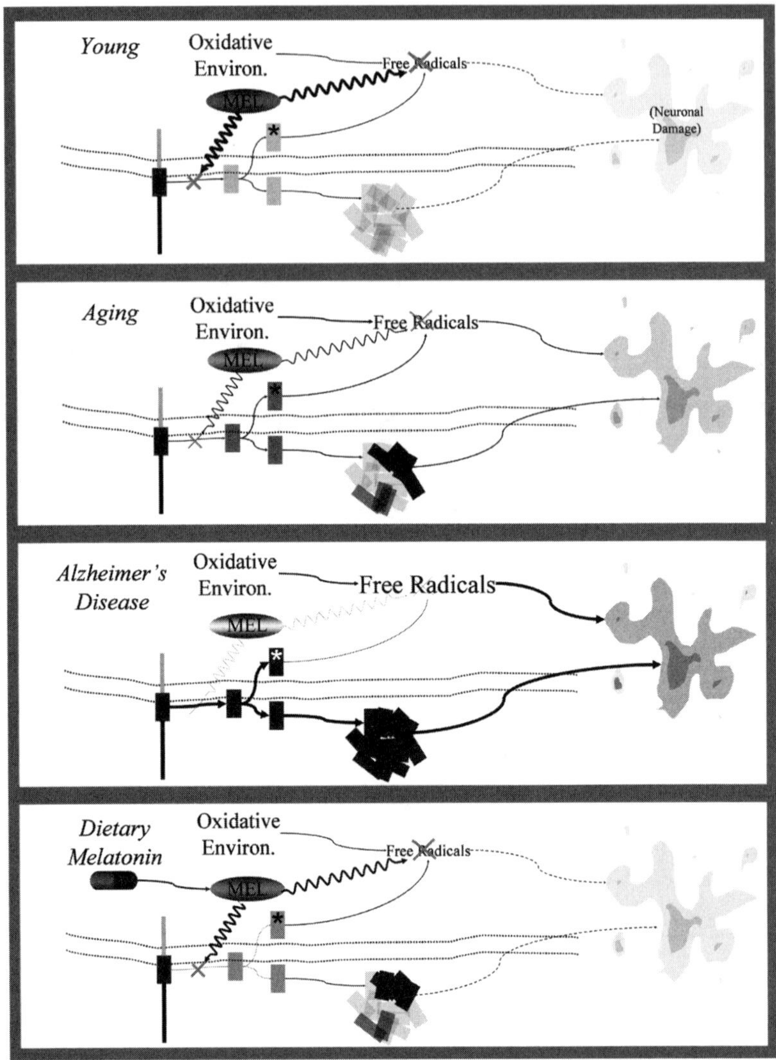

Frontispiece [in color online]: Schematic of putative effects of melatonin and oral melatonin supplementation on Alzheimer's disease (AD)–related nerve cell damage. MEL in ellipse represents endogenous melatonin; intensity of color represents tissue levels of the hormone. Small blue rectangles are the AD–associated amyloid β peptide (Aβ). Light intensity indicates soluble form and lack of aggregation. Deep color indicates formation into amyloid plaque. In young individuals, melatonin levels are sufficient to prevent toxic Aβ formation and formation of highly active Aβ* radicals. In addition, melatonin counteracts free radicals in general. Inhibition indicated with wavy arrows, intensity of arrows indicating level of inhibition. Lack of amyloid plaque and lower oxidation result in low levels of neuronal damage. Melatonin levels decrease as an individual ages, permitting more Aβ formation and formation of some amyloid plaque. In addition, oxidative species, such as free radicals, are less inhibited. More neuronal damage results. In Alzheimer's disease, melatonin levels are severely increased, permitting widespread formation of amyloid plaque, generation of high levels of Aβ* radicals and other oxidative species, and resulting in high levels of neuronal degeneration. Oral/dietary supplementation with melatonin increases tissue melatonin levels to age-normal or even higher amounts, inhibiting (and potentially reversing) amyloid plaque formation and free radical damage, thereby reducing neuronal damage. Figure based on the work in this volume by Lahiri and colleagues (pp. 216–230).

ANNALS OF THE NEW YORK ACADEMY OF SCIENCES
Volume 1035

PROTECTIVE STRATEGIES FOR NEURODEGENERATIVE DISEASES

Edited by Debomoy K. Lahiri

The New York Academy of Sciences
New York, New York
2004

Library of Congress Cataloging-in-Publication Data

Protective strategies for neurodegenerative diseases / edited by Debomoy K. Lahiri.
   p.; cm. — (Annals of the New York Academy of Sciences; v. 1035)
 Includes bibliographical references and index.
 ISBN 1-57331-529-X (cloth: alk. paper) — ISBN 1-57331-530-3 (pbk.: alk. paper)
 1. Nervous system—Degeneration—Prevention—Congresses.
 [DNLM: 1. Neurodegenerative Diseases—drug therapy. 2. Neurodegenerative
Diseases—prevention & control. 3. Anti-Inflammatory Agents—therapeutic use.
4. Antioxidants—therapeutic use. 5. Models, Animal. 6. Neuroprotective
Agents—therapeutic use. WL 359 P967 2004] I. Lahiri, Debomoy K. II. Series.
 Q11.N5 vol. 1035
 [RC394.D35]
 500 s—dc22
 [616.8

                                                                                  2004027338

ANNALS OF THE NEW YORK ACADEMY OF SCIENCES
Volume 1035
December 2004

PROTECTIVE STRATEGIES FOR NEURODEGENERATIVE DISEASES

Editor
DEBOMOY K. LAHIRI

Advisory Panel
STEPHEN C. BONDY AND JOE MARWAH

This volume is the result of the **Seventh International Conference on Protective Strategies for Neurodegenerative Diseases**, which was held August 14–18, 2004, at the University of British Columbia in Vancouver, British Columbia, Canada.

CONTENTS

Preface: Current Research Trend on Neurodegeneration, Neuroinflammation, and Neuroprotection. *By* DEBOMOY K. LAHIRI ix

Part I. Alzheimer's Disease

Targeting Amyloid-Degrading Enzymes as Therapeutic Strategies in Neurodegeneration. *By* ANTHONY J. TURNER, LILIA FISK, AND NATALIA N. NALIVAEVA 1

Effect of Hypoxia/Ischemia and Hypoxic Preconditioning/Reperfusion on Expression of Some Amyloid-Degrading Enzymes. *By* NATALIA N. NALIVAEVA, LILIA FISK, EKATERINA G. KOCHKINA, SVETLANA A. PLESNEVA, IGOR A. ZHURAVIN, EVA BABUSIKOVA, DUSAN DOBROTA, AND ANTHONY J. TURNER 21

The Integrated Role of Desferrioxamine and Phenserine Targeted to an Iron-Responsive Element in the APP-mRNA 5′-Untranslated Region. *By* AMANDA VENTI, TONY GIORDANO, PAUL EDER, ASHLEY I. BUSH, DEBOMOY K. LAHIRI, NIGEL H. GREIG, AND JACK T. ROGERS 34

BACE1 Gene Expression and Protein Degradation. *By* WEIHUI ZHOU, HONG QING, YIGANG TONG, AND WEIHONG SONG 49

Part II. Antioxidants and NSAIDs as Neuroprotective Strategies

NSAID and Antioxidant Prevention of Alzheimer's Disease: Lessons from *In Vitro* and Animal Models. *By* GREG M. COLE, TAKASHI MORIHARA, GISELLE P. LIM, FUSHENG YANG, AYNUN BEGUM, AND SALLY A. FRAUTSCHY 68

Microglia as a Potential Bridge between the Amyloid β-Peptide and Tau. *By* MASASHI KITAZAWA, TRITIA R. YAMASAKI, AND FRANK M. LaFERLA 85

Part III. Inflammation and Neurodegenerative Diseases

Inflammation and the Degenerative Diseases of Aging. *By* PATRICK L. MCGEER AND EDITH G. MCGEER 104

Inflammation, Neurodegenerative Diseases, and Environmental Exposures. *By* AREZOO CAMPBELL 117

Induction of Serine Racemase by Inflammatory Stimuli Is Dependent on AP-1. *By* SHENGZHOU WU AND STEVEN W. BARGER 133

Part IV. Complement and Neurodegenerative Diseases

Neuroprotection from Complement-Mediated Inflammatory Damage. *By* AMOD P. KULKARNI, LAURIE A. KELLAWAY, DEBOMOY K. LAHIRI, AND GIRISH J. KOTWAL 147

Vaccinia Virus Complement Control Protein Reduces Inflammation and Improves Spinal Cord Integrity Following Spinal Cord Injury. *By* DAVID N. REYNOLDS, SCOTT A. SMITH, YI P. ZHANG, QIU MENGSHENG, DEBOMOY K. LAHIRI, DANTE J. MORASSUTTI, CHRISTOPHER B. SHIELDS, AND GIRISH J. KOTWAL 165

Part V. Melatonin and Neuroprotection

Melatonin Relieves the Neural Oxidative Burden that Contributes to Dementias. *By* RUSSEL J. REITER, DUN-XIAN TAN, AND MIGUEL A. PAPPOLLA 179

Retardation of Brain Aging by Chronic Treatment with Melatonin. *By* S. C. BONDY, D. K. LAHIRI, V. M. PERREAU, K. Z. SHARMAN, A. CAMPBELL, J. ZHOU, AND E. H. SHARMAN 197

Melatonin, Metals, and Gene Expression: Implications in Aging and Neurodegenerative Disorders. *By* DEBOMOY K. LAHIRI, DEMAO CHEN, PREETI LAHIRI, JACK T. ROGERS, NIGEL H. GREIG, AND STEPHEN BONDY 216

Part VI. Parkinson's Disease

The Degeneration of Dopamine Neurons in Parkinson's Disease: Insights from Embryology and Evolution of the Mesostriatocortical System. *By* PHILIPPE VERNIER, FREDERIC MORET, SOPHIE CALLIER, MARINA SNAPYAN, CHRISTOPHE WERSINGER, AND ANITA SIDHU 231

The Role of α-Synuclein in Both Neuroprotection and Neurodegeneration.
    By ANITA SIDHU, CHRISTOPHE WERSINGER, CHARBEL E-H. MOUSSA,
    AND PHILIPPE VERNIER   250

Blockade of PKCδ Proteolytic Activation by Loss of Function Mutants
    Rescues Mesencephalic Dopaminergic Neurons from Methylcyclo-
    pentadienyl Manganese Tricarbonyl (MMT)–Induced Apoptotic Cell
    Death. *By* V. ANANTHARAM, M. KITAZAWA, C. LATCHOUMYCANDANE,
    A. KANTHASAMY, AND A. G. KANTHASAMY   271

Part VII. Therapeutic Strategies and Pharmacological Manipulation

New Therapeutic Strategies and Drug Candidates for Neurodegenerative
    Diseases: p53 and TNF-α Inhibitors, and GLP-1 Receptor Agonists.
    By NIGEL H. GREIG, MARK P. MATTSON, TRACYANN PERRY, SIC L.
    CHAN, TONY GIORDANO, KUMAR SAMBAMURTI, JACK T. ROGERS,
    HAIM OVADIA, AND DEBOMOY K. LAHIRI   290

Nicotinic Receptor Modulation for Neuroprotection and Enhancement of
    Functional Recovery Following Brain Injury or Disease. *By* J. R. PAULY,
    C. M. CHARRIEZ, M. V. GUSEVA, AND S. W. SCHEFF.   316

Pharmacological Manipulation of Brain Kynurenine Metabolism.
    By JOHN F. REINHARD, JR.   335

Cooperative Ideas about Cooperative Strategies. *By* STEVEN W. BARGER   350

Index of Contributors   355

Financial assistance was received from:

• NATIONAL INSTITUTES OF HEALTH
• VANCOUVER BIOMEDICAL HEALTH RESEARCH FOUNDATION

Preface: Current Research Trend on Neurodegeneration, Neuroinflammation, and Neuroprotection

DEBOMOY K. LAHIRI

*Departments of Psychiatry and of Medical and Molecular Genetics,
Institute of Psychiatric Research, Indiana University School of Medicine,
Indianapolis, Indiana 46202, USA*

The Seventh International Conference on Protective Strategies for Neurodegenerative Diseases was held on August 14–18, 2004, at the University of British Columbia, Vancouver, in Canada. For the seventh consecutive year, the conference was organized by selected scientists from academia and industry and supported by the Vancouver BioMedical Health Research Foundation and the National Institutes of Health. The focus of this year's conference was on various protective and therapeutic strategies for neurodegenerative disorders, such as Alzheimer's disease (AD) and Parkinson's disease (PD). The conference discussed how both the progression of neurodegenerative processes and their potential amelioration may be influenced by a variety of intrinsic and exogenous factors. Such factors included anti-inflammatory agents, melatonin, metals, growth factors, and dietary supplements. The goal of this meeting was to bring together a critical mass of scientists to discuss research findings involving both nutritional and pharmacological strategies for slowing of normal brain aging and its pathological variants, such as AD and PD. The speakers were selected because of their significant contributions and expertise in the field. The expectation was that new concepts concerning neurodegenerative disease and its mitigation would emerge. This goal was met as is apparent from the papers in this volume of the *Annals of the New York Academy of Sciences* series.

The presentations covered a rapidly growing field of neurodegeneration, inflammation, neuroprotection, and therapeutic strategies. The book is divided into seven discrete sections based on the following themes, although there are some overarching concepts across all the papers and sections. The first section deals with AD, with emphasis on the role of amyloid peptides. The second section discusses the potential of antioxidants and nonsteroidal anti-inflammatory drugs (NSAIDs) as neuroprotective agents. The third section concerns the inflammatory pathways that are common to most of the neurodegenerative diseases. The fourth section highlights the role of complement pathway in neurodegenerative disorders. The fifth section discusses the neuroprotective properties of melatonin. The sixth section provides insight into PD, with an emphasis on the role of dopaminergic neurons and the α-synuclein protein.

Address for correspondence: Debomoy K. Lahiri, Ph.D., Indiana University School of Medicine, 791 Union Drive, Indianapolis, IN 46202. Voice: 317-274-2706; fax: 317-274-1365.
dlahiri@iupui.edu

Ann. N.Y. Acad. Sci. 1035: ix–xiii (2004). © 2004 New York Academy of Sciences.
doi: 10.1196/annals.1332.022

The final section summarizes potentially therapeutic strategies in the treatment of these diseases. Highlights of the conference are summarized below.

One of the major hallmarks of AD is brain deposition of the amyloid β-peptide (Aβ), which results from proteolysis of the beta-amyloid precursor protein (APP) by β- and γ-secretases. Aβ is regarded by many as a central point of neurodegeneration leading to AD. At least three major aspects concerning AD were discussed. The first issue was related to the amyloid-degrading enzymes that cleave Aβ itself, thus preventing the accumulation of potentially toxic Aβ peptides. The second aspect was related to lowering the precursor protein, APP, as this ultimately gives rise to Aβ peptides. The final presentation was related to the β-secretase or β-APP-cleaving enzyme (BACE) that cleaves APP to Aβ peptides, resulting in their subsequent oligomerization and deposition into senile plaques.

Turner and colleagues discussed the merits of targeting amyloid-degrading enzymes as therapeutic strategies in neurodegeneration. They summarized the role of three major molecules in amyloid turnover: neprilysin (NEP), endothelin converting enzyme (ECE), and insulin-degrading enzyme (IDE), all of which are zinc metallo-peptidases. They reported that reduction in expression levels of some of these proteases in aging might predispose to the development of AD. Thus, increasing their levels by gene delivery or pharmacological means could be neuroprotective. In a related topic, Nalivaeva and coworkers discussed the effect of hypoxia/ischemia on expression of some amyloid-degrading enzymes. This work is relevant because both ischemia and hypoxia have been shown to play key roles in AD pathogenesis; however, their exact role in the disease process, such as on APP metabolism, is poorly understood. Studies from the authors' laboratory suggest that oxygen deprivation results in increased APP expression and decreased β-secretase activity in the brain. There is also a decrease in the expression of NEP and ECE-1 after hypoxia. Notably, it was suggested that preconditioning to mild hypoxia could have a neuroprotective effect restoring, in particular, APP, β-secretase, NEP, and ECE-1 to their control values.

In the context of downregulation of APP levels, Venti and colleagues discussed the role of the APP-mRNA 5′-untranslated region (5′UTR) on APP expression, particularly that of an iron-responsive element (IRE). The authors reported an RNA-based screen for small APP 5′UTR binding molecules to identify leads that limit APP translation and thereby Aβ peptide production. They showed that the APP 5′UTR directed drugs, desferrioxamine (Fe3+ chelator), tetrathiolmobdylate (Cu2+ chelator), and dimercaptopropanol (Pb2+, Hg2+ chelator), each suppressed APP holoprotein expression (and lowered Aβ peptide secretion). This suppression was also reported using a novel anticholinesterase drug, phenserine. Thus, it provided "proof of concept" for this strategy to target the APP 5′UTR sequence to identify "anti-amyloid" drugs. The approach on regulating secretase enzymes, such as BACE, is also gaining considerable attention. BACE1, the major -secretase involved in cleaving APP, has been identified as a type 1 membrane–associated aspartyl protease. Zhou and colleagues described BACE1 gene expression and protein degradation. BACE1 gene expression is controlled by a TATA-less promoter and regulated by the transcription factor Sp1, which plays an important role in regulation of BACE1 to process APP generating Aβ. They also reported that BACE1 protein is ubiquitinated and that the degradation of BACE1 proteins and APP processing are regulated by the ubiquitin-proteasome pathway.

Cole and colleagues presented new data on the utility of NSAIDs and antioxidants in preventing AD. They described conventional and unconventional NSAIDs, antioxidants, and combined approaches in cell culture and animal models for AD, including aging. They also showed that the unconventional NSAID/antioxidant curcumin is effective in lowering oxidative damage, cognitive deficits, synaptic marker loss, and amyloid burden. Curcumin has immunomodulatory properties, simultaneously inhibiting cytokine and microglial activation indices related to neurotoxicity. In a parallel study, Kitazawa and colleagues discussed inflammation as a critical component of AD pathogenesis. This involves activation of both microglia and astrocytes. Microglia may act as a bridge between the $A\beta$ peptide and tau. They reviewed the interesting molecular mechanisms of inflammatory responses in AD brain, animal models, and current therapies using NSAIDs, antioxidants, and immunotherapy as neuroprotective strategies for AD.

In addition to the amyloid pathway, inflammatory processes were another area of focus in this conference. Both oxidative damage and inflammation are elevated in brains of AD patients, but their pathogenic significance remains unclear.

McGeer and McGeer enlightened how chronic inflammation is associated with a broad spectrum of neurodegenerative diseases of aging, including amyotrophic lateral sclerosis, AD, and PD. They pointed out that inflammation is a two-edged sword; at low levels it promotes healing, but at high, sustained levels it can seriously damage host tissue. This latter phenomenon was described as autotoxicity so as to distinguish it from autoimmunity. Analysis of mRNA levels of inflammatory mediators suggests that the intensity of inflammation is considerably higher in AD hippocampus and in PD substantia nigra than in osteoarthritic joints. Full therapeutic doses of NSAIDs, or combinations of anti-inflammatory agents, may be needed to achieve neurological benefits.

Campbell stressed the point that the etiology of neurodegenerative disorders is multifactorial and consists of interactions among aging, environmental factors, and genetic predisposition. Innate immune responses in the CNS may be enhanced by environmental exposures leading to neurodegeneration. Environmental factors, such as aluminum, lipopolysaccharide (LPS), and particulate matter present in air pollution, can trigger inflammatory events in the CNS. These factors may enhance existing, age-related inflammation in the CNS and thus accelerate neuronal senescence.

Wu and Barger showed that proinflammatory stimuli utilize a signal transduction pathway, culminating in AP-1 transcription factor activation to induce expression of serine racemase (SRace). The interest in this enzyme is because inflammatory stimuli such as $A\beta$ could elevate steady-state mRNA levels for SRace, perhaps leading to inappropriate glutamatergic stimulation under conditions of inflammation. However, the mechanism is not clearly understood.

Kulkarni and colleagues discussed strategies of neuroprotection from complement-mediated inflammatory damage. Complement plays an important role in the etiology of most of the neuroinflammatory disorders. Neuroprotective agents, such as free radical scavengers, could potentially modulate inflammation. In this context, a multifunctional protein, vaccinia virus complement control protein (VCP), may play a pivotal role in the treatment of several neuroinflammatory disorders. VCP is known to inhibit cytokines and chemokines and both complement pathways that are involved in inflammation. Following the same theme, Reynolds and colleagues showed that VCP reduces inflammation, which results in improvement of the spinal cord integrity following spinal cord injury. Thus, complement inhibitors such as VCP can serve as neuroprotective agents in inflammation associated with several neurodegenerative disorders.

The role of melatonin as a potentially neuroprotective agent was the main theme of one section of the conference. Reiter and colleagues summarized recent research on the beneficial actions of melatonin within the CNS. They reported that melatonin treatment may relieve the neural oxidative burden associated with dementias. They proposed that multiple functions of melatonin and its metabolites as ubiquitously acting direct free radical scavengers and indirect antioxidants may provide significant neural protection against aging and other neurodegenerative disorders.

Bondy and colleagues emphasized the issue of functional decline during aging. Slowing the process of functional decline in the aging brain is relevant to both non-pathological senescence and a broad range of neurodegenerative diseases. One of the ideas supported by their data is that supplementation with dietary melatonin may ameliorate both oxidative damage and inflammatory activity associated with senescence.

In parallel to this work, Lahiri and colleagues integrated the role of melatonin, metal ions, and gene expression in aging and neurodegenerative disorders. Melatonin can interact with metals and, in some cases, neutralizes their toxic effects. Levels of melatonin decrease with aging in mice, and its dietary supplementation results in a significant rise in levels of melatonin in different tissues. Elevated brain melatonin levels were associated with a significant reduction in levels of toxic cortical Aβ of both 40- and 42-amino-acid forms. Dietary melatonin supplementation may slow the neurodegenerative changes associated with brain aging, and the depletion of melatonin in the brain of aging mice may, in part, account for these undesirable changes.

In addition to AD, several presentations are related to PD, which is, to a large extent, specific to the human species. Vernier and colleagues described some insights on the degeneration of dopamine neurons in PD from the perspective of ontogeny and phylogeny of the mesostriatocortical system. Studying from the evolutionary context, they suggested that the peculiar phenotype of the dopamine mesencephalic neurons, which has been selected during vertebrate evolution and reshaped in the human lineage, may make these neurons particularly susceptible to oxidative stress and, thus, to the specific changes associated with PD. Regarding the mechanistic aspect of PD, Sidhu and colleagues reviewed the role of α-synuclein in both neuro-protection and neurodegeneration. The primary property of the wild-type form of this protein may be neuroprotection and this may get lost in familial PD-linked mutations. Disruption of the neuroprotective effects of α-synuclein could initiate the observed neurotoxicity of α-synuclein in dopaminergic neurons leading to PD. Another important theme discussed is that environmental factors also play a great role in PD. Anantharam and colleagues focused on the molecular mechanism of environmental toxins in neurodegeneration. They showed that a blockade of protein kinase C-delta (PKCδ) proteolytic activation rescues mesencephalic dopaminergic neurons from MMT-induced apoptotic cell death. This suggests that PKCδ may serve as an attractive therapeutic target in Parkinson-related neurological diseases.

Regarding therapeutic interventions, Greig and colleagues outlined new strategies and drug candidates for neurodegenerative diseases. Neurodegenerative disorders may result from the aberrant action of several biochemical pathways and targets. To retard the neurodegenerative process, they proposed specific targets important within the pathological cascade. Such targets include the cytokine, such as TNF-α; the intracellular protein and transcription factor, p53; and the glucagon-like peptide-1 (GLP-1) receptor. These sites offer testable drug targets for different neurodegenerative disorders.

Pauly and colleagues described how alteration of nicotinic receptor modulation could be utilized for neuroprotection and enhancement of functional recovery following brain injury. Animal and human studies that investigated possible neuroprotective actions of nicotine and other nicotinic receptor agents were reviewed. In a similar approach, Reinhard proposed pharmacological manipulation of brain kynurenine metabolism. Inhibition of kynurenine metabolism may allow the amino acid to be converted to kynurenic acid, a neuroprotective antagonist of excitatory amino acid receptors. Finally, Barger summarized the discussion on several cooperative ideas, particularly on intellectual property issue, current research funding status, and limitations of public and private funding.

The foregoing description is merely a glimpse of what was presented in this meeting and cannot do full justice to the breadth of the sessions and program in what was a truly exciting gathering. The original aim of the conference was to identify the "points of convergence" of a variety of age-related and neurodegenerative diseases. To achieve this goal, scientists discussed their recent data from all aspects in order to generate novel strategies for future research and therapy. This was the unique and productive part of the meeting. The consensus in the meeting was that all these current research efforts should lead to a better understanding of the pathobiochemical processes that occur in neurodegenerative brains in order to effectively develop novel drug targets to prevent their occurrence. On that positive note, the next meeting to be held in Vancouver in August 2005 is eagerly anticipated.

I thank the Vancouver BioMedical Health Research Foundation and the National Institutes of Health for their financial support and the New York Academy of Sciences for publishing the proceedings. I would like to extend my special thanks to Stephen Bondy and Joe Marwah for their invaluable advice and support. I also thank Tapati Lahiri for her help and encouragement in this project. Finally, I express a word of gratitude to the University of British Columbia for providing an excellent venue for the meeting.

Targeting Amyloid-Degrading Enzymes as Therapeutic Strategies in Neurodegeneration

ANTHONY J. TURNER, LILIA FISK, AND NATALIA N. NALIVAEVA

Proteolysis Research Group, School of Biochemistry and Microbiology, University of Leeds, Leeds LS2 9JT, United Kingdom

ABSTRACT: The levels of amyloid β-peptides (Aβ) in the brain represent a dynamic equilibrium state as a result of their biosynthesis from the amyloid precursor protein (APP) by β- and γ-secretases, their degradation by a team of amyloid-degrading enzymes, their subsequent oligomerization, and deposition into senile plaques. While most therapeutic attention has focused on developing inhibitors of secretases to prevent Aβ formation, enhancing the rate of Aβ degradation represents an alternative and viable strategy. Current evidence both *in vivo* and *in vitro* suggests that there are three major players in amyloid turnover: neprilysin, endothelin converting enzyme(s), and insulin-degrading enzyme, all of which are zinc metallopeptidases. Other proteases have also been implicated in amyloid metabolism, including angiotensin-converting enzyme, and plasmin but for these the evidence is less compelling. Neprilysin and endothelin converting enzyme(s) are homologous membrane proteins of the M13 peptidase family, which normally play roles in the biosynthesis and/or metabolism of regulatory peptides. Insulin-degrading enzyme is structurally and mechanistically distinct. The regional, cellular, and subcellular localizations of these enzymes differ, providing an efficient and diverse mechanism for protecting the brain against the normal accumulation of toxic Aβ peptides. Reduction in expression levels of some of these proteases following insults (e.g., hypoxia and ischemia) or aging might predispose to the development of Alzheimer's disease. Conversely, enhancement of their levels by gene delivery or pharmacological means could be neuroprotective. Even a relatively small enhancement of Aβ metabolism could slow the inexorable progression of the disease. The relative merits of targeting these enzymes for the treatment of Alzheimer's disease will be reviewed and possible side-effects of enhancing their activity evaluated.

KEYWORDS: amyloid β peptide; Alzheimer's disease; amyloid β-degrading enzymes; endothelin-converting enzyme; insulin-degrading enzyme; neprilysin; neurodegeneration; plasmin

INTRODUCTION

Alzheimer's disease (AD) is one of the most devastating neurodegenerative disorders in humans. It involves progressive accumulation of β-amyloid peptide

Address for correspondence: Professor Anthony J. Turner, School of Biochemistry and Microbiology, University of Leeds, Leeds, LS2 9JT, UK. Voice: +44-113-343-2987; fax: +44-113-343-3157.

a.j.turner@leeds.ac.uk

Ann. N.Y. Acad. Sci. 1035: 1–20 (2004). © 2004 New York Academy of Sciences.
doi: 10.1196/annals.1332.001

(Aβ) deposits, loss of neurons, cognitive deficit, and death. Genetic mutations that increase the production or stability of these proteins result in accelerated and more severe forms of the disease. Accumulation of Aβ peptide has been accepted as one of the major pathological features of AD. A strong correlation between Aβ deposition and AD development has been confirmed by many cases of early-onset familial AD, where gene mutations alter Aβ production and processing.[1,2] The involvement of amyloid peptides in the development of AD has been summarized by Hardy and Selkoe.[3] Understanding the mechanism by which Aβ pathologically accumulates in the brain and forms the plaques is crucial and can provide suggestions for development of therapeutic strategies for the treatment of AD.

APP AND Aβ PRODUCTION AND ACCUMULATION

Aβ, the pathogenic agent for AD, is a physiological metabolite constantly produced and catabolized in the brain. It is formed from a constituent membrane-bound protein, amyloid precursor protein (APP). Accumulation and aggregation of Aβ is the primary cause of AD, inducing an inflammatory response followed by neuritic injury, hyperphosphorylation of tau protein, and formation of fibrillary tangles, leading to neuronal dysfunction and cell death. The importance of Aβ production is debatable: has it an irreplaceable physiological function or does it only represent a metabolic pathway of APP degradation?[4] In this context, there is evidence that Aβ can regulate the activity of voltage-dependent Ca^{2+} channels[5] as well as being able to enhance GTPase activity in neurons,[6] which might affect long-term potentiation.[4]

Production of Aβ depends initially on the availability of APP, which exists as several isoforms of 695, 751, and 770 amino acids residues, respectively. APP is an integral membrane protein with a large ectodomain, a single membrane-spanning domain, and a short cytosolic domain. APP is cleaved by selective proteases (α-, β-, and γ-secretase) into various fragments. Members of the ADAM (a disintegrin and metalloprotease) family are the main candidates for α-secretase, especially ADAM 10.[7] The action of α-secretase results in production of a soluble APP (sAPPα) and theoretically should prevent generation of Aβ peptide. This process has been shown to be inhibited by peptide-hydroxamates such as batimastat[8] and upregulated by agonists of muscarinic cholinergic receptors—carbachol and muscarine.[9–11] It is also upregulated by phorbol esters.[12] A moderate neuronal overexpression of ADAM10 in mice transgenic to human APP reduced the formation of Aβ and prevented their deposits in plaques. In contrast, expression of a mutant inactive ADAM10 led to an increase in a number and size of amyloid plaques in the brain of the same transgenic mice.[13] Activation of α-secretase is considered as one of the potential therapeutic strategies for AD.[1]

Formation of amyloidogenic Aβ requires the activity of β- and γ-secretases. A detailed and updated review of this process has recently been provided by Mattson.[14] Recently, the molecules responsible for these proteolytic activities have been identified. The main β-secretase activity is believed to belong to the novel transmembrane aspartic protease, β-site APP-cleaving enzyme 1 (BACE1; also called Asp2 and memapsin 2). BACE1 exhibits all the functional properties of β-secretase and initiates formation of Aβ.[15] Subsequently a protease homologous to BACE1, BACE2, has also been identified and characterized.[16] Therapeutically, BACE1 provides an attractive drug target for AD. BACE knockout mice do not form Aβ and appear to be healthy.[17] However, new endogenous substrates are being discovered for BACE1 and so a certain caution is appropriate. Several approaches have been undertaken to find an effective inhibitor of human β-secretase activity, mostly in the field of peptidomimetic, noncleavable substrate analogues. The strategies of BACE mRNA recognition and its downregulation based on the antisense action of small inhibitory nucleic acids (siNAs) are also under consideration. These include antisense oligonucleotides, catalytic nucleic acids (ribozymes and deoxyribozymes), and small interfering RNAs (siRNAs).[18]

There is still no fully convincing agreement about the nature of γ-secretase, but the consensus is that presenilins (PSs) are involved in amyloidogenic processing of APP. PSs were discovered during a search for genetic mutations that cause early-onset familial AD. PSs and signal peptide peptidase (SPP) comprise a novel protease family of integral membrane proteins that may utilize a catalytic mechanism similar to classical aspartic proteinases, such as pepsin, renin, and cathepsin D (for review, see Martoglio and Golde).[19] The defining features of the PSs and SPP are their ability to cleave substrate polypeptides within a transmembrane region. It requires the presence of two active site aspartate residues in adjacent membrane-spanning regions and a conserved PAL motif near their COOH-terminus. PSs appear to be the catalytic subunit of multiprotein complexes that possess γ-secretase activity.[20] The cleavage of APP by γ-secretase results in formation of Aβ peptide fragments with 40, 42, and 43 amino acids, suggesting the existence of multiple variations of APP cleavage by γ-secretase. $A\beta_{40}$ is the most abundant form, while $A\beta_{42}$ is more toxic, less soluble and tends to form deposits.[21]

Membrane topology studies show that mutations of APP in the transmembrane domain dramatically affect the ratio of $A\beta_{40}/A\beta_{42}$.[22] The mechanism by which PS and APP mutations cause abnormal production of longer Aβ isoforms has not been clarified so far. A promising approach for the treatment of AD by inhibiting γ-secretase cleavage has some limitations because PS-1 knockout mice had developmental abnormalities and failed to survive.[23]

Besides the catalytic subunit PS-1, three additional subunits, nicastrin (NCT), APH-1, and PEN-2 have been identified.[24] The γ-secretase complex mediates the little understood pathway of regulated intramembrane proteolysis (protein RIPing).[25]

As was shown in numerous studies, Aβ induces neuronal death as well as activation of caspases, the effectors of apoptosis. Synapses are believed to be the main site for the neurodegenerative processes during AD. Exposure of cultured hippocampal neurons to Aβ increases the level of protease-activated receptor (PAR4) in cortical synaptosomes and in dendrites.[26] PAR4 induces mitochondrial alterations and activation of caspases. Moreover, in response to depolarization and exposure to Aβ, the levels of cytoplasmic calcium are drastically elevated in cortical synaptosomes from transgenic mice (mutants of presenilin-1) in comparison to nontransgenic mice expressing wild-type presenilin-1.

Despite numerous studies supporting the amyloid hypothesis of Alzheimer's disease (amyloid peptides as solely neurotoxic for neurons and brain tissue), current scientific evidence leaves little doubt that Aβ also has an essential role at the synapse and in synaptic structure-functional plasticity, which underlie learning and memory.[4] Therefore, the change of Aβ biology and accumulation of Aβ in Alzheimer's disease may represent a physiological mechanism to compensate for impaired brain structure or function similar to elevation of hemoglobin levels in individuals suffering altitude sickness.[27] These considerations should be also taken into account in developing the therapeutic strategies for AD.

CLEARANCE

Aβ occurs at much higher levels in the brain than in the periphery. Aβ_{40} was found to average 9.7 ng/mL in AD cerebrospinal fluid (CSF) and only 0.14 ng/mL in plasma, while Aβ_{42} was found to average 0.61 ng/mL in AD CSF and only 0.009 ng/mL in the plasma.[28] The 69-fold difference reflects the balance between the production and breakdown of Aβ peptides in the brain compared with the peripheral organs. Accumulation of excess amounts of Aβ in the brain was shown to be prevented by its drainage from the extracellular space by perivascular pathways.[29] Moreover, there are recently discovered biochemical pathways of elimination of Aβ. Until recently, production of Aβ in the brain and other tissues was thought to be an irreversible process, leading in the case of their disruption, to amyloidogenic diseases. However, in the last few years, several proteases, such as neprilysin (NEP), insulin-degrading enzyme (IDE; insulysin), endothelin-converting enzymes (ECE-1 and ECE-2), and plasmin have been found to be capable of degrading of Aβ *in vitro* and *in vivo*.[30,31] Pathological downregulation of these enzymes could predispose to accumulation of Aβ and the development of AD. Thus, a possible therapeutic approach for treatment of AD might be a chronic upregulation of these proteinases, either pharmacologically or through a gene therapy approach. Here, we give an overview of the current knowledge of the main enzymes capable of degrading amyloid peptides (FIGS. 1 and 2).

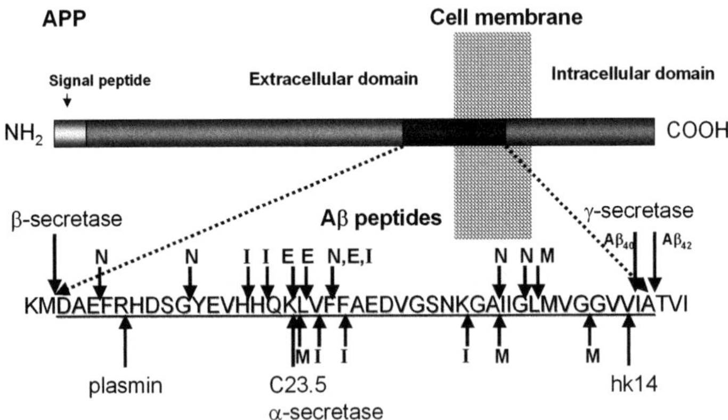

FIGURE 1. The sites of cleavage of the amyloid β-peptide by amyloid-degrading enzymes. Aβ is formed from APP through the consecutive actions of β- and γ-secretases. The Aβ peptide of 40 or 42 amino acids is cleaved at multiple sites by: N, NEP; I, IDE; E, ECE; M, MMP-9; and plasmin. C23.5 and hk14 represent recombinant antibody fragments screened for amyloid-degrading activity.[108]

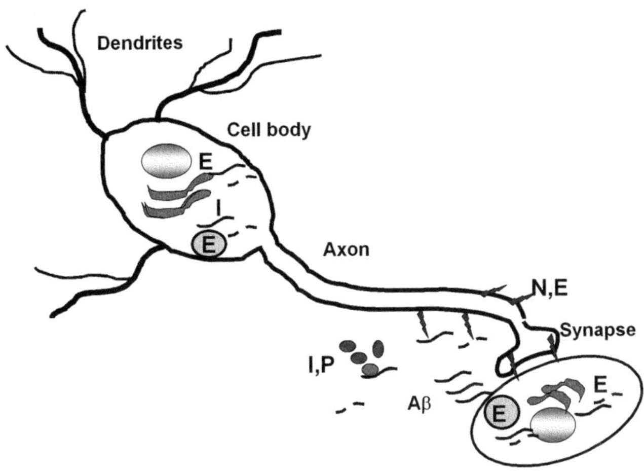

FIGURE 2. The neuronal localization of the Aβ-degrading enzymes. NEP is an axonal and synaptic membrane protein. ECE is located in multiple compartments including the trans-Golgi network, secretory vesicles, and the plasma membrane. IDE is mainly located in the cytosol, but is also secreted from neurons. Plasmin is an extracellular proteinase. All contribute to the efficient removal of the amyloid peptide.

AMYLOID-DEGRADING ENZYMES

Neprilysin

NEP (neutral endopeptidase-24.11 or neprilysin, EC 3.4.24.11) is a zinc metalloprotease originally discovered as a kidney enzyme that degraded peptide hormones.[32] It is also known as enkephalinase because of its ability to cleave enkephalins and terminate peptidergic neurotransmission.[33,34] It is a 93-kDa glycosylated ectoenzyme, a membrane-bound protein whose active site faces the extracellular space.[35] NEP is identical to CD10, a protein used as a marker of common acute lymphoblastic leukemia (CALLA).[36–38] NEP cleaves peptide bonds of small regulatory peptides at their hydrophobic amino acid residues.[32] NEP has wide regulatory activity and degrades a variety of bioactive peptides, such as opioid peptides, tachykinins (substance P), atrial natriuretic peptides, bombesin-like peptides, chemotactic peptides, and adrenocorticotropin hormone (ACTH).[32,39] NEP is involved in many physiological processes, such as cardiovascular regulation, inflammation, neuropeptide metabolism, cell migration, and proliferation.[32,38,40] The key role of NEP in degrading physiologically active peptides coupled with its ability to catabolize Aβ is further indirect evidence for the view of Koudinov and Berezov[4] that the amyloid peptide is a biologically relevant metabolite.

In humans, the NEP gene is located on chromosome 3, spans more than 80 kb and contains 24 miniexons.[41] NEP is a highly conserved protein. There are only six non-conservative changes in the 742 amino acids of the human and rat NEPs.[42] NEP has been detected in the central nervous system and in peripheral tissues, particularly in the membranes of the brush-border epithelial cells of intestine and kidney, lung, testis, prostate, synovium cells, neutrophils, chondrocytes, thymocytes, and in several epithelial and endocrine cells.[42–45]

Among other peptides, NEP was recently shown to be capable of degrading Aβ peptides, which could make it an important player in the effort to create therapies for AD.[46] NEP deficiency in mice results in a defect in the metabolism of endogenous $A\beta_{(1\text{-}40)}$ and $A\beta_{(1\text{-}42)}$ in a gene dose-dependent manner that suggests that partial downregulation of NEP activity may contribute to AD development by promoting Aβ accumulation.[47] It was also found that NEP was able to degrade not only monomeric, but also oligomeric forms of $A\beta_{(1\text{-}40)}$ and $A\beta_{(1\text{-}42)}$.[48,49] NEP mRNA and protein levels were found to be decreased in AD brain compared to age-matched controls.[50]

Previously, it was shown that NEP is expressed in the brain at relatively low levels.[35] While NEP consists of about 4% of all brush-border proteins in the kidney, in the brain its expression is 1,000 times lower.[51] A clear decrease in NEP levels in the aging brain was observed in the hippocampal formation of mice, when the NEP level was reduced by 20% at 132 weeks compared to the 10-week group.[52] Analyzing expression of NEP in the rat brain cortex, we found that it decreases significantly starting after one month of postnatal life and is practically undetectable in the aged individuals.[53] However, in the striatum, a brain area where amyloid peptide does not accumulate, NEP levels increase with age.[54] The overall reduction of NEP levels during the lifespan, and especially in neurites around β-amyloid plaques, has been reported by Apelt and colleagues.[55] They observed an upregulation of NEP in plaque-surrounding reactive astrocytes and suggested that plaque-mediated astrogliosis may also play a role in Aβ degradation. Thus, there is a significant amount of data confirming that NEP is able to degrade Aβ and NEP downregulation with age can play an important role in development of AD. Some studies have shown an association of the NEP gene to the late-onset AD, whereas others have not.[56–58] Further studies are required with larger cohorts to establish whether or not such associations are relevant.

Recently a homologue of NEP, namely neprilysin 2 (NEP2), was discovered and in the brain shown to be restricted mainly to developing and differentiated fields of the CNS. Unlike NEP and ECE-1, which are broadly expressed in the CNS and periphery, NEP2 was found to be almost exclusively expressed only in selected populations of neurons and in the spinal cord. The only peripheral areas where expression of NEP2 was detected were the pituitary and choroid plexuses. NEP2 was also found capable of degrading Aβ[48] and its distinct localization from NEP suggests that, together with ECE-1, it may be better poised to catabolize Aβ as it is more abundantly expressed in the areas relevant to AD pathology.[59]

Insulin-Degrading Enzyme

Besides NEP, insulin-degrading enzyme (IDE) has been suggested as another major candidate for Aβ degradation.[60] IDE (or insulysin) is a zinc metallopeptidase and a member of the inverzincin family of zinc proteinases. IDE is primarily located in the cytosol but it is also found in peroxisomes.[61] A fraction of the enzyme can be found in the plasma membrane[62,63] as well as in a secreted form.[64] A recent report has shown that alternative translation initiation generates a mitochondrial isoform of IDE that may cleave targeting sequences of mitochondrial proteins.[65] IDE cleaves its substrates at hydrophobic and basic residues, but it is not strictly sequence-specific. It has been proposed that the specificity of the enzyme is dictated by conformational features of the substrate and its size (preference for larger peptides).[61] IDE has an ability to degrade *in vitro* a wide range of physiological substrates, including insulin, and has physiological functions in addition to insulin metabolism.

A role for IDE in Aβ removal was originally suggested by Kurochkin and Goto[66] (reviewed by Kurochkin[67] and pursued by Selkoe and colleagues[64]). The hypothesis that reduced IDE activity may contribute to Aβ accumulation in the brain was supported by Perez and colleagues.[68] In a comparative study of IDE activity in fractions from AD brain and age-matched controls a significant decrease in Aβ degrading activity in the AD brain was revealed. Transgenic overexpression of IDE or NEP in neurons significantly reduces brain Aβ levels, slows down or completely prevents amyloid plaque formation and its associated cytopathology, and rescues premature lethality present in APP transgenic mice.[69]

A number of studies have linked AD pathology with insulin metabolism and action. Insulin and insulin-like growth factors (IGFs), which play a role in learning and memory, were also suggested to be involved in the pathogenetic pathways leading to AD.[70] Moreover, impaired glucose metabolism is one of the characteristic events in the pathology of AD.[71] It was demonstrated that insulin receptors are upregulated in AD brains but have defective signal transduction. In addition, it was shown that Aβ blocked insulin modulation of APP proteolytic processing and the release of sAPPα in Chinese hamster ovary (CHO) cells transfected with insulin receptors.[72]

$A\beta_{(1\text{-}40)}$ and $A\beta_{(1\text{-}42)}$ peptides were also shown to reduce insulin binding to its receptor as well as receptor autophosphorylation. The observed decrease in the affinity of insulin binding to the insulin receptor was independent of the receptor concentration. In contrast, reversed Aβ peptide (40-1) did not reduce insulin binding or insulin receptor autophosphorylation, which could suggest that $A\beta_{(1\text{-}40)}$ and $A\beta_{(1\text{-}42)}$ are direct competitive inhibitors of insulin binding and action.[73]

There is a clear association between hyperinsulinemia, diabetes, and AD and a possible common mechanism of disease development is now under investigation. Studies on genetically modified mice showed that IDE (−/−) deficiency results in a >50% decrease in Aβ degradation in both brain membrane fractions and primary neuronal cultures with a similar deficit in insulin degradation in the liver.[74] The IDE (−/−) mice showed an increased cerebral accumulation of endogenous Aβ and had hyperinsulinemia and glucose intolerance (as in diabetes mellitus type 2).

Other evidence of involvement of IDE in Aβ degradation was reported by Farris and colleagues.[75] They showed that endogenously secreted $A\beta_{(1\text{-}40)}$ and $A\beta_{(1\text{-}42)}$ are significantly elevated in primary neuronal cultures from rats with IDE missense mutations. These animals provide a model of type 2 diabetes mellitus (DM2) suggesting that partial loss-of-function mutations in IDE cause development of DM2 and also impair neuronal regulation of Aβ levels.

Epidemiological studies suggested that a non–insulin-dependent DM2 is associated with an increased risk of AD. Ho and colleagues[76] showed that diet-induced insulin resistance promoted $A\beta_{(1\text{-}40)}$ and $A\beta_{(1\text{-}42)}$ peptide generation in the brain. This was accomplished by an increased γ-secretase activity and decreased IDE activity. An observed functional decrease of insulin receptor (IR)–mediated signal transduction in the brain was caused by decreased IR β-subunit autophosphorylation and reduced phosphatidylinositol 3 (PI3)-kinase/AKT/protein kinase (PK)–B in these same brain regions. AKT/PKB had an inhibitory effect on glycogen synthase kinase (GSK)–3α activity. Previously it has been shown that GSK-3α promotes Aβ generation. A decrease in GSK-3α and GSK-3β phosphorylation (an index of GSK activation) correlated with generation of the C-terminal fragment of amyloid precursor protein. All this suggests that insulin resistance may be an underlying mechanism responsible for the observed increased relative risk for AD neuropathology and suggests that IR signaling can influence Aβ production in the brain.

Recent experiments have demonstrated that IDE is involved in clearance of intracellular Aβ. Usually little Aβ peptide is found intracellularly but when APP is overexpressed in cells, Aβ$_{(1-42)}$ has been found in the ER. Under normal conditions the misfolded proteins (and others substrates for ER-associated degradation [ERAD]) are translocated to the cytosol, where they are degraded by proteasomes. However, it was shown that Aβ degradation might happen by two distinctive pathways: proteasome dependent and proteasome independent. RNA interference experiments showed that proteasome-independent degradation involves the action of IDE.[77] At lower expression levels Aβ would be degraded in the same way as other ERAD substrates (proteasome-dependent pathway) and it becomes a substrate for the normally unused IDE pathway only because the first pathway was saturated.

A decreased cortical glucose utilization (particularly in the hippocampus and entorhinal cortex) caused by insulin dysregulation might contribute to AD pathology. It was shown that increased oxidative stress can be responsible for the formation of advanced glycation end-products, increased tau phosphorylation, and neurofibrillary tangle formation and increased Aβ aggregation through inhibition of insulin-degrading enzyme.[78]

Genetic variations within or extremely close to the IDE gene can contribute both to the disease risk and the severity of AD.[79] Linkage studies have identified a large (>60 Mb) region on chromosome 10q that segregates with AD. A 276-kb linkage disequilibrium block spans three genes including IDE. Consistent risk alleles and haplotypes were obvious across the study, with effects in some cases as large as that of the ε4 allele of APOE.

Genetic studies undertaken in France[80] and in Japan[56] have found no evidence for IDE gene polymorphism and susceptibility to early- or late-onset AD. In contrast, another study by Blomqvist and colleagues.[81] suggested there was the equivalent presence of detrimental and protective alleles to AD and Parkinson disease (PD).

Despite little evidence of a genetic connection in IDE gene mutations and AD, there is ample data confirming its involvement in Aβ degradation. The upregulation of protein levels and/or increasing activity of IDE and its selectivity to Aβ may be another therapeutic approach to AD. Likewise, factors leading to downregulation of IDE could predispose to AD.

Endothelin-Converting Enzyme

Another candidate for Aβ degradation is endothelin converting enzyme (ECE). ECE is a homologue of NEP, demonstrating about 37% amino acid identity in the rat protein. ECE-1 is a membrane-bound metalloprotease that catalyzes the conversion of big endothelin into vasoactive endothelins. A significant structural difference between NEP and ECE is that ECE-1 exists as a disulfide-linked dimer. Another difference between these two enzymes is their sensitivity to inhibitors. Nanomolar concentrations of thiorphan and phosphoramidon (PR) inhibit NEP, whereas ECE-1 is inhibited only at micromolar concentrations of PR and is insensitive to thiorphan. ECE-1 is expressed at high levels in endothelial cells. It is also present in a variety of other cells. In smooth muscle cells it is associated with α-actin filaments.[82] It is also found in neurons and glia in the brain and is localized both intra- and extracellularly.[83] This difference in distribution is explained by the existence of several isoforms of ECE-1, which correspond to an alternative splicing of a single gene localized on chromosome 1.[84] At the present time four isoforms of ECE-1 have been reported. Although the relative levels of the isoform mRNA species vary between human tissues, ECE-1c mRNA is generally the predominant isoform message. There are distinct subcellular localizations for the four isoforms: whereas ECE-1a, ECE-1c, and ECE-1d proteins are localized mainly at the cell surface, ECE-1b was found to be intracellular and showed significant co-localization with a marker protein for the trans-Golgi network.[85] There are no significant differences in the catalytic properties between them, so it was suggested that intracellular ECE-1 localized in Golgi and vesicles might be involved in processing of big endothelin whereas cell-surface ECE-1 may metabolize other regulatory peptides.[86]

A gene encoding an ECE-like protein (ECE-2) was described by Emoto and Yanagisawa.[87] ECE-2 protein is mainly localized in the brain and has low abundance in endothelial and smooth muscle cells. It has 59% identity with ECE-1, but an acidic pH optimum and is practically inactive at neutral pH. ECE-2 is localized in the secretory compartments and is likely to be involved in protein processing.

Evidence that ECE is capable of degrading amyloid-β peptide was first provided by Eckman and colleagues.[88] They showed that overexpression of ECE-1 in Chinese hamster ovary cells, lacking endogenous ECE activity, reduced extracellular Aβ concentration by up to 90%. This effect was completely abolished by treatment with the metalloproteinase inhibitor phosphoramidon. Recombinant soluble ECE-1 was capable of hydrolyzing synthetic Aβ_{40} and Aβ_{42} *in vitro* at multiple sites. In a further study it was reported that the levels of both Aβ_{40} and Aβ_{42} were significantly increased in mice with reduced ECE-1 activity. Eckman and colleagues[89] compared ECE heterozygous and knock-out mice and showed that the concentration of Aβ peptides in the brain of these animals was elevated in comparison with control littermates in a gene-dependent manner.

Plasmin

Plasmin is a serine proteinase derived from an inactive zymogen, plasminogen, as a result of the action of serine proteinases called plasminogen activators. It degrades many components of the extracellular matrix[90] and in the blood it acts primarily as a thrombolytic enzyme. In the brain the plasminogen system was shown to be involved in numerous functions, such as neuronal plasticity,[91] long-term potentiation via degradation of laminin,[92] learning and memory.[93] Activation of the plasminogen system in the brain was demonstrated after focal cerebral ischemia.[94] This plasminogen activation was observed within several days after the insult, suggesting its contribution to extracellular matrix disruption, secondary hemorrhage, and brain edema in subacute stages of ischemic stroke. Levels of plasmin were shown to be decreased in the brain of AD patients and especially in the hippocampus.[95,96]

The role of plasmin in the pathology of AD is unknown but there are several observations manifesting its role in catabolism of amyloid peptide.[95,97] Purified plasmin was shown to degrade Aβ with physiologically relevant efficiency, that is, approximately one tenth the rate of plasmin on fibrin.[98] Mass spectral analyses showed that plasmin cleaves Aβ at multiple sites. Electron microscopy confirms that plasmin degrades Aβ fibrils. Moreover, exogenously added plasmin blocks Aβ neurotoxicity.[99]

Plasmin has been shown to associate with the cholesterol-enriched membrane microdomains (lipid rafts,)[100] which also appear to favor the formation of the amyloid peptide.[101,102] These observations provide cell biological correlates of the observed effects of cholesterol on the pathology of AD (see above).

Studies by Kingston and colleagues[103] showed that assembled forms of Aβ can stimulate the enzymatic activity of tissue plasminogen activator (tPA) *in vitro*. Plasmin produced by tPA-mediated plasminogen activation specifically cleaves Aβ in a manner such that it enhances the β-sheet secondary properties of the peptide. This in turn leads to enhanced stimulation of tPA activity and more robust plasminogen activation. Such a feedback mechanism could lead to excessive proteolysis in the vessel wall contributing to hemorrhagic stroke.[97] More recently it was confirmed that aggregated, but not nonaggregated, Aβ increases the level of the mRNAs encoding tPA and urokinase-type plasminogen activator (uPA).

Recently several research groups reported a familial AD locus on chromosome 10.[104] uPA was also found to be located within this locus.[105] These authors have also demonstrated that a combination of uPA and plasminogen, but neither alone, inhibited Aβ toxicity, reduced Aβ depositions, and diminished fibrillogenesis.

Other

There may well be other enzymes that can metabolize the amyloid peptide *in vivo*. Two candidates that have been shown to do this *in vitro* are angiotensin-converting enzyme (ACE)[106] and matrix metalloproteinase-9 (MMP-9).[107] There is, however, no reported functional correlation of these activities with AD pathology.

Recently, two light-chain antibody fragments that had proteolytic activity against Aβ have been identified by Rangan and colleagues.[108] One of these proteins had an α-secretase–like activity and produced 1-16 and 16-40 fragments of Aβ, while another demonstrated carboxypeptidase-like activity cleaving sequentially from the carboxyl terminal of Aβ. Additionally it was shown that cleavage of Aβ40 by hk14, the light-chain antibody having carboxypeptidase-like activity, alters aggregation of Aβ and neutralizes any cytotoxic effects of the peptide. Cleavage of Aβ40 with c23.5, the light chain having α-secretase–like cleavage, substantially increases the aggregation rate of Aβ. However, it does not show any corresponding increase in cytotoxicity. These results demonstrate that antibody fragment mediated proteolytic degradation of Aβ peptide can be a potential therapeutic route to control Aβ aggregation and toxicity *in vivo*. These results also suggest that increasing α-secretase activity as a therapeutic route must be approached with some caution because this can lead to a substantial increase in aggregation.[109]

Glucagon-like peptide–1 (GLP-1) was suggested as another factor contributing to reduction of the levels of endogenous Aβ.[110] Localization of GLP-1 receptor in the brain of humans and rodents correlated with the central role of this peptide in regulation of food intake. Stimulation of neuronal GLP-1 receptors were also shown to regulate neuronal plasticity and survival. GLP-1 and its natural analogue exendin-4, were found to reduce endogenous levels of Aβ in mouse brain and to reduce levels of APP in neurons. Because GLP-1 receptor is coupled to the cAMP second messenger pathway this peptide affects a number of therapeutic targets associated with AD and might be beneficial for developing a new treatment strategy.

AMYLOID LEVELS ARE DYNAMIC

The data provided in this review clearly demonstrate that amyloid metabolism is a complex system involving numerous participants and regulating production, clearance, and catabolism of Aβ. This complex system must be taken into account when the strategy for the treatment of AD is considered. Better understanding of the functioning of the system in normally developed brain and under various pathologies will help us elucidate the pathology of AD. An organism is affected by various factors over the course of its life that affects its development and functioning, which leads to modulation of Aβ metabolism.

FACTORS AFFECTING Aβ BALANCE

Age

Normal brain aging is accompanied by numerous changes in the brain structure and functions and results in reductions in cognitive functions and memory, as well as in development of various disorders of old age. Apart from biochemical changes with age, the brain undergoes significant morphological changes with age. Some brain structures demonstrate more significant morphological changes than others and result in a functional deficit. For example, it was demonstrated that normal aging is accompanied by hippocampal atrophy and is associated with mild memory impairment. The degree of the atrophy was found to be related with the age and was more pronounced in males.[111]

Normal brain aging is associated with a degree of functional impairment of neuronal activity that results in a reduction in memory and cognitive functions. This is related not only with the aging of the nervous cells and impairment of their metabolism leading to cell death, but also with accumulation of a number of chemical compounds that interfere with normal biochemical processes. Impairment of lipid metabolism and accumulation of products of lipid peroxidation appears to be toxic to the brain and also leads to the pathological changes in membranes of the cells affecting efficiency of functioning of channels and membrane-bound enzyme complexes.[112]

There are hypotheses linking the aging of the brain with disruption of its calcium homeostasis. The "Ca^{2+} hypothesis of aging" tries to address the problems of age-induced changes in synaptic plasticity of neuronal cells. In a recent review by Toescu and Verkhratsky[113] the analysis of the data to date demonstrated that these changes are ultimately determined by changes in the metabolic status of the aged neurons. In this context, it appears that the changes in mitochondrial status and function are of primary importance. Accumulation of Aβ in the aging brain is one of the factors of impaired neuronal activity. It induces membrane-associated oxidative stress, resulting in perturbed ceramide and cholesterol metabolism, which in turn triggers a neurodegenerative cascade that leads to clinical disease.[114]

In the normal brain, production of Aβ is balanced by its elimination from the extracellular space by perivascular pathways.[115] The pattern of deposition of Aβ in senile plaques and in cerebral amyloid angiopathy (CAA) suggests that Aβ accumulates in pericapillary and periarterial interstitial fluid drainage pathways of the brain. This can also be a result of failure of drainage of Aβ along periarterial pathways within the brain and leptomeninges due to aging of cerebral arteries. Since there is a strong correlation between cerebrovascular diseases and development of AD, therapies to increase elimination of Aβ from the brain might be considered as one of the possible ways to control or prevent development of AD. Moreover, the extent to which cerebrovascular diseases prevent removal of Aβ from the aging human brain needs to be considered in the development of antibody therapy for AD.[29]

Abnormal posttranslational protein modifications are also recognized as a common age-related phenomenon that may produce dysfunctional structural proteins and enzymes. A variety of proteins, including enzymes, can be substrates of oxidative damage in AD brains.[116] Several studies have shown that 4-hydroxynonenal (HNE), a byproduct of lipid peroxidation that can form covalent adducts with proteins through histidine and lysine residues, is increased in AD and may contribute to a cytopathological effect observed as a consequence of oxidative stress.[117] Sayre and colleagues[118] have shown that HNE-modified proteins are increased not only in neurofibrillary tangle–bearing neurons, but also in "normal" pyramidal neurons in AD. Wang and colleagues[119] have shown that NEP also undergoes HNE modification with age and that the ratio of oxidized to total NEP was greater in AD than in controls.

Age-related deficit of Aβ-degrading enzymes can be one of the factors of Aβ accumulation in the brain. As we have already discussed, expression of NEP is reduced in the brain of adult animals compared to younger individuals, which can testify to a specific role of NEP in the development of the nervous system. Similarly, the levels of activity of IDE in the rat brain were shown to be maximal on the thirteenth day of postnatal development. This was unique for CNS and differed remarkably from the time-course in liver and kidney, suggesting that insulin and IDE have a growth-promoting role in the developing rat brain.[120]

Reduced plasmin activity in Alzheimer's brain was suggested to be related to the changes in the membrane composition of neuronal cells. It was demonstrated that membranes of AD patients had a mild, but significant reduction in cholesterol and anomalous lipid raft microdomains. This was accompanied by the loss of raft-enriched proteins, including plasminogen-binding and plasminogen-activating molecules.[96,100] Interestingly, the survival prognosis of elder patients who had suffered ischemic stroke was also found to depend on the level of brain cholesterol. Short-term mortality was higher in older patients with low total cholesterol levels, independent of a large number of other factors.[121] Low levels of cholesterol were also observed in the white matter of AD patients with no changes in total fatty acid contents.[122]

Brain hypoxia is one of the most common complications resulting from impaired brain metabolism and circulation and can affect animals and humans at various stages of their life. It is well known that prenatal hypoxia causes dramatic changes in the developmental profile and behavioral characteristics of animals and is one of the most common reasons for mental retardation and cognitive deficit in children.[123] In later life, brain hypoxia affects both behavioral and cognitive abilities of individuals and leads to various neuropathologies.[124] There is ample evidence that ischemia, and especially ischemic stroke, may contribute to the pathogenesis of AD. Although there are numerous epidemiological studies suggesting that risk factors for stroke are associated with AD, the molecular mechanisms by which ischemia and hypoxia may be associated with AD are unclear. Analyzing the effect of acute prenatal hypoxia on the thirteenth day of gestation, we have demonstrated that expression both of NEP and ECE were reduced in the cortex of hypoxic animals within the first month after birth compared to control animals. Preconditioning to mild hypoxia was found to restore these parameters, suggesting its neuroprotective properties.[53]

There are studies demonstrating involvement of tPA in response to the ischemic insult. A surge in tPA activity was found around the blood vessels in the area of ischemic penumbra. This tPA interacts with the blood-brain barrier, causing an increase in its permeability and allowing penetration of matrix metalloproteinases (in particular of MMP-9) and other harmful substances from the blood into the brain. Moreover, tPA seems to act through an interaction with low-density lipoprotein receptor–related protein as an endogenous regulator of cerebrovascular permeability, not only under pathological but also physiologic conditions.[125] Taking into account the role of plasmin in Aβ catabolism, there might be a direct link between the episodes of ischemia and Aβ catabolism.

THERAPEUTIC APPROACHES

Taking into account available data and the results of our own studies, it is reasonable to suggest that upregulation of Aβ-degrading enzymes could be a viable therapeutic approach for treatment of AD. Leading research groups are already working on this problem by exploiting various techniques. Thus, using a recombinant adeno-associated viral vector-mediated gene transfer Iwata and coworkers[126] demonstrated axonal transport of NEP to presynaptic sites. This gene transfer abolished the increase in Aβ levels in the hippocampal formations of NEP-deficient mice and also reduced the increase in young mutant APP transgenic mice. At later stages, Aβ levels in the hippocampal formation contralateral to the vector-injected side were also significantly reduced as a result of transport of NEP from the ipsilateral side. In both sides, soluble Aβ was degraded more efficiently than insoluble Aβ. Amyloid deposition in aged mutant APP transgenic mice was remarkably decreased. In another study, a lentiviral vector expressing human neprilysin was tested in transgenic mouse models of amyloidosis. It was found that unilateral intracerebral injection of Lenti-Nep reduced Aβ deposits by half compared to the untreated side.[127] Furthermore, Lenti-Nep ameliorated neurodegenerative alterations in the frontal cortex and hippocampus of these transgenic mice.

While a gene therapy approach might be viable in selectively raising neuronal levels of NEP (or other Aβ-degrading enzymes), an alternative approach might be

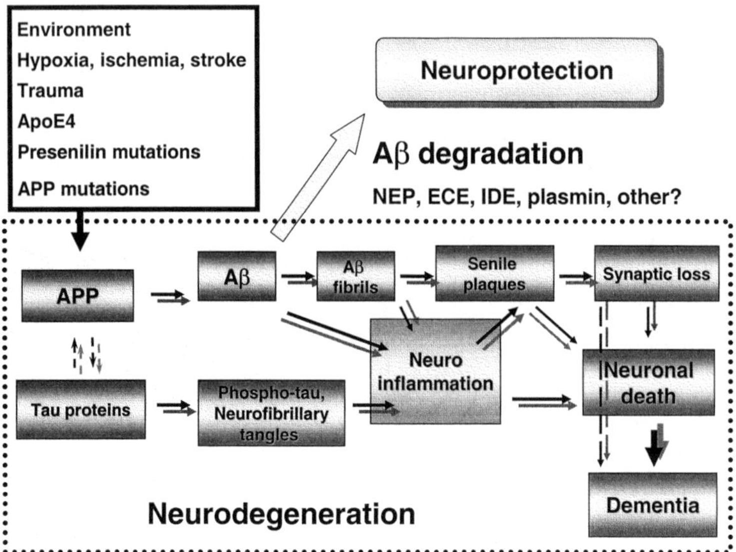

FIGURE 3. Schematic of the routes to neurodegeneration and the neuroprotection provided by the enzymatic degradation of the Aβ peptide by degrading enzymes such as NEP, ECE, and IDE.

pharmacological upregulation of NEP. Indeed, one recent report has shown that green-tea extract has precisely that effect[128] and a systematic screening for NEP regulators may prove worthwhile.

In conclusion, the discovery that amyloid peptide levels are dynamic as a result of proteolytic degradation has opened up new therapeutic avenues (FIG. 3). Targeting the relevant enzymes might be a simple and inexpensive approach to AD treatment, particularly since a small enhancement in degrading activity should retard significantly the abnormal peptide accumulation in the brain and the associated cognitive decline.

ACKNOWLEDGMENTS

This work was supported by the U.K. Medical Research Council, the Wellcome Trust, and the Royal Society. L. Fisk is the recipient of the Krebs Memorial Scholarship from The Biochemical Society.

REFERENCES

1. LICHTENTHALER, S.F. & C. HAASS. 2004. Amyloid at the cutting edge: activation of α-secretase prevents amyloidogenesis in an Alzheimer disease mouse model. J. Clin. Invest. **113:** 1384–1387.
2. HARDY, J. 2004. Toward Alzheimer therapies based on genetic knowledge. Annu. Rev. Med. **55:** 15–25.

3. HARDY, J. & D. SELKOE. 2002. The amyloid hypothesis of Alzheimer's disease: progress and problems on the road to therapeutics. Science **297:** 353–356.

4. KOUDINOV, A.R. & T.T. BEREZOV. 2004. Alzheimer's amyloid-β (Aβ) is an essential synaptic protein, not neurotoxic junk. Acta Neurobiol. Exp. (Wars) **64:** 71–79.

5. MACMANUS, A. *et al.* 2000. Enhancement of $^{45}Ca^{2+}$ influx and voltage-dependent Ca^{2+} channel activity by β-amyloid-(1-40) in rat cortical synaptosomes and cultured cortical neurons. Modulation by the proinflammatory cytokine interleukin-1β. J. Biol. Chem. **275:** 4713–4718.

6. MOLNAR, Z. *et al.* 2004. Enhanced G-protein activation by a mixture of Aβ(25-35), Aβ(1-40/42) and zinc. J. Neurochem. **89:** 1215–1223.

7. LAMMICH, S. *et al.* 1999. Constitutive and regulated α-secretase cleavage of Alzheimer's amyloid protein by a disintegrin metalloprotease. Proc. Natl. Acad. Sci. USA **96:** 3922–3927.

8. PARVATHY, S. *et al.* 1998. Alzheimer's amyloid precursor protein α-secretase is inhibited by hydroxamic acid-based zinc metalloprotease inhibitors: similarities to the angiotensin converting enzyme secretase. Biochemistry **37:** 1680–1685.

9. BUXBAUM, J.D. *et al.* 1992. Cholinergic agonists and interleukin 1 regulated processing and secretion of the Alzheimer β/A4 amyloid protein precursor. Proc. Natl. Acad. Sci. USA **89:** 10075–10078.

10. ALLINSON, T.M. *et al.* 2003. ADAMs family members as amyloid precursor protein α-secretases. J. Neurosci. Res. **74:** 342–352.

11. CANET-AVILES, R.M. *et al.* 2002. Muscarine enhances soluble amyloid precursor protein secretion in human neuroblastoma SH-SY5Y by a pathway dependent on protein kinase C(α), src-tyrosine kinase and extracellular signal-regulated kinase but not phospholipase C. Brain Res. Mol. Brain Res. **102:** 62–72.

12. ZHU, G. *et al.* 2001. Protein kinase C ε suppresses Aβ production and promotes activation of α-secretase. Biochem. Biophys. Res. Commun. **285:** 997–1006.

13. POSTINA, R. *et al.* 2004. A disintegrin-metalloproteinase prevents amyloid plaque formation and hippocampal defects in an Alzheimer disease mouse model. J. Clin. Invest. **113:** 1456–1464.

14. MATTSON, M. 2004. Pathways towards and away from Alzheimer's disease. Nature **430:** 631–639.

15. VASSAR, R., & M. CITRON. 2000. Aβ-generating enzymes: recent advances in β- and γ-secretase search. Neuron **27:** 419-422.

16. VASSAR, R. 2004. BACE1: the β-secretase enzyme in Alzheimer's disease. J. Mol. Neurosci. **23:** 105–114.

17. LUO, Y. *et al.* 2001. Mice deficient in BACE1, the Alzheimer's β-secretase, have normal phenotype and abolished β–amyloid generation. Nat. Neurosci. **4:** 231–232.

18. NAWROT, B. 2004. Targeting BACE with small inhibitory nucleic acids—a future for Alzheimer's disease therapy? Acta Biochim. Pol. **51:** 431–444.

19. MARTOGLIO, B. & T.E. GOLDE. 2003. Intramembrane-cleaving aspartic proteases and disease: presenilins, signal peptide peptidase and their homologs. Hum. Mol. Genet. **12:** R201–R206.

20. DE STROOPER, B. 2003. Aph-1, Pen-2, and nicastrin with presenilin generate an active γ-secretase complex. Neuron **38:** 9–12.

21. EL-AGNAF, O.M. *et al.* 2000. Oligomerization and toxicity of β-amyloid-42 implicated in Alzheimer's disease. Biochem. Biophys. Res. Commun. **273:** 1003–1007.

22. LICHTENTHALER, S.F. *et al.* 1999. Mechanism of the cleavage specificity of Alzheimer's disease γ-secretase identified by phenylalanine-scanning mutagenesis of the transmembrane domain of the amyloid precursor protein. Proc. Natl. Acad. Sci. USA **96:** 3053–3058.

23. SHEN, J. *et al.* 1997. Skeletal and CNS defects in presenilin-1-deficient mice. Cell **89:** 629–639.

24. SHIROTANI, K. *et al.* 2004. Identification of distinct γ-secretase complexes with different APH-1 variants. J. Biol. Chem. Jul 30 [Epub ahead of print].

25. HELDIN, C.H & J. ERICSSON. 2001. Signal transduction. RIPping tyrosine kinase receptors apart. Science **294:** 2111–2113.

26. MATTSON, M.P. *et al.* 2001. Neurodegenerative disorders and ischemic brain diseases. Apoptosis **6:** 69–81.

27. LEE, H.-G. *et al.* 2004, Challenging the amyloid cascade hypothesis: senile plaques and amyloid-β as protective adaptations to Alzheimer disease. Ann. N.Y. Acad. Sci. **1019:** 1–4.
28. MEHTA, P.D. *et al.* 2001. Amyloid β protein 1-40 and 1-42 levels in matched cerebrospinal fluid and plasma from patients with Alzheimer disease. Neurosci. Lett. **304:** 102–106.
29. WELLER, R.O. *et al.* 2002. Cerebrovascular disease is a major factor in the failure of elimination of Aβ from the aging human brain. Ann. N.Y. Acad. Sci. **977:** 162–168.
30. CARSON, J.A. & A.J. TURNER. 2002. β-Amyloid catabolism: role for neprilysin (NEP) and other metallopeptidases? J. Neurochem. **81:** 1–8.
31. LEISSRING, M.A. *et al.* 2003. Kinetics of amyloid β-protein degradation determined by novel fluorescence- and fluorescence polarization-based assays. J. Biol. Chem. **278:** 37314–37320.
32. TURNER, A.J. & K. TANZAWA. 1997. Mammalian membrane metallopeptidases: NEP, ECE, KELL, and PEX. FASEB J. **11:** 355–364.
33. MATSAS, R., A.J. KENNY & A.J. TURNER. 1986. An immunohistochemical study of endopeptidase-24.11 ("enkephalinase") in the pig nervous system. Neuroscience **18:** 991–1012.
34. TURNER, A.J. 1990. Neuropeptide signalling and cell-surface peptidases. Adv. Second. Messenger Phosphoprotein Res. **24:** 467–471.
35. SALES, N. *et al.* 1991. Neutral endopeptidase 24.11 in rat peripheral tissues: comparative localization by "ex vivo" and "in vitro" autoradiography. Regul. Pept. **33:** 209–222.
36. LETARTE, M. *et al.* 1988. Common acute lymphocytic leukemia antigen is identical to neutral endopeptidase. Exp. Med. **168:** 1247–1253.
37. LeBIEN, T.W. & R.T. McCORMACK. 1989. The common acute lymphoblastic leukemia antigen (CD10)-emancipation from a functional enigma. Blood **73:** 625–635
38. SHIPP, M.A. *et al.* 1991. CD10/neutral endopeptidase 24.11 hydrolyzes bombesin-like peptides and regulates the growth of small cell carcinomas of the lung. Proc. Natl. Acad. Sci. USA **88:** 10662–10666.
39. DUVAUX-MIRET, O. *et al.* 1992. Immunosuppression in the definitive and intermediate hosts of the human parasite Schistosoma mansoni by release of immunoreactive neuropeptides. Proc. Natl. Acad. Sci. USA **89:** 778–781.
40. HARRISON, N.K. *et al.* 1995. Effects of neuropeptides on human lung fibroblast proliferation and chemotaxis. Lung Cell. Mol. Physiol. **12:** L278–L283.
41. ROQUES, B.P. *et al.* 1993. Neutral endopeptidase 24.11: Structure, inhibition, and experimental and clinical pharmacology. Pharmacol. Rev. **45:** 87–146.
42. ERDOS, E.G. & R.A. SKIDGEL. 1989. Neutral endopeptidase 24.11 (enkephalinase) and related regulators of peptide hormones. FASEB J. **3:** 145–151.
43. CONNELLY, J.C. *et al.* 1985. Neutral endopeptidase 24.11 in human neutrophils: cleavage of chemotactic peptide. Proc. Natl. Acad. Sci. USA **82:** 8737–8741.
44. MAPP, P.I. *et al.* 1992. Localization of the enzyme neutral endopeptidase to the human synovium. J. Rheumatol. **19:** 1838–1844.
45. PIERART, M.E. *et al.* 1988. Effect of human endopeptidase 24.11 ("enkephalinase") on IL-1-induced thymocyte proliferation activity. J. Immunol. **140:** 3808–3811.
46. IWATA, N. *et al.* 2000. Identification of the major Aβ1-42-degrading catabolic pathway in brain parenchyma: suppression leads to biochemical and pathological deposition. Nat Med. **6:** 143–150.
47. SAITO, T. *et al.* 2003. Alzheimer's disease, neuropeptides, neuropeptidase, and amyloid-β peptide metabolism. Sci. Aging Knowledge Environ. **3:** PE1.
48. SHIROTANI, K. *et al.* 2001. Neprilysin degrades both amyloid β peptides 1-40 and 1-42 most rapidly and efficiently among thiorphan- and phosphoramidon-sensitive endopeptidases. J. Biol. Chem. **276:** 21895–21901.
49. KANEMITSU, H. *et al.* 2003. Human neprilysin is capable of degrading amyloid β peptide not only in the monomeric form, but also the pathological oligomeric form. Neurosci. Lett. **350:** 113–116.
50. YASOJIMA, K. *et al.* 2001. Reduced neprilysin in high plaque areas of Alzheimer brain: a possible relationship to deficient degradation of β-amyloid peptide. Neurosci. Lett. **297:** 97–100.

51. BARNES, K., A.J. TURNER & A.J. KENNY. 1992. Membrane localization of endopeptidase-24.11 and peptidyl dipeptidase A (angiotensin converting enzyme) in the pig brain: a study using subcellular fractionation and electron microscopic immunocytochemistry. J. Neurochem. **58:** 2088–2096.
52. IWATA, N. *et al.* 2002. Region-specific reduction of Aβ-degrading endopeptidase, neprilysin, in mouse hippocampus upon aging. J. Neurosci. Res. **70:** 493–500.
53. NALIVAEVA, N.N. *et al.* 2004. Effects of prenatal hypoxia on expression of amyloid precursor protein and metallopeptidases in the rat brain. Lett. Peptide Sci. **10:** 455–462.
54. NALIVAEVA, N.N. *et al.* 2004. Effect of hypoxia/ischaemia and hypoxic preconditioning/reperfusion on expression of some amyloid degrading enzymes. Ann. N.Y. Acad. Sci. This volume.
55. APELT, J., K. ACH & R. SCHLIEBS. 2003. Ageing-related downregulation of neprilysin, a putative β-amyloid-degrading enzyme, in transgenic Tg2576 Alzheimer-like mouse brain is accompanied by an astroglial upregulation in the vicinity of β-amyloid plaques. Neurosci. Lett. **339:** 183–186.
56. SAKAI, A. *et al.* 2004. Association of the neprilysin gene with susceptibility to late-onset Alzheimer's disease. Dement. Geriatr. Cogn. Disord. **17:** 164–169.
57. LILIUS, L. *et al.* 2003. No association between polymorphisms in the neprilysin promoter region and Swedish Alzheimer's disease patients. Neurosci. Lett. **337:** 111–113.
58. ODA, M. *et al.* 2002. Dinucleotide repeat polymorphisms in the neprilysin gene are not associated with sporadic Alzheimer's disease. Neurosci. Lett. **320:** 105–107.
59. FACCHINETTI, P. *et al.* 2003. Ontogeny, regional and cellular distribution of the novel metalloprotease neprilysin 2 in the rat: a comparison with neprilysin and endothelin-converting enzyme-1. Neuroscience **118:** 627–639.
60. LEISSRING. M.A. *et al.* 2003. Enhanced proteolysis of β-amyloid in APP transgenic mice prevents plaque formation, secondary pathology, and premature death. Neuron **40:** 1087–1093.
61. DUCKWORTH, W.C., R.G. BENNETT & F.G. HAMEL. 1998. Insulin degradation: progress and potential. Endocr. Rev. **19:** 608–624.
62. SETA, K.A. & R.A. ROTH. 1997. Overexpression of insulin degrading enzyme: cellular localization and effects on insulin signaling. Biochem. Biophys. Res. Commun. **231:** 167–171.
63. VEKRELLIS, K. *et al.* 2000. Neurons regulate extracellular levels of amyloid β-protein via proteolysis by insulin-degrading enzyme. J. Neurosci. **20:** 1657–1665.
64. QIU, W.Q. *et al.* 1998. Insulin-degrading enzyme regulates extracellular levels of amyloid β-protein by degradation. J. Biol. Chem. **273:** 32730–32738.
65. LEISSRING, M.A. *et al.* 2004. Alternative translation initiation generates a novel isoform of insulin-degrading enzyme targeted to mitochondria. Biochem. J. [Epub ahead of print.]
66. KUROCHKIN, I.V. & S. GOTO. 1994. Alzheimer's β-amyloid peptide specifically interacts with and is degraded by insulin degrading enzyme. FEBS Lett. **345:** 33-37.
67. KUROCHKIN, I.V. 2001. Insulin-degrading enzyme: embarking on amyloid destruction. Trends Biochem. Sci. **26:** 421–425.
68. PEREZ, A. *et al.* 2000. Degradation of soluble amyloid β-peptides 1-40, 1-42, and the Dutch variant 1-40Q by insulin degrading enzyme from Alzheimer disease and control brains. Neurochem. Res. **2:** 247–255.
69. LEISSRING, M.A. *et al.* 2003. Enhanced proteolysis of β-amyloid in APP transgenic mice prevents plaque formation, secondary pathology, and premature death. Neuron **40:** 1087–1093.
70. DORE, S. *et al.* 1997. Distribution and levels of [^{125}I]IGF-I, [^{125}I]IGF-II and [^{125}I]insulin receptor binding sites in the hippocampus of aged memory-unimpaired and -impaired rats. Neuroscience **80:** 1033–1040.
71. BIGL, M. *et al.* 2003. Cortical glucose metabolism is altered in aged transgenic Tg2576 mice that demonstrate Alzheimer plaque pathology. J. Neural. Transm. **110:** 77-94.
72. LING, X. *et al.* 2002. Amyloid β antagonizes insulin promoted secretion of the amyloid β protein precursor. J. Alzheimers Dis. **4:** 369–374.
73. XIE, L. *et al.* 2002. Alzheimer's β-amyloid peptides compete for insulin binding to the insulin receptor. J. Neurosci. **22:** RC221.

74. FARRIS, W. *et al.* 2003. Insulin-degrading enzyme regulates the levels of insulin, amyloid β-protein, and the β-amyloid precursor protein intracellular domain in vivo. Proc. Natl. Acad. Sci. USA **100**: 4162–4167.
75. FARRIS, W. *et al.* 2004. Partial loss-of-function mutations in insulin-degrading enzyme that induce diabetes also impair degradation of amyloid β-protein. Am. J. Pathol. **164**: 1425–1434.
76. HO, L. *et al.* 2004. Diet-induced insulin resistance promotes amyloidosis in a transgenic mouse model of Alzheimer's disease. FASEB J. **18**: 902–904.
77. SCHMITZ, A. *et al.* 2004. Endoplasmic reticulum-localized amyloid β-peptide is degraded in the cytosol by two distinct degradation pathways. Traffic **5**: 89–101.
78. GROSSMAN, H. 2003. Does diabetes protect or provoke Alzheimer's disease? Insights into the pathobiology and future treatment of Alzheimer's disease. CNS Spectr. **8**: 815–823.
79. PRINCE, J.A. *et al.* 2003. Genetic variation in a haplotype block spanning IDE influences Alzheimer disease. Hum. Mutat. **22**: 363–371.
80. BOUSSAHA, M. *et al.* 2002. Polymorphisms of insulin degrading enzyme gene are not associated with Alzheimer's disease. Neurosci. Lett. **329**: 121–123.
81. BLOMQVIST, M.E. *et al.* 2004. Sequence variation in the proximity of IDE may impact age at onset of both Parkinson disease and Alzheimer disease. Neurogenetics **5**: 115–119.
82. BARNES, K. & A.J. TURNER. 1999. The endothelin converting enzyme is located on α-actin filaments in smooth muscle cells. Cardiovasc. Res. **42**: 814–822.
83. BARNES, K & A.J. TURNER. 1997. The endothelin system and endothelin-converting enzyme in the brain: molecular and cellular studies. Neurochem. Res. **22**: 1033–1040.
84. VALDENAIRE, O., E. ROHRBACHER & M.G. MATTEI. 1995. Organization of the gene encoding the human endothelin-converting enzyme (ECE-1). J. Biol. Chem. **270**: 29794–2978.
85. SCHWEIZER, A. *et al.* 1997. Human endothelin-converting enzyme (ECE-1): three isoforms with distinct subcellular localizations. Biochem. J. **328**: 871–877.
86. HOANG, M.V. & A.J. TURNER. 1997. Novel activity for endothelin-converting enzyme: hydrolysis of bradykinin. Biochem. J. **327**: 23–26.
87. EMOTO, N. & M. YANAGISAWA. 1995. Endothelin-converting enzyme-2 is a membrane-bound, phorphoramidon-sensitive metalloprotease with acidic pH optimum. J. Biol. Chem. **270**: 15262–15268.
88. ECKMAN, E.A., D.K. REED & C.B. ECKMAN. 2001. Degradation of the Alzheimer's amyloid β peptide by endothelin-converting enzyme. J. Biol. Chem. **276**: 24540–24548.
89. ECKMAN, E.A. *et al.* 2003. Alzheimer's disease β-amyloid peptide is increased in mice deficient in endothelin-converting enzyme. J. Biol. Chem. **278**: 2081-2084.
90. WERB, Z. 1997. ECM and cell surface proteolysis: regulating cellular ecology. Cell **91**: 439–442.
91. TSIRKA, S.E., A.D. ROGOVE & S. STRICKLAND. 1996. Neuronal cell death and tPA. Nature **384**: 123–124.
92. NAKAGAMI, Y. *et al.* 2000. Laminin degradation by plasmin regulates long-term potentiation. J. Neurosci. **20**: 2003–2010.
93. MADANI, R., S. NEF & J.D. VASSALLI. 2003. Emotions are building up in the field of extracellular proteolysis. Trends Mol. Med. **9**: 183–185.
94. PFEFFERKORN, T. *et al.* 2000. Plasminogen activation in experimental permanent focal cerebral ischemia. Brain Res. **882**: 19–25.
95. LEDESMA, M.D. *et al.* 2000. Brain plasmin enhances APP α-cleavage and Aβ degradation and is reduced in Alzheimer's disease brains. EMBO Rep. **1**: 530–535.
96. LEDESMA, M.D. *et al.* 2003. Raft disorganization leads to reduced plasmin activity in Alzheimer's disease brains. EMBO Rep. **4**: 1190–1196.
97. VAN NOSTRAND, W.E. & M. PORTER. 1999. Plasmin cleavage of the amyloid β-protein: alteration of secondary structure and stimulation of tissue plasminogen activator activity. Biochemistry **38**: 11570–11576.
98. TUCKER, H.M. *et al.* 2000. The plasmin system is induced by and degrades amyloid-β aggregates. J. Neurosci. **20**: 3937–3946.
99. TUCKER, H.M. *et al.* 2000. Tissue plasminogen activator requires plasminogen to modulate amyloid-β neurotoxicity and deposition. J. Neurochem. **75**: 2172–2177.

100. LEDESMA, M.D. *et al.* 2003. Proteomic characterisation of neuronal sphingolipid-cholesterol microdomains: role in plasminogen activation. Brain Res. **987:** 107–116.
101. EHEHALT, R. *et al.* 2003. Amyloidogenic processing of the Alzheimer β-amyloid precursor protein depends on lipid rafts. J. Cell Biol. **160:** 113–123.
102. CORDY, J.M. *et al.* 2003. Exclusively targeting β-secretase to lipid rafts by GPI-anchor addition up-regulates β-site processing of the amyloid precursor protein. Proc. Natl. Acad. Sci. USA **100:** 11735–11740.
103. KINGSTON, I.B., M.J.M. CASTRO & S.A. ANDERSON. 1995. In vitro stimulation of tissue-type plasminogen activator by Alzheimer amyloid β-peptide analogues. Nat. Med. **1:** 138–142.
104. ERTEKIN-TANER, N. *et al.* 2000. Linkage of plasma Aβ42 to a quantitative locus on chromosome 10 in late-onset Alzheimer's disease pedigrees. Science **290:** 2303–2304.
105. TUCKER, H.M., M. KIHIKO-EHMANN & S. ESTUS. 2002. Urokinase-type plasminogen activator inhibits amyloid-β neurotoxicity and fibrillogenesis via plasminogen. J. Neurosci. Res. **70:** 249–255.
106. HU, J. *et al.* 2001. Angiotensin-converting enzyme degrades Alzheimer amyloid β-peptide (Aβ); retards Aβ aggregation, deposition, fibril formation; and inhibits cyto-toxicity. J. Biol. Chem. **276:** 47863–47868.
107. BACKSTROM, J.R. *et al.* 1996. Matrix metalloproteinase-9 (MMP-9) is synthesized in neurons of the human hippocampus and is capable of degrading the amyloid-β peptide (1–40). J. Neurosci. **16:** 7910–7919.
108. RANGAN, S.K. *et al.* 2003. Degradation of β-amyloid by proteolytic antibody light chains. Biochemistry **42:** 14328–14334.
109. LIU, R. *et al.* 2004. Proteolytic antibody light chains alter β-amyloid aggregation and prevent cytotoxicity. Biochemistry **43:** 9999–10007.
110. PERRY, T.A. & N.H. GREIG. 2004. A new Alzheimer's disease interventive strategy: GLP-1. Curr. Drug Targets **5:** 565–571.
111. GOLOMB, J. *et al.* 1993. Hippocampal atrophy in normal aging. An association with recent memory impairment. Arch. Neurol. **50:** 967–973.
112. MONTINE, T.J. *et al.* 2002. Lipid peroxidation in aging brain and Alzheimer's disease. Free Radic. Biol. Med. **33:** 620–626.
113. TOESCU, E.C. & A. VERKHRATSKY. 2004. Ca^{2+} and mitochondria as substrates for deficits in synaptic plasticity in normal brain aging. J. Cell. Mol. Med. **8:** 181–190.
114. CUTLER, R.G. *et al.* 2004. Involvement of oxidative stress-induced abnormalities in ceramide and cholesterol metabolism in brain aging and Alzheimer's disease. Proc. Natl. Acad. Sci. USA **101:** 2070–2075.
115. WELLER, R.O. *et al.* 2000. Cerebral amyloid angiopathy: accumulation of Aβ in interstitial fluid drainage pathways in Alzheimer's disease. Ann. N.Y. Acad. Sci. **903:** 110–117.
116. BUTTERFIELD, D.A. *et al.* 2002. Evidence of oxidative damage in Alzheimer's disease brain: central role for amyloid β-peptide. Trends Mol. Med. **7:** 548–554.
117. LAUDERBACK, C.M. *et al.* 2001. The glial glutamate transporter, GLT-1, is oxidatively modified by 4-hydroxy-2-nonenal in the Alzheimer's disease brain: the role of Aβ1–42. J. Neurochem. **78:** 413–416.
118. SAYRE, L.M. *et al.* 1997. 4-Hydroxynonenal-derived advanced lipid peroxidation end products are increased in Alzheimer's disease. J. Neurochem. **68:** 2092–2097.
119. WANG, D.S. *et al.* 2003. Oxidized neprilysin in aging and Alzheimer's disease brains. Biochem. Biophys. Res. Commun. **310:** 236–241.
120. REISER, M. *et al.* 1987. Proteolytic degradation of insulin and glucagon in rat brain during ontogenesis. Acta Histochem. **82:** 35–39.
121. ZULIANI, G. *et al.* 2004. Low cholesterol levels are associated with short-term mortality in older patients with ischemic stroke. J. Gerontol. A. Biol. Sci. Med. Sci. **59:** 293–297.
122. ROHER, A.E. *et al.* 2002. Increased A β peptides and reduced cholesterol and myelin proteins characterize white matter degeneration in Alzheimer's disease. Biochemistry **37:** 11080–11090.
123. NYAKAS, C., B. BUWALDA & P.G. LUITEN. 1996. Hypoxia and brain development. Prog. Neurobiol. **49:** 1–51.
124. DOLINAK, D., C. SMITH & D.I. GRAHAM. 2000. Global hypoxia per se is an unusual cause of axonal injury. Acta Neuropathol. (Berl.) **100:** 553–560.

125. YEPES, M. & D.A. LAWRENCE. 2004. Tissue-type plasminogen activator and neuroserpin: a well-balanced act in the nervous system? Trends Cardiovasc. Med. **14:** 173–180.
126. IWATA, N. *et al.* 2004. Presynaptic localization of neprilysin contributes to efficient clearance of amyloid-β peptide in mouse brain. J. Neurosci. **24:** 991–998.
127. MARR, R.A. *et al.* 2003. Neprilysin gene transfer reduces human amyloid pathology in transgenic mice. J. Neurosci. **23:** 1992–1996.
128. LEVITES, Y. *et al.* 2003. Neuroprotection and neurorescue against Aβ toxicity and PKC-dependent release of nonamyloidogenic soluble precursor protein by green tea polyphenol (−)-epigallocatechin-3-gallate. FASEB J. **17:** 952–954.

Effect of Hypoxia/Ischemia and Hypoxic Preconditioning/Reperfusion on Expression of Some Amyloid-Degrading Enzymes

NATALIA N. NALIVAEVA[a,b] LILIA FISK,[a] EKATERINA G. KOCHKINA,[b] SVETLANA A. PLESNEVA,[b] IGOR A. ZHURAVIN,[b] EVA BABUSIKOVA,[c] DUSAN DOBROTA,[c] AND ANTHONY J. TURNER[a]

[a]*School of Biochemistry and Microbiology, University of Leeds, Leeds LS2 9JT, United Kingdom*

[b]*Institute of Evolutionary Physiology and Biochemistry, RAS, 194223 Saint Petersburg, Russia*

[c]*Department of Biochemistry, Jessenius Faculty of Medicine, Comenius University, 036 01 Martin, Slovak Republic*

ABSTRACT: Alzheimer's disease (AD) is linked to certain common brain pathologies (e.g., ischemia, stroke, and trauma) believed to facilitate its development and progression. One of the logical approaches to this problem is to study the effects of ischemia and hypoxia on the metabolism of amyloid precursor protein, which plays one of the key roles in the pathogenesis of AD. This involves an analysis of (1) proteases, which participate in proteolysis of amyloid precursor protein either by the nonamyloidogenic route (α-secretase) or the amyloidogenic pathway and lead to formation of toxic β-amyloid peptides (β- and γ-secretases) and (2) several metallopeptidases that might play a role in degradation of β-amyloid peptide ($A\beta$). The study of the effects of prenatal hypoxia and acute hypoxia in adult animals allowed us to conclude that oxygen deprivation results not only in an increase of amyloid precursor protein expression in the brain but also in a decrease in the activity of α-secretase. In some brain structures involved in AD pathology (the cortex and striatum), we also observed a decrease in the expression of two of the $A\beta$ degrading enzymes, neprilysin and endothelin-converting enzyme, after hypoxia. A decrease in expression of these metalloproteases was also observed in the model of four-vessel occlusion ischemia in rats with their restoration to the control levels after reperfusion. Preconditioning to mild hypoxia both in the prenatal period and in adults appeared to have a neuroprotective effect restoring, in particular, the levels of amyloid precursor protein, activity of α-secretase, and expression of neprilysin and endothelin-converting enzyme to their control values.

KEYWORDS: amyloid precursor protein; α-secretase; Alzheimer's disease; endothelin-converting enzyme; hypoxia; ischemia; metallopeptidases; neprilysin; preconditioning; reperfusion

Address for correspondence: Dr. Natalia N. Nalivaeva, School of Biochemistry and Microbiology, University of Leeds, Leeds LS2 9JT, United Kingdom. Voice: +44-113-343-2987; fax: +44-113-343-3157.

n.n.nalivaeva@leeds.ac.uk

Ann. N.Y. Acad. Sci. 1035: 21–33 (2004). © 2004 New York Academy of Sciences.
doi: 10.1196/annals.1332.002

INTRODUCTION

Brain ischemia and associated hypoxia are among the most common complications resulting from impaired brain circulation and metabolism, which can affect animals and humans at various stages of their life. Ischemic stroke is the third leading cause of death in Western countries, after heart disease and cancer.[1] Brain hypoxia affects both behavioral and cognitive abilities of individuals and leads to various neuropathologies.[2] There is strong association between cerebrovascular diseases and Alzheimer's disease (AD). The strongest evidence for this connection is that patients with cerebrovascular disease or vascular dementia will often bear AD pathology at autopsy even when there was no clinical pre-existing AD.[3] While small vascular lesions may not significantly influence the cognitive decline in patients with AD, the frequent cerebrovascular lesions may play an important role in determining the presence and severity of AD.[4–6] While brain ischemia and stroke are considered age-related diseases, chronic prenatal and neonatal hypoxia is the most common complication in children, affecting individuals during their entire life.[7]

There are several animal models of ischemia and hypoxia widely used for biochemical studies. The animal models of ischemia appeared to be a valuable scientific tool due to their "reproducibility, replicability and control on confounding variables".[8] The striking similarity of the rodent genome to the human genome makes animal models even more versatile and permits analysis of the genes involved in the hypoxic/ischemic response of the brain. Using DNA microarray techniques it was demonstrated that 28 ischemia-hypoxia response genes were upregulated and 6 downregulated in the brain of rats subjected to focal ischemia. These genes included immediate-early genes, heat-shock proteins, antioxidative enzymes, trophic factors, and genes involved in RNA metabolism, inflammation, and cell signaling.[9] Animal models of prenatal hypoxia have been useful for the testing of potential neuroprotective agents, especially when conducted with concurrent physiological monitoring.[10] Using the model of normobaric prenatal hypoxia in rats, it was shown that hypoxia on the thirteenth day of gestation (1) results in significant changes in the activity of enzymes involved in the biogenesis of cyclic nucleotides and transmembrane ion transport and (2) affects the cholinergic system of the brain, especially of the cortex and striatum, in postnatal ontogenesis of animals.[11] It was also demonstrated that expression of amyloid precursor protein (APP) and formation of its soluble fragment sAPPα were affected by prenatal hypoxia during the entire lifespan of animals.[12]

Although there have been some attempts to assess the factors by which ischemia and stroke are associated with AD (for review, see Bazan and colleagues[13]), the molecular mechanisms of this phenomenon are still unclear. There are data suggesting that amyloid metabolism is affected by ischemia and hypoxia and that an increased level of APP is a part of the acute adaptive response of the brain to hypoxia.[14] Ischemic-reperfusion brain injury was shown to induce overexpression of APP in reactive astrocytes, with expression peaking at 7 days and 6 months after the insult.[15] It has been shown that combined treatment with both Aβ and hypoxia significantly decreases the number of neuronal cells and increases the number of TUNEL-positive cells going through apoptosis.[16] Transient ischemia followed by reperfusion was shown to result in an increase of the Kunitz protease inhibitor-bearing isoforms of APP (KPI-APP) with a decrease of the APP_{695} isoform, which lacks the KPI domain.[17] It was suggested that the KPI domain of APP could inhibit proteases and prevent normal processing of APP. This would result in an inhibition of production of sAPP, which is reported to play a neuroprotective role against ischemic injury in the brain.[18] This was supported by the observations of Ho and colleagues,[19] who demonstrated that expression of the KPI-domain reduces cleavage by α-secretase. Thus, overexpression of the longer APP isoforms under hypoxia/ischemia could lead to neuronal pathology through decreased production of sAPP and, as a result, increased production of neurotoxic Aβ by alternative processing of APP.[20] Increased Aβ formation under chronic hypoxic conditions was also shown to disturb calcium homeostasis in cortical astrocytes which may lead to cell death and brain pathology.[21]

Generation of reactive oxygen species (ROS) and reactive nitrogen species represent a complex cascade of events occurring during ischemia and stroke.[22] Accumulated ROS was shown to deteriorate amyloid metabolism and lead to accumulation of Aβ in the brain.[23] ROS-induced formation of protofibrils and aggregates of Aβ resulted in neuronal cell dysfunction and cell death.[24] It was recently demonstrated that S-nitrosothiols (SNOs) play the key role in cellular responses to hypoxia.[25] S-nitrosylation was shown to activate metalloproteinases and, in particular, matrix metalloproteinases (MMPs) that, via an extracellular proteolysis pathway, lead to neuronal cell death.[26] Since major enzymes participating in APP metabolism appear to be metalloproteinases (e.g., α-secretase), this observation strengthens even more the link between hypoxia and amyloid-related brain pathology.

Accumulation of Aβ in the normal brain might be prevented by its drainage from the extracellular space via perivascular pathways. It was shown that under certain pathologies, e.g., cerebral amyloid angiopathy (CAA), Aβ accumulates in the walls of arteries of both the cortex and meninges.[27] The pattern of deposition of Aβ in senile plaques and in CAA suggests that Aβ accumulates in pericapillary and periarterial drainage pathways. It is possible that under conditions of ischemia the drainage of Aβ will be affected to a certain extent.

Alternatively to drainage, Aβ can be eliminated from the extra- and intracellular space via its degradation. Recently it was demonstrated that there is a range of enzymes capable of degrading Aβ (for review, see Carson and Turner).[28] Among them are several metallopeptidases, including neprilysin (NEP, neutral endopeptidase-24.11),[29] its homologue, endothelin-converting enzyme (ECE-1)[30] and insulin-degrading enzyme (IDE),[31] which were shown to abolish Aβ accumulation and its pathogenic effects both *in vitro* and *in vivo*. NEP is also one of the major endopeptidases responsible for the inactivation of enkephalins and substance P in the brain.[32] In the carotid body it plays an important role in maintaining levels of this neurotransmitter critical to transduction of hypoxic stimuli.[33,34] In the brain, intrastriatal administration of phosphoramidon, a dual inhibitor of NEP and ECE-1, resulted in a significantly increased infarct volume to hypoxia with a significant attenuation of cerebral blood flow.[35] However, intrastriatal administration of a selective NEP inhibitor, thiorphan, had no effect either on cerebral blood flow or infarct volume induced by the hypoxic challenge, suggesting that phosphoramidon-sensitive ECE-1 is functionally active in the modulation of cerebral blood flow in rats undergoing hypoxia.[35] Involvement both of NEP and ECE-1 in the hypoxic response and degradation of Aβ make them an important target for reducing the damaging effect of hypoxia on Aβ accumulation and development of the neuropathology.

In the present paper, we present the data on the effects of hypoxia and ischemia on amyloid metabolism in the brain of rats subjected to acute hypoxia or global transient ischemia. For this we analyzed levels of expression of APP and its soluble fragment sAPPα, as well as expression of two Aβ-degrading enzymes (NEP and ECE-1). We also compared the effect of hypoxic preconditioning and reperfusion after ischemia on the analyzed parameters.

METHODS

Hypoxia

The experiments were performed using Wistar female and male rats. In the prenatal hypoxia paradigm, pregnant female rats were subjected to normobaric hypoxia on 13–14 days of gestation (the period of active proliferation of neuroblasts and the beginning of migration of nervous cells) as described previously.[11] Hypoxic conditions were mimicked in a special chamber (100 L in volume) equipped with systems of thermoregulation, ventilation, CO_2 absorption, and gas analysis. To create hypoxic conditions, the content of oxygen in the chamber was decreased linearly from 21% to 7% during the first 10 min by substitution with helium and then was maintained at this level (7%) for 3 hours. Concentration of CO_2 in the chamber was not higher than 0.1% and the temperature was kept at 22°C. Female rats from the control group were kept during the same period of time in the same room in a cage under normal oxygen content. In some experiments pregnant rats were preconditioned to hypoxia (15% O_2, 2 h) on days 10, 11, and 12 of gestation. The newborn animals were kept after birth under standard vivarium conditions and were used for biochemical analysis on postnatal days 5, 11, 20, 30, and 300.

In the acute adult hypoxia paradigm, Wistar male rats at the age of 10 months were used. Experimental animals were subjected to hypoxia as described above. Preconditioning to hypoxia was performed by the same scheme. Animals were taken for biochemical analysis 35 min and 24 h after acute hypoxia.

For biochemical experiments animals were sacrificed by decapitation and the sensorimotor cortex and striatum were dissected from the brain according to a stereotaxic atlas.[36] There were a minimum of five animals in each experimental group.

Ischemia

Forebrain ischemia was induced in Wistar male rats by the four-vessel occlusion method as described by Pulsinelli and colleagues.[37] The rats were surgically prepared under halothane anesthesia by permanently occluding the vertebral arteries. The carotid arteries were exposed and loops of silastic tubing were placed loosely around them to allow rapid subsequent exposure of these vessels. On the next day the carotid arteries were located again and occluded with artery clamps. Ischemia was reversed after 15 min by removing the clamps. Following the given reperfusion period (2 h), rats were sacrificed and decapitated. The right and left brain hemispheres without the basal ganglia and hippocampi were used for the analysis of the proteins of interest. There were three animals in each experimental group.

All experiments on animals were performed under the legal protocols on animal protection and welfare.

Preparation of the Samples

Analysis of the proteins of interest was performed either in the low-salt soluble or membrane (detergent-soluble) fractions of the brain samples, which were obtained following the protocol described in Nalivaeva and colleagues.[12] To obtain these fractions the brain tissue was cleared of the blood vessels and homogenized in 1 mL of 0.02 M Tris-HCl (pH 7.5), 0.01 M $MgCl_2$, and 0.05 M NaCl and centrifuged at 500,000*g* for 10 min in a Beckman model TL100 tabletop ultracentrifuge. The supernatant was collected and considered the low-salt soluble fraction. The pellet was resuspended in 1 mL of 0.01 M phosphate buffer (pH 7.4) with 1% Triton X-100, incubated on ice for 1 h and centrifuged as above for 10 min to generate the detergent-soluble fraction. The amount of protein in the fractions obtained was analyzed by the routine bicinchoninic acid (BCA) protein assay using the BCA kit (Sigma). For further immunoblotting analysis the fractions were lyophilized and dissolved to a final concentration of 2 mg/mL in the sample buffer containing 125 mM Tris, 2% w/vol SDS, 20% vol/vol glycerol, 2 mM EDTA, 2 mM EGTA, 5 µg/mL leupeptin, 5 µg/mL pepstatin A, 10 µg/mL aprotinin, (pH 6.8) with 1% bromophenol blue and 10% β-mercaptoethanol when required.

Immunoblotting

Samples containing equal amounts of protein (40–90 µg) were resolved on SDS-polyacrylamide gels and blotted onto poly(vinylidene) difluoride membranes (Immobilon P, Millipore). Membranes were probed with adequate primary antibody, as shown below, followed by a secondary horseradish peroxidase-conjugated antibody (1:2,000 dilution). Membranes were washed for 30 min with Tris-buffered saline pH 7.6 containing 0.1% (vol/vol) Tween 20 and proteins of interest were detected with the enhanced chemiluminescent detection system (Amersham Pharmacia Biotech Limited, Bucks., U.K.).

Analysis of APP and sAPP was performed using the selective antibody 22C11; ECE-1, Mab 32 (AEC32-236) (Dr. K. Tanzawa, Tokyo, Japan); NEP, polyclonal rabbit anti-rat antibody (USBiological); actin, anti-actin (20-33) IgG fraction of antiserum developed in rabbit (Sigma); and horseradish peroxidase-linked secondary antibody was from Amersham Biosciences (U.K.). Sample loading was monitored either by actin or by staining the PVDF membranes with 0.1% Ponceau S (Sigma) in 5% acetic acid (vol/vol). Quantification of the bands was performed by laser scanning densitometry using Bio-Rad Multi-AnalistTM/PC software, Version 1.1.1 (Bio-Rad, Hemel Hempstead, U.K.).

All biochemical experiments were performed at least in triplicate and the statistical analysis was performed using the *t* test.

RESULTS AND DISCUSSION

Effect of Acute Hypoxia and Ischemia on APP and sAPP

To evaluate the effect of impaired oxygen supply on the levels of APP and its soluble fragment sAPP we performed the analysis of low-salt–soluble fractions (containing sAPP) and detergent-soluble (containing membrane bound APP) fractions from the brain hemispheres of rats subjected to global transient ischemia and from the cortex of rats subjected to acute normobaric hypoxia. The data obtained demonstrated that both hypoxia and ischemia resulted in elevation of the levels of APP in the brain (FIGS. 1 and 2). In the case of 15-min global transient ischemia this elevation both in the right and left hemispheres was twofold compared to control values, which was comparable with the degree of increase of APP levels observed in the cortex immediately (35 min) and 24 h after acute hypoxia. The levels of APP were found to return practically to their control values after 2-h reperfusion. It suggests that reoxygenation of the brain leads to restoration of normal metabolism at least at the level of APP expression.

Analysis of sAPP revealed a different character of reaction of the brain to reduced oxygen supply at the level of the cortex and cerebral hemispheres (FIGS. 1 and 2). In the cortex, we observed a significant decrease of the production of sAPP both 35 min and 24 h after acute hypoxia, while global transient ischemia resulted in a marked

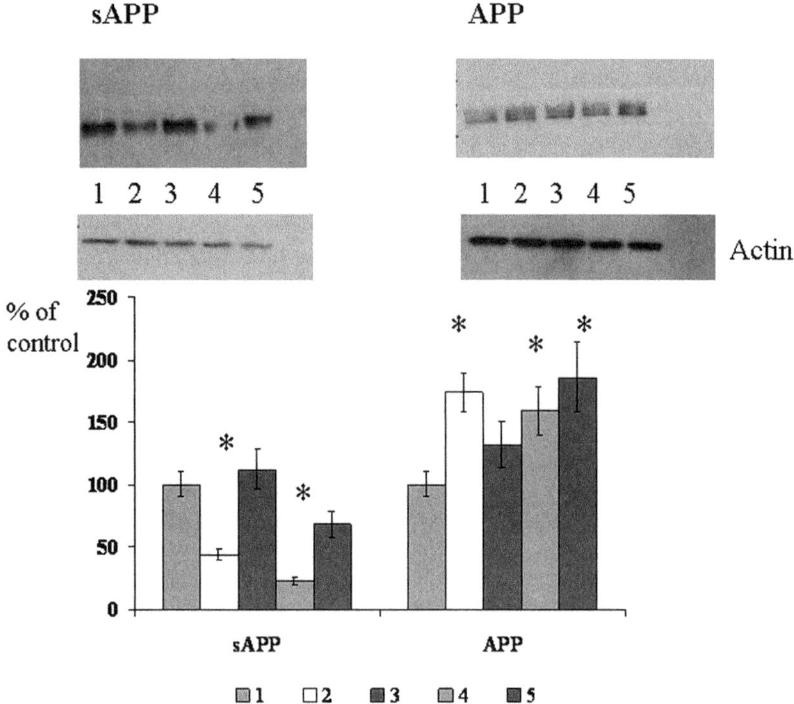

FIGURE 1. Analysis of the effect of acute hypoxia and hypoxic preconditioning on the levels of APP and sAPP in the hemispheres of 10-month-old rats. (1) Control, (2) 35 min after hypoxia, (3) 35 min after hypoxia with preconditioning, (4) 24 h after hypoxia, (5) 24 h after hypoxia with preconditioning. Western blot: APP and sAPP analyzed with monoclonal antibody 22C11. The chart represents the densitometric analysis of the blots. Loading of samples was monitored either by actin (in case of membrane-bound APP) or by staining the membranes with Ponceau S (in case of sAPP, data not shown). Ordinate in arbitrary units in % compared to control. *$P < .05$, compared to control.

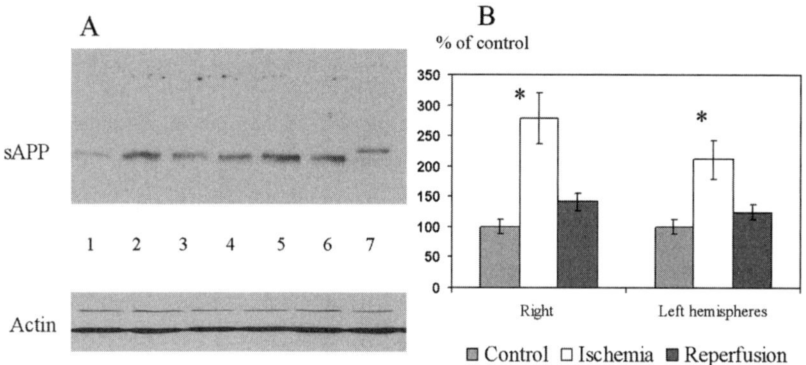

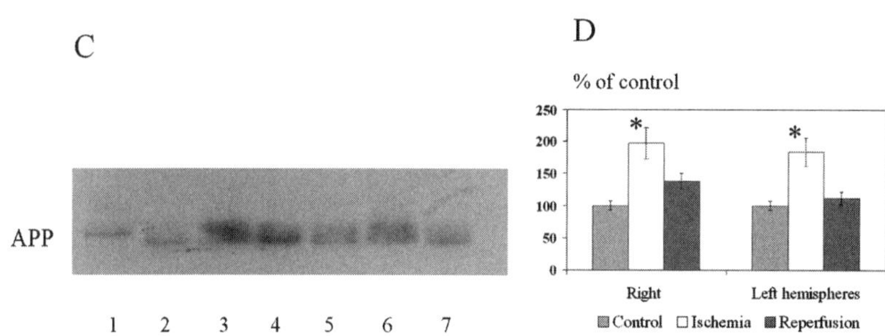

FIGURE 2. Effect of global transient ischemia on sAPP (**A**) and APP (**C**) in the right and left hemispheres of rat brain. (1) Control rat (right hemisphere), (2) ischemia 15 min, (3) reperfusion for 2 h, (4) control rat (left hemisphere), (5) ischemia 15 min, (6) reperfusion 2 h, (7) positive control (APP$_{751}$ from SH-SY5Y neuroblastoma cells). Western blot: APP and sAPP analyzed with monoclonal antibody 22C11. Loading of samples was monitored by the levels of actin. (**B** and **D**) Data of the densitometry of the bands. Ordinate is arbitrary units in % compared to control. *$P < .05$, compared to control.

increase of sAPP in the cerebral hemispheres. This difference in the observed characteristics might be a result of a specific reaction of different types of neuronal cells in the brain structures composing cerebral hemispheres and the cortex. On the other hand, this also might be a result of the time of the episode of oxygen deprivation. In the case of acute hypoxia animals were subjected to reduced oxygen content (7% external pO_2 and approximately 1.7% pO_2 within the brain cortex) for a longer period of time (3 h) than in the case of ischemia (15 min), although in the latter case blood and oxygen supply to the brain were totally blocked. Similarly to APP levels, the levels of sAPP in the brain hemispheres practically returned to control values after reperfusion. Along with the increased levels of membrane-bound APP, the decrease in the production of sAPP observed in the cortex can testify to a reduced α-secretase-like activity in this brain structure under conditions of acute hypoxia. These data correlate with our previous observation of a decreased α-secretase-like activity in the SMC of rats subjected to prenatal hypoxia at various stages of postnatal life.[12]

Analyzing the effect of preconditioning to mild hypoxia before the episode of acute hypoxia, we have found that it had a remarkable effect on the levels of sAPP observed 35 min and 24 h after hypoxia. In both cases, the levels of the soluble form of APP in the brain cortices of animals subjected to hypoxia with preconditioning (lines 3 and 5) were much higher than just after acute hypoxia only (lines 2 and 4, Fig. 1). The neuroprotective effect of hypoxic preconditioning was reported earlier by Wick and colleagues, who suggested that vascular endothelial growth factor (VEGF) and its receptor (VEGFR-2) are involved in neuronal survival mediated by hypoxic preconditioning.[38] Liu and coworkers also reported neuroprotective effects of hypoxic preconditioning on transient focal ischemia-reperfusion injuries in rat brain. They observed that preconditioning to hypoxia resulted in attenuated cortical infarction and protected the brain against oxidative damages caused by reoxygenation.[39] More recently, Hellweg and colleagues also demonstrated that expression of APP mRNA increased upon repetitive inhibition of oxidative phosphorylation with 3-nitropropionate (an inhibitor of mitochondrial complex II, nine treatments at 2-day intervals), but remained at control levels after nine *in vivo* treatments at 4-day intervals.[40] Our data provide additional evidence that a neuroprotective effect of preconditioning might also involve an α-secretase-like metalloproteinase and production of sAPP, the neuroprotective effect of which on memory and cell proliferation has been reported by other authors.[41,42]

Effect of Ischemia on Expression of Aβ-Degrading Enzymes

Since their discovery, the enzymes capable of degrading Aβ[28] have become an important target in the studies of AD pathology. Using the model of ischemia in rats we also analyzed its effect on expression at the level of protein products of two major Aβ-degrading enzymes, namely NEP and ECE-1. The data of these experiments are presented in Figure 3. The data obtained have clearly demonstrated that global transient ischemia resulted in a dramatic decrease in the levels of ECE-1 detected in the detergent-soluble fraction of rat brain hemispheres (Fig. 3, lines 2 and 5). Reperfusion of the brain for 2 h led to restoration of the levels of expression of this metalloproteinase in the brain hemispheres back to control amount (lines 3 and 6). Levels of NEP were also found to be reduced in the brain hemispheres after ischemia and partially restored after reperfusion (Fig. 3). Decreased levels of cerebral NEP and ECE are reported here for the first time and further study is now underway to elucidate which brain areas and type of cells are responsible for this phenomenon. However, taken together, the data of this part of the study and the data of the analysis of expression of APP allow us to suggest that ischemia and the accompanying hypoxia in general might result in a shift of the balance of amyloid metabolism towards elevated production of Aβ. In case of chronic hypoxia or repeated ischemic stroke, this might underlie accumulation of toxic Aβ fibrils, neuronal death, and development of dementia of Alzheimer's type.

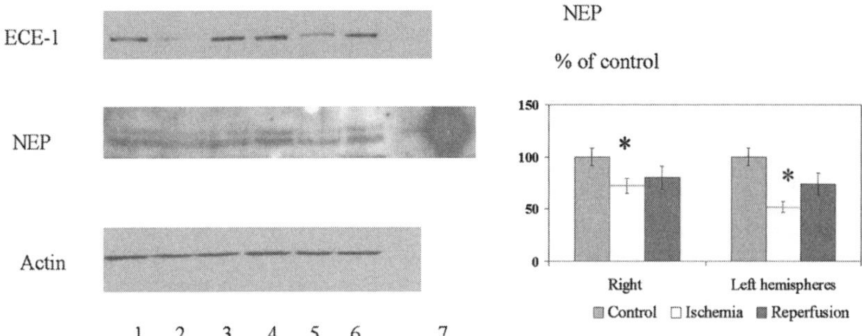

FIGURE 3. Effect of transient global ischemia on NEP and ECE-1 in the rat brain. (1) Control rat (right hemisphere), (2) ischemia 15 min, (3) reperfusion for 2 h, (4) control rat (left hemisphere), (5) ischemia 15 min, (6) reperfusion 2 h, (7) positive control, NEP from rat kidney. The chart represents the densitometric analysis of the NEP levels revealed by immunoblotting. Ordinate is arbitrary units in % compared to control. $*P < .05$, compared to control.

Effect of Prenatal Hypoxia on NEP in the Striatum of Rats

As we showed previously, prenatal hypoxia significantly affected production of APP in the sensorimotor cortex (SMC) observed at various periods of postnatal life.[12] The postnatal levels of APP were found to be higher than in control animals. Moreover, secretion of the soluble form of APP (sAPP) by α-secretase was found to be the most active on day 30 of postnatal development and there was a significant decrease in the production of sAPP after prenatal hypoxia. NEP was found to be expressed in the cortex of rats only at the early stages of postnatal development and it was barely detectable in adult rats. In animals subjected to prenatal hypoxia we observed a decrease in the levels of NEP in the SMC.[12] Developing this study, we have found that in the rat striatum the expression of NEP was lowest on the fifth day of postnatal life, but increased steadily from day 11 to the end of the first month of postnatal development and then did not change with age (FIG. 4A). Prenatal hypoxia resulted in a decrease in the levels of expression of NEP in the striatum in later life, the most significant decrease being observed on day 30 of postnatal life (FIG. 4B). Similar to our data obtained in the SMC of rats,[12] preconditioning to mild hypoxia in the prenatal period attenuated the effect of acute hypoxia, to which animals were subjected on day 13.5 of gestation. The levels of NEP observed in the striatum of animals after hypoxic preconditioning were similar to those in the controls. The effect of hypoxic preconditioning in the prenatal period on restoration of the decreased expression of NEP both in the cortex and striatum of the developing is in accordance with the data of literature on the neuroprotective effect of preconditioning on the immature brain.[43,44]

The data presented here and our previous data support the hypothesis that NEP deficiency might be a reason for Aβ accumulation in the cortex, but not in the striatum of AD patients, since expression of this metallopeptidase in the striatum remains at significantly high levels even in old age. Apelt and colleagues[45] also reported an

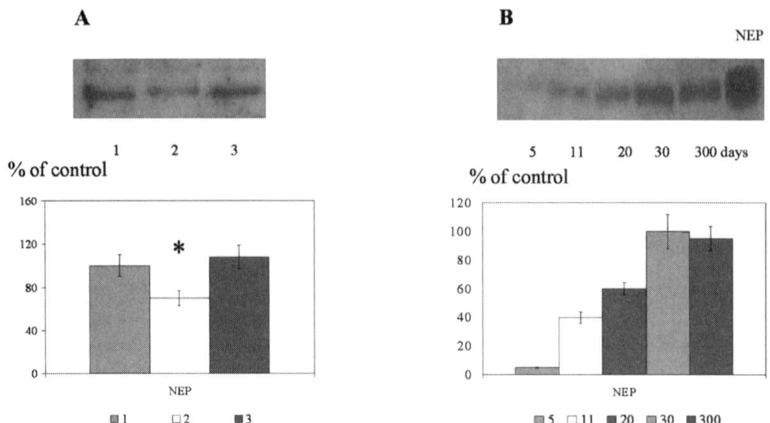

FIGURE 4. Effect of acute prenatal hypoxia (3 h, 7% O_2) on 13.5th day of gestation (E13.5) and preconditioning to mild hypoxia (2 h, 15% O_2) on the levels of NEP in the striatum of rats on postnatal day 30 (**A**). (1) Control, (2) after prenatal hypoxia on E13.5, (3) after prenatal hypoxia on E13.5 with preconditioning on E10, 11, and 12 (see *Methods*). (**B**) Levels of expression of NEP in the striatum at different periods of postnatal life (5–300 days) of control animals. NEP is positive control from rat kidney. Western blot: NEP analyzed with rabbit anti-rat polyclonal antibodies (US Biological). Loading of the samples was monitored by staining the PVDF membranes with Ponceau S. Charts represent the data of the densitometry of the bands revealed by immunoblotting. Ordinate is arbitrary units in % compared to control. *$P < .05$, compared to control.

overall reduction of NEP levels over the course of a lifetime, especially in neurites around β-amyloid plaques. The literature suggests that upregulation of NEP activity in the brain might be a viable therapeutic approach for treatment of AD. However, the age-dependent pattern of NEP expression in the brain cortex demonstrated in our studies and by other groups suggests that this might have some limitations in older individuals and should be done at a relatively young age to prevent accumulation of Aβ and formation of plaques. This suggestion is supported by the data of Mohajieri and colleagues,[46] who demonstrated that neuronal upregulation of NEP led to a decrease in Aβ levels only in the brain of young transgenic mice expressing AD-causing APP mutation (SwAPP) and had no effect in aged mice with pre-existing plaque pathology.

CONCLUSIONS

The data reported here provide new evidence supporting the hypothesis that amyloid metabolism is affected by hypoxia and ischemia and that increased production of APP and a deficit of the activity of Aβ-degrading enzymes might be amongst the reasons underlying the link between ischemia and AD. Accumulation of Aβ in the hypoxic brain might be also a result of an imbalance between APP processing via nonamyloidogenic (α-secretase) and amyloidogenic (β- and γ-secretase) pathways.

Although upregulation of α-secretase pathway and inhibition of β- and γ-secretase have been widely tested as possible therapeutic targets for treatment of AD, they have certain limitations.[47,48] Upregulation of the enzymes that degrade APP might be a more feasible approach to AD treatment. Some studies of the neuroprotective effects of natural biologically active compounds[49] allow us to hope that there might be inexpensive ways to slow down the process of plaque formation or its prevention. On the other hand, the neuroprotective effect of hypoxic preconditioning, although not fully understood, might be another way to protect the brain against pathological processes. While delivery of some drugs to the brain may be difficult because of the blood-brain barrier, hypoxic preconditioning can protect the brain without any barrier via stimulating its own molecular mechanisms.

ACKNOWLEDGMENTS

This work was supported by INTAS-01-245, The Biochemical Society (to L. Fisk), The Royal Society, and RBRF-02-04-49385.

REFERENCES

1. CAMARATA, P.J., R.C. HEROS & R.E. LATCHAW. 1994. "Brain attack": the rationale for treating stroke as a medical emergency. Neurosurgery **34:** 144–157.
2. DOLINAK, D., C. SMITH & D.I. GRAHAM. 2000. Global hypoxia per se is an unusual cause of axonal injury. Acta Neuropathol. (Berl.) **100:** 553–560.
3. KALARIA, R.N. 2000. The role of cerebral ischemia in Alzheimer's disease. Neurobiol. Aging **21:** 321–330.
4. JELLINGER, K.A. 2002. The pathology of ischemic-vascular dementia: An update. J. Neurol. Sci. **203-204:** 153–157.
5. BRETELER, M.M. 2000. Vascular risk factors for Alzheimer's disease: an epidemiologic perspective. Neurobiol. Aging **21:** 153–160.
6. ESIRI, M.M. *et al.* 1999. Cerebrovascular disease and threshold for dementia in the early stages of Alzheimer's disease. Lancet **354:** 919–920.
7. NYAKAS, C., B. BUWALDA & P.G. LUITEN. 1996. Hypoxia and brain development. Prog. Neurobiol. **49:** 1–51.
8. GINSBERG, M.D. 2003. Adventures in the pathophysiology of brain ischemia: penumbra, gene expression, neuroprotection: the 2002 Thomas Willis Lecture. Stroke **34:** 214–223.
9. SCHMIDT-KASTNER, R. *et al.* 2002. DNA microarray analysis of cortical gene expression during early recirculation after focal brain ischemia in rat. Brain Res. Mol. Brain Res. **108:** 81–93.
10. FROEN, J.F. *et al.* 2002. Interleukin-10 reverses acute detrimental effects of endotoxin-induced inflammation on perinatal cerebral hypoxia-ischemia. Brain Res. **942:** 87–94.
11. LAVRENOVA, S.M., N.N. NALIVAEVA & I.A. ZHURAVIN. 2003. Activity of acetylcholinesterase in the motor-sensory cortex in early ontogenesis of rats exposed to prenatal hypoxia. J. Evol. Biochem. Physiol. **39:** 203–210.
12. NALIVAEVA, N.N. *et al.* 2004. Effects of prenatal hypoxia on expression of amyloid precursor protein and metallopeptidases in the rat brain. Lett. Peptide Sci. **10:** 455–462.
13. BAZAN, N.G., R. PALACIOS-PELAEZ & W.J. LUKIW. 2002. Hypoxia signaling to genes: significance in Alzheimer's disease. Mol. Neurobiol. **26:** 283–298.
14. BAIDEN-AMISSAH, K. *et al.* 1998. Expression of amyloid precursor protein (β-APP) in the neonatal brain following hypoxic ischaemic injury. Neuropathol. Appl. Neurobiol. **24:** 346–352.
15. PLUTA, R. 2002. Astroglial expression of the β-amyloid in ischemia-reperfusion brain injury. Ann. N.Y. Acad. Sci. **977:** 102–108.

16. EGASHIRA, N. *et al.* 2002. Hypoxia enhances beta-amyloid-induced apoptosis in rat cultured hippocampal neurons. Jpn. J. Pharmacol. **90:** 321–327.
17. KIM, H.S. *et al.* 1998. Post-ischemic changes in the expression of Alzheimer's APP isoforms in rat cerebral cortex. NeuroReport **9:** 533–537.
18. SMITH-SWINTOSKY, V.L. *et al.* 1994. Secreted forms of β-amyloid precursor protein protect against ischemic brain injury. J. Neurochem. **63:** 781–784.
19. HO, L., K. FUKICHI & S.G. YOUNKIN. 1996. The alternatively spliced Kunitz protease inhibitor domain alters amyloid protein precursor processing and amyloid β protein production in cultured cells. J. Biol. Chem. **271:** 30929–30934.
20. MATTSON, M.P. 1994. Secreted forms of β-amyloid precursor protein protect against ischemic brain injury. J. Neurochem. **63:** 781–784.
21. SMITH, I.F. *et al.* 2003. Hypoxic remodelling of Ca^{2+} mobilization in type I cortical astrocytes: involvement of ROS and pro-amyloidogenic APP processing. J. Neurochem. **88:** 869–877.
22. BEHL, C. & B. MOOSMANN. 2002. Oxidative nerve cell death in Alzheimer's disease and stroke: antioxidants as neuroprotective compounds. Biol. Chem. **383:** 521–536.
23. SMITH, J.V. & Y.J. LUO. 2003. Elevation of oxidative free radicals in Alzheimer's disease models can be attenuated by *Ginkgo biloba* extract EGb 761. Alzheimer's Dis. **4:** 287–300.
24. TABNER, B.J. *et al.* 2001. Production of reactive oxygen species from aggregating proteins implicated in Alzheimer's disease, Parkinson's disease and other neurodegenerative diseases. Curr. Top. Med. Chem. **1:** 507–517.
25. LIPTON, S.A. 2001. Nitric oxide and respiration. Nature **413:** 118–121.
26. GU, Z. *et al.* 2002. S-nitrosylation of matrix metalloproteinases: signaling pathway to neuronal cell death. Science **297:** 1186–1190.
27. WELLER, R.O. *et al.* 2000. Cerebral amyloid angiopathy: accumulation of Aβ in interstitial fluid drainage pathways in Alzheimer's disease. Ann. N.Y. Acad. Sci. **903:** 110–117.
28. CARSON, J. A. & A.J. TURNER. 2002. β-amyloid catabolism: role for neprilysin (NEP) and other metallopeptidases? J. Neurochem. **81:** 1–8.
29. IWATA, N. *et al.* 2000. Identification of the major Abeta1-42-degrading catabolic pathway in brain parenchyma: suppression leads to biochemical and pathological deposition. Nat. Med. **6:** 143–150.
30. ECKMAN, E.A. *et al.* C.B. 2003. Alzheimer's disease beta-amyloid peptide is increased in mice deficient in endothelin-converting enzyme. J. Biol. Chem. **278:** 2081–2084.
31. VEKRELLIS, K. *et al.* 2000. Neurons regulate extracellular levels of amyloid β-protein via proteolysis by insulin-degrading enzyme. J. Neurosci. **20:** 1657–1665.
32. MATSAS, R. *et al.* 1985. The metabolism of neuropeptides. Endopeptidase-24.11 in human synaptic membrane preparations hydrolyses substance P. Biochem. J. **228:** 487–492.
33. KUMAR, G.K. 1997. Peptidases of the peripheral chemoreceptors: biochemical, immunological, in vitro hydrolytic studies and electron microscopic analysis of neutral endopeptidase-like activity of the carotid body. Brain Res. **748:** 39–50.
34. GRASEMANN, H. *et al.* 1999. Targeted deletion of the neutral endopeptidase gene alters ventilatory responses to acute hypoxia in mice. J. Appl. Physiol. **87:** 1266–1271.
35. PARK, L. & J. THORNHILL. 2001. Phosphoramidon-sensitive endothelin-converting enzymes modulate cerebral blood flow and neural damage of hypoxic rats. Neurosci. Lett. **301:** 95–98.
36. FIFKOVA, E. *et al.*, Eds. 1967. Electrophysiological Methods in Biological Research, pp. 653–695. Academia. Prague.
37. PULSINELLI, W.A., D.E. LEVY & T.E. DUFFY. 1983. Cerebral blood flow in the four-vessel occlusion rat model. Stroke **14:** 832–834.
38. HELLWEG, R. *et al.* 2003. Neuroprotection and neuronal dysfunction upon repetitive inhibition of oxidative phosphorylation. Exp. Neurol. **183:** 346–354.
39. WICK, A. *et al.* 2002. Neuroprotection by hypoxic preconditioning requires sequential activation of vascular endothelial growth factor receptor and Akt. J. Neurosci. **22:** 6401–6407.

40. LIN, A.M. *et al.* 2003. Hypoxic preconditioning prevents cortical infarction by transient focal ischemia-reperfusion. Ann. N.Y. Acad. Sci. **993:** 168–178.
41. BOUR, A. *et al.* 2004. A secreted form of the β-amyloid precursor protein (sAPP695) improves spatial recognition memory in OF1 mice. Neurobiol. Learn. Mem. **81:** 27–38.
42. CAILLE, I. *et al.* 2004. Soluble form of amyloid precursor protein regulates proliferation of progenitors in the adult subventricular zone. Development **131:** 2173–2181.
43. GIDDAY, J.M. *et al.* 1994. Neuroprotection from ischemic brain injury by hypoxic preconditioning in the neonatal rat. Neurosci. Lett. **168:** 221–224.
44. VANNUCCI, R.C., J. TOWFIGHI & S.J. VANNUCCI. 1998. Hypoxic preconditioning and hypoxic-ischemic brain damage in the immature rat: pathologic and metabolic correlates. J. Neurochem. **71:** 1215–220.
45. APELT, J., K. ACH & R. SCHLIEBS. 2003. Ageing-related downregulation of neprilysin, a putative β-amyloid-degrading enzyme, in transgenic Tg2576 Alzheimer-like mouse brain is accompanied by an astroglial upregulation in the vicinity of β-amyloid plaques. Neurosci. Lett. **339:** 183–186.
46. MOHAJERI, M.H. *et al.* 2004. Anti-amyloid activity of neprilysin in plaque-bearing mouse models of Alzheimer's disease. FEBS Lett. **562:** 16–21.
47. LICHTENTHALER, S.F. & C. HAASS. 2004. Amyloid at the cutting edge: activation of α-secretase prevents amyloidogenesis in an Alzheimer disease mouse model. J. Clin. Invest. **113:** 1384–1387.
48. HARDY, J. & D. SELKOE. 2002. The amyloid hypothesis of Alzheimer's disease: progress and problems on the road to therapeutics. Science **297:** 353–356.
49. LEVITES, Y. *et al.* 2003. Neuroprotection and neurorescue against Aβ toxicity and PKC-dependent release of nonamyloidogenic soluble precursor protein by green tea polyphenol (−)-epigallocatechin-3-gallate. FASEB J. **17:** 952–954.

The Integrated Role of Desferrioxamine and Phenserine Targeted to an Iron-Responsive Element in the APP-mRNA 5′-Untranslated Region

AMANDA VENTI,[a] TONY GIORDANO,[b] PAUL EDER,[a] ASHLEY I. BUSH,[a] DEBOMOY K. LAHIRI,[c] NIGEL H. GREIG,[d] AND JACK T. ROGERS[a]

[a]*Genetics and Aging Research Unit, Department of Psychiatry, Massachusetts General Hospital East, Charlestown, Massachusetts 02129, USA*

[b]*Department of Molecular Biology and Biochemistry, Louisiana State University, Shreveport, Louisiana 71130, USA*

[c]*Department of Psychiatry, Institute of Psychiatric Research, Indiana University School of Medicine, Indianapolis, Indiana 46202, USA*

[d]*National Institute on Aging, Baltimore, Maryland 21224, USA*

ABSTRACT: The Alzheimer's amyloid precursor protein (APP) is the metalloprotein that is cleaved to generate the pathogenic Aβ peptide. We showed that iron closely regulated the expression of APP by 5′-untranslated region (5′-UTR) sequences in APP mRNA. Iron modulated APP holoprotein expression by a pathway similar to iron control of the translation of the ferritin-L and -H mRNAs by iron-responsive elements in their 5′-UTRs. APP gene transcription is also responsive to copper deficit where the Menkes protein depleted fibroblasts of copper to suppress transcription of APP through metal regulatory and copper regulatory sequences upstream of the APP 5′ cap site. APP is a copper-zinc metalloprotein and chelation of Fe^{3+} by desferrioxamine and Cu^{2+} by clioquinol appeared to provide effective therapy for the treatment of AD in limited patient studies. We have introduced an RNA-based screen for small APP 5′-UTR binding molecules to identify leads that limit APP translation (but not APLP-1 and APLP-2) and amyloid Aβ peptide production. A library of 1200 drugs was screened to identify lead drugs that limited APP 5′-UTR–directed translation of a reporter gene. The efficacy of these leads was confirmed for specificity in a cell-based secondary assay to measure the steady-state levels of APP holoprotein relative to APLP-1/APLP-2 by Western blotting. Several chelators were identified among the APP 5′-UTR directed leads consistent with the presence of an IRE stem-loop in front of the start codon of the APP transcript. The APP 5′-UTR–directed drugs—desferrioxamine (Fe^{3+} chelator), tetrathiomolybdate (Cu^{2+} chelator), and dimercaptopropanol (Pb^{2+} and Hg^{2+} chelator)—each suppressed APP holoprotein expression (and lowered Aβ peptide secretion). The novel anticholinesterase phenserine also provided "proof of concept" for our strategy to target the APP 5′-UTR sequence to identify "anti-amyloid" drugs. We further

Address for correspondence: Jack Rogers, Ph.D., Genetics and Aging Research Unit, Department of Psychiatry (HMS Neuroscience), MGH (East), Charlestown, MA 02129. Voice: 617-726-8838. jrogers@partners.org

Ann. N.Y. Acad. Sci. 1035: 34–48 (2004). © 2004 New York Academy of Sciences.
doi: 10.1196/annals.1332.003

defined the interaction between iron chelation and phenserine action to control APP 5′-UTR–directed translation in neuroblastoma (SY5Y) transfectants. Phenserine was most efficient to block translation under conditions of intracellular iron chelation with desferrioxamine suggesting that this anticholinesterase operated through an iron (metal)–dependent pathway at the APP 5′-UTR site.

KEYWORDS: amyloid precursor protein (APP); Alzheimer's disease; iron-responsive elements

INTRODUCTION

Overview

Genetic and biochemical evidence has linked the biology of metals (Fe, Cu, and Zn) to Alzheimer's disease (AD). Alleles in the hemochromatosis gene accelerate the onset of disease by five years.[1] This finding has certainly validated interest in the model wherein metals (iron) accelerate the course of AD. Biochemical measurements demonstrated elevated levels of copper zinc and iron in the brains of AD patients.[2]

Supporting this concept, an iron-responsive element (IRE) was an active RNA regulatory domain in the 5′-untranslated region (5′-UTR) of the AD amyloid precursor protein (APP) transcript. A novel IL-1–responsive acute-box RNA enhancer was shown to be present between this IRE stemloop and in front of the start codons in the APP mRNA and ferritin mRNA.[3] Our purpose has been to define the function of the newly discovered APP mRNA IRE in the context of IL-1–dependent translation of APP holoprotein (FIG. 1). Like the iron storage protein ferritin, APP is a neuroprotective metalloprotein. This fact is consistent the presence of an active IRE in the 5′-UTR of the APP transcript.

Posttranscriptional Regulation of the APP Transcript

Cytokines, which are physiologically relevant to AD, change the efficiency of APP mRNA translation and APP mRNA stability by signaling through RNA sequences. By this route, APP gene expression is increased at the posttranscriptional level to generate more template potentially for the deposition of more amyloid Aβ peptide.[4] Two *cis*-acting elements in the APP 3′-UTR regulate the stability of the precursor transcript. TGF-β induces a 68 kD protein to bind to an 81nt motif and thus stabilize the APP mRNA.[5] Also, addition of serum growth factors overrides the action of another 3′-UTR element, a 29-base sequence (2285–2313), that normally destabilizes APP mRNA in endothelial cells (and peripheral blood lymphocytes)[6] (FIG. 1).

In astrocytes, we reported that APP gene expression was upregulated by IL-1 at the translational level.[3] Upregulation occurs through 5′-UTR sequences by a pattern of gene expression similar to that for the universal iron storage protein, ferritin.[7] This is in keeping with the findings of de Sauvage and colleagues who reported that polyadenylation site selection in the APP mRNA 3′-UTR is critical for efficient translation in *Xenopus* oocytes.[8] The longer 3.3 kb APP mRNA was found to be translated threefold more efficiently than the shorter 3.042 kb transcript.

Mbella and colleagues then observed that these 3′-UTR sequences enhanced APP mRNA translation in mammalian (Chinese hamster ovary) cells, and more closely mapped two guanosine residues that are crucial for this action.[9] These authors used RNA-electrophoretic mobility shift assays to determine that a translational repressor protein interacts with the shorter transcript.[9] However, the presence of the 258 nucleotide poly(A) regulatory region (PAR) (nt +3042 to +3300) removes binding of this APP mRNA repressor and facilitates longer APP mRNA translation.[9] We concluded that APP 3′-UTR sequences operate in conjunction with the APP 5′-UTR to establish the post-transcriptional control of APP gene expression (and Aβ production).

Posttranscriptional Control of Gene Expression via IREs

IREs are involved in the posttranscriptional regulation of several genes that control intracellular iron homeostasis. The AD brain harbors dysregulated binding of iron-related proteins (IRPs) to IREs,[10] an event that would be predicted to have implications for the expression of IRE controlled genes. Certainly the generic IRE RNA stemloop may be an important site to cause mis-regulation of these key proteins during the course of AD. The absence of IRP-2, which controls iron homeostasis, was associated with mis-regulated iron metabolism and ferritin translation and TfR mRNA stability in both the gut mucosa and the central nervous system.[11] Like ferritin, the other transcripts that encode active IREs in their 5′-UTR include: (1) the mRNA for erythroid aminoluvenyl synthase (eALAS) (eALAS is the rate-limiting enzyme that controls heme biosynthesis in the mitochondria of red blood cells[12,13]), (2) transferrin (Tf) mRNA translation as activated by binding of IRPs to the 5′-UTR of the Tf transcript. Transferrin transports iron throughout the bloodstream to tissues,[14] (3) IREG-1 (ferriportin) mRNA, which is responsible for iron efflux from the duodenum into the bloodstream and macrophage iron efflux,[15,16] and (4) APP mRNA is the most recently characterized member of the family of genes that encodes a functional IRE (Rogers *et al.*, 2002).

Like the transferrin receptor, the divalent metal ion transporter (DMT-1) is known to be regulated by an IRE in its 3′-UTR as one of the alternatively spliced DMT-1 transcripts.[17] DMT-1 is responsible for uptake of iron and other divalent cations from the gut into the bloodstream into enterocytes.[18]

The APP Transcript Encodes a Functional 5′-UTR IRE

The AD APP transcript encodes a functional IRE in its 5′-UTR. Using the "Gap" sequence alignment program (GCGDefs, University of Wisconsin),[19] we reported an overall 67% sequence identity between APP 5′-UTR sequences (+51 to +94) and the 44 nt IRE in H-ferritin mRNA (+12 to +59) (Rogers *et al.*, 2002). Two clusters within this APP 5′-UTR IRE-Type II domain showed >70% identity with the ferritin IRE sequences. First, an 18 base sequence in APP mRNA (+51 to +66) was found to be 72% similar to 5′ half of the H mRNA IRE (+12 to +29). Second, APP sequences (+82 to +94) (a 13 base cluster) were found to be 76% identical to the loop domain of ferritin IRE (+43 to +55). The IRE alignment shown in FIGURE 2 demonstrated that the IRE-Type II sequence in the APP 5′-UTR (+51 to +94) was sited immediately upstream of the IL-1–responsive acute box domain in the APP 5′-UTR (+100 to −146).

This IRE-Type II in the 5' of APP mRNA was fully functional as assessed by multiple, separate transfection assays.[19] RNA gel-shift experiments showed that the mutant version of the APP 5'-UTR cRNA probe no longer binds to IRP.[19] Using RNA electrophoretic mobility shift assays, we performed many controls to demonstrate that IRP-1 specifically binds to the stemloop that is predicted to fold from APP 5'-UTR sequences.[19] Our preliminary data also confirmed that IRP-2 selectively interacted with the APP 5'-UTR to the same extent as originally observed for IRP-1. We concluded that IRPs interact selectively with the APP transcript. These data provided strong genetic support for an integral role for the involvement APP holoprotein in iron metabolism. The fact that IRP-1/IRP-2 are the cognate APP 5'-UTR binding partners will prove useful for screening novel lead compounds that limit APP translation, particularly if IRP-1 and IRP-2 expression can be functionally linked to APP expression.

APP 5'-UTR as Drug Target

Of significance, the APP 5'-UTR is a pivotal riboregulator of the amount of APP translated in response to IL-1[20] and iron.[19] Iron levels and IL-1 regulate translation of APP through the 5'-UTR (APP 5'-UTR) of the precursor transcript.[3] Aβ peptide is cleaved from the APP to fibrilize and to form the plaque, which is an underpinning pathological hallmark of AD. We, therefore, reasoned that drugs that interact with the APP 5'-UTR could well be useful drug candidates for AD therapeutics.

Our goal has been to screen a drug library for APP 5'-UTR–directed compounds that limit APP translation and ultimately amyloid–Aβ-peptide output from neuronal cell culture systems. The APP 5'-UTR folds into a stable RNA secondary structure (Gibbs free energy: $\Delta G = -54.9$ kcal/ mol),[21] and APP 5'-UTR sequences were found to be different to typical eukaryotic mRNAs such as FMR mRNA (Fragile X syndrome). In this regard, FMR 5'-UTR sequences are structured[22] and conform to the "Kozak model" by suppressing 40S ribosome translation scanning.[23] Instead, the APP 5'-UTR increases baseline translation of reporter mRNAs.[19]

Since the APP 5'-UTR was responsive to both metals and IL-1 we predicted that drug screens to the APP 5'-UTR would lead to identification of novel metal chelators and nonsteroidal antiinflammatory drugs as therapeutic agents for AD.[24] A transient transfection–based assay was employed to screen a library of 1,200 FDA pre-approved drugs (FDA drugs), and we identified 17 drug "hits" that >95% suppressed translation of the hybrid APP 5'-UTR–luciferase transcript in neuroblastoma (SY5Y) transfectants (*N*=5). Our drug hits were commonly used FDA drugs in more than five distinct classes of drugs.[24] These classes were (1) blockers of receptor-ligand interactions, (2) bacterial antibiotics, (3) statins, (4) metal chelators, (5) mutagens, and (6) detergents. During a secondary screen we validated 6 of the 17 hits for their capacity to selectively reduce luciferase expression translationally driven from the APP 5'-UTR but maintain co-expression of GFP with an internally controlled viral internal ribosome entry site in a dicistronic screening construct (pJR1). For this purpose SY5Y neuroblastoma cells were stably transfected with the pJR1. The FDA drugs dimercaptopropanol, paroxetine, azithromycin, quinoline-gluconate, tamsulosin, and atorvastatin each suppressed luciferase reporter mRNA translation via the 146 nt APP 5'-UTR sequence.[24]

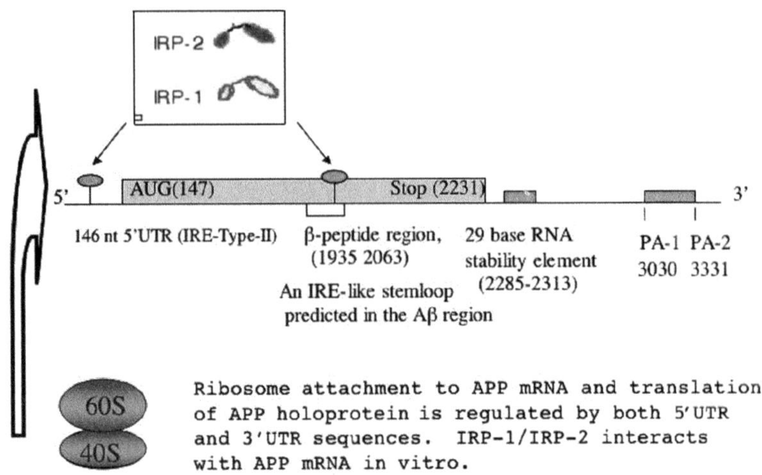

FIGURE 1. Posttranscriptional regulatory domains mapped to the APP transcript. The 3-kb APP transcript is controlled at the level of message translation by the action of 5'-UTR[19] and 3'-UTR regulatory domains. The 3'-untranslated region is alternatively poly-adenylated and the longer APP transcript is translated more efficiently than the shorter transcript.[8,9] A 29 nt RNA destabilizing element was mapped to the 3'-UTR of APP mRNA.[6]

Phenserine and Desferrioxamine: Proof-of-Concept Drugs

The iron chelator desferrioxamine and the anticholinesterase inhibitor phenserine were identified as two "proof of concept" drugs that limited of APP 5'-UTR–directed enhancement of translation. Each drug reduced APP holoprotein expression by suppressing translation of the Aβ-amyloid precursor concomitant to APP 5'-UTR–directed enhancement. Phenserine is a anticholinesterase inhibitor that exemplifies a novel class of small molecules (of known therapeutic function) that provide a second bonus therapeutic action to block APP 5'-UTR–directed translation of APP in astrocytoma and neuroblastoma cell lines and in rats.[25,31] Our strategy to perform RNA-based drug screens directed to the APP 5'-UTR was based on previous experiments that showed that APP holoprotein expression was regulated predominantly at the translational level by IL-1 (inflammation) and iron.[19,26,27]

In this report, we investigated the mechanism by which the anticholinesterase inhibitor phenserine suppressed APP 5'-UTR–directed translation of the mRNA encoding APP. Previously, phenserine was shown to decrease translation of APP holoprotein leading to a therapeutic reduction of Aβ-peptide secretion.[31] Here, we found that phenserine alone only exerted a repression of APP 5'-UTR–driven translation when present at high dose, but that phenserine was more effective as a APP translation blocker in the presence of background iron chelation. Using a neuroblastoma cell line model, phenserine and desferrioxamine acted synergistically to suppress APP 5'-UTR–directed translation.

MATERIALS AND METHODS

Constructs Used to Study the Action of APP 5′-UTR and APP 3′-UTR Sequencers

The map of the 146 nucleotide APP 5′-UTR shows subregions of the APP 5′-UTR region (+51 to 94) that exhibited significant sequence identity to the ferritin IRE (FIG. 2). This sequence was designated as an IRE-Type II.[19] We have generated three new constructs (FIG. 2B). The pAS-1 construct encodes the 90 nt *Sma*I-*Nru*I APP 5′-UTR fragment inserted immediately upstream of the luciferase reporter gene start codon (*Hind*III and *Nco*I sites in pGL-3). This 90 nucleotide sequence harbors the IL-1–responsive and basal RNA regulatory sequences in APP mRNA.[3] The pGAL construct encodes the complete 146 nucleotide 5′-UTR of the APP gene inserted in between the *Hind*III and *Nco*I sites in front of the luciferase gene in the pGL-3 vector (FIG. 1). This construct transcribes a hybrid luciferase reporter that encodes the 90 nt element, but also an additional upstream 55 nucleotides immediately downstream from the 5′ cap site of APP mRNA. The pGALA construct transcribes a hybrid luciferase mRNA with the 146 nt APP 5′-UTR sequence element inserted in front of the luciferase reporter gene start codon. However, the pGALA construct also harbors an additional 1.2 kb of APP 3′-UTR sequences downstream from the stop codon.[9,19] The pGALA construct was prepared by cloning the complete 1.2 kb APP 3′-UTR into a convenient *Xba*I site in pGAL construct.[19]

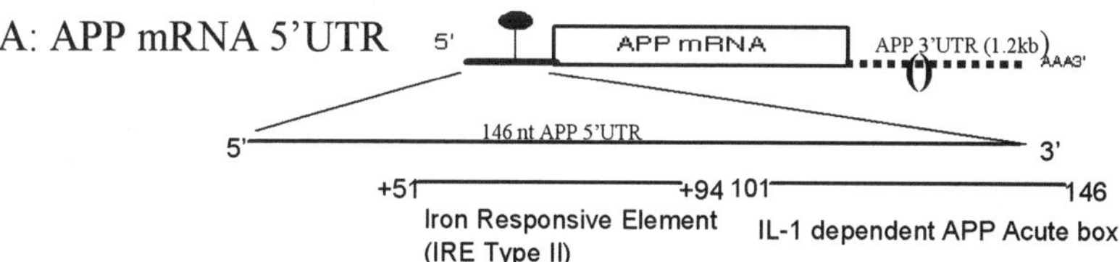

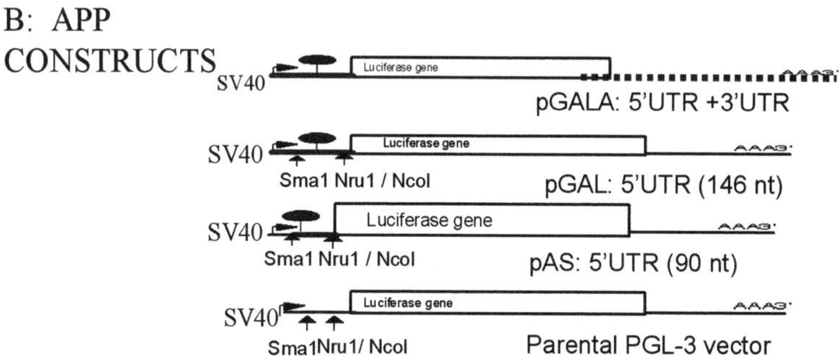

FIGURE 2. (**A**) Regulatory domains that influence APP translation by iron and IL-1. (**B**) Constructs used to map phenserine and desferrioxamine regulatory domains in the APP 5′-UTR. The luciferase expression constructs, pAS (90 base *Sma*I-*Nru*I fragment of the APP 5′-UTR), pGAL (full-length APP 5′-UTR), and pGALA (APP 5′- and 3′-UTR), are derived from pGL3 (Promega, Madison, WI).

Transfections

Neuroblastoma cells were transfected with 10 µg DNA from the constructs and were cotransfected with 5 µg DNA from a construct that expresses green fluorescent protein (GFP). Luciferase and GFP reporter genes were expressed from an SV40 promoter. Transfections were performed in the presence of lipofectamine-2000 according to manufacturers instructions (Gibco). In the experiments shown in FIGURES 3–5, neuroblastoma cells (SY5Y) were grown in separate flasks (100 mm^2). Each flask was then transfected (12 h) with either pGL-3, pGAL, or pGALA and co-transfected with pGFP. The transfected cells were subsequently passaged equally into 96-well flasks to be exposed to drugs for 48 h (N=5 for each treatment).

Drug Treatment

Phenserine (50 mM stock in PBS) and desferrioxamine (50 mM stock in PBS), were each diluted into 2 mL DMEM (without fetal calf serum) for 1 h at 37°C to maximize solubility at the concentrations indicated in figure legends. At each individual concentration, compounds were multi-pipetted in 100 µL volumes into 96-wells (three to four identical wells of transfected cells growing at 80% confluence for 48 h) (N=6 for phenserine and desferrioxamine). After the treatment with each compound, cell viability was established by a microscopic examination of each well. Relative live-cell GFP gene expression was established for transfectants in each well of the 96-well plates by reading at 480/509 nm wavelength (GFP) using an automated Wallac 1420 multilabel counter. After obtaining a GFP readout, the transfectants in each 96-well plate were lysed in 50 µL Reporter Lysis Buffer (Promega, Madison, WI). Luciferase assays were performed over 15 sec using the Walac 1420 counter.

In the experiments shown in FIGURES 3–5 the pAS, pGAL, pGALA, and pGL-3 transfectants were grown in triplicate rows on 96-well plates, and were exposed to (1) desferrioxamine (concentrations of 10 µM and 100 µM) and (2) phenserine (concentration of 10 µM) and (3) phenserine and desferrioxamine (concentration of 10 µM). These experiments investigated the requirement of reduced background intracellular iron levels before observing effective inhibition of APP mRNA translation by phenserine.

Assay for Aβ Production in B3 Lens Epithelial Cells

Cells were treated by APP 5′-UTR–directed drugs as previously described by Morse and colleagues.[27] Conditioned medium was collected from drug- and untreated human B3 cells. Aβ(1–40) and Aβ(1–42) levels were measured using a standard sandwich ELISA assay where 2G3 and 21F12 antibodies captured Aβ(1–40) and Aβ(1–42), respectively, and 266B antibody was used for detection.

RESULTS

Several APP 5′-UTR–Directed Drugs Were Identified as Primary and Secondary Chelators

We identified that several FDA compounds that limited APP 5′-UTR–directed translation were metal chelators. This result was consistent with the presence of a bona fide IRE that was shown to be active in the 5′-UTR of the APP transcript. Western blot analysis provided a secondary assay of five APP 5′-UTR–directed FDA drugs (with chelation activity) that were active to limit the steady-state levels of intracellular APP holoprotein in neuroblastoma (SY5Y) cells.[27] The list of APP 5′-UTR–directed compounds is shown in TABLE 1 as dimercaptopropanol (Hg^{2+} and Pb^{2+} chelator), desferrioxamine (Fe^{3+} chelator), tetrathiomolybdate (Cu^{2+} chelator), phenserine (anticholinesterase inhibitor), and paroxetine (selective serotonin reuptake inhibitor), each of which limited Aβ-peptide secretion.

The Effect of APP 5′-UTR–Directed Drugs Leads to Limited Aβ Peptide Production

We tested the capacity of dimercaptopropanol, desferrioxamine, tetrathiomolybdate, phenserine, and paroxetine (APP 5′-UTR–screened drugs that reduced translation of APP holoprotein) to limit secreted Aβ peptide levels. For this purpose, lens epithelial cells (B3) were an excellent endogenous cell line since B3 cells generate greater levels of basal Aβ relative to neuroblastoma cells. ELISA data (TABLE 1) showed that paroxetine lowered Aβ peptide secretion into the conditioned medium of lens B3 cells by up to 50% after a 4-day treatment (15 μM paroxetine). Treatment with dimercaptopropanol also reduced Aβ(1–40) and Aβ(1–42) levels by 30% to 50% relative to untreated B3 cells (72-h treatment of the cells). We also showed that paroxetine reduced Aβ peptide levels by 50% in B3 cells.[27] In the primary screen of our FDA drug library, another serotonin re-uptake blocker, Prozac, did not limit APP 5′-UTR–directed translation. Therefore other selective serotonin reuptake inhibitors (SSRIs) that are unrelated to paroxetine in chemical structure are unlikely to reduce Aβ secretion.

In sum, our current results showed that drugs that lowered APP holoprotein translation (i.e., paroxetine and dimercaptopropanol) also reduced the secretion of Aβ(1–40) and Aβ(1–42). Phenserine lowered APP holoprotein levels by 30% and Aβ peptide levels by 33% in neuroblastoma cells.[31] A three-week trial demonstrated an 68% reduction of Aβ(1–40) and a 58% reduction of Aβ(1–42) in the brains of mice injected daily for 3 weeks (TABLE 1). Phenserine was administered intraperitoneally at 2.5 mg/kg daily for 3 weeks (Dr. Nigel Greig, National Institute on Aging). Desferrioxamine reduced Aβ peptide secretion for B3 epithelial cells and SY5Y cells (TABLE 1) (Rogers and Payton, in preparation).

Desferrioxamine Facilitated Phenserine-Dependent Suppression of APP 5′-UTR–Driven Translation

Phenserine and desferrioxamine were designated as "proof of concept" drugs for a protocol to screen for small molecules to limit the translation of APP holoprotein (and Aβ peptide output) after their initial identification by screening drug libraries for compounds against the APP 5′-UTR target (RNA targeting the translation of an endogenous pathogenic gene). In this report, we tested how these two compounds interacted with respect to APP 5′-UTR–directed translation of a luciferase reporter using a transfection-based assay. Phenserine was previously shown to suppress APP holoprotein translation through 5′-UTR sequences in the precursor transcript.[31] Therefore, we characterized the interaction of phenserine and desferrioxamine

TABLE 1. Capacity of APP 5′-UTR directed FDA drugs to limit Aβ peptide output

FDA drug	Inhibition of Aβ peptide production	Action as a metal chelator
Dimercaptopropanol	0.01 μM DMP = 36% reduction/B3 cells	Hg^{2+} and Pb^{2+} chelator
Desferrioxamine	30 μM DFO = >30% reduction/SY5Y cells	Fe^{3+} chelator ($K_d = 10^{-21}$ M)
Tetrathiomolybdate	Not measured	Cu^{2+} chelator
Phenserine	50 μM Ps = 33% reduction/SK-N-SH cells	An anticholinesterase inhibitor that also cooperated with desferrioxamine to limit IRE action in the 5′-UTR of APP mRNA (Figs. 3–5)
Paroxetine (Paxil™, Px)	10 μM Px = 50% reduction/B3 cells	SSRI that also modulated the steady-state levels of TfR mRNA[27]

acting through the complete 146 base APP 5′-UTR and the 90 nt *Sma*I-*Nru*I segment of the APP 5′-UTR. We also tested the interaction of APP 5′-UTR and 3′-UTR sequences to confer phenserine- and desferrioxamine-specific translational block.

The experiments in FIGURES 3–5 determined whether phenserine suppressed APP 5′-UTR–driven expression by utilizing iron as a cofactor. APP 5′-UTR sequences encode a functional IRE (IRE-Type II).[19] Transfection data using luciferase constructs showed that 10 μM phenserine had no effect on APP 5′-UTR–driven translation conferred to a luciferase reporter mRNA (FIGS. 3-5). However APP 5′-UTR–specific constructs showed that the combined addition of phenserine with the iron chelator desferrioxamine (10 μM) exerted a greater inhibitory action to suppress APP 5′-UTR–driven luciferase mRNA translation than was observed for each drug separately. This pattern was reproduced for the three constructs that expressed chimeric APP UTR-luciferase transcripts as pAS (90 nt element), pGAL (APP 5′UTR) and pGALA (APP 5′-UTR and 3′-UTR) (FIG. 2). As a key experimental control, the luciferase gene expressed from the parental PGl-3 vector (no APP sequences) was unresponsive to desferrioxamine in SY5Yneuroblastoma transfectants ($N = 6$).[19] The presence of 3′-UTR sequences generated a greater level of suppression of luciferase mRNA translation in response to desferrioxamine (FIG. 5). Western blot experiments will be employed to evaluate whether phenserine and desferrioxamine in combination might reduce APP holoprotein synthesis to a degree greater than each drug separately.

DISCUSSION

This report describes new experiments to demonstrate that a novel anticholinesterase inhibitor (phenserine) operated to suppress APP 5′-UTR–directed translation of a transfected luciferase reporter mRNA via an iron-dependent pathway. Future targeted mutagenesis of the APP 5′UTR will characterize whether the +51 to +94 domain in APP mRNA (IRE-Type II)) accounts for translational repression of the Aβ

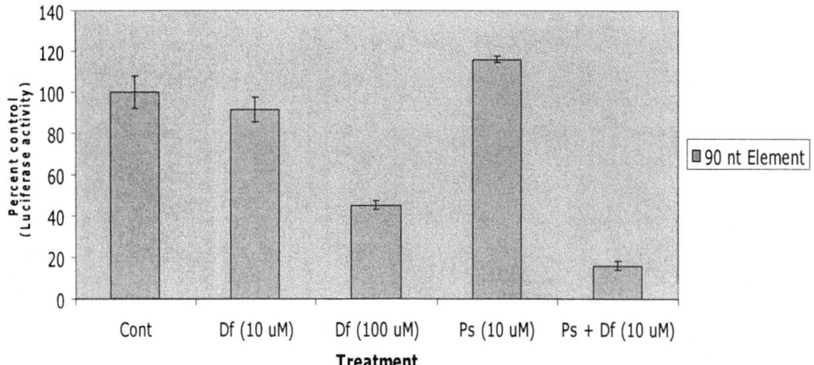

FIGURE 3. Neuroblastoma cells were transfected with the pAS-1 construct (APP 5′-UTR 90 nt *Sma*I-*Nru*I element) (FIG. 2). After transfection (12 h) with lipofectamine (Gibco) cells were passaged equally into 96-well plates and treated for 48 h in triplicate with the following: Untreated cells (cont), 10 μM desferrioxamine, 100 μM desferrioxamine, 10 μM phenserine, 10 μM cocktail of phenserine and desferrioxamine. After drug treatment, lysates were prepared from the cells and were assessed for luciferase activity. Representative lysates from the two sets of transfectants were assayed for β-galactosidase activity and found to display equal activity within each transfection experiment. (Representative data $N = 6$, as in FIGURES 4 and 5.)

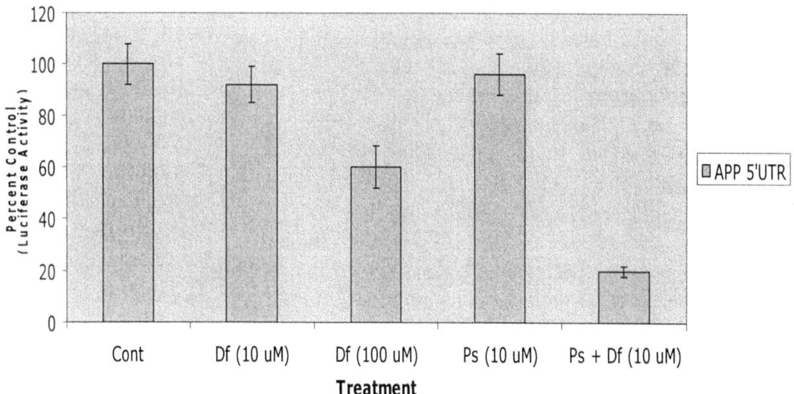

FIGURE 4. Neuroblastoma cells were transfected with the pGAL construct (full-length 146 nt APP 5′-UTR) (FIG. 2). After transfection (12 h) with lipofectamine (Gibco) cells were passaged equally into 96-well plates and treated for 48 h in triplicate with the following: Untreated cells (cont), 10 μM desferrioxamine, 100 μM desferrioxamine, 10 μM phenserine, 10 μM cocktail of phenserine and desferrioxamine. After drug treatment, derivative lysates were assessed for luciferase activity.

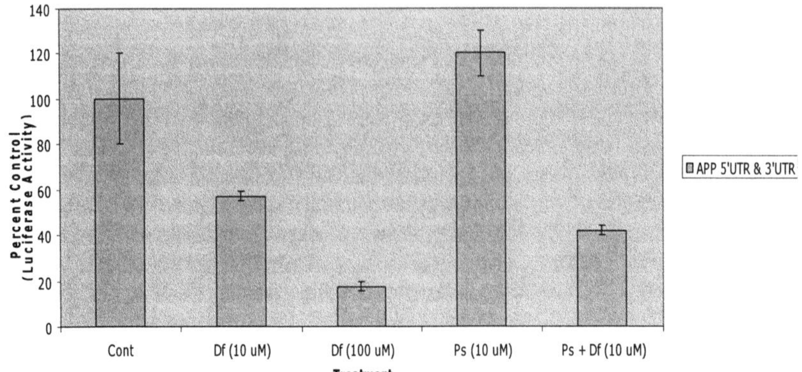

FIGURE 5. Neuroblastoma cells were transfected with the pGALA construct (APP 5′-UTR and 3′-UTR) (FIG. 2). After transfection (12 h) with lipofectamine (Gibco) cells were passaged equally into 96-well plates and treated for 48 h in triplicate with the following: Untreated cells (cont), 10 μM desferrioxamine, 100 μM desferrioxamine, 10 μM phenserine, 10 μM cocktail of phenserine and desferrioxamine. After drug treatment, derivative lysates were assessed for luciferase activity.

precursor by phenserine and the extent to which coding sequences and the APP 3′-UTR is involved. Certainly the identification of two metal chelators (dimercaptopropanol and desferrioxamine) as APP 5′-UTR–directed compounds that lowered APP holoprotein levels, but left APLP-1 levels unchanged (therapeutic action), was consistent with the presence of an IRE in the 5′-UTR of the APP transcript but not in the 5′-UTRs of the APLP-1 and APLP-2 transcripts.

Using the SY5Y neuroblastoma cells as a model phenserine did not limit APP 5′-UTR activity at concentrations lower than a 10 μM drug dose. However desferrioxamine cooperatively facilitated phenserine to suppress APP 5′-UTR–directed translation (10 μM each compound in the cell culture medium for 48 h) (FIGS. 3–5). These data suggest that the mechanism for the action of this anticholinesterase may be to suppress APP 5′-UTR–conferred regulation of APP expression by a pathway that depends on threshold intracellular iron levels.

Phenserine was shown to inhibit APP 5′-UTR activity independently of MAP kinase and PI3 kinase pathways.[31] The most compelling and testable model is that phenserine operated through the conserved IRE element (+51 to +94) in the APP 5′-UTR. Certainly, the potential capacity of phenserine and desferrioxamine to cooperatively suppress APP translation through APP 5′-UTR sequences suggests that this AChE inhibitor also targets the APP IRE (Type II) domain. Interestingly 10 μM phenserine alone did not influence the translation of the chimeric Luc/5′-UTR/3′-UTR transcript in the presence of the 1 kb 3′-UTR of APP transcript. These experiments suggested that phenserine-specific translational inhibition might also be the consequence of other *cis*-regulatory domains in the APP transcript.

The data in FIGURE 5 demonstrated that the desferrioxamine action to limit APP translation appeared to be the result of a translational interaction between the 5′- and 3′-ends of the APP transcript. Iron chelation with desferrioxamine appeared to be most effective in the presence of both APP 5′-UTR and 3′-UTR sequences (compare the transfection data in FIGURES 3-5). These experiments suggested that the IRE in the APP 5′-UTR interacts with the 3′-UTR when most effectively repressing luciferase reporter mRNA translation in transfection-based studies.[28] Clearly, the interaction between 5′-UTR and 3′-UTR sequences is required for effective translation of most eukaryotic mRNAs.[28]

IRP-1 and IRP-2 are known to modulate intracellular iron homeostasis by controlling ferritin-L and –H mRNA translation and transferrin receptor mRNA stability.[29] In this regard, IRP-1 is a *cis*-aconitase in addition to being a well-known ferritin mRNA IRE-binding protein (and APP 5′-UTR binding protein). However, IRP-1 selectively binds to the IRE-Type II in the APP mRNA.[19] Therefore, APP mRNA translation may be decreased under conditions of intracellular iron chelation via APP 5′-UTR sequences, likely by an altered interaction with between the APP 5′-UTR and IRP-1/IRP-2.[19]

We propose that phenserine might interfere with binding of IRP-1 to the APP 5′-UTR to explain the mechanism by which the anticholinesterase inhibitor suppresses the translation of the transfected chimeric APP 5′-UTR luciferase transcript. The known enzyme inhibitory action of phenserine toward the active site cleft of anticholinesterases may be re-directed to the active site cleft of IRP-1. This IRP-1 cleft region regulates translational control of ferritin and APP mRNAs and the RNA binding activity of IRP-1 is an interconvertable event in response to iron levels.[29] In future experiments, phenserine might be tested for its capacity to influence the *cis*-aconitase activity of IRP-1, an event leading to reduced translation of APP mRNA with beneficial therapeutic consequences. Of interest, physiological levels of iron in the brains of transgenic mice may be relatively lower than the iron concentration in tissue culture medium (DMEM supplemented with 10% fetal calf serum at the 40 μM level of serum iron). Thus the presence of lower brain iron levels may provide an explanation for the fact that phenserine is effective in transgenic mice, as was the case when tissue culture experiments were performed in the presence of 10 μM desferrioxamine (FIGS. 3–5).

DRUG SELECTIVITY AND APP 5′-UTR–DIRECTED SCREENS

RNA-based therapeutics underpin the mechanism of action of the common antibiotics, erythromycin and tetracycline.[30] We investigated the mechanism by which the anticholinesterase inhibitor, phenserine, suppressed translation of the mRNA encoding APP.[31] Phenserine decreases translation of APP holoprotein leading to a therapeutic reduction of Aβ-peptide secretion.[31] This cholinesterase inhibitor exemplifies a novel class of small molecules (of known therapeutic function) that provide a second bonus therapeutic action to block APP 5′-UTR–directed translation of APP in astrocytoma and neuroblastoma cell lines[31] and in rats.[25]

In future screens, we will include a selectivity control to ensure specificity wherein chosen drugs will have to be counter-screened against the 5′-UTRs of APLP-1 and APLP-2 transcripts.[32,33] A sufficiently specific therapeutic anti-amyloid compound would be expected to leave expression of the related APLP-1 and APLP-2 genes unchanged before the drug could be tested *in vivo* as a therapeutic agent for AD. Limiting APP expression would be predicted to have low negative physiological impact because APLP-1 and APLP-2 should provide functional redundancy for APP as illustrated the viability of APP knockout mice.[33]

We propose that the APP 5′-UTR target will prove very useful to identify novel therapeutic candidate drugs. The APP 5′-UTR is a valid target that is unique to the APP transcript but also encodes IL-1, TGF-β, and iron-responsive domains. Therefore drugs targeted to this APP 5′-UTR should include both new chelators and nonsteroidal antiinflammatory drugs in addition to other drug classes as was reported by our pilot screen of a small library of FDA drugs. Larger novel (non-FDA) libraries of combinatorial low molecular weight compounds can also be screened for their capacity to block 5′-UTR–dependent translation of APP holoprotein (and hence Aβ peptide production).

CONCLUSIONS CONCERNING METALS AND METAL-DEPENDENT TRANSLATION

There is a marked increase in the steady-state levels of metals (iron, copper, and zinc) in the AD brain that would be predicted to contribute to toxic gene expression patterns with deleterious consequences for neuronal survival.[2] Certainly APP mRNA translational control by iron and APP gene transcriptional control by copper[34] each provide new genetic support for the model that APP is a metalloprotein expressed to detoxify metal controlled oxidative stress (neuroprotective framework). Both extracellular amyloid plaques and intracellular neurofibrillary tangles are the predominant pathological features characterizing the clinical onset of AD (both early and late onset). A proximal pathological feature of AD is the formation of neurofibrillary tangles by Tau even though mutations to the Tau gene cause hereditary fronto-temporal dementia.[35,36] Iron (Fe^{3+}) binds with hyperphosphorylated Tau.[37] Inhalation of aluminum dust was observed to cause a mild cognitive disorder that might be a prelude to AD among foundry workers in northern Italy.[38] However, the chromosome 21 gene encoding APP remains central to our understanding the progression of Alzheimer's disease and is a central target for developing therapeutic agents. APP is a metalloprotein of neuroprotective function that is significantly regulated by changed intracellular levels of copper and iron.

ACKNOWLEDGMENTS

J.T.R. greatly appreciates the support of Professor Rudolph Tanzi. This work was supported by grants from the National Institutes of Health (AG21081) and the Alzheimer's Association to J.T.R. and grants from the National Institutes of Health (AG18379 and AG18884) and the Alzheimer's Association to D.K.L.

REFERENCES

1. SAMPIETRO, M. *et al.* 2001. The hemochromatosis gene affects the age of onset of sporadic Alzheimer's disease. Neurobiol Aging **22:** 563–568.
2. LOVELL, M.A. *et al.* 1998. Copper, iron and zinc in Alzheimer's disease senile plaques. J. Neurol. Sci. **158:** 47–52.

3. ROGERS, J.T. *et al.* 1999. Translation of the alzheimer amyloid precursor protein mRNA is up- regulated by interleukin-1 through 5′-untranslated region sequences. J. Biol. Chem. **274**: 6421–6431.

4. RAJAGOPALAN, L.E. & J.S. MALTER. 2000. Growth factor-mediated stabilization of amyloid precursor protein mRNA is mediated by a conserved 29-nucleotide sequence in the 3′-untranslated region. J. Neurochem. **74**: 52–59.

5. AMARA, F.M. *et al.* 1999. TGF-beta(1), regulation of alzheimer amyloid precursor protein mRNA expression in a normal human astrocyte cell line: mRNA stabilization. Brain Res. Mol. Brain Res. **71**: 42–49.

6. ZAIDI, S.H. & J.S. MALTER. 1994. Amyloid precursor protein mRNA stability is controlled by a 29-base element in the 3′-untranslated region. J. Biol. Chem. **269**: 24007–4013.

7. ROGERS, J.T. 1996. Ferritin translation by interleukin-1: the role of sequences upstream of the start codons of the heavy and light subunit genes. Blood **87**: 2525–2537.

8. DE SAUVAGE, F., V. KRUYS, O. MARINX, *et al.* 1992. Alternative polyadenylation of the amyloid protein precursor mRNA. EMBO J. **11**: 3099–3103.

9. MBELLA, E.G. *et al.* 2000. A GG nucleotide sequence of the 3′ untranslated region of amyloid precursor protein mRNA plays a key role in the regulation of translation and the binding of proteins. Mol. Cell Biol. **20**: 4572–4579.

10. PINERO, D.J., J. HU & J.R. CONNOR. 2000. Alterations in the interaction between iron regulatory proteins and their iron responsive element in normal and Alzheimer's diseased brains [In Process Citation]. Cell. Mol. Biol. (Noisy-Le-Grand) **46**: 761–776.

11. LAVAUTE, T. *et al.* 2001. Targeted deletion of the gene encoding iron regulatory protein-2 causes misregulation of iron metabolism and neurodegenerative disease in mice. Nat. Genet. **27**: 209–214.

12. MELOFORS, O., B. GOOSSEN, B. JOHANSSON, *et al.* 1993. Translational control of 5-aminolevulinate synthase mRNA by iron-responsive elements in erythroid cells. J. Biol. Chem. **268**: 5974-5978.

13. COX, T.C. *et al.* 1991. Human erythroid 5-aminolevulinate synthase: promoter analysis and identification of an iron-responsive element in the mRNA. EMBO J. **10**: 1891–1902.

14. COX, L.A. & G.S. ADRIAN. 1993. Post-transcriptional regulation of chimeric human transferrin genes by iron. Biochemistry **32**: 4738–4745.

15. CHUNG, J., D.J. HAILE & M. WESSLING-RESNICK. 2004. Copper-induced ferroportin-1 expression in J774 macrophages is associated with increased iron efflux. Proc. Natl. Acad. Sci. USA **101**: 2700–2705.

16. KNUTSON, M.D. *et al.* 2003. Iron loading and erythrophagocytosis increase ferroportin 1 (FPN1) expression in J774 macrophages. Blood **102**: 4191–4197.

17. GUNSHIN, H. *et al.* 2001. Iron-dependent regulation of the divalent metal ion transporter. FEBS Lett. **509**: 309–316.

18. GUNSHIN, H. *et al.* 1997. Cloning and characterization of a mammalian proton-coupled metal-ion transporter. Nature **388**: 482–488.

19. ROGERS, J.T. *et al.* 2002. An iron-responsive element type II in the 5′-untranslated region of the Alzheimer's amyloid precursor protein transcript. J. Biol. Chem. **277**: 45518–45528.

20. NILSSON, L., J. ROGERS & H. POTTER. 1998. The essential role of inflammation and induced gene expression in the pathogenic pathway of Alzheimer's disease. Front. Biosci. **3**: 436–446.

21. ZUKER, M. 1989. On finding all suboptimal foldings of an RNA molecule. Science **244**: 48–52.

22. FENG, Y. *et al.* 1995. Translational suppression by trinucleotide repeat expansion at FMR1. Science **268**: 731–734.

23. SVITKIN, Y.V. *et al.* 2001. The requirement for eukaryotic initiation factor 4A (elF4A) in translation is in direct proportion to the degree of mRNA 5′ secondary structure. RNA **7**: 382–394.

24. ROGERS, J.T., P.S. EDER, X. HUANG *et al.* 2002. Alzheimer's disease drug discovery targeted to the APP mRNA 5′-untranslated region. J. Mol. Neurosci. **19**: 77–82.

25. HAROUTUNIAN, V. *et al.* 1997. Pharmacological modulation of Alzheimer's beta-amyloid precursor protein levels in the CSF of rats with forebrain cholinergic system lesions. Brain Res. Mol. Brain Res. **46**: 161–168.

26. PAYTON, S. *et al.* 2003. Drug discovery targeted to the Alzheimer's APP mRNA 5'-untranslated region: the action of paroxetine and dimercaptopropanol. J. Mol. Neurosci. **20:** 267–275.
27. MORSE, L. *et al.* 2004. FDA pre-approved drugs targeted to the translational regulation and processing of the amyloid precursor protein. J. Mol. Neurosci. **24:** 129–136.
28. CHEN, C.Y. & P. SARNOW. 1995. Initiation of protein synthesis by the eukaryotic translational apparatus on circular RNAs. Science **268:** 415–417.
29. THOMSON, A.M., J.T. ROGERS & P.J. LEEDMAN. 1999. Iron-regulatory proteins, iron-responsive elements and ferritin mRNA translation. Int. J. Biochem. Cell Biol. **31:** 1139–1152.
30. PORSE, B.T. *et al.* 1999. UV-induced modifications in the peptidyl transferase loop of 23S rRNA dependent on binding of the streptogramin B antibiotic, pristinamycin IA. RNA **5:** 585–595.
31. SHAW, K.T. *et al.* 2001. Phenserine regulates translation of beta-amyloid precursor protein mRNA by a putative interleukin-1 responsive element, a target for drug development. Proc. Natl. Acad. Sci. USA **98:** 7605–7610.
32. WASCO, W. *et al.* 1993. Isolation and characterization of APLP2 encoding a homologue of the Alzheimer's associated amyloid beta protein precursor. Nat. Genet. **5:** 95–100.
33. VON KOCH, C.S. *et al.* 1997. Generation of APLP2 KO mice and early postnatal lethality in APLP2/APP double KO mice. Neurobiol. Aging **18:** 661–669.
34. BELLINGHAM, S.A. *et al.* 2004. Copper depletion down-regulates expression of Alzheimer's disease amyloid-beta precursor protein gene. J. Biol. Chem. In press.
35. KOSIK, K. *et al.* 2002. Discovery of compounds that will prevent tau pathology. J. Mol. Neurosci. **19:** 261–266.
36. LU, M. & K. KOSIK. 2001. Competition for microtubule-binding with dual expression of tau missense and splice isoforms. Mol. Biol. Cell. **12:** 171–184.
37. SHIN, R. *et al.* 2003. A novel trivalent cation chelator Feralex dissociates binding of aluminum and iron associated with hyperphosphorylated tau of Alzheimer's disease. Brain Res. **961:** 139–146.
38. POLIZZI, S. *et al.* 2002. Neurotoxic effect of aluminum among foundry workers and Alzheimer's disease. Neurotoxicology **23:** 761–774.

BACE1 Gene Expression and Protein Degradation

WEIHUI ZHOU, HONG QING, YIGANG TONG, AND WEIHONG SONG

Department of Psychiatry, Brain Research Center, University of British Columbia, Vancouver, BC V6T 1Z3, Canada

ABSTRACT: Deposition of amyloid β protein in the brain is the major pathological feature of Alzheimer's disease. Amyloid β protein is generated from β-amyloid precursor protein by β-secretase and γ-secretase. Proteolytic processing of amyloid precursor protein at the β site by BACE1 is essential to generate amyloid β protein. BACE1, the major β-secretase involved in cleaving amyloid precursor protein, has been identified as a type 1 membrane–associated aspartyl protease. In this study, we found that *BACE1* gene expression is controlled by a TATA-less promoter. *BACE1* gene expression is tightly regulated at the transcriptional level and the transcription factor Sp1 plays an important role in regulation of BACE1 to process amyloid precursor protein generating amyloid β protein. Furthermore, we found that BACE1 protein is ubiquitinated, and the degradation of BACE1 proteins and amyloid precursor protein processing are regulated by the ubiquitin-proteasome pathway.

KEYWORDS: BACE1; β-amyloid precursor protein; amyloid β-protein; Alzheimer's disease; transcriptional regulation; proteasomal degradation

INTRODUCTION

Alzheimer's disease (AD) is the most common neurodegenerative disorder leading to dementia.[1] It accounts for two-thirds of all cases of dementia and its prevalence increases with age. AD affects about 10% of the population over the age of 65. Recent molecular genetic studies have shown that four genes confer susceptibility to AD: amyloid precursor protein (APP) gene on chromosome 21;[2–6] Apo E gene on chromosome 19;[1,7–10] presenilin 1 (PS1) on chromosome 14;[11–15] and presenilin 2 (PS2) on chromosome 1.[16–18] Autosomal dominant inheritance of AD can arise from mutations of APP, PS1, or PS2. These mutations alter the processing of APP, giving rise to increased production of amyloid β protein (Aβ), particularly a 42-amino-acid form of Aβ with a high propensity for plaque formation, implicating a role for altered APP processing in the pathogenesis of familial AD.[19–23]

Deposition of Aβ in the brain is a central pathological feature of AD. Aβ is derived from APP, a type 1 transmembrane protein. APP is processed by three enzymes: α-, β-, and γ-secretases. In the normal condition, the majority of APP

Address for correspondence: Dr. Weihong Song, Department of Psychiatry, University of British Columbia, Vancouver, BC V6T 1Z3, Canada. Voice: 604-822-8019; fax: 604-822-7756. weihong@interchange.ubc.ca

Ann. N.Y. Acad. Sci. 1035: 49–67 (2004). © 2004 New York Academy of Sciences. doi: 10.1196/annals.1332.004

proteins undergo a non-amyloidogenic pathway, where α-secretase cleaves APP first within the Aβ domain to generate a secreted form of APP (sAPPα) and C83, precluding Aβ generation. In the amyloidogenic pathway APP is first cleaved by BACE1 to generate a secreted form of APP (sAPPβ) and a 99-residue membrane-associated fragment (C99). C99 is subsequently cleaved by γ-secretase to generate Aβ and CTFγ fragments.

Proteolytic processing of APP at the β site is essential to generate Aβ. BACE (or BACE1) has been identified as a type 1 membrane–associated aspartyl protease of 501 amino acids.[24–27] It cleaves APP at the major β site to generate C99 and at a minor glu-11 site to release a lower level of a C89 fragment. The majority of BACE1 is located in Golgi and endosomal compartments. BACE1 undergoes a complex set of posttranslational modifications during its maturation. Pro-BACE1 is cleaved by furin and other members of the furin family of convertases to remove the 24-amino-acid N-terminal region of the pro-peptide within the trans-Golgi network (TGN).[28–31] The 24-amino-acid prodomain is required for the efficient exit of pro-BACE1 from the endoplasmic reticulum.[28–31] Prodomain processing of BACE2 is autocatalytic.[32] Mature BACE1 has four N-glycosylation sites at Asn153, 172, 223, and 354, and the β-secretase activity is dependent on the extent of N-glycosylation.[30,33–35] The cytoplasmic domain of BACE1 and its phosphorylation are required for efficient maturation and its intracellular trafficking through the TGN and endosomal system.[30,35,36] Suppression of BACE1 by siRNA reduced APP βCTF and Aβ production in primary cortical neurons derived from both wild-type and the Swedish APP mutant transgenic mice.[37] BACE1-KO mice have abolished Aβ generation, but exhibit a normal phenotype without any observed developmental deficits.[38–40] Furthermore, disruption of BACE1 gene rescues memory deficits and cholinergic dysfunction in Tg2576 Swedish APP mutant transgenic mice.[41] These results suggest that therapeutic inhibition of BACE1 is a valid therapeutic target for AD.

To examine the molecular mechanisms underlying the transcriptional regulation of BACE1 gene expression and its role in AD pathogenesis, we have cloned and functionally characterized the *BACE1* gene promoter region. We found that the *BACE1* gene is tightly regulated at the transcriptional level and transcription factor Sp1 plays a significant role in regulating the *BACE1* gene expression. In this report, we also demonstrate for the first time that BACE1 is ubiquitinated and BACE1 protein and APP processing is regulated by the ubiquitin-proteasome pathway.

EXPERIMENTAL METHODS

BACE1 Gene Promoter Luciferase Reporter Chimeric Plasmids and BACE1 cDNA Constructs

A primer corresponding to BACE1 gene coding sequence (5′-cacaagcttcatccacagcaggagccagg) was first used to amplify the 5′ upstream region of BACE1 gene from a human fetus brain genomic library (Clontech) using 5′ genome walking strategy. A series of deletion plasmids were generated to contain various 5′ upstream fragments of the BACE1 in front of the luciferase reporter gene in pGL3-basic expression vector.[42] To generate pB1P-H-mut1Sp1 and pB1P-H-mut2Sp1, site-directed mutagenesis by PCR was used. Primer BACE1-932mut1Sp1, 5′-

ccgctcgagcattttgggaggccgacgtg**ttg**ggatcatttgaggccag-3′ or primer BACE1-932mut2Sp1, 5′-ccgctcgagcattttgggaggccgacgt**attgta**atcatttgaggccag-3′, and primer BACE1-292r, 5′-cacaagcttccaccataatccagctcg-3′ were used to amplify the BACE1 promoter fragment H with mutated Sp1 binding site at −910 bp. A human BACE1 cDNA was cloned into pcDNA4 (Invitrogen) with mycHis tag fused at the C-terminus of BACE1 (pBACE-mycHis). BACE1 cDNA was also cloned into pEGFP-N2 vector (BD Biosciences) to generate pBACE-EGFP plasmid with an enhanced green fluorescent protein EGFP fused at the C-terminus of BACE1 protein. A ubiquitin plasmid pHis-Ubi without myc tag was derived from pCW-7.[43] APP C99 and C83 cDNA were amplified by PCR and then cloned into pcDNA3 vector (Invitrogen) to generate mammalian expression plasmid pAPP-C99 and pAPP-C83.

Cell Culture and Transfection

HEK293 cells, neuroblastoma SH-SY5Y cells, Sp1-WT cells, and Sp1-KO cells were cultured in Dulbecco's modified Eagle's medium (DMEM) containing 10% fetal bovine serum (FBS), 1 mM sodium pyruvate, 2 mM L-glutamine, 50 U/mL penicillin G sodium, and 50 µg/mL streptomycin sulfate (Invitrogen). PC12 cells were seeded on collagen-coated plates and cultured in RPMI-1640 medium supplemented with 5% horse serum and 10% FBS. 20E2 cell line is a Swedish mutant APP stable HEK cell line. B2 cell line contains the stably transfected BACE1 in HEK 293 cells, and 2EB2 cell line has both the Swedish mutant APP and BACE1 stably transfected in HEK cells. The stable cell lines were maintained in complete DMEM media supplemented with 100 µg/mL Zeocin. For transient transfection, cells were grown to approximately 70% confluence and transfected with plasmids using LipofectAMINE2000 (Invitrogen) according to the manufacturer's instructions. The cells were harvested 48 h following transfection.

Luciferase Assay

Cells were grown to approximately 70% confluence and transfected with 2 µg plasmid DNA/35-mm plate using LipofectAMINE2000 Reagent (Invitrogen). The pCH110 β-galactosidase expression plasmid was cotransfected to normalize for transfection efficiency. Cells were harvested 48 h after transfection and lysed in either 200 µL of 1× Reporter Lysis Buffer (Promega) for luciferase activity assay or RIPA-DOC buffer (1% Triton X100, 1% sodium deoxycholate, 0.1% sodium dodecyl sulfate, 0.15 M NaCl, 0.05 M Tris-HCl, pH 7.2) supplemented with protease inhibitors (Complete, Boehringer Mannheim). The luciferase assay was performed according to the protocol for the Luciferase Assay System (Promega) and the relative light intensity was measured using a luminometer (Fluoroskan Ascent, Thermo-Lab Systems) to reflect the luciferase activity. For the β-galactosidase assay, 25 µL of cell lysate was used, in addition to 25 µL of 1X Reporter Lysis Buffer and 50 µL of 2× Assay Buffer (Promega). β-Galactosidase activity was determined by measuring the level of the hydrolysis product of O-nitro-β-D-galactopyranoside (Sigma) at a wavelength of 405 nm (Multiskan Ascent, ThermoLab System) and then converting to units of β-galactosidase enzyme based on a standard. The luciferase activity was normalized according to the β-galactosidase activity and expressed as relative luciferase unit (RLU) to reflect the promoter activity.

Immunohistochemical Staining, Immunoprecipitation, and Immunoblotting

For immunostaining assay, HEK 293 cells were seeded on coverslips and transfected with pBACE-EGFP and pCW-7 plasmid. The transfected cells were fixed with prewarmed fixing solution (4% paraformaldehyde, 0.12 M sucrose) at room temperature for 20 min, then permeabilized with prewarmed 0.1% Triton X-100 in phosphate-buffered saline (PBS) at room temperature for 30 min. The cells were then blocked with 5% bovine serum albumin (BSA) before incubation with a rabbit anti-ubiquitin primary antibody. Cy3-conjugated anti-rabbit secondary antibody (Jackson ImmunoResearch, Inc.) and Hoechst 33258 were used to detect ubiquitin and nucleus, respectively. Cells were sealed in the mount medium (Biomedia Corp.) on slides and subjected to fluorescent microscopic analysis with a Carl Zeiss Axiovert-200 microscope. For immunoblotting, myc-tagged BACE1 proteins were detected using mouse monoclonal anti-myc antibody 9E10 or rabbit polyclonal anti-BACE1 antibody 208. APP and APP-CTFs were detected using rabbit polyclonal anti-APP C-terminus antibody C20. For immunoprecipitation, cells were lysed in NP-40 buffer (10 mM HEPES, pH 7.5, 142.4 mM KCl, 5 mM $MgCl_2$, 1 mM EGTA and 1% NP-40) on ice. The immunoprecipitates were then analyzed by 4–20% Tris-glycine gel with a detecting antibody for coimmunoprecipitation. For pulse-chase analysis, the radiolabeled proteins in SDS-PAGE gels were detected and quantitated by Instant-Imager (Packard Bioscience Company). Rabbit anti-Sp1 polyclonal antibody (Sp1-ab2, Active Motif) raised against the full-length Sp1 protein was used to detect Sp1 expression. Internal control β-actin expression was analyzed using monoclonal anti–β-actin antibody AC-15 (Sigma). Aβ was analyzed by 10–20% Tris-Tricine gel with monoclonal antibody 4G8 and 6E10 (Signet). Aβ40/42 was also measured by Sandwich ELISA assay with β-amyloid 1-40 or 1-42 colorimetric ELISA kit (Biosource International, Inc) according to the manufacturer's instructions.

RESULTS

Molecular Cloning of the Human BACE1 Gene Promoter

The 5′ upstream region of BACE1 gene was amplified with PCR from a human fetus brain genomic library (Clontech) using 5′ genome walking strategy. This region contained a 2,668-bp fragment of the 5′ flanking region and the first exon of the *BACE1* gene.[42] Sequence analysis revealed that the *BACE1* gene has a complex transcriptional unit. It lacks typical CAAT and TATA boxes and contains a GC-rich region with 71% of GC content between the transcription start site and the first codon and 62% around the transcription start site. Computer-based transcription factor binding site search revealed that this 2.6-kb 5′ flanking region contains several putative regulatory elements, such as a GC box, HSF-1, PU-box, AP1, AP2, and lymphokine response binding sites. To determine if the 2,668-bp fragment of genomic DNA contains the promoter of the *BACE1* gene, we subcloned the fragment into a promoterless luciferase gene reporter plasmid vector pGL3-basic. pB1P-A plasmid is constructed to contain 2.1-kb 5′-UTR from −1944 to +292 of the BACE1 gene upstream of the luciferase reporter gene. Compared with an empty vector control, pB1P-A transfected cells have significant luciferase activity. This indicated that the 2.1-kb fragment contains the functional promoter region of the human *BACE1* gene.

Sp1 Regulates the BACE1 Gene Transcription

To examine the *cis*-acting regulatory elements in the upstream region of the minimal promoter, deletion plasmids were made to contain various fragments between −1,944 bp to −619 bp. We found that the region between −932 bp to −896 bp contains a putative Sp1 binding site. Gel shift assay identified a Sp1 binding element located at −911 bp and deletion of Sp1 binding element from the *BACE1* gene promoter resulted in a significant decrease in luciferase expression from 195.47±33.01 to 40.82±11.06 RLU (pB1P-I) in PC12 cells (*P*<.001) (FIG. 1A). Further deletion of 139 bp (pB1P-J) drastically increased the promoter activity to 337.49±82.25 RLU in PC12 cells (FIG. 1A) (*P*<.001 relative to pB1P-I and *P*>.05 relative to pB1P-H). To further confirm this Sp1 binding element's function, we abolished the Sp1 site of pB1P-H by generating two Sp1-binding site mutant plasmids, changing three nucleotides of Sp1 core binding sequence from **GGGCGG** to **GTTGGG** to generate pB1P-H-mut1Sp1 (Mutant-1), and six nucleotides of Sp1 consensus binding sequence from **GGGCGG** to **ATTGTA** to generate pB1P-H-mut2Sp1 (Mutant-2). These mutations markedly inhibited the BACE1 promoter activity to 57.66±1.83% (Mutant-1) and 52.90±2.66% (Mutant-2), respectively (*P*<.001), and there was no significant change in promoter activity between the Mutant-1 and Mutant-2 plasmids (*P*>.05) (FIG. 1B). We then performed an assay to determine if this binding element biologically responded to the transcription factor Sp1 in the transcriptional regulation of the human *BACE1* gene. Plasmid pB1P-H containing 1.2 kb of the *BACE1* gene promoter fragment was cotransfected into HEK293T cells with pCGN-Sp1, a mammalian plasmid vector to express transcription factor Sp1 (FIG. 1C). Overexpression of Sp1 had no effect on the luciferase activity in the control cells transfected with empty vector. However, the luciferase activity increased dramatically in cells cotransfected pB1P-H with Sp1, a fourfold increase compared to the non-Sp1 transfected cells (435.74±24.99% and 100±3.56%, respectively, *P*<.001) (FIG. 1D). Overexpression of Sp1 had no significant upregulatory effect on the luciferase activity in the cells transfected with pB1P-I, a Sp1-binding element deletion plasmid (49.36±8.17% in the Sp1-transfected cells and 33.12±4.86% in the non–Sp1-transfected cells, *P*>.05). These data demonstrated that the Sp1 site is necessary and sufficient for the 34-bp fragment's upregulatory effect on the BACE1 transcription. To further examine the role Sp1 plays in the regulation of the *BACE1* gene transcription, cells were transfected with pB1P-H and treated with a Sp1 binding inhibitor, mithramycin A. The treatment of mithramycin A resulted in a significant reduction of the BACE1 promoter activity in a dose-dependent and time-dependent manner. Addition of 25 nM, 75 nM, and 125 nM of mithramycin A for 48 h decreased the promoter activity to 89.10±1.40%, 52.75±1.74%, and 38.02±4.24%, respectively (*P*<.001 by ANOVA) (FIG. 1E), and 125 nM mithramycin A treatment for 16 h and 48 h inhibited the promoter activity to 79.55±6.12% and 38.02±4.24%, respectively (*P*<.001 by ANOVA) (FIG. 1F). Further analysis of the RT-PCR results showed that the endogenous mRNA level of the *BACE1* gene was significantly reduced in Sp1-KO cells (58.55±7.40%) relative to Sp1-WT cells (*P*<.001).[42] These results indicate that Sp1 plays an important role in the transcriptional regulation of the human *BACE1* gene.

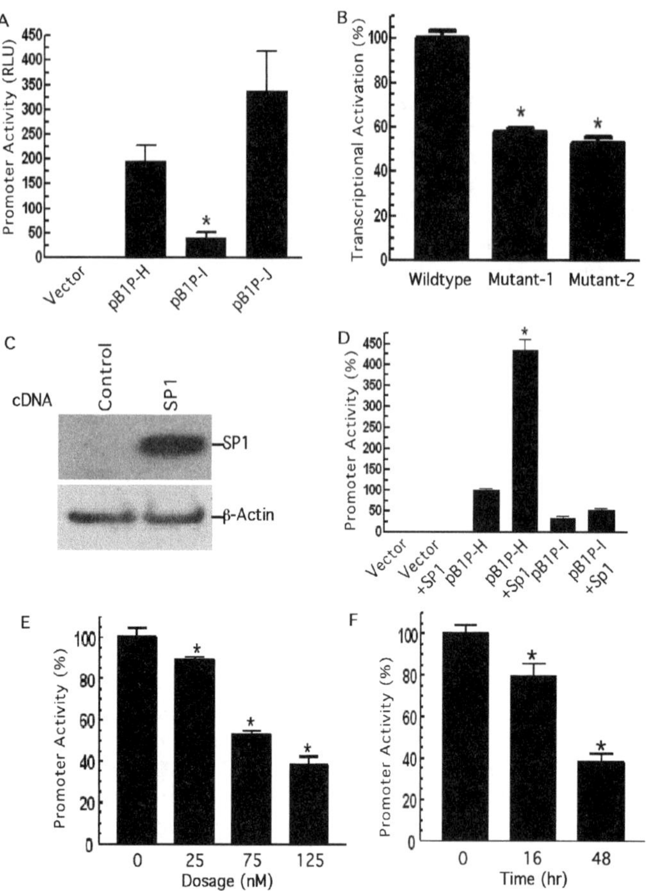

FIGURE 1. Sp1 potentiates the *BACE1* gene transcription. (**A**) The fragment of −932 to +292 bp or −896 to +292 bp from the BACE1 promoter was cloned into pGL3-Basic to generate Sp1-containing or Sp1-absent plasmids, pB1P-H or pB1P-I, respectively. PC12 cells were transfected with plasmid pB1P-H, pB1P-I, pB1P-J, and empty vector control. Luciferase activity was measured at 72 h by a luminometer and expressed in relative luciferase units (RLU). β-Galactosidase activity was used to normalize transfection efficiency. The values represent mean ± SEM, *N*=3–6. *$P<.001$ relative to pB1P-H and pB1P-J by ANOVA with post-hoc Newmann-Keuls test. (**B**) Plasmid pB1P-H (wild-type), pB1P-H-mut1Sp1 (Mutant-1), and pB1P-H-mut1Sp1 (Mutant-2) were transfected into HEK293T cells and the promoter activity was measured. *N*=3, * $P<.001$. (**C**) Sp1 protein was robustly expressed in pCGN-Sp1 transfected cells and β-actin was used as an internal protein control. (**D**) Transcriptional activation of the BACE1 promoter is potentiated by Sp1. Empty vector, Sp1-binding site containing BACE1 promoter plasmid pB1P-H and Sp1-binding site absent BACE1 promoter plasmid pB1P-I were cotransfected with Sp1 expression plasmid pCGN-Sp1 into cells. Overexpression of Sp1 significantly increases the pB1P-H BACE1 promoter activity by more than fourfold and has no significant effect on pB1P-I and control plasmid. *N*=3, * $P<.001$. (**E, F**) Inhibition of the BACE1 promoter activity by mithramycin A. The BACE1 promoter construct pB1P-H was transfected in HEK293T cells. The transfected

Sp1 Facilitates BACE1 Cleavage of APP and Aβ

Proteolytic processing of APP by BACE1 at its β site is essential for generating Aβ. To determine if Sp1's regulatory effect on the BACE1 gene transcription eventually affects its downstream event, i.e., APP processing to generate Aβ, we analyzed the protein levels of BACE1, APP C99 (the major BACE1 cleavage product) in the Swedish-mutant APP695 stably-expressed HEK293 cells transfected with Sp1 cDNA and the cells treated with mithramycin A as well as the control cells (FIG. 2A). Sp1 overexpression significantly increased the level of BACE1 protein and its cleavage product, APP C99 fragment, and the production of Aβ, relative to control cells. In contrast, mithramycin A, the Sp1-binding inhibitor, markedly reduced the generation of BACE1 protein, APP C99 and Aβ. Quantitative analysis (FIG. 2B) showed that Sp1 overexpression slightly increased APP expression ($127.45\pm5.23\%$) and Mithramycin decreased APP levels ($87.46\pm1.75\%$) relative to control ($P>.05$). However, Sp1 overexpression resulted in marked increases of the levels of BACE1 to $184.94\pm7.11\%$, APP C99 to $212.27\pm12.21\%$, and Aβ to $215.67\pm15.06\%$, relative to control cells, and mithramycin A caused significant reduction of the levels of BACE1 to $49.77\pm7.06\%$, APP C99 to $20.76\pm9.25\%$, and Aβ to $55.76\pm4.29\%$, relative to control cells ($P<.001$) (FIG. 2B). β-Actin protein was used as internal control and its level in cell lysates showed no change in either Sp1-overexpressed cells or mithramycin A–treated cells, compared to control cells. Thus, Sp1 affects APP processing to generate Aβ by regulating BACE1 gene expression at its transcription level and subsequently, its protein production.

Proteasome Inhibitors Markedly Reduced the Degradation of BACE1 Protein

To investigate if the degradation of BACE1 protein is regulated by the ubiquitin-proteasome pathway, neuroblastoma SH-SY5Y cells were treated with the highly specific proteasome inhibitor lactacystin and BACE1 protein levels were analyzed by immunoblotting. Endogenous BACE1 protein was detected by 208, a polyclonal antibody raised in a rabbit against BACE1 C-terminus. Lactacystin markedly increased endogenous BACE1 protein level in SH-SY5Y cells (FIG. 3A). Lactacystin treatment also significantly increased the level of BACE1 protein in BACE1 cDNA transiently transfected SH-SY5Y cells (FIG. 3B). Lactacystin increased BACE1 protein levels in a dose- (FIG. 3C) and time-dependent (FIG. 3D) manner in BACE1 cDNA stably transfected B2 cells.[44] These results suggested that inhibition of the ubiquitin-proteasome pathway by lactacystin decreased the degradation of BACE1 in both neuronal and non-neuronal cells. To further examine if BACE1 degradation is regulated by the ubiquitin-proteasome pathway, B2 cells were treated with other proteasome inhibitors. *N*-Acetyl-L-leucinyl-L-leucinyl-L-methional (ALLM), *N*-acetyl-L-leucinyl-L-leucinyl-L-norleucinal (ALLN), and *N*-carbobenzoxyl-L-leucinyl-

---

cells were treated with vehicle solution control or mithramycin A for 48 h at 25, 75, or 125 nM (**E**) for dosage-dependent assay or with mithramycin A at 125 nM for 16 or 48 h for time-course assay (**F**). Cells were harvested at the same transfection endpoint and luciferase activity was measured and expressed as mean±SEM percent of control promoter activity. *$P<.01$ relative to control by ANOVA with post-hoc Newmann-Keuls test. (From *Molecular and Cellular Biology*, 2004, **24**: 864–874. Reprinted with permission.)

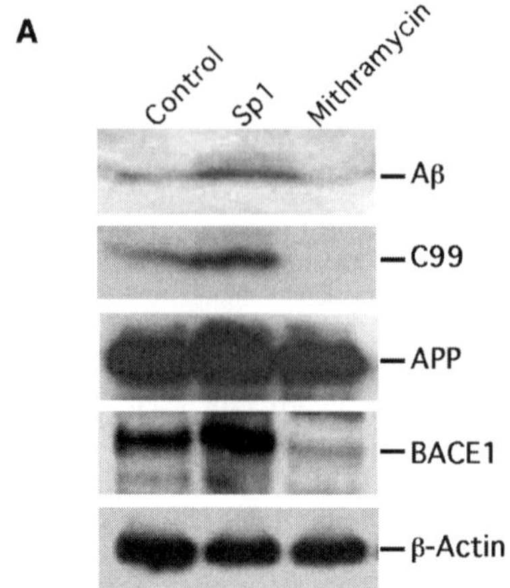

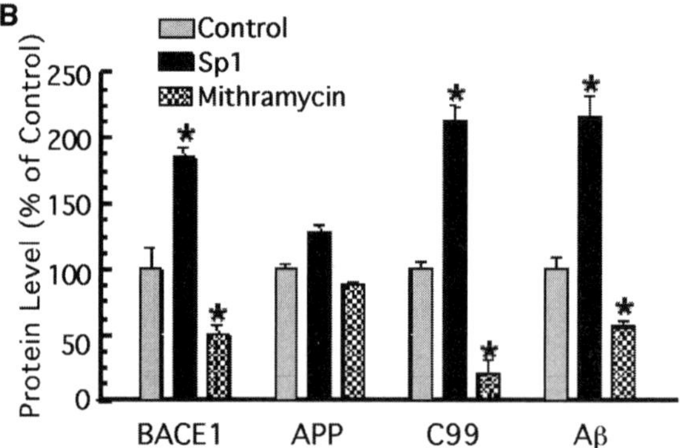

FIGURE 2. Sp1 increases BACE1 protein generation, β-secretase cleavage of APP, and Aβ production. (**A**) Swedish mutant APP stably expressed HEK293 cells were transfected with pCGN-Sp1 plasmid (Sp1) or without Sp1 transfection (Control) and treated with mithramycin A at 125 nM (Mithramycin) for 48 hours. Western blot analysis was performed to detect Aβ, APP C99, full-length APP, BACE1, and β-actin. Monoclonal anti β-actin antibody (AC-15) was used to detect β-actin and BACE1 protein level was detected by rabbit polyclonal BACE1 antibody LK-16. To detect APP C99, the major BACE1 cleavage product, cell lysates were analyzed by 10–20% Tris-Tricine gel with 6E10 antibody. For Aβ detection, conditioned media were first immunoprecipitated with Aβ antibody 4G8 and immunoblot assay was then performed to analyze the precipitates on 10–20% Tris-Tricine gel with monoclonal antibody 6E10. Note that overexpression of Sp1 increases BACE1 protein and subsequently affects APP processing at β-site, while inhibition of Sp1 binding by mithramycin A has an opposite effect. No significant changes were detected in β-actin and full-length APP levels. (**B**) Quantitative analysis of the generation of Aβ, APP C99, full-length APP, and BACE1. Values are means ± S.E.M. and *N*=3. The protein levels are expressed as a percentage of the levels in control cells. *$P<.001$ relative to controls by ANOVA with post-hoc Newmann-Keuls test. (From *Molecular and Cellular Biology*, 2004, **24:** 864–874. Reprinted with permission.)

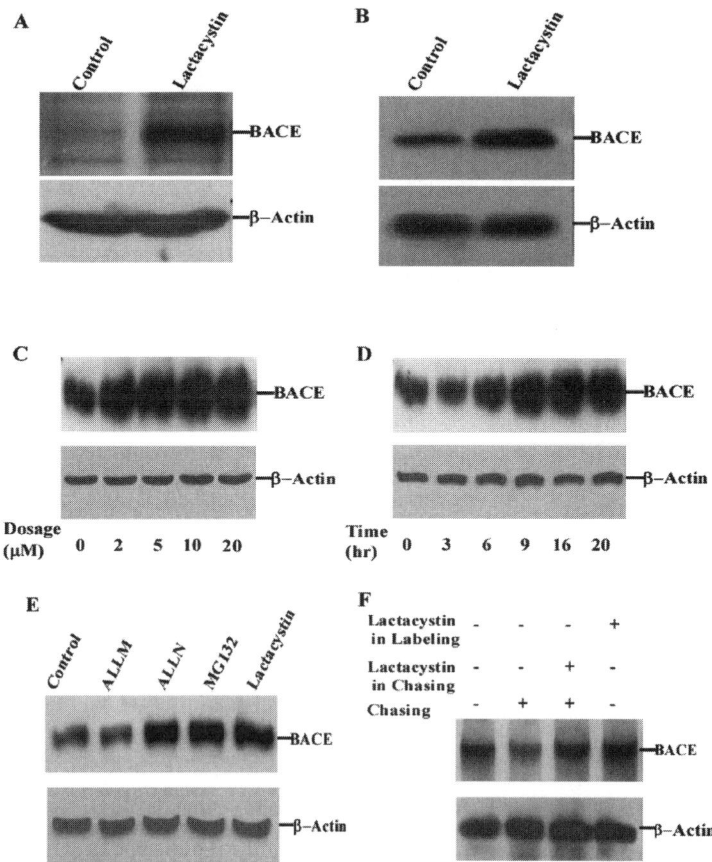

FIGURE 3. Proteasome inhibitors inhibit BACE1 protein degradation. **(A)** Neuroblastoma SH-SY5Y cells were treated with 10 µM lactacystin for 9 h and endogenous BACE protein was detected by antibody 208. **(B)** Plasmid pBACE-mycHis was transiently transfected into SH-SY5Y cells using Lipofectamine 2000. The transfected cells were treated with 10 µM lactacystin for 9 h and harvested at 48-h time point. BACE proteins were detected by monoclonal anti-myc antibody 9E10. **(C)** BACE cDNA stably transfected B2 cells were treated with vehicle solution control or lactacystin for 9 h at 2, 5, 10, or 20 µM for dosage-dependent assay, or with lactacystin at 10 µM for 0–20 h for time-course assay **(D)** 9E10 antibody was used to detect BACE1 and monoclonal anti β-actin antibody (AC-15) was used to detect β-actin. Lactacystin treatment markedly increased BACE protein levels and had no effect on β-actin. **(E)** B2 cells were treated with vehicle solution control, ALLM (25 µM), ALLN (25 µM), MG132 (5 µM), or lactacystin (10 µM) for 9 hours. The irreversible synthetic proteasome inhibitor lactacystin and reversible peptide aldehyde ALLN and MG132 increased BACE protein levels, while ALLM, non-proteasome protease inhibitor, had no effect on BACE protein level. β-Actin was not affect by the treatments. **(F)** Pulse-chase experiment was performed to examine the proteasomal degradation of BACE. B2 cells were incubated with ^{35}S-methionine and ^{35}S-cysteine labeling media for 9 h, and then replaced with nonradioactive chasing media. Proteins from cell lysates were immunoprecipitated with 9E10 and analyzed on 4~20% gradient Tris-Glycine gels. The gels were dried and subject to autoradiography. (Adapted by permission from *The FASEB Journal*, 2004, **18:** 1571–1573.)

L-leucinyl-L-leucinal (MG-132) are a group of peptide aldehydes.[45] Like lactacystin, ALLN and MG-132 specifically inhibited protein degradation by the proteasome. In contrast, ALLM, a non–proteasome-specific protease inhibitor, had little effect on the ubiquitin-proteasome pathway in intact cells. FIGURE 3E showed that ALLN, and MG-132 significantly increased BACE1 protein levels relative to control in B2 cells. However, ALLM did not affect BACE1 proteolysis. These findings suggested that the proteasome inhibitors upregulated the BACE1 protein levels by inhibiting the ubiquitin-proteasome pathway. To investigate if the turnover of BACE1 protein is regulated by the ubiquitin-proteasome pathway, a pulse-chase experiment was performed. B2 cells were metabolically radiolabeled with the media containing ^{35}S-methionine and ^{35}S-cysteine and then incubated with fresh media containing excessive amount of nonradioactive methionine and cysteine. The radiolabeled BACE1 proteins were immunoprecipitated with 9E10 antibody and analyzed on 4~20% gradient Tris/glycine gels. FIGURE 3F showed that without proteasome inhibitor treatment the newly synthesized BACE1 proteins were degraded and the turnover rate was 53.63±5.49% for 9-h chasing time ($P<.001$ relative to control). In contrast, addition of lactacystin in the chasing media increased the BACE1 protein levels to 109.77±2.92% from 53.63±5.49% in the non-lactacystin treatment in the chasing media ($P<.001$), and the levels of BACE1 protein in the cells treated with chasing media containing lactacystin for 9 h were similar to that in the cells without chasing and lactacystin treatment ($P<.05$), indicating that the turnover of the newly synthesized radiolabeled BACE1 protein was inhibited. Furthermore, addition of lactacystin in labeling media increased the radiolabeled BACE1 protein level to 124.37±4.43% ($P<.05$ relative to control). Lactacystin treatment had no effect on β-actin. These data demonstrated that the degradation of BACE1 was inhibited by lactacystin through the blockage of the ubiquitin-proteasome pathway.

BACE1 Ubiquitination

An immunohistochemical staining assay was performed to investigate if BACE1 protein colocalized with ubiquitin protein. HEK293 cells were transfected with pBACE-EGFP and myc-tagged ubiquitin plasmid pCW-7[43] (FIG. 4A). BACE1-EGFP fusion protein was detected by the green fluorescent signal. The myc-tagged ubiquitin was immunostained with 9E10 antibody. The merged image showed that the green fluorescent BACE1 proteins colocalized with the red fluorescent ubiquitin proteins. To examine the interaction between BACE1 and ubiquitin, B2 cells were transiently transfected with ubiquitin expression plasmid pHis-UBi. FIGURE 4B showed that the high molecular weight BACE1 complexes were generated in the cells treated with lactacystin or transfected with pHis-Ubi, indicating that BACE1 protein was polyubiquitinated. To confirm the ubiquitination of BACE1 protein, co-immunoprecipitation assay was performed. HEK293 cells were transfected with pBACE-EGFP, pCW-7, or a combination of both plasmids. The cell lysates were immunoprecipitated with anti-EGFP antibody to pull down BACE1-EGFP fusion protein. The immunoprecipitates were immunoblotted with 9E10 to detect myc-tagged ubiquitin. The anti-EGFP antibody immunoprecipitating samples from either pBACE-EGFP transfected cells or myc-ubiquitin pCW-7 transfected cells contained no myc-ubiquitin. However, high molecular weight BACE1-ubi molecules were detected by 9E10 in the anti-EGFP antibody immunoprecipitating samples from the

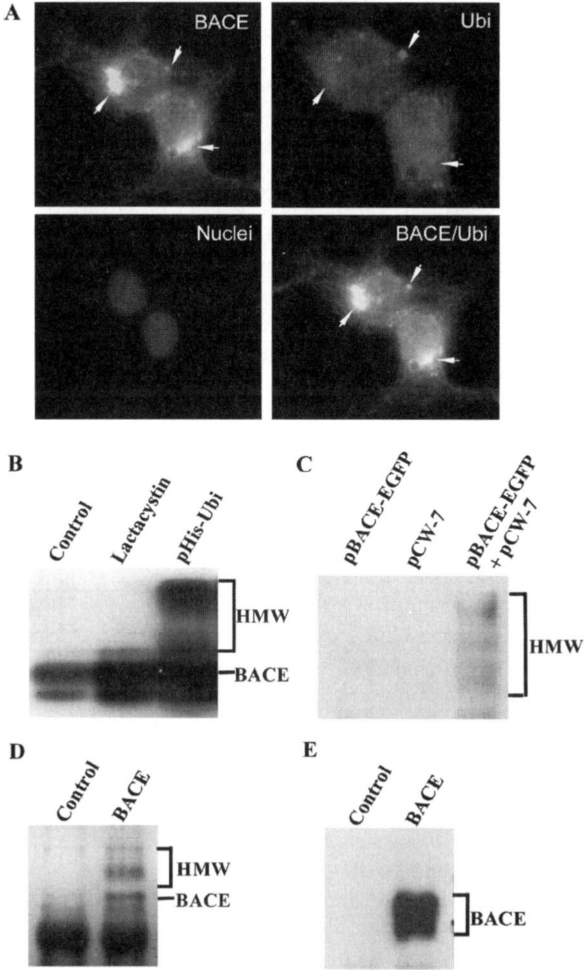

FIGURE 4. BACE ubiquitination. (**A**) Colocalization of BACE and ubiquitin. HEK293 cells were transfected with pBACE-EGFP and myc-tagged ubiquitin plasmid pCW-7. Expression of BACE-EGFP fusion protein was indicated by the green fluorescent signal (*upper left panel*) and myc-tagged ubiquitin was immunostained with 9E10 antibody (*upper right panel*). Hoechst staining was used to detect nucleus (*lower left panel*). (*Lower right panel*) Superimposed images showing the colocalization of BACE and ubiquitin. *Arrows* indicate the examples of the colocalized proteins. (**B**) B2 cells were treated with lactacystin or transfected with ubiquitin protein plasmid pHis-Ubi. BACE proteins were detected by 9E10. Lactacystin treatment and ubiquitin plasmid transfection generated high molecular weight (HMW) BACE complex. (**C**) HEK293 cells were transfected with pBACE-EGFP, pCW-7, or combination of both plasmids. The cell lysates were immunoprecipitated with anti-EGFP antibody to pull down BACE-EGFP fusion protein, followed by Western blot analysis with 9E10 to detect myc-tagged ubiquitin in the BACE-EGFP-containing immunoprecipitates. Co-immunoprecipitation of BACE and ubiquitin was detected. The cell lysates from HEK

cells transfected with both BACE1-EGFP and myc-ubiquitin cDNA, indicating the co-immunoprecipitation of BACE1 and ubiquitin (FIG. 4C). A reverse co-immuno-precipitation assay was performed to further confirm the ubiquitination of BACE1 proteins. HEK 293 cells and myc-tagged BACE1 stably expressing B2 cells were lysed with NP-40 lysis buffer and the cell lysates were immunoprecipitated with anti-ubiquitin antibody. The samples were then analyzed by immunoblotting with either anti-BACE1 antibody 208 (FIG. 4D) or anti-myc antibody 9E10 (FIG. 4E) to detect BACE1 protein. BACE1 was only detected in the cells transfected with myc-tagged BACE1 plasmid, but not the control HEK293 non-transfected cells. These results clearly demonstrated that BACE1 was ubiquitinated.

Regulation of APP Processing and Aβ Generation by the Ubiquitin-Proteasome Pathway

To further examine if proteasomal degradation of BACE1 had any effect on APP proteolytic processing at the β-secretase site and on Aβ production, β-secretase cleavage product, APP C99, in cell lysates and Aβ levels in conditioned media were analyzed. In 2EB2 cells expressing Swedish mutant APP and BACE1, the major β-secretase cleavage product APP C99 production and minor Glu-11 β-secretase cleavage product APP C89 were markedly increased by treatment with lactacystin compared to control (FIG. 5A). To examine if this proteasomal inhibition of BACE1 degradation affected Aβ generation, Aβ ELISA analysis was performed. The Swedish mutant APP stably transfected 20E2 cells were treated with lactacystin and Aβ and the conditioned media were captured by anti-hAβ mAB directed to the N-terminus of Aβ proteins. Aβ40 and Aβ42 were detected by rabbit antibodies specific to Aβ40 and Aβ42 (BioSource International, Inc, Camarillo, CA). Lactacystin treatment increased the levels of Aβ40 generation to 132.05±3.85% relative to control ($P<.001$) and the levels of Aβ42 from 6.80±0.25% in control to 24.75±0.26% ($P<.001$) (FIG. 5B). Similar results were also obtained by using neuroblastoma SH-SY5Y cells (FIG. 5C). Aβ40 production was increased by 156.08±0.70% ($P<.01$) in lactacystin treated cells, and Aβ42 production was doubled in the treated cells (38.08±0.86%) relative to control cells (19.06±0.76%) ($P<.001$). Thus, the proteasomal inhibitor, lactacystin, not only regulates the β-secretase cleavage of APP, but also affects the Aβ production.

DISCUSSION

Aβ is the principal component of senile neuritic plaques in the brain of AD. Proteolytic processing of APP at the β site by BACE1, the major APP β-secretase *in vivo*, is essential to generate Aβ.[24–27] *BACE1* gene expression is tightly regulated and it

---

293 cells and myc-tagged BACE stably expressing B2 cells were immunoprecipitated with anti-ubiquitin antibody followed by immunoblotting with either anti-BACE antibody 208 (**D**) or anti-myc antibody 9E10 (**E**) to detect BACE proteins. BACE was detected in the samples pulled down by anti-ubiquitin antibody. (Reprinted by permission from *The FASEB Journal*, 2004, **18:** 1571–1573.)

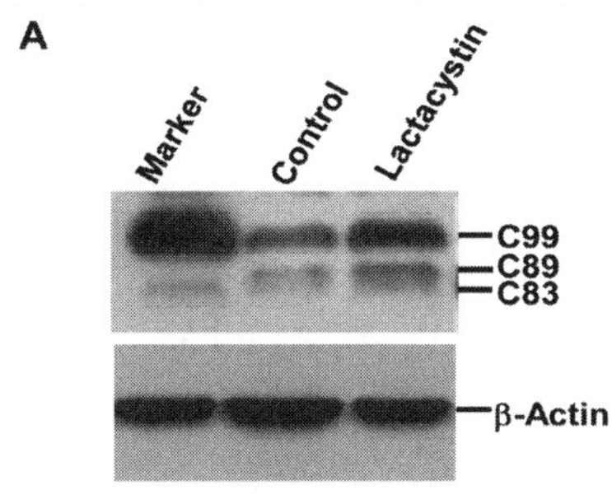

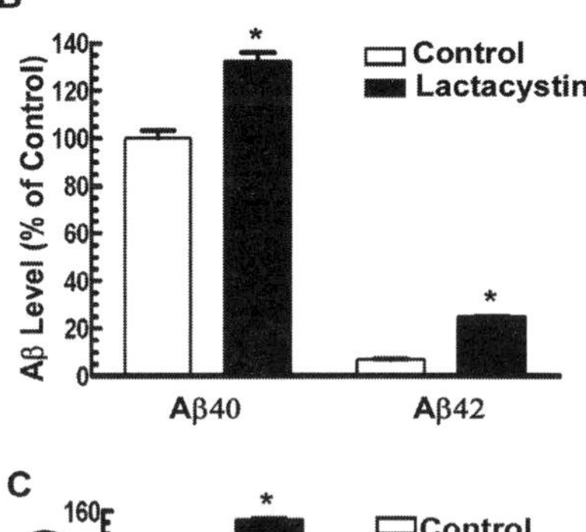

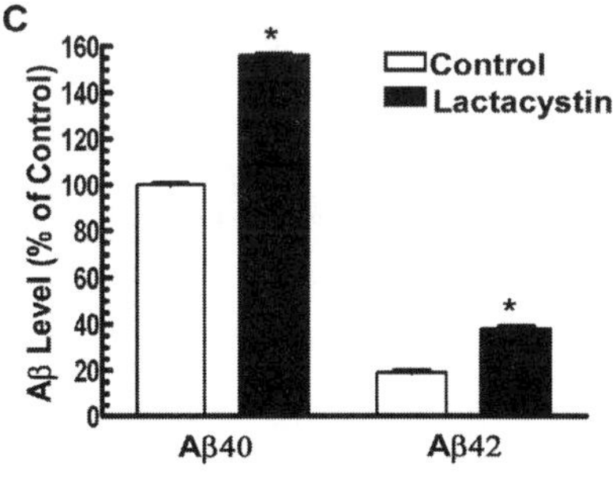

FIGURE 5. Regulation of APP processing and Aβ generation by the ubiquitin-proteasome pathway. **(A)** 2EB2 cells were incubated with 10 µM lactacystin for 9 hours. Cell lysates were analyzed by 16% Tris-Tricine gel with C20 to detect APP C-terminal fragments and AC-15 to detect β-actin. pAPP-C99 was transfected into cells and the expressed C99 protein was used as the marker. **(B)** 20E2 cells, the Swedish mutant APP stably transfected cells and **(C)** neuroblastoma SH-SY5Y cells were treated with lactacystin at 10 µM for 9 hours. The conditioned media was harvested and Aβ40 and Aβ42 were quantitated by sandwich ELISA. The values represent mean ± S.E.M., *N*=4. **P*<.01 relative to control by ANOVA with post-hoc Newmann-Keuls test. Values are means ± SEM (*N*=3). (Reprinted by permission from *The FASEB Journal*, 2004, **18**: 1571–1573.)

shows tissue specificity with its enzymatic activity mainly in central nervous system.[24,46] Expression is not under the control of activated glia-derived cytokines or growth factors.[47] BACE1 is expressed at the highest levels in the pancreas and also at high levels in the brain.[27] Tissue-specific expression of BACE1 is very important for normal APP processing and dysregulation of BACE1 expression may play a role in AD pathogenesis.[42] In order to define the molecular mechanism by which *BACE1* gene expression is regulated, we cloned and characterized 2.6 kb 5'-UTR of the human *BACE1* gene. Sequence analysis showed that the *BACE1* promoter, unlike most type II eukaryotic gene promoters, does not contain a TATA and CAAT box in this region and has a high GC content. This TATA-less and high GC feature of *BACE1* gene, similar to APP gene,[48] resembles many housekeeping gene promoters.[49] The 5' flanking region has various possible transcription factor binding elements such as a GC box, AP1, AP2, PU box, and lymphokine responsive site. It shows that *BACE1* gene expression is tightly regulated at the transcription level.[42,50] Furthermore, we show that transcription factor Sp1 plays a significant role in regulating the *BACE1* gene expression. Our study provides the first information on the molecular mechanism by which the human *BACE1* gene expression is regulated.

Many housekeeping and tissue-specific genes contain functionally important Sp1 binding sites. Sp1 is one of the first identified eukaryotic transcription factors and contains three Cys-His zinc finger motifs.[51,52] Sp1 has been shown to play an important role in the regulation of the expression of many genes. Its C-terminal domain interacts with other transcription factors in a synergistic manner, which controls gene expression in time and space.[53] Sp1 is required for normal embryonic development and Sp1-null embryos have severe developmental abnormality and die at an early embryonic stage (around E11).[54,55] To investigate if the *BACE1* gene is one of the downstream Sp1 target genes in physiological condition, overexpression and gene knockout experiments were used. Overexpression of Sp1 protein significantly facilitates the BACE1 promoter activity, while lack of endogenous Sp1 protein in Sp1-KO cells markedly reduced the transcriptional activation of the BACE1 gene. Moreover, the endogenous BACE1 mRNA level was also reduced in these Sp1-KO cells. The β-secretase cleavage of APP is essential for generating Aβ. Our study indicates that Sp1 controls the *BACE1* gene expression at the transcriptional level and in turn regulates APP processing to generate Aβ. Overexpression of Sp1 facilitates BACE1 enzymatic activity by increasing BACE1 protein generation, which leads to a higher level of Aβ production, while inhibition of Sp1 binding by mithramycin A downregulates BACE1 expression to a lower level of Aβ generation. These results definitively demonstrate that Sp1 regulates the *BACE1* gene expression *in vivo* and the human *BACE1* gene is one of the Sp1 downstream target genes.

AD pathogenesis is believed to be multifactorial. Although genetic analysis has failed to uncover either coding sequence mutations in the open reading frame of BACE1 or genetic linkage or allelic association of BACE1 with AD in the patients with familial AD,[56,57] increased β-secretase activity was reported in some FAD brains[58] and nearly threefold greater expression level of BACE1 in the cortex of sporadic AD patients versus age-matched controls.[59] To further investigate how BACE1 protein level is regulated at the posttranslational level, we examine the role of ubiquitin-proteasome pathway in BACE1 degradation. The ubiquitin-proteasome pathway has been implicated in the pathogenesis of neurodegenerative disorders such as Parkinson's disease, Alzheimer's disease, and to a lesser extent normal aging of the brain.[43,60–64] The ubiquitin-proteasome pathway is also involved in the early stages of Wallerian degeneration of local axons, which is a common pathological feature of many neurodegenerative diseases and peripheral neuropathies.[65] The proteasome selectively degrades multiple substrates that are important in maintaining neuronal homeostasis, including the catabolism of oxidized, damaged, and aggregated proteins.[65–67] In AD, the activity of the proteasome was significantly decreased in the parahippocampal gyrus, the superior and middle temporal gyri, and the inferior parietal lobe of AD brains. These regions show severe degenerative alterations in AD. Frameshift mutations of ubiquitin-B were found in AD brains.[63] This mutant ubiquitin-B gene expresses aberrant ubiquitin-B proteins (+1 proteins) (UBB+1) in the carboxyl terminus. The +1 proteins were not found in young control patients. This type of transcript mutation is likely an important factor in the widely occurring non-familial early- and late-onset forms of Alzheimer's disease. UBB+1 lacks the capacity to ubiquitinate, and overexpression of UBB+1 in neuroblastoma cells significantly induces nuclear fragmentation and cell death. These results suggest that the ubiquitin-proteasome degradation machinery is involved in the pathogenesis of AD.[63,64]

In this study, our data indicate that BACE1 is ubiquitinated and clearly demonstrate that blocking the ubiquitin-proteasome pathway will inhibit BACE1 degradation. The proteasomal inhibition of BACE1 degradation led to increased production of BACE1 enzymatic activity, more β-cleavage product C99, and increased both Aβ40 and Aβ42 in neuronal and non-neuronal cells. It has been reported that degradation of APP CTFs were also mediated by the proteasome pathway[68–70] and Aβ itself also inhibits the proteasome complex.[71] Inhibition of the turnover of the APP-C99 fragment potentiated Aβ generation.[72] Our data are consistent with this report and the inhibition of the BACE1 turnover by the proteasome inhibitors partly contributes to the increased level of Aβ generation.

One of the pharmaceutical strategies in AD therapy is to reduce Aβ production by either inhibiting β-secretase or γ-secretase activity. Studies indicate that inhibition of γ-secretase may have a potential severe side effect. Presenilin-KO inhibited not only γ-secretase cleavage of APP to generate Aβ, but also Notch signaling, which resulted in severe developmental abnormalities in mice.[73–76] However, mice deficient in BACE1 develop normally without any detectable physiological defects.[38–40] *BACE1* gene knockout in mice resulted in a marked reduction in Aβ formation,[38–40] while overexpression of human BACE1 in the Swedish mutant APP transgenic mice significantly increased brain levels of Aβ at a steady-state,[77] suggesting that BACE1 plays an essential role in the amyloidogenic pathway in AD pathogenesis and is a good therapeutic target for AD treatment. BACE1 is predominantly expressed in hippocampal neurons, the cerebral cortex, and the cerebellar granular layer.[46,78] During ontogeny, BACE1 expression shifts from widespread synthesis throughout the body prenatally to a tissue specific pattern postnatally.[46]

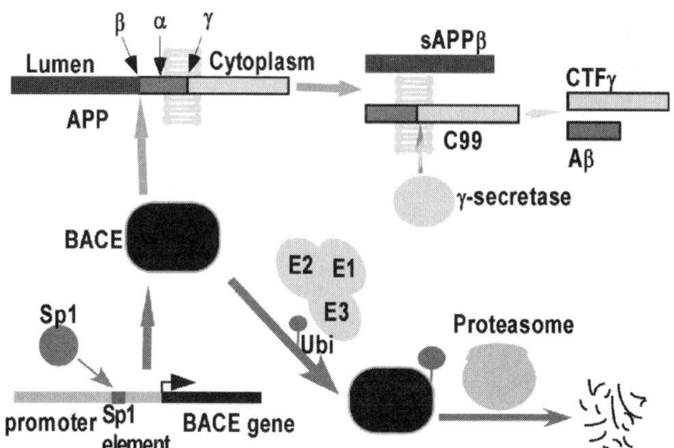

FIGURE 6. Regulation of BACE1 gene expression and protein degradation. APP is processed by three different enzymes: α-, β-, and γ-secretase. BACE1, the major APP β-secretase *in vivo*, is essential enzyme to cleave APP to generate Aβ. Transcription factor Sp1 plays an important role in regulating BACE1 gene transcription and the degradation of BACE is mediated by the ubiquitin-proteasome pathway.

Future study will determine what part of the BACE1 promoter contains the cis-acting element responsible for its neuronal tissue-specific expression pattern and identify transcription factors that may work synergistically with Sp1 in the transcriptional regulation of *BACE1* gene, as well as the possible *BACE1* gene dysregulation in AD patients. Our finding of BACE1 degradation mediated by the ubiquitin-proteasome pathway suggests that BACE1 protein homeostasis is well controlled at both transcriptional and translational levels (FIG. 6). Dysregulation at either BACE1 gene transcription or/and posttranslational modification might constitute an important event in the pathogenesis of certain AD cases.

ACKNOWLEDGMENTS

This work was supported by Canadian Institutes of Health Research (CIHR), Jack Brown and Family Alzheimer's Research Foundation, and Michael Smith Foundation for Health Research (W.S.). W.S. is the holder of the Canada Research Chair in Alzheimer's Disease. W.Z. was the recipient of the Arthur & June Willms Fellowships and Y.T. was the recipient of the Michael Smith Foundation for Health Research Post Doctoral Fellowship. W.Z. and H.Q. contributed equally to this work.

REFERENCES

1. ALZHEIMER, A. 1907. Uber eine eigenartige erkrangung der hirnrinde. All. Z. Psychiat. Psych. Gerichtl. Med. **64:** 146–148.
2. KANG, J. *et al.* 1987. The precursor of Alzheimer's disease amyloid A4 protein resembles a cell-surface receptor. Nature **325:** 733–736.
3. TANZI, R.E. *et al.* 1987. Amyloid beta protein gene: cDNA, mRNA distribution, and genetic linkage near the Alzheimer locus. Science **235:** 880–884.
4. GOLDGABER, D. *et al.* 1987. Characterization and chromosomal localization of a cDNA encoding brain amyloid of Alzheimer's disease. Science **235:** 877–880.
5. ST. GEORGE-HYSLOP, P.H. *et al.* 1987. The genetic defect causing familial Alzheimer's disease maps on chromosome 21. Science **235:** 885–890.
6. ROBAKIS, N.K. *et al.* 1987. Molecular cloning and characterization of a cDNA encoding the cerebrovascular and the neuritic plaque amyloid peptides. Proc. Natl. Acad. Sci. USA **84:** 4190–4194.
7. STRITTMATTER, W.J. *et al.* 1993. Apolipoprotein E: high-avidity binding to beta-amyloid and increased frequency of type 4 allele in late-onset familial Alzheimer disease. Proc. Natl. Acad. Sci. USA **90:** 1977–1981.
8. STRITTMATTER, W.J. *et al.* 1993. Binding of human apolipoprotein E to synthetic amyloid beta peptide: isoform-specific effects and implications for late-onset Alzheimer disease. Proc. Natl. Acad. Sci. USA **90:** 8098–8102.
9. SCHMECHEL, D.E. *et al.* 1993. Increased amyloid beta-peptide deposition in cerebral cortex as a consequence of apolipoprotein E genotype in late-onset Alzheimer disease. Proc. Natl. Acad. Sci. USA **90:** 9649–9653.
10. CORDER, E.H. *et al.* 1993. Gene dose of apolipoprotein E type 4 allele and the risk of Alzheimer's disease in late onset families. Science **261:** 921–923.
11. SHERRINGTON, R. *et al.* 1995. Cloning of a gene bearing missense mutations in early-onset familial Alzheimer's disease. Nature **375:** 754–760.
12. LI, J., J. MA & H. POTTER. 1995. Identification and expression analysis of a potential familial Alzheimer disease gene on chromosome 1 related to AD3. Proc. Natl. Acad. Sci. USA **92:** 12180–12184.
13. MULLAN, M. *et al.* 1992. A locus for familial early-onset Alzheimer's disease on the long arm of chromosome 14, proximal to the alpha 1-antichymotrypsin gene. Nat. Genet. **2:** 340–342.

14. ST. GEORGE-HYSLOP, P. *et al.* 1992. Genetic evidence for a novel familial Alzheimer's disease locus on chromosome 14. Nat. Genet. **2:** 330–334.
15. SCHELLENBERG, G.D. *et al.* 1992. Genetic linkage evidence for a familial Alzheimer's disease locus on chromosome 14. Science **258:** 668–671.
16. LEVY-LAHAD, E. *et al.* 1995. A familial Alzheimer's disease locus on chromosome 1. Science **269:** 970–973.
17. LEVY-LAHAD, E. *et al.* 1995. Candidate gene for the chromosome 1 familial Alzheimer's disease locus. Science **269:** 973–977.
18. ROGAEV, E.I. *et al.* 1995. Familial Alzheimer's disease in kindreds with missense mutations in a gene on chromosome 1 related to the Alzheimer's disease type 3 gene. Nature **376:** 775–778.
19. CITRON, M. *et al.* 1992. Mutation of the beta-amyloid precursor protein in familial Alzheimer's disease increases beta-protein production. Nature **360:** 672–674.
20. GOATE, A. *et al.* 1991. Segregation of a missense mutation in the amyloid precursor protein gene with familial Alzheimer's disease. Nature **349:** 704–706.
21. CITRON, M. *et al.* 1997. Mutant presenilins of Alzheimer's disease increase production of 42-residue amyloid beta-protein in both transfected cells and transgenic mice. Nat. Med. **3:** 67–72.
22. SUZUKI, N. *et al.* 1994. An increased percentage of long amyloid beta protein secreted by familial amyloid beta protein precursor (beta APP717) mutants. Science **264:** 1336–1340.
23. SCHEUNER, D. *et al.* 1996. Secreted amyloid beta-protein similar to that in the senile plaques of Alzheimer's disease is increased in vivo by the presenilin 1 and 2 and APP mutations linked to familial Alzheimer's disease. Nat. Med. **2:** 864–870.
24. VASSAR, R. *et al.* 1999. Beta-secretase cleavage of Alzheimer's amyloid precursor protein by the transmembrane aspartic protease BACE. Science **286:** 735–741.
25. HUSSAIN, I. *et al.* 1999. Identification of a novel aspartic protease (Asp 2) as beta-secretase. Mol. Cell Neurosci. **14:** 419–427.
26. SINHA, S. *et al.* 1999. Purification and cloning of amyloid precursor protein beta-secretase from human brain. Nature **402:** 537–540.
27. YAN, R. *et al.* 1999. Membrane-anchored aspartyl protease with Alzheimer's disease beta-secretase activity. Nature **402:** 533–537.
28. BENJANNET, S. *et al.* 2001. Post-translational processing of beta-secretase (beta-amyloid-converting enzyme) and its ectodomain shedding. The pro- and transmembrane/cytosolic domains affect its cellular activity and amyloid-beta production. J. Biol. Chem. **276:** 10879–10887.
29. BENNETT, B.D. *et al.* 2000. A furin-like convertase mediates propeptide cleavage of BACE, the Alzheimer's beta -secretase. J. Biol. Chem. **275:** 37712–37717.
30. CAPELL, A. *et al.* 2000. Maturation and pro-peptide cleavage of beta-secretase. J. Biol. Chem. **275:** 30849–30854.
31. CREEMERS, J.W. *et al.* 2001. Processing of beta-secretase by furin and other members of the proprotein convertase family. J. Biol. Chem. **276:** 4211–4217.
32. HUSSAIN, I. *et al.* 2001. Prodomain processing of Asp1 (BACE2) is autocatalytic. J. Biol. Chem. **276:** 23322–23328.
33. CHARLWOOD, J. *et al.* 2001. Characterization of the glycosylation profiles of Alzheimer's beta-secretase protein Asp-2 expressed in a variety of cell lines. J. Biol. Chem. **276:** 16739–16748.
34. HANIU, M. *et al.* 2000. Characterization of Alzheimer's beta-secretase protein BACE. A pepsin family member with unusual properties. J. Biol. Chem. **275:** 21099–21106.
35. HUSE, J.T. *et al.* 2000. Maturation and endosomal targeting of beta-site amyloid precursor protein-cleaving enzyme: the Alzheimer's disease beta-secretase. J. Biol. Chem.**275:** 33729–33737.
36. WALTER, J. *et al.* 2001. Phosphorylation regulates intracellular trafficking of beta-secretase. J. Biol. Chem. **276:** 14634–14641.
37. KAO, S.-C. *et al.* 2004. BACE1 Suppression by RNA interference in primary cortical neurons. J. Biol. Chem. **279:** 1942–1949.
38. LUO, Y. *et al.* 2001. Mice deficient in BACE1, the Alzheimer's beta-secretase, have normal phenotype and abolished beta-amyloid generation. Nat. Neurosci. **4:** 231–232.

39. CAI, H. *et al.* 2001. BACE1 is the major beta-secretase for generation of Abeta peptides by neurons. Nat. Neurosci. **4:** 233–234.
40. ROBERDS, S.L. *et al.* 2001. BACE knockout mice are healthy despite lacking the primary [beta]-secretase activity in brain: implications for Alzheimer's disease therapeutics. Hum. Mol. Genet. **10:** 1317–1324.
41. OHNO, M. *et al.* 2004. BACE1 deficiency rescues memory deficits and cholinergic dysfunction in a mouse model of Alzheimer's disease. Neuron **41:** 27–33.
42. CHRISTENSEN, M.A. *et al.* 2004. Transcriptional regulation of BACE1, the beta-amyloid precursor protein beta-secretase, by Sp1. Mol. Cell Biol. **24:** 865–874.
43. WARD, C. L., S. OMURA & R. R. KOPITO. 1995. Degradation of CFTR by the ubiquitin-proteasome pathway. Cell **83:** 121–127.
44. QING, H. *et al.* 2004. Degradation of BACE by the ubiquitin-proteasome pathway. FASEB J. **18:** 1571–1573.
45. JENSEN, T.J. *et al.* 1995. Multiple proteolytic systems, including the proteasome, contribute to CFTR processing. Cell **83:** 129–135.
46. MARCINKIEWICZ, M. & N.G. SEIDAH. 2000. Coordinated expression of [beta]-amyloid precursor protein and the putative [beta]-secretase BACE and [alpha]-secretase ADAM10 in mouse and human brain. J. Neurochem. **75:** 2133–2143.
47. SATOH, J. & Y. KURODA. 2000. Amyloid precursor protein beta-secretase (BACE) mRNA expression in human neural cell lines following induction of neuronal differentiation and exposure to cytokines and growth factors. Neuropathology **20:** 289–296.
48. SONG, W. & D.K. LAHIRI. 1998. Molecular cloning of the promoter of the gene encoding the rhesus monkey beta-amyloid precursor protein: structural characterization and a comparative study with other species. Gene **217:** 151–164.
49. BASLER, K. *et al.* 1986. Scrapie and cellular PrP isoforms are encoded by the same chromosomal gene. Cell **46:** 417–428.
50. GE, Y.W. *et al.* 2004. Functional characterization of the 5′ flanking region of the BACE gene: identification of a 91 bp fragment involved in basal level of BACE promoter expression. FASEB J. **18:** 1037–1039.
51. DYNAN, W.S. & R. TJIAN. 1983. Isolation of transcription factors that discriminate between different promoters recognized by RNA polymerase II. Cell **32:** 669–680.
52. LETOVSKY, J. & W. DYNAN. 1989. Measurement of the binding of transcription factor Sp1 to a single GC box recognition sequence. Nucl. Acids. Res. **17:** 2639–2653.
53. LI, R. *et al.* 1991. Direct interaction between Sp1 and the BPV enhancer E2 protein mediates synergistic activation of transcription. Cell **65:** 493–505.
54. BOUWMAN, P. *et al.* 2000. Transcription factor Sp3 is essential for post-natal survival and late tooth development. EMBO J. **19:** 655–661.
55. MARIN, M. *et al.* 1997. Transcription factor Sp1 is essential for early embryonic development but dispensable for cell growth and differentiation. Cell **89:** 619–628.
56. CRUTS, M. *et al.* 2001. Amyloid beta secretase gene (BACE) is neither mutated in nor associated with early-onset Alzheimer's disease. Neurosci. Lett. **313:** 105–107.
57. NICOLAOU, M. *et al.* 2001. Mutations in the open reading frame of the beta-site APP cleaving enzyme (BACE) locus are not a common cause of Alzheimer's disease. Neurogenetics **3:** 203–206.
58. RUSSO, C. *et al.* 2000. Presenilin-1 mutations in Alzheimer's disease. Nature **405:** 531–532.
59. HOLSINGER, R.M. *et al.* 2002. Increased expression of the amyloid precursor beta-secretase in Alzheimer's disease. Ann. Neurol. **51:** 783–786.
60. GIASSON, B.I. & V.M. LEE. 2003. Are ubiquitination pathways central to Parkinson's disease? Cell **114:** 1–8.
61. KELLER, J.N., K.B. Hanni & W.R. Markesbery. 2000. Impaired proteasome function in Alzheimer's disease. J. Neurochem. **75:** 436–439.
62. LOPEZ SALON, M. *et al.* 2000. Defective ubiquitination of cerebral proteins in Alzheimer's disease. J. Neurosci. Res. **62:** 302–310.
63. VAN LEEUWEN, F.W. *et al.* 1998. Frameshift mutants of beta amyloid precursor protein and ubiquitin-B in Alzheimer's and Down patients. Science **279:** 242–247.
64. DE VRIJ, F.M. *et al.* 2001. Mutant ubiquitin expressed in Alzheimer's disease causes neuronal death. FASEB J. **15:** 2680–2688.

65. ZHAI, Q. *et al.* 2003. Involvement of the ubiquitin-proteasome system in the early stages of wallerian degeneration. Neuron **39:** 217–225.
66. GRUNE, T., T. REINHECKEL & K.J. DAVIES. 1997. Degradation of oxidized proteins in mammalian cells. FASEB J. **11:** 526–534.
67. TANAKA, K. & T. CHIBA. 1998. The proteasome: a protein-destroying machine. Genes Cells **3:** 499–510.
68. NUNAN, J. *et al.* 2003. Proteasome-mediated degradation of the C-terminus of the Alzheimer's disease beta-amyloid protein precursor: effect of C-terminal truncation on production of beta-amyloid protein. J. Neurosci. Res. **74:** 378–385.
69. NUNAN, J. *et al.* 2001. The C-terminal fragment of the Alzheimer's disease amyloid protein precursor is degraded by a proteasome-dependent mechanism distinct from gamma-secretase. Eur. J. Biochem. **268:** 5329–5336.
70. SKOVRONSKY, D.M. *et al.* 2000. A distinct ER/IC gamma-secretase competes with the proteasome for cleavage of APP. Biochemistry **39:** 810–817.
71. ODDO, S. *et al.* 2004. Abeta immunotherapy leads to clearance of early, but not late, hyperphosphorylated tau aggregates via the proteasome. Neuron **43:** 321–332.
72. VERDILE, G. *et al.* 2000. Inhibiting amyloid precursor protein C-terminal cleavage promotes an interaction with presenilin 1. J. Biol. Chem. **275:** 20794–20798.
73. DE STROOPER, B. *et al.* 1999. A presenilin-1-dependent gamma-secretase-like protease mediates release of Notch intracellular domain. Nature **398:** 518–522.
74. SHEN, J. *et al.* 1997. Skeletal and CNS defects in Presenilin-1-deficient mice. Cell **89:** 629–639.
75. SONG, W. *et al.* 1999. Proteolytic release and nuclear translocation of Notch-1 are induced by presenilin-1 and impaired by pathogenic presenilin-1 mutations. Proc. Natl. Acad. Sci. USA **96:** 6959–6963.
76. WONG, P.C. *et al.* 1997. Presenilin 1 is required for Notch1 and DII1 expression in the paraxial mesoderm. Nature **387:** 288–292.
77. BODENDORF, U. *et al.* 2002. Expression of human beta-secretase in the mouse brain increases the steady-state level of beta-amyloid. J. Neurochem. **80:** 799–806.
78. IRIZARRY, M.C., J.J. LOCASCIO & B.T. HYMAN. 2001. [beta]-Site APP cleaving enzyme mRNA expression in APP transgenic mice: Anatomical overlap with transgene expression and static levels with aging. Am. J. Pathol. **158:** 173–177.

NSAID and Antioxidant Prevention of Alzheimer's Disease

Lessons from *In Vitro* and Animal Models

GREG M. COLE,[a,b,c,d] TAKASHI MORIHARA,[a,c] GISELLE P. LIM,[a,c]
FUSHENG YANG,[a,c] AYNUN BEGUM,[a,c] AND SALLY A. FRAUTSCHY[a,b,c,d]

[a]*Greater Los Angeles Veterans Affairs Healthcare System,* [b]*Geriatric Research,
Education and Clinical Center, Sepulveda, California 91343, USA*

Departments of [c]*Medicine and* [d]*Neurology, University of California,
Los Angeles, California 90095, USA*

ABSTRACT: Both oxidative damage and inflammation are elevated in brains of
Alzheimer's disease (AD) patients, but their pathogenic significance remains
unclear. The reduced AD risk associated with high intake of both nonsteroidal
anti-inflammatory drugs (NSAIDs) and antioxidants suggests causal roles, but
clinical trials in AD patients have yielded only limited or negative results. To
test the potential efficacy and mechanisms of candidate approaches, we have
explored conventional and unconventional NSAIDs, antioxidants, and combined NSAID/antioxidants in cell culture and animal models for AD (including
aging APPsw transgenic mice and soluble $A\beta$ rodent infusion models). The
conventional NSAID ibuprofen has the strongest epidemiological support. At
sustainable doses designed to mimic protective consumption in the epidemiology, ibuprofen reduces amyloid accumulation but suppresses a surprisingly
limited subset of inflammatory markers in APPsw transgenic mice. Both $A\beta$
production (APP, β- and γ-secretases) and post-production pathways (those
affecting $A\beta$ aggregation or clearance: e.g., IL-1 or α1ACT) are potentially involved in ibuprofen and other NSAID anti-AD activities. The post-production
pathways are predictably shared with other seemingly protective NSAIDs, including naproxen that do not lower $A\beta42$ *in vitro*. Using clinically feasible
dosing, brain levels of NSAIDs appear too low to implicate a number of
pharmacological dose targets that have been demonstrated *in vitro*. Ibuprofen
did not suppress microglial markers related to phagocytosis. The putative anti-
inflammatory omega-3 fatty acid DHA had a profound impact on pathogenesis
but did not lower inflammation, while vitamin E was surprisingly ineffective in
reducing oxidative damage or amyloid in the aged APPsw mouse. In contrast,
the unconventional NSAID/antioxidant curcumin was effective, lowering oxidative damage, cognitive deficits, synaptic marker loss, and amyloid deposition.
Curcumin proved to be immunomodulatory, simultaneously inhibiting cytokine
and microglial activation indices related to neurotoxicity, but increasing an
index of phagocytosis. Curcumin directly targeted $A\beta$ and was also effective in
other models, warranting further preclinical and clinical exploration.

Address for correspondence: Greg M. Cole, Greater Los Angeles Healthcare System, Veterans
Administration Medical Center, 16111 Plummer St., Bldg. 7, Room A102, North Hills, CA
91343. Voice: 818-891-7711, ext. 9949; fax: 818-895-5835.
gmcole@ucla.edu

Ann. N.Y. Acad. Sci. 1035: 68–84 (2004). © 2004 New York Academy of Sciences.
doi: 10.1196/annals.1332.005

KEYWORDS: interleukin-1β; α-1-antichymotrypsin; docosahexaenoic acid; ibuprofen

INTRODUCTION

Acquittal in Clinical Trials and the Case against Oxidative Damage and Inflammation

There is no doubt that the usual suspects of oxidative damage[1–4] and inflammation[5–7] are present early and throughout Alzheimer's disease (AD) pathogenesis. Both have long rap sheets as toxic effectors in chronic degenerative diseases and are implicated by thick dossiers on AD versus control brains. Further evidence, suggesting possible causal roles, comes from epidemiological studies that repeatedly show reduced AD risk with higher intake of antioxidants[8–10] or non-steroidal anti-inflammatory drugs (NSAIDs).[11–13] However, one requires more than a circumstantial case to prove whether either or both of these suspected perpetrators are minor accomplices or actually guilty of playing important causal roles in AD pathogenesis. Strong DNA (genetic) evidence may add strong credence to causality, so despite holes in the amyloid cascade hypothesis, data on autosomal dominant familial AD mutations influencing β-amyloid would maintain that amyloid β peptide 1-42 (Aβ42) causes the disease. Although there is no genetic evidence for oxidation as causal process, there are suggestions, some controversial, of increased association of multiple inflammatory gene alleles (α1ACT, IL-1β, TNFα, IL-6, IL-10)[14–20] and α2-macroglobulin[21] with increased sporadic AD risk. This suggests that, like ApoE alleles, inflammatory processes may modulate age of onset and risk in sporadic AD, but will not exert a powerful enough drive to cause autosomal dominant AD. Nevertheless, factors delaying the onset of sporadic AD may have profound impact because it is estimated that a 10-year delay would reduce the number of cases by 75%. Overall, the evidence from pathology and epidemiology, implicating oxidative damage and inflammation in AD has been strong enough to support clinical trials in AD patients using antioxidant, vitamin E, and several NSAIDs (naproxen, COX-2 inhibitors). Unfortunately, despite some promising data from several small trials, the results from large clinical trials have failed to show that either vitamin E or NSAIDs can slow cognitive decline and AD progression. On the grounds of these negative trial data alone, one might be tempted to dismiss the case against oxidative damage and inflammation as mediators of the disease.

Convicted by Preclinical Data?

Before we conclude that oxidative damage and inflammation should simply be acquitted, we need to explore the evidence provided by preclinical *in vitro* and *in vivo* studies. Do these studies provide support for the conviction that oxidative damage and inflammation play important causal roles in the AD? Will their effective treatment help prevent or delay disease onset?

CNS INFLAMMATION INDUCES OXIDATIVE DAMAGE, AN IMPORTANT MEDIATOR OF Aβ AGGREGATES AND OLIGOMER TOXICITY

While cytotoxic T cells, autoimmune antibodies, and high inflammatory cytokine levels may be important effectors in peripheral inflammatory conditions, the CNS inflammation in AD is primarily characterized by reactive microglia, IL-1, and complement factors.[7] Apart from the role of activation of the complement pathway, which should be considered separately, reactive oxygen species (ROS) produced by activated microglia are perhaps the most obvious toxic effectors with central nervous system (CNS) inflammation. In principle, activated macrophages and microglia induce NADPH oxidase and iNOS to produce a respiratory burst of relatively diffusible superoxide and NO that combine focally and at some distance, to produce the highly reactive effector germicidal, peroxynitrite. Other ROS, for example, myeloperoxidase-derived hypochlorite may also contribute to toxicity, but these toxins are less clearly implicated. Consistent with this, the principal neurotoxins induced by Aβ aggregates stimulate microglia activation *in vitro*, require iNOS stimulation and appear to be peroxynitrite radicals,[22,23] responsible for extensive damage in AD.[3] Although more controversial, Aβ aggregates may also promote oxidative damage via direct effects including induction of hydrogen peroxide production in neuronal cell lines and primary neurons,[2] catalysis via iron or copper binding,[24] or even peptidyl radicals.[25] Overall, these results argue for some potential for treatments that target the specific inflammatory factors and Aβ species, causing oxidative damage in AD.

WHAT ARE THE RELEVANT TARGETS OF OXIDATIVE DAMAGE AND INFLAMMATION?

Synaptic and Postsynaptic Targets

Neuron death is not the only index of damage induced by Aβ-induced inflammatory ROS. One relevant very recent example comes from Montine's group who finds that intracerebroventricular administration of a bolus of LPS to mice results in marked dendritic regression within 24 h that is dependent on CD14, iNOS, COX-2, PGE2, and EP-1 receptors.[26,27] Remarkably, the dendritic deficits occur in the absence of any neuron loss and are transient, as demonstrated by a full reversal one week later. Another example is provided by administration of small Aβ oligomers that produce very rapid deficits in long-term potentiation (LTP) *in vitro*[28] or *in vivo*.[29] Knockout mice and pharmacological data show that these Aβ aggregate–induced deficits are dependent on iNOS and NADPH oxidase induction and can be inhibited by catalase and superoxide dismutase, consistent with a microglia-mediated peroxynitrite attack.[30] These results are also entirely consistent with experiments from our group showing that chronic intracerebroventricular infusion of Aβ can induce selective loss of postsynaptic markers, including drebrin, NR2B, and PSD-95, which can be blocked by the combined NSAID–antioxidant curcumin.[31] Similarly, microarray analysis shows small but significant alterations in postsynaptic mRNAs involved in synaptic plasticity in amyloid-laden aging APPsw × PS1 mutant transgenic mice that have Aβ-dependent cognitive deficits.[32] Our own recent data, discussed below, also support synaptic and largely postsynaptic attacks in APPsw mice mediated by amyloid and oxidative damage, which can be modulated by dietary factors.

Unsaturated Fatty Acids

The CNS is a fatty tissue loaded with polyunsaturated fatty acids that are extremely vulnerable to oxidative attack by lipid peroxidation. While hydroxyl radicals have a plethora of targets, the danger of lipid peroxidation is that it is an autocatalytic feed-forward process, generating lipid peroxides that initiate more lipid peroxidation. Because of this, lipid peroxidation is likely to occur in localized bursts. Global measures of lipid peroxidation that include relatively uninvolved sites may obscure or dilute the severity of focal damage. In addition to being sites of Aβ generation and accumulation, neurons and synapses are highly enriched in long chain unsaturated fatty acids, and one of the most vulnerable is the omega-3 fatty acid, docosahexaenoic acid (DHA, C22:6 (n-3)) because of its six double bonds. DHA is primarily neuronal. The large increases in oxidized DHA (F4-isoprostanes or neuroprostanes) in AD[33] are a good index of the oxidative attack on neurons that may result in focal DHA depletion.

Reduced DHA intake (from fish) is a risk factor for AD that could be easily remedied with supplements. Most laboratory chow is enriched in DHA and other omega-3 fatty acids that may limit the effects of familial AD genes in mouse models. APPsw mice on a DHA-depleting diet showed elevated oxidative damage in conjunction with transgene-dependent reductions in brain DHA levels. These changes were accompanied by large (≥80%) losses of postsynaptic proteins like the actin-regulatory protein drebrin, which is known to be reduced in AD.[34] DHA-depleting chow not only exaggerated APPsw transgene-dependent focal postsynaptic caspase-cleaved actin and postsynaptic deficits, but also induced presumably Aβ-dependent defects in the neuroprotective PI3-kinase pathway in mice. The insulin-signaling PI3-kinase pathway appears to be induced by APP transgene overexpression and has been invoked as one explanation for limited neurodegeneration in APP transgenics.[35]

Because free radicals are notoriously reactive, their targets are typically proximal neighbors including proteins, lipids, DNA, RNA, and small molecule targets. While all of these targets show evidence of increased oxidative modification in AD,[25,36–38] low-level damage is either repairable or circumvented by redundancy. For example, unlike dividing cells where unrepaired nuclear DNA damage can lead to replicating carcinogenic mutations, neurons in AD may be able to sustain and accumulate high levels of unrepaired DNA damage in redundant or non-coding regions (including strand breaks detectable by TUNEL[39]) without rapidly dying. This DNA damage accumulates prior to tangles and is associated with protein nitration.[40] Most RNA or protein damage is either effectively repaired or managed by normal turnover or surveillance and targeting by defenses like the heat shock system. Proteasomal degradation, which is very effective, can fail when overwhelmed by protein aggregates. Not surprisingly, most age-related neurodegenerative diseases involve protein aggregates that circumvent the degradation processes and accumulate.

Protein Aggregation Is Seeded by Oxidative Damage–Driven Dimerization

In addition to the prominent extracellular Aβ deposits, AD has intraneuronal aggregates of phosphorylated tau (tangles/curly fibers), α-synuclein (Lewy pathology), and actin/ cofilin (Hirano pathology), as well as intraneuronal Aβ. The initial dimerization step in the protein aggregation process appears likely to be driven by an oxidative damage step. For example, synuclein pathology is heavily nitrated[41] and promoted by tyrosine dimerization[42] and by peroxynitrite generation *in vitro*.[43] Similarly, prior to autophosphorylation, the initial tau dimerization is promoted by cysteine oxidation and disulfide crosslinking[44,45] or fatty acid oxidation.[46] Another aging and AD pathology, Hirano body accumulation, appears to involve cofilin dimerization with analogous disulfide mediated dimer or oligomer formation.[47] Finally, even Aβ dimerization occurs early during aging[48] and can be promoted or stabilized by metals with oxidation and dityrosine crosslinking.[49,50] In all of these cases, the rate-limiting early seeding events in intracellular aggregate formation would theoretically be promoted by oxidative damage related to inflammation, aging, and/or environmental risk factors, favoring the formation of rare seeding events. For example, synuclein aggregates may be initiated after short-term exposure to MPTP, rotenone, or other mitochondrial toxins, while tau aggregates may be initiated by head injury earlier in life. After oxidant-mediated aggregate seeding has been fully initiated and stabilized, one can hypothesize that monomer will deposit onto existing seeds in the presence of basal levels of monomer. Seeding may occur even in the absence of continued exposure to initiating pathological stimuli or pathologically elevated levels of monomer production. One corollary hypothesis is that antioxidant or NSAID intervention should occur early and will be relatively ineffective in reducing subsequent monomer addition steps.

Signal Transduction Pathways

Toxic forms of aggregated Aβ applied to neurons and neuronal cell lines in primary culture are reported to stimulate signal transduction pathways including FAK, Fyn, PK-C, PI3-K, JNK, GSK3β, and ERK.[51–57] Similarly, toxic soluble Aβ oligomer species are reported to bind to synaptic and postsynaptic sites coincident with PSD-95[58] and block the induction of LTP.[59] COX-2 on the postsynaptic side appears to play some important role in synaptic plasticity through pathways that are not fully understood,[60] suggesting that low doses of COX inhibitors may be able to limit pro-oxidant or Aβ oligomer effects on LTP and cognitive deficits, while high doses of COX inhibitors will actually block LTP. Recent data from Ashe and collaborators suggest that NSAIDs can effectively reduce cognitive deficits in Tg2576 mice through COX-2 inhibitory activity in the absence of direct effects on Aβ accumulation.[61] This property could be shared by other NSAID cyclooxygenase inhibitors, like naproxen, to the extent that they are capable of entering the brain and suppressing prostaglandin production.

IBUPROFEN AND OTHER CONVENTIONAL CYCLOOXYGENASE-INHIBITING NSAIDs AND AMYLOID REDUCTION

The first over-the-counter NSAID, ibuprofen, was most widely used and has the strongest epidemiological support of any single NSAID for reducing AD risk. How does it work? Ibuprofen may have multiple targets (FIG. 1). (Tau pathology has not yet been tested as a target for NSAIDs.) Strong data identify glial-mediated neurodegeneration, COX-2 in neurons, and excitotoxic neurodegeneration as NSAID

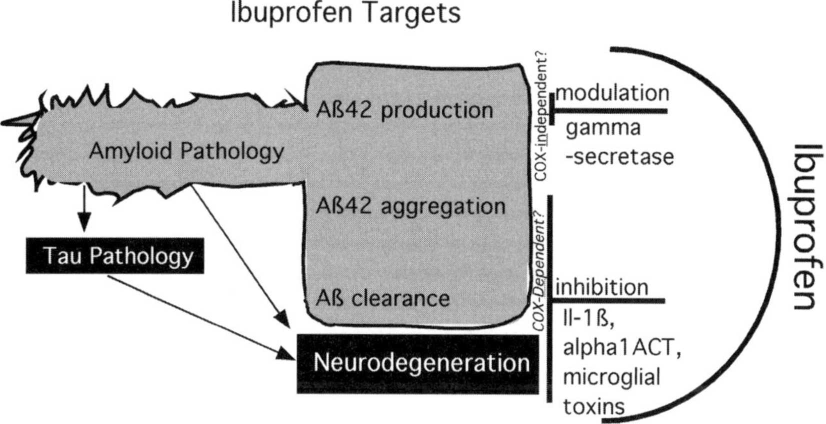

FIGURE 1. Ibuprofen may influence more than one target in AD pathogenesis. While tau remains an untested target, experimental data support neurodegeneration mediated by COX-2-sensitive excitotoxicity and microglial toxin production as plausible neuroprotective pathways. In addition, ibuprofen limits amyloid accumulation (TABLE 1), which may be due to reduced production of Aβ42 via modulation of γ-secretase or reduced production of IL-1β and downstream targets including pro-amyloidogenic α1ACT. Inhibition of pro-oxidants could also reduce amyloid aggregation, but in our models ibuprofen did not reduce oxidative damage or iNOS.

targets. These theories would predict that the neurodegeneration and synapse loss occurring throughout the clinical decline phase of AD should be limited by anti-inflammatory treatment, resulting in slowed progression. However, to date, the clinical trial evidence is against a strong NSAID effect on clinical progression, but consistent with far greater NSAID efficacy in reducing AD risk when NSAIDs were used longer than two years before assessment. Instead, the epidemiology from the twin sibling studies suggests that, like ApoE genotype, the primary NSAID effect is on age of onset leading to a 10-year delay in onset and risk reduction in 75% of NSAID users.[62] Age of onset is known to be accelerated by APP and presenilin mutations that increase Aβ42 production and by ApoE4 genotype, which is known to influence Aβ clearance and deposition. Therefore it was reasonable to wonder whether NSAIDs could also delay onset and reduce risk by influencing Aβ accumulation.

At sustainable doses designed to mimic apparently protective NSAID consumption in the epidemiology, ibuprofen reduces amyloid accumulation[63] but suppresses a surprisingly limited subset of inflammatory markers in APPsw transgenic mice, notably IL-1β and downstream murine ACT mRNA, but not iNOS, macrosialin, C1q, CD11b, or CD11c mRNA (Morihara and colleagues, submitted for publication). The latter two markers are upregulated on phagocytic microglia suggesting that at this dose, ibuprofen does not suppress microglial phagocytosis and amyloid clearance, although ibuprofen dosing was high enough to be anti-inflammatory. Several groups have been able to observe the amyloid-lowering impact of ibuprofen or related NSAIDs *in vivo*, but not all NSAID experiments have produced significant reductions in amyloid (TABLE 1).

TABLE 1. Results from various research groups

Research group	Mice	Drug and dose	Paradigm (start to finish, age in months)	Reported effects on Aβ42 *in vitro*	Amyloid pathology *in vivo*	Other pathology
Lim *et al.*,[63] 2001	Tg2576	Ibuprofen 375 ppm	10–16	Reduce	Plaque 56%, SDS-insoluble Aβ 39%	
Lim *et al.*,[64] 2002	Tg2576	Ibuprofen 375 ppm	13–16	Reduce	Ent cortex plaque	
Jantzen *et al.*,[65] 2002	Tg2576, PS1, M146L	Ibuprofen 375 ppm	7–12	Reduce	Aβ load (IHC) 20–25%	
		NCX-2216 (nitro-NSAIDs) 375 ppm	7–12	Probably reduce?	Aβ load (IHC) 40–45%, Congo red 35–40%	Microglial activation
		Celecoxib (COX-2) 175 ppm	7–12	Increase	NS trend, Aβ load (Aβ-ir plaques 15–20%)	
Staufenbiel *et al.*,[66] 2002	APP23	Ibuprofen 60 mg/kg	10.7–13.7	Reduce	NS effect	
Dedeoglu *et al.*,[67] 2002	Tg2576	Ibuprofen 100 mg/kg	16–19	Reduce	Total Aβ plaque area, Aβ42 plaque area	
Yan *et al.*,[68] 2003	Tg2576	Ibuprofen 375 ppm	11–15	Reduce	SDS-sol Aβ42 & 40, formic acid–sol Aβ42 & 40, NS trend, plaques 60%	
Volmar *et al.*,[69] 2002	PSAPP	NS-398 (COX-2) 20 mg/kg ip	3–6	Increase	Thioflavin S, 4G8-ir plaque	GFAP
Quinn *et al.*,[70] 2003	Tg2576	Indomethacin 56 µg/day or 2.2 mg/kg/day	12–20	Reduce	Plaque, only in hippo	PGE2
Eriksen *et al.*,[71] 2003	Tg2576	Ibuprofen 375 ppm	8–16	Reduce	Insoluble Aβ40 & Aβ42	
		R-Flurbiprofen 67 ppm	8–16	Reduce	Insoluble Aβ40 & Aβ42	
Pratico *et al.*,[72] 2003	Tg2576	Indomethacin 10 mg/L	8–15	Reduce	Aβ40, Aβ42	PGE2
		Nimesulide (COX-2) 40 mg/L	8–15	?	Aβ	PGE2
Kotilinek *et al.*,[61] 2001	Tg2576	Ibuprofen 375 ppm	11.5–13	Reduce	NS trend, Aβ40	

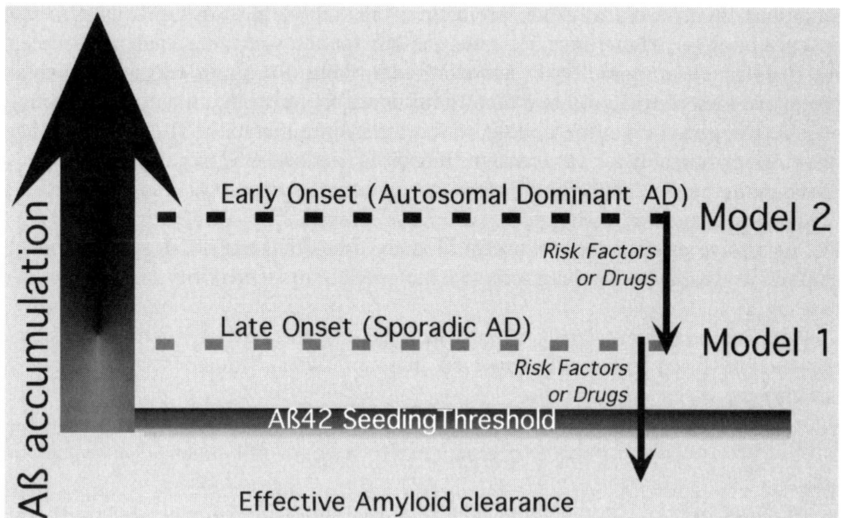

FIGURE 2. Seeding threshold model for amyloid reduction. A threshold for Aβ initial aggregation and onset limiting seeding is hypothesized to be defined by the balance of Aβ1-42 production and clearance mechanisms. If the Aβ42 production level is close to this seeding threshold (as is likely the case with late onset sporadic AD) an AD risk factor, drug, or other treatment that modestly lowers or raises Aβ42 production or clearance may have a profound effect on the onset of amyloid deposition. If the production level is significantly above the seeding threshold (as is the case with one or more powerful autosomal dominant AD mutations), the onset will be earlier and relatively impervious to the same small changes in Aβ production or clearance that influence AD risk in sporadic AD.

Among the possible explanations for the differing amyloid reduction results are the variable timing of the interventions and the more aggressive nature of some of the models. In general, as illustrated in FIGURE 2, one can assume that Aβ42 production rates need to reach some threshold set by clearance and aggregation rates before amyloid will accumulate. If the higher Aβ42 is over this hypothetical threshold, the earlier rate-limiting seeding occurs. The kinetics of aggregation argues that seeding is the rate-limiting event and thus, early intervention to prevent seeding is most likely to be effective. Aβ burden could be much less sensitive to treatments occurring after the exponential growth phase (~10–16 months in Tg2576 mice) when amyloid deposition is presumably fully seeded. In transgenic mice, very high levels of APP expression and autosomal dominant mutations that increase total Aβ (Swedish) or Aβ42 (London or PS1) are needed to drive Aβ42 over the threshold for deposit formation. Early APP transgenic models failed because APP expression was less than two times the expression of endogenous murine APP and insufficient for aggregation. Aβ42 aggregate seeding determines the age of onset and is supported by acceleration of deposition with injection of preformed aggregates.[73] In the newer generations of transgenic models employing multiple autosomal dominant AD mutations, high levels of Aβ42 production result in deposit accumulation in the absence of aging. These mice are better models for autosomal dominant early onset AD than late onset sporadic AD. More or less by definition, prevalent environmental protective factors will not dramatically influence the outcome in autosomal dominant AD where you get the disease if you inherit the mutation. Thus, models that drive Aβ, presumably 42, far above the threshold needed for aggregation may not respond to factors that are efficacious in less aggressive sporadic AD models. Further, while quite useful for testing potent secretase inhibitors or anti-aggregation agents, the aggressive models are less useful to study drugs that target the age-dependent changes in clearance or aggregation that may pertain to the majority of sporadic AD cases.

Both Aβ production (APP, β- and γ-secretases) and post-production pathways (IL-1>α1ACT are potentially involved in ibuprofen and other NSAID anti-AD activities.

γ-Secretase Modulation

A subset of NSAIDs including ibuprofen (but not naproxen and COX-2 inhibitors) can selectively lower Aβ42 production without inhibiting total Aβ or NOTCH *in vitro* or *in vivo*.[74,75] This important result has led to the discovery of selective Aβ42 lowering agents that do not suppress total γ-secretase activity and other substrate pathways, such as notch signaling. While this is undoubtedly a highly significant result relevant to new drug discovery, it remains unclear that conventional NSAID dosing can be maintained at high enough levels to limit Aβ42 production *in vivo*. We confirmed that selective Aβ42 reduction can be achieved *in vitro* with high (>100 μM) doses of R-enantiomers of ibuprofen and flurbiprofen, which have limited COX inhibitory activity.[76] Whereas in the rodent models, R-flurbiprofen can be converted to the more toxic COX inhibiting S-flurbiprofen, this conversion is limited in humans and high doses are better tolerated. Using clinically feasible dosing, brain levels of NSAIDs are typically in the range predicted to inhibit COX, but at less than 5 μM, are too low to implicate a number of pharmacological dose targets like NFκB and PPARγ and possibly γ-secretase. Not all groups have reported success in lowering Aβ42 with ibuprofen or similar NSAIDs *in vivo*. Whether or not modulation of γ-secretase with sustainable NSAID treatment results in lower Aβ42 and increased Aβ1-38 in relevant *in vivo* models is difficult to determine solely on the basis of measuring levels of Aβ42. This is because the Aβ42 peptide is prone to aggregate and aggregate clearance mechanisms involving astrocytes and microglia may also be influenced by NSAIDs. Additional measurements of Aβ1-38 by mass spectroscopy, ELISA or other methods after acute and chronic *in vivo* NSAID treatments in multiple models should help resolve this currently controversial issue.

Inhibition of BACE1 Expression

There is a strong argument for increased cytokines, notably IL-1 in AD.[77] IL-1 may impact amyloid production because the principal β-secretase, BACE1, can be induced in IFN-γ–primed neuronal cells by the pro-inflammatory cytokines, IL-1β or TNFα, and the BACE1 induction can be blocked by treatment with ibuprofen or PPARγ agonists.[78] We can confirm these *in vitro* results but have not observed *in vivo* reductions in BACE1 with chronic ibuprofen (Morihara and colleagues, unpublished observations). Similarly, oxidative damage can induce BACE1 in human neuronal NT2 cells by activating JNK and p38,[79] suggesting that both oxidative damage and inflammation may increase focal BACE1 expression in AD. Based on that hypothesis, we have tested the antioxidant and NSAID curcumin and found it to be a very effective inhibitor of pro-inflammatory cytokine-induced BACE expression *in vitro* and *in vivo* (Morihara *et al.*, in preparation).

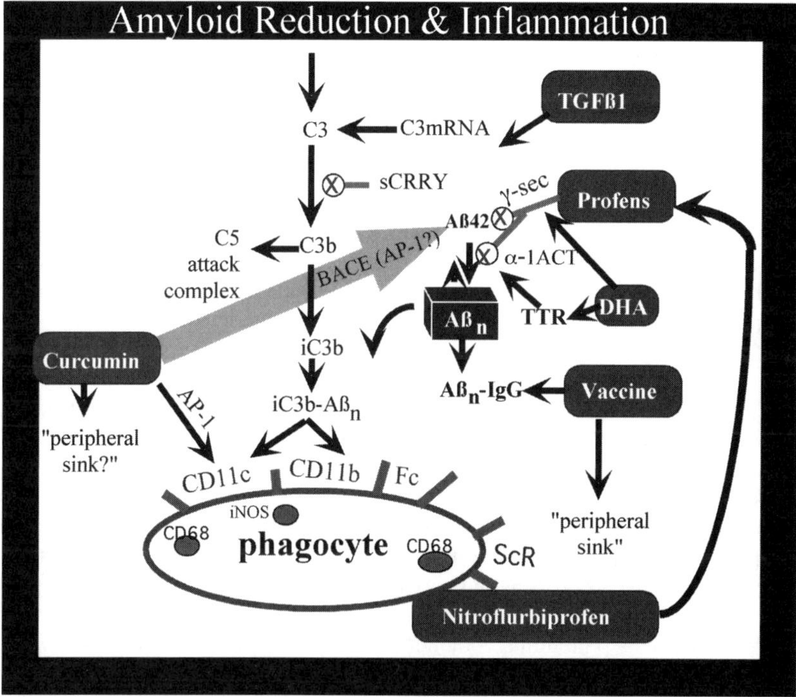

FIGURE 3. Amyloid reduction related to inflammation. As demonstrated by Wyss-Coray and collaborators, TGFβ1 stimulation of complement C3 can promote Aβ aggregate (Aβ$_n$) opsonization by C3B and iC3b fragments and their clearance by CD11b and CD11c receptors on microglia or other monocytic lineage phagocytes. The amyloid vaccine antibodies reduce Aβ aggregates by directly binding to them, promoting Fc-mediated amyloid clearance and functioning as a "peripheral sink." NSAID profens (ibuprofen, flurbiprofen, etc.) can act on γ-secretase to reduce Aβ42 production and also reduce IL-1–mediated pro-amyloidogenic α1ACT. Nitroflurbiprofen has the additional property of activating microglia and apparent clearance. Curcumin can bind directly to Aβ aggregates, limit their production and possibly act as a "peripheral sink". Curcumin can also suppress JNK activation and potentially suppress inflammation or oxidative damage induced BACE1 and γ-secretase activity. Curcumin also suppresses iNOS/pro-oxidant production and CD11b while promoting phagocytic markers CD11c and CD68 (macrosialin).

THE OMEGA-3 FATTY ACID DHA HAS BOTH NEUROPROTECTIVE AND ANTI-AMYLOID EFFECTS

Depletion or replacement of the putative anti-inflammatory omega-3 fatty acid DHA had a profound impact on AD pathogenesis from 17–22 months in aged Tg2576 mice. DHA depletion increased drebrin and other postsynaptic marker losses (PI3-K p85a subunit, and phosphoBAD), oxidative damage, and caspase activation; while DHA repletion rescued these in aged Tg2576 mice.[34] DHA also reduced amyloid burden and Aβ levels.[80] In contrast, dietary omega-3 fatty acids and DHA did not lower the presynaptic synaptophysin or inflammatory cytokines or influence ApoE or GFAP levels in our Tg2576 experiments. Brain DHA loss in the model was APP-transgene–dependent and presumably driven by oxidation of DHA by Aβ aggregates. Our results support a DHA role in modulating insulin signaling via PI3-kinase and levels of its p85α subunit. DHA depletion aggravated cognitive deficits in the Morris water maze in Tg2576 mice, while DHA supplementation was protective.[34] Relevant DHA and fish oil mechanisms may include the observed effects on PI3-K and downstream pathways, modulation of secretase activities via membrane fluidity changes, induction of anti-amyloidogenic transthyretin,[81] and metabolism to potent neuroprotective compounds.[82] Like fish oil, DHA can be taken as a supplement at high doses with few side effects and both are likely protective against vascular disease, one of the major contributors to age-related dementia. Collectively, these data suggest that fish oil and more specifically DHA, may be clinically useful for AD treatment or prevention and, like the amyloid vaccine, profen NSAIDs, and curcumin may reduce amyloid by influencing more than one target (FIG. 3).

COMBINED ANTIOXIDANT NSAID AND CURCUMIN TARGETS Aβ PATHOGENESIS AT MULTIPLE SITES

If oxidative damage and damage to neuroprotective molecules like DHA are relevant to AD pathogenesis, antioxidants would be expected to provide some protection. In our hands, neither ibuprofen nor vitamin E supplements were effective in controlling protein carbonyls as an index of oxidative damage, but other groups have some evidence for protection with these agents. In contrast, the unconventional NSAID–antioxidant curcumin combination was remarkably effective—lowering oxidized proteins, inflammatory cytokines, activated microglial markers iNOS and CD11b, cognitive deficits, postsynaptic marker loss, and amyloid accumulation.[83,84]

As shown in FIGURE 4, curcumin has the potential to suppress the AD pathogenic cascade at multiple sites. Curcumin is not only a potent antioxidant,[85] but an effective inhibitor of the inflammatory cytokines COX-2 and iNOS, via inhibition of JNK kinase–mediated AP-1 transcription.[86] As reviewed above, cytokines, JNK, COX-2, and iNOS are all implicated in Aβ toxicity or Aβ-induced AD pathogenesis. Curcumin can block JNK *in vitro* and may also limit inflammation and oxidative damage induction of BACE1[79] or γ-secretase activity.[87] Curcumin proved to be immunomodulatory, simultaneously inhibiting cytokine and microglial activation indices related to neurotoxicity, but increasing mRNA and immunostaining for several markers of phagocytic microglia (Morihara, unpublished data). As previously reviewed, curcumin resembles the amyloid binding dye Congo Red, binds and labels

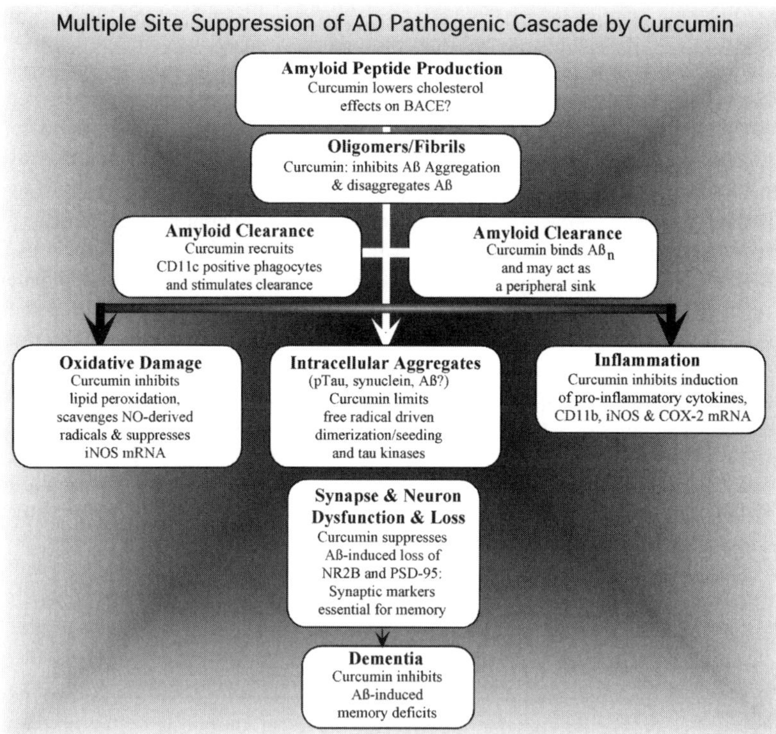

FIGURE 4. Multiple site suppression of the AD pathogenic cascade by curcumin. Curcumin's cholesterol-lowering ability and JNK inhibition may reduce Aβ production and inhibit its toxicity. Like Aβ antibodies, curcumin directly inhibits Aβ aggregate formation and promotes aggregate dissolution. The compound can also bind to $A\beta_n$ and promote clearance by microglia or possibly as a peripheral sink. Unlike antibodies, curcumin directly suppresses lipid peroxidation and COX-2, CD11b, iNOS, and pro-inflammatory cytokine expression. By limiting oxidative damage directly or from inflammation, curcumin should block intracellular protein aggregate seeding at the initial dimerization step. In our models, this multi-step interference in AD pathogenic mechanisms protects against synaptic marker loss and memory deficits.

plaques *in vitro* and *in vivo*, and inhibits amyloid aggregation *in vitro* and *in vivo*.[84] More recent data show that curcumin also inhibits oligomer formation and oligomer-dependent Aβ toxicity *in vitro* (Yang and colleagues, submitted for publication). Whether part of curcumin's anti-amyloid activity *in vivo* is due to its anti-aggregation activity is difficult to establish since the compound has multiple anti-amyloid actions including antioxidant and cholesterol lowering activity[83,84] and possible suppression of BACE1 induction. Curcumin is an amyloid-binding compound whose peripheral blood and tissue levels are higher in the gastrointestinal tract than in the brain.[88] Thus, it is conceivable that, like Congo Red, gelsolin, and anti-Aβ antibodies, curcumin may also act as a "peripheral sink." Because curcumin effectively inhibits iNOS expression *in vitro*,[89,90] *in vivo*,[91,92] and in the CNS (our data), it should be able to suppress key aspects of the Aβ response that are iNOS-dependent, including microglial neurotoxin production[26] and LTP inhibition.[30]

CONCLUDING REMARKS

Based on its strong anti-carcinogenic activity, curcumin has undergone extensive preclinical toxicology and clinical testing and has a very favorable safety profile.[86,93] Based on its potential for intervention at multiple targets in AD pathogenesis, its ready availability and inexpensive cost, clinical trials in mild to moderate AD patients under an FDA-approved Investigational New Drug (IND) study have been initiated by our colleagues at the UCLA Alzheimer Center (Drs. J. Cummings and J. Ringman). Clinical trials are the final judge and jury for any drug, but the case for a successful intervention based on the epidemiology of risk reduction will inevitably be better for prevention Epidemiology tells us who got the disease, not what affects the rate of progression or efficacy in any given symptomatic stage. The evidence from epidemiology and preclinical trials argues strongly for a combined and synergistic role of inflammation and oxidative damage in driving AD pathogenesis at early stages that should be addressed with combined antioxidant and NSAID treatments.

ACKNOWLEDGMENTS

This work was supported by AG13471, NS43946, VA Merit, and Alzheimer Association (G.M.C.). The authors declare that they have no competing financial interest.

REFERENCES

1. BEHL, C., J. DAVIS, G.M. COLE, *et al.* 1992. Vitamin E protects nerve cells from amyloid β-protein toxicity. Biochem. Biophys. Res. Commun. **186:** 944–950.
2. BEHL, C., J.B. DAVIS, R. LESLEY, *et al.* 1994. Hydrogen peroxide mediates amyloid β-protein toxicity. Cell **77:** 817–827.
3. SMITH, M.A., P.L. RICHEY HARRIS, L.M. SAYRE, *et al.* 1997. Widespread peroxynitrite-mediated damage in Alzheimer's disease. J. Neurosci. **17:** 2653–2657.
4. PAPPOLLA, M.A., M.A. SMITH, T. BRYANT-THOMAS, *et al.* 2002. Cholesterol, oxidative stress, and Alzheimer's disease: expanding the horizons of pathogenesis. Free Radic. Biol. Med. **33:** 173–181.
5. McGEER, P.L., H. AKIYAMA, S. ITAGAKI, *et al.* 1989. Immune system response in Alzheimer's Disease. Can. J. Neurol. Sci. **16:** 516–527.
6. ROGERS, J., S. WEBSTER, L. LIH-FEN, *et al.* 1996. Inflammation and Alzheimer's disease pathogenesis. Neurobiol. Aging **17:** 681–686.
7. AKIYAMA, H., S. BARGER, S. BARNUM, *et al.* 2000. Inflammation and Alzheimer's disease. Neurobiol Aging **21:** 383–421.
8. ZANDI, P.P., J.C. ANTHONY, A.S. KHACHATURIAN, *et al.* 2004. Reduced risk of Alzheimer disease in users of antioxidant vitamin supplements: the Cache County Study. Arch. Neurol. **61:** 82–88.
9. MORRIS, M.C., D.A. EVANS, J.L. BIENIAS, *et al.* 2002. Dietary intake of antioxidant nutrients and the risk of incident Alzheimer disease in a biracial community study. J. Am. Med. Assoc. **287:** 33230–33237.
10. ENGELHART, M.J., M.I. GEERLINGS, A. RUITENBERG, *et al.* 2002. Dietary intake of antioxidants and risk of Alzheimer disease. J. Am. Med. Assoc. **287:** 3223–3229.

11. STEWART, W.F., C. KAWAS, M. CORRADA, *et al.* 1997. Risk of Alzheimer's disease and duration of NSAID use. Neurology **48:** 626–632.
12. ZANDI, P.P., J.C. ANTHONY, K.M. HAYDEN, *et al.* 2002. Reduced incidence of AD with NSAID but not H2 receptor antagonists: the Cache County Study. Neurology **59:** 880–886.
13. IN T' VELD, B.A., A. RUITENBERG, A. HOFMAN, *et al.* 2001. Nonsteroidal anti-inflammatory drugs and the risk of Alzheimer's disease. N. Engl. J. Med. **345:** 1515–1521.
14. KAMBOH, M.I., D.K. SANGHERA, R.E. FERRELL, *et al.* 1995. APOE*4-associated Alzheimer's disease risk is modified by α1-antichymotrypsin polymorphism. Nat. Genet. **10:** 486–488.
15. NICOLL, J.A., R.E. MRAK, D.I. GRAHAM, *et al.* 2000. Association of interleukin-1 gene polymorphisms with Alzheimer's disease. Ann. Neurol. **47:** 365–368.
16. GRIMALDI, L.M., V.M. CASADEI, C. FERRI, *et al.* 2000. Association of early onset Alzheimer's disease with an interleukin-1 alpha gene polymorphism. Ann. Neurol. **47:** 361–365.
17. MRAK, R.E. & W.S. GRIFFIN. 2000. Interleukin-1 and the immunogenetics of Alzheimer disease. J. Neuropathol. Exp. Neurol. **59:** 471–476.
18. LUEDECKING, E.K., S.T. DEKOSKY, H. MEHDI, *et al.* 2000. Analysis of genetic polymorphisms in the transforming growth factor-beta1 gene and the risk of Alzheimer's disease. Hum. Genet. **106:** 565–569.
19. MCGEER, P.L. & E.G. MCGEER. 2001. Polymorphisms in inflammatory genes and the risk of Alzheimer disease. Arch. Neurol. **58:** 1790–1792.
20. AROSIO, B., D. TRABATTONI, L. GALIMBERTI, *et al.* 2004. Interleukin-10 and interleukin-6 gene polymorphisms as risk factors for Alzheimer's disease. Neurobiol. Aging **25:** 1009–1015.
21. BLACKER, D., M.A. WILCOX, N.M. LAIRD, *et al.* 1998. Alpha-2 macroglobulin is genetically associated with Alzheimer's [see comments]. Nat. Genet. **19:** 357–360.
22. MEDA, L., M.A. CASSATELLA, G.I. SZENDREL, *et al.* 1995. Activation of microglial cells by β-amyloid protein and interferon-γ. Nature **374:** 647–650.
23. XIE, Z., M. WEI, T.E. MORGAN, *et al.* 2002. Peroxynitrite mediates neurotoxicity of amyloid beta-peptide1-42- and lipopolysaccharide-activated microglia. J. Neurosci. **22:** 3484–3492.
24. OPAZO, C., X. HUANG, R.A. CHERNY, *et al.* 2002. Metalloenzyme-like activity of Alzheimer's disease beta-amyloid. Cu-dependent catalytic conversion of dopamine, cholesterol, and biological reducing agents to neurotoxic H(2)O(2). J. Biol. Chem. **277:** 40302–40308.
25. BUTTERFIELD, D.A. 2002. Amyloid beta-peptide (1-42)-induced oxidative stress and neurotoxicity: implications for neurodegeneration in Alzheimer's disease brain: a review. Free Radic. Res. **36:** 1307–1313.
26. MILATOVIC, D., S. ZAJA-MILATOVIC, K.S. MONTINE, *et al.* 2003. Pharmacologic suppression of neuronal oxidative damage and dendritic degeneration following direct activation of glial innate immunity in mouse cerebrum. J. Neurochem. **87:** 1518–1526.
27. MONTINE, T.J., D. MILATOVIC, R.C. GUPTA, *et al.* 2002. Neuronal oxidative damage from activated innate immunity is EP2 receptor-dependent. J. Neurochem. **83:** 463–470.
28. CHEN, Q.S., B.L. KAGAN, Y. HIRAKURA, *et al.* 2000. Impairment of hippocampal long-term potentiation by Alzheimer amyloid beta-peptides. J. Neurosci. Res. **60:** 65–72.
29. WALSH, D.M., I. KLYUBIN, J.V. FADEEVA, *et al.* 2002. Naturally secreted oligomers of amyloid beta protein potently inhibit hippocampal long-term potentiation in vivo. Nature **416:** 535–539.
30. WANG, Q., M.J. ROWAN & R. ANWYL. 2004. Beta-amyloid-mediated inhibition of NMDA receptor-dependent long-term potentiation induction involves activation of microglia and stimulation of inducible nitric oxide synthase and superoxide. J. Neurosci. **24:** 6049–6056.
31. FRAUTSCHY, S.A., W. HU, S.A. MILLER, *et al.* 2001. Phenolic anti-inflammatory antioxidant reversal of Aβ-induced cognitive deficits and neuropathology. Neurobiol. Aging **22:** 991–1003.

32. DICKEY, C.A., J.F. LORING, J. MONTGOMERY, *et al.* 2003. Selectively reduced expression of synaptic plasticity-related genes in amyloid precursor protein + presenilin-1 transgenic mice. J. Neurosci. **23:** 5219–5226.
33. MONTINE, K.S., J.F. QUINN, J. ZHANG, *et al.* 2004. Isoprostanes and related products of lipid peroxidation in neurodegenerative diseases. Chem. Phys. Lipids **128:** 117–124.
34. CALON, F., G.P. LIM, F. YANG, *et al.* 2004. Docosahexaenoic acid protects from dendritic pathology in an Alzheimer's disease mouse model. Neuron **43**(5): 633–645.
35. STEIN, T.D. & J.A. JOHNSON. 2002. Lack of neurodegeneration in transgenic mice overexpressing mutant amyloid precursor protein is associated with increased levels of transthyretin and the activation of cell survival pathways. J. Neurosci. **22:** 7380–7388.
36. SMITH, M.A., L.M. SAYRE, V.M. MONNIER, *et al.* 1996. Oxidative post-translational modifications in Alzheimer disease. Mol. Chem. Neuropathol. **28:** 41–48.
37. SAYRE, L.M., D.A. ZELASKO, P.L.R. HARRIS, *et al.* 1997. 4-hydroxynonenal-derived advanced lipid peroxidation end products are increased in Alzheimer's disease. J. Neurochem. **68:** 2092–2097.
38. NUNOMURA, A., G. PERRY, G. ALIEV, *et al.* 2001. Oxidative damage is the earliest event in Alzheimer disease. J. Neuropathol. Exp. Neurol. **60:** 759–767.
39. YANG, F., X. SUN, W. BEECH, *et al.* 1998. Antibody to caspase-cleaved actin detects apoptosis in differentiated neuroblastoma and neurons and plaque associated neurons and microglia in Alzheimer's disease. Am. J. Pathol. **152:** 379–389.
40. SU, J.H., G.M. DENG & C.W. COTMAN. 1997. Neuronal DNA damage precedes tangle formation and is associated with up-regulation of nitrotyrosine in Alzheimer's disease brain. Brain Res. **774:** 193–199.
41. DUDA, J.E., B.I. GIASSON, Q. CHEN, *et al.* 2000. Widespread nitration of pathological inclusions in neurodegenerative synucleinopathies. Am. J. Pathol. **157:** 1439–1445.
42. TAKAHASHI, T., H. YAMASHITA, T. NAKAMURA, *et al.* 2002. Tyrosine 125 of alpha-synuclein plays a critical role for dimerization following nitrative stress. Brain Res. **938:** 73–80.
43. PAXINOU, E., Q. CHEN, M. WEISSE, *et al.* 2001. Induction of alpha-synuclein aggregation by intracellular nitrative insult. J. Neurosci. **21:** 8053–8061.
44. BHATTACHARYA, K., K.B. RANK, D.B. EVANS, *et al.* 2001. Role of cysteine-291 and cysteine-322 in the polymerization of human tau into Alzheimer-like filaments. Biochem. Biophys. Res. Commun. **285:** 20–26.
45. GUTTMANN, R.P., A.C. ERICKSON & G.V. JOHNSON. 1995. Tau self-association: stabilization with a chemical cross-linker and modulation by phosphorylation and oxidation state. J. Neurochem. **64:** 1209–1215.
46. GAMBLIN, T.C., M.E. KING, J. KURET, *et al.* 2000. Oxidative regulation of fatty acid–induced tau polymerization. Biochemistry **39:** 14203–14210.
47. PFANNSTIEL, J., M. CYRKLAFF, A. HABERMANN, *et al.* 2001. Human cofilin forms oligomers exhibiting actin bundling activity. J. Biol. Chem. **276:** 49476–49484.
48. ENYA, M., M. MORISHIMA-KAWASHIMA, Y. SHINKAI, *et al.* 1999. Appearance of sodium dodecyl sulfate-stable amyloid β-protein (Aβ) dimer in the cortex during aging. Am. J. Pathol. **154:** 271–279.
49. YOBURN, J.C., W. TIAN, J.O. BROWER, *et al.* 2003. Dityrosine cross-linked Abeta peptides: fibrillar beta-structure in Abeta(1-40) is conducive to formation of dityrosine cross-links but a dityrosine cross-link in Abeta(8-14) does not induce beta-structure. Chem. Res. Toxicol. **16:** 531–535.
50. ATWOOD, C.S., G. PERRY, H. ZENG, *et al.* 2004. Copper mediates dityrosine cross-linking of Alzheimer's amyloid-beta. Biochemistry **43:** 560–568.
51. TAKASHIMA, A., K. NOGUCHI, K. SATO, *et al.* 1993. tau protein kinase I is essential for amyloid β-protein-induced neurotoxicity. Proc. Natl. Acad. Sci. USA **90:** 7789–7793.
52. LAMBERT, M.P., A.K. BARLOW, B.A. CHROMY, *et al.* 1998. Diffusible, nonfibrillar ligands derived from Aβ1-42 are potent central nervous system neurotoxins. Proc. Natl. Acad. Sci. USA **95:** 6448–6453.
53. KUPERSTEIN, F. & E. YAVIN. 2003. Pro-apoptotic signaling in neuronal cells following iron and amyloid beta peptide neurotoxicity. J. Neurochem. **86:** 114–125.
54. ZHANG, C., H.E. QIU, G.A. KRAFFT, *et al.* 1996. A beta peptide enhances focal adhesion kinase/Fyn association in a rat CNS nerve cell line. Neurosci. Lett. **211:** 187–190.

55. ZHANG, C., H.E. QIU, G.A. KRAFFT, *et al.* 1996. Protein kinase C and F-actin are essential for stimulation of neuronal FAK tyrosine phosphorylation by G-proteins and amyloid beta protein. FEBS Lett. **386:** 185–188.
56. DANIELS, W.M., J. HENDRICKS, R. SALIE, *et al.* 2001. The role of the MAP-kinase superfamily in beta-amyloid toxicity. Metab. Brain Dis. **16:** 175–185.
57. MINOGUE, A.M., A.W. SCHMID, M.P. FOGARTY, *et al.* 2003. Activation of the c-Jun N-terminal kinase signaling cascade mediates the effect of amyloid-beta on long term potentiation and cell death in hippocampus: a role for interleukin-1beta? J. Biol. Chem. **278:** 27971–27980.
58. GONG, Y., L. CHANG, K.L. VIOLA, *et al.* 2003. Alzheimer's disease-affected brain: presence of oligomeric A beta ligands (ADDLs) suggests a molecular basis for reversible memory loss. Proc. Natl. Acad. Sci. USA **100:** 10417–10422.
59. WANG, Q., D.M. WALSH, M.J. ROWAN, *et al.* 2004. Block of long-term potentiation by naturally secreted and synthetic amyloid beta-peptide in hippocampal slices is mediated via activation of the kinases c-Jun N-terminal kinase, cyclin-dependent kinase 5, and p38 mitogen-activated protein kinase as well as metabotropic glutamate receptor type 5. J. Neurosci. **24:** 3370–3378.
60. CHEN, C., J.C. MAGEE & N.G. BAZAN. 2002. Cyclooxygenase-2 regulates prostaglandin E2 signaling in hippocampal long-term synaptic plasticity. J. Neurophysiol. **87:** 2851–2857.
61. KOTILNEK, L.A., Q. WANG, M.A.L.G.P. WESTERMAN, *et al.* 2004. NSAIDs improve amyloid beta protein-induced deficits in memory and synaptic plasticity. Neurobiol. Aging **25:** S580(P4–368).
62. BREITNER, J.C.S., K.A. WELSH, M.J. HELMS, *et al.* 1995. Delayed onset of Alzheimer's disease with nonsteroidal anti-inflammatory and histamine H2 blocking drugs. Neurobiol. Aging **16:** 523–530.
63. LIM, G.P., F. YANG, T. CHU, *et al.* 2000. Ibuprofen suppresses plaque pathology and inflammation in a mouse model for Alzheimer's Disease. J. Neurosci. **20:** 5709–5714.
64. LIM, G.P., F. YANG, T. CHU, *et al.* 2001. Ibuprofen effects on Alzheimer pathology and open field activity in APPsw transgenic mice. Neurobiol. Aging **22:** 983–981.
65. JANTZEN, P.T., K.E. CONNOR, G. DiCARLO, *et al.* 2002. Microglial activation and beta-amyloid deposit reduction caused by a nitric oxide-releasing nonsteroidal anti-inflammatory drug in amyloid precursor protein plus presenilin-1 transgenic mice. J. Neurosci. **22:** 2246–2254.
66. STAUFENBIEL, M., E. WIESLI, T. ZIGERLI, *et al.* 2002. Chronic ibuprofen does alter Aβ in the APP23 mouse. Neurobiol. Aging **23:** S414.
67. DEDEOGLU, A., D.F. SIWEK, K. KORMIER, *et al.* 2002. Ibuprofen preferentially reduces Aβ(1-42) deposition in amyloid precursor protein transgenic mice. Soc. Neurosci. **28:** 483.4.
68. YAN, Q., J. ZHANG, H. LIU, *et al.* 2003. Anti-inflammatory drug therapy alters beta-amyloid processing and deposition in an animal model of Alzheimer's disease. J. Neurosci. **23:** 7504–7509.
69. VOLMAR, C.H., J.T. ROACH, D. PARIS, *et al.* 2002. Improved behavior and increased cerebral blood flow by COX-2 and p38 MAPK inhibitors in the PSAPP transgenic mouse model. Soc. Neurosci. **28.**
70. QUINN, J., T. MONTINE, J. MORROW, *et al.* 2003. Inflammation and cerebral amyloidosis are disconnected in an animal model of Alzheimer's disease. J. Neuroimmunol. **137:** 32–41.
71. ERIKSEN, J.L., M.M. NICOLLE, S. PRESCOTT, *et al.* 2003. Chronic treatment of transgenic mice with ρ-flurbiprofen. Soc. Neurosci. **29:** 295.22.
72. PRATICO, D., Y. YAO, K. URYU, *et al.* 2003. Opposite effects of indomethacin and nimesulide on Aβ levels and amyloid deposition in a transgenic mouse model of Alzheimer amyloidosis. Soc. Neurosci. **29:** 20.4.
73. WALKER, L.C., F. BIAN, M.J. CALLAHAN, *et al.* 2002. Modeling Alzheimer's disease and other proteopathies in vivo: is seeding the key? Amino Acids **23:** 87–93.
74. WEGGEN, S., J.L. ERIKSEN, P. DAS, *et al.* 2001. A subset of NSAIDs lower amyloidogenic Abeta42 independently of cyclooxygenase activity. Nature **414:** 212–216.

75. ERIKSEN, J.L., S.A. SAGI, T.E. SMITH, *et al.* 2003. NSAIDs and enantiomers of flurbiprofen target gamma-secretase and lower Abeta 42 in vivo. J. Clin. Invest. **112:** 440–449.
76. MORIHARA, T., T. CHU, O. UBEDA, *et al.* 2002. Selective inhibition of Aβ42 production by NSAID R-enantiomers. J. Neurochem. **83:** 1–4.
77. GRIFFIN, W.S. & R.E. MRAK. 2002. Interleukin-1 in the genesis and progression of and risk for development of neuronal degeneration in Alzheimer's disease. J. Leukoc. Biol. **72:** 233–238.
78. SASTRE, M., I. DEWACHTER, G.E. LANDRETH, *et al.* 2003. Nonsteroidal anti-inflammatory drugs and peroxisome proliferator-activated receptor-gamma agonists modulate immunostimulated processing of amyloid precursor protein through regulation of beta-secretase. J. Neurosci. **23:** 9796–9804.
79. TABATON, M. 2004. Oxidative stress and beta-APP proteolytic processing. Neurobiol. Aging **25:** S69 (S4-02-03).
80. LIM, G.P., F. CALON, F. YANG, *et al.* 2004. Omega-3 fatty acid enriched diet reduces amyloid in an Alzheimer's disease mouse model. Neurobiol. Aging **25:** S570.
81. PUSKAS, L.G., K. KITAJKA, C. NYAKAS, *et al.* 2003. Short-term administration of omega 3 fatty acids from fish oil results in increased transthyretin transcription in old rat hippocampus. Proc. Natl. Acad. Sci. USA. In press.
82. MUKHERJEE, P.K., V.L. MARCHESELLI, C.N. SERHAN, *et al.* 2004. Neuroprotectin D1: a docosahexaenoic acid-derived docosatriene protects human retinal pigment epithelial cells from oxidative stress. Proc. Natl. Acad. Sci. USA **101:** 8491–8496.
83. LIM, G.P., T. CHU, F. YANG, *et al.* 2001. The curry spice curcumin reduces oxidative damage and amyloid pathology in an Alzheimer transgenic mouse. J. Neurosci. **21:** 8370–8377.
84. COLE, G.M., F. YANG, G.P. LIM, *et al.* 2003. A rationale for curcuminoids for the prevention or treatment of Alzheimer's disease. Curr. Med. Chem. Immun. Endocr. Metab. Agents **3:** 15–25.
85. VENKATESAN, P. & M.N.A. RAO. 2000. Structure-activity relationships for the inhibition of lipid peroxidation and the scavenging of free radicals by synthetic symmetrical curcumin analogues. J. Pharm. Pharmacol. **52:** 1123–1128.
86. AGGARWAL, B.B., A. KUMAR & A.C. BHARTI. 2003. Anticancer potential of curcumin: preclinical and clinical studies. Anticancer Res. **23:** 363–398.
87. LIAO, Y.-F., B.-J. WANG, H.-T. CHEN, *et al.* 2004. Gamma-secretase-mediated cleavage of amyloid precursor protein is stimulated by the cytokine-elicited activation of a JNK-dependent MAPK pathway. Neurobiol. Aging **25:** S180(P1–295).
88. PAN, M.H., T.M. HUANG & J.K. LIN. 1999. Biotransformation of curcumin through reduction and glucuronidation in mice. Drug Metab. Dispos. **27:** 486–494.
89. BROUET, I. & H. OHSHIMA. 1995. Curcumin, an anti-tumour promoter and anti-inflammatory agent, inhibits induction of nitric oxide synthase in activated macrophages. Biochem. Biophys. Res. Commun. **206:** 533–540.
90. PAN, M.H., S.Y. LIN-SHIAU & J.K. LIN. 2000. Comparative studies on the suppression of nitric oxide synthase by curcumin and its hydrogenated metabolites through down-regulation of IkappaB kinase and NFkappa B in macrophages. Biochem. Pharmacol. **60:** 1665–1676.
91. CHAN, M.M., H.I. HUANG, M.R. FENTON, *et al.* 1998. In vivo inhibition of nitric oxide synthase gene expression by curcumin, a cancer preventive natural product with anti-inflammatory properties. Biochem. Pharmacol. **55:** 1955–1962.
92. CHAN, M.M., H.I. HUANG, M.R. FENTON, *et al.* 1998. In vivo inhibition of nitric oxide synthase gene expression by curcumin, a cancer preventive natural product with anti-inflammatory properties. Biochem. Pharmacol. **55:** 1955–1962.
93. KELLOFF, G.J., J.A. CROWELL, E.T. HAWK, *et al.* 1996. Strategy and planning for chemopreventive drug development: clinical development plan: curcumin. J. Cell. Biochem. Suppl. **26:** 72–85.

Microglia as a Potential Bridge between the Amyloid β-Peptide and Tau

MASASHI KITAZAWA, TRITIA R. YAMASAKI, AND FRANK M. LaFERLA

Laboratory of Molecular Neuropathogenesis, Department of Neurobiology and Behavior, University of California, Irvine, Irvine, California 92697-4545, USA

ABSTRACT: Inflammation is a critical component of the pathogenesis of Alzheimer's disease (AD), consisting of the activation of both microglia and astrocytes. Activated microglia and reactive astrocytes are found in and around extraneuronal amyloid-β plaques and are thought to facilitate the clearance of these deposits from the brain parenchyma. However, mounting evidence indicates that chronic activation of microglia, presumably via the secretion of cytokines and reactive molecules, may exacerbate plaque pathology as well as enhance the hyperphosphorylation of tau and the subsequent development of neurofibrillary tangles. Thus, suppression of microglial activity in AD brain has been considered as a potential treatment of AD and may slow the disease progression. Along these lines, anti-inflammatory drugs, particularly non-steroidal anti-inflammatory drugs (NSAIDs), lessen the effects of AD pathology. In this review, we discuss the molecular mechanism of inflammatory responses in AD brain as well as animal models, and current therapies using NSAIDs, antioxidants, and immunotherapy as neuroprotective strategies for AD.

KEYWORDS: interleukins; p38-MAPK; NSAID; antioxidant; immunotherapy

INTRODUCTION

Alzheimer's disease (AD), the most common cause of dementia in the elderly, is marked by a progressive degeneration of limbic and cortical brain structures, mainly in the temporal lobe. Approximately 4.5 million people in the United States are currently afflicted with this disorder, and the number is expected to rise sharply in future years due to the increase in the elderly population, which represents the fastest growing segment in our society.[1] It is estimated that nearly 13–16 million people will suffer from AD by 2050 and, among those, nearly 13% of individuals over age 65 may be affected.[1,2] Most AD cases are sporadic, with multiple risk factors, such as aging, environmental stress, and diet, suggested to play critical pathogenic roles. The remaining AD cases, which account for 5–10% of total AD cases, are rare, but inherited from one generation to the next and are referred to as familial AD (FAD).

Address for correspondence: Frank M. LaFerla, Ph.D., Laboratory of Molecular Neuropathogenesis, Department of Neurobiology and Behavior, University of California, Irvine, 1109 Gillespie Neuroscience Research Facility, Irvine, CA 92697-4545. Voice: 949-824-1232; fax: 949-824-7356.

laferla@uci.edu

Ann. N.Y. Acad. Sci. 1035: 85–103 (2004). © 2004 New York Academy of Sciences.
doi: 10.1196/annals.1332.006

TABLE 1. Genes associated with FAD and effects on Aβ formation

Gene	Locus	Number of mutations	AD (%)	FAD (%)	Age of onset	Effect on Aβ	Trait
βAPP	21	11	<0.1	2–3	60s	↑ Aβ formation	Autosomal dominant
PS1	14	76+	<2	~50	16–62	↑ Aβ42	Autosomal dominant
PS2	1	6	<0.1	<1	60+	↑ Aβ42	Autosomal dominant
ApoE ε4 allele	19	–	~40%	–	60+	↑ Aβ ↑ deposits	Risk factor

NOTE: Four major genes associated with familial Alzheimer's disease (FAD) are listed. Mutations in amyloid-β precursor protein (βAPP), presenilin-1 (PS1), and presenilin-2 (PS2) are autosomal dominant in FAD and increase the total Aβ production. Among them, presenilin mutations account for the majority of early-onset FAD as well as total cases of FAD. However, FAD is rare among all AD cases. On the other hand, the ε4 allele of ApoE is considered to be a risk factor for AD. However, individuals who possess this allele do not necessarily develop AD in their life time.

Mutations in the amyloid precursor protein (APP), presenilin 1 (PS1), and presenilin 2 (PS2) genes cause autosomal dominant FAD (for review[3]). These mutations are known to increase formation of total amyloid-β (Aβ) levels (TABLE 1) (for review[4]). Typically, FAD patients develop the disease much earlier than those with the sporadic form. In addition, those individuals harboring the ε4 allele of apolipoprotein E (ApoE) have a 20–90% increased risk for AD,[5] and recent data suggest that the molecular mechanism may involve an interaction between Aβ and ApoE.

There are two major neuropathological hallmarks of AD: extraneuronal amyloid plaques and neurofibrillary tangles (NFTs). Amyloid plaques are mainly composed of insoluble Aβ fragments, whereas NFTs consist of aggregates of hyperphosphorylated tau protein. These two insoluble protein aggregates are believed to play critical roles in the neurodegenerative process. However, the exact molecular mechanisms by which they cause neurodegeneration remain to be definitely established. In addition, there are other critical changes that occur in the AD brain, including cell loss, synapse loss, and inflammation. Inflammation is not unique to AD, but occurs in other neurodegenerative disorders, such as Parkinson's disease, Pick's disease, multiple sclerosis, and viral encephalitis.[6,7] The inflammatory response in AD is characterized by activated microglia and reactive astrocytes.[8] Numbers of extraneuronal amyloid plaques are associated with activated microglia and reactive astrocytes, which have long been thought to be a reaction (i.e., secondary response) to amyloid. However, growing evidence suggests that microglia may also exacerbate the pathogenesis of AD, especially by facilitating the progression of NFTs. Thus, suppressing the inflammatory reaction may attenuate NFT pathology and lessen the disease progression. In this review, we discuss the role that microglia play in response to amyloid plaques and NFTs, and the possible therapeutic approaches targeting microglia.

INFLAMMATORY RESPONSES AND ALZHEIMER'S DISEASE

Inflammatory responses within the brain are mainly carried out by activated microglia and reactive astrocytes. Microglia were first identified as brain phagocytes in 1919.[9] In the normal brain, they are generally ramified in their resting state. In this stage, microglia do not produce any pro-inflammatory or reactive oxygen/nitrogen molecules (for review[10]). However, following pathological and/or traumatic insults, microglia become activated and assume an amoeboid morphology and increase in size. In addition, certain receptors are upregulated in activated microglia. These activated microglia can be detected by various antibodies and lectins including Mac-1/CD11b, HLA-DR, CD45, RCA-1, and F4/80.[8] Once activated, microglia phagocytose foreign substances and release pro-inflammatory molecules, such as cytokines that include interleukins (ILs), interferons (INFs), tumor necrosis factors (TNFs), and growth factors that further activate other inflammatory responses and thus potentiate the cycle. Activated microglia also generate and secrete reactive oxygen and nitrogen species (ROS/RNS) to attack and remove foreign substances. This process could further exacerbate the degenerative condition as oxidative stress has been suggested to contribute to Aβ neuropathology. It is likely that activated microglia are a major source of ROS in the AD brain, further highlighting the potential molecular mechanism by which microglia inadvertently enhance disease progression. Thus, inhibiting microglia and/or scavenging ROS could have therapeutic efficacy for treating AD (see below for more detail).

Postmortem Studies

Activated microglia and reactive astrocytes are commonly observed in postmortem AD brains.[11] Increased cell surface expression of major histocompatibility complex (MHC) class II, a conventional marker for microglia, and glial fibrillary acidic protein (GFAP), a specific marker for reactive astrocytes, have been observed in the AD brain.[12,13] Notably, activated microglia and reactive astrocytes tend to localize around fibrillar amyloid plaques; thus amyloid plaques may be viewed as foreign substances in the brain and thereby trigger these inflammatory responses. In the AD brain, activated microglia as well as reactive astrocytes have been shown to contain Aβ fragments, providing evidence of phagocytic degradation of Aβ.[14,15] The clearance of Aβ plaques by microglial phagocytosis is further supported by several other studies. Both fibrillar and soluble Aβ injected into rat striatum were cleared by microglial activity. Other *in vitro* studies also reveal that clearance occurs through a phagocytic mechanism.[16–18] Rogers and colleagues observed that microglia isolated from the AD brain were capable of scavenging aggregated Aβ peptides in a few weeks.[19] Additionally, clearance of Aβ plaques was recently reported by locally activated microglia in AD brain.[20] Frackowiak and colleagues, however, conducted ultrastructural analysis of phagocytic activity of microglia and found very limited effectiveness of microglia in degrading amyloid fibrils, but rather the amyloid fibrils were stored in deep infoldings of cell membranes.[21] On the other hand, astrocytes may more effectively degrade amyloid fibrils by phagocytic activity. The migration of astrocytes into Aβ plaques is promoted by the presence of monocyte chemoattractant protein-1 (MCP-1),[22] a chemokine that is released by activated microglia surrounding Aβ plaques in AD brain.[23] As a result, astrocytes are recruited to Aβ plaques and further contribute to degradation and clearance of plaques, which has been demonstrated in several *in vitro* studies.[24,25]

A recent study demonstrated that activated microglia associated with Aβ plaques may partially serve to facilitate maturation of fibrillar Aβ plaques.[26] It remains unresolved as to whether Aβ found in microglia is the result of their phagocytic activity or a consequence of their own processing of APP to Aβ.[27–29] The sum of a vast literature on the role of microglia activation suggests that they have some benefit for clearing Aβ plaques, but that their chronic activation may inadvertently cause further destruction and neuropathological changes in the AD brain.[30,31] Interestingly, Di-Patre and Gelman observed that activated microglia in the hippocampus of AD brain are more diffuse and not correlated with senile plaques.[32] In this study, however, numbers of activated microglia are closely related with numbers of NFT-containing neurons, indicating that inflammatory responses may play an important role in the pathogenesis of tau hyperphosphorylation. We will further discuss this later in this review.

As microglia become activated, elevated levels of cytokines are detected in the AD brain. Selected cytokines have been found: IL-1α, IL-1β, IL-6, TNFα, CXC-R2, CC-R3, CC-R5, and TGF-β are all elevated in AD brain.[8,33–35] Isolated microglia from postmortem AD and control (non-demented) patients' brain tissue exhibit different cytokine expression profiles following exposure to Aβ peptides. Compared to control brain tissue, microglia from the AD brain show significantly increased expression of IL-1β following exposure to Aβ.[36] Further, in peripheral monocytes, blood-borne precursors of microglia, increased levels of TNF-α, IL-1β, IL-6, IL-8, and IL-12 have been reported following exposure to Aβ peptides.[37] These results strongly suggest that Aβ peptides and/or plaques initiate the activation of microglia and subsequent release of pro-inflammatory molecules in the AD brain.

Although various interleukins have been shown to be elevated in AD brain, the physiological and pathological function of these interleukins may differ. Increased levels of IL-1α are found in early stages of AD and studies indicate that microglia-induced IL-1α may play an important role in plaque evolution from diffuse forms of Aβ.[38] Furthermore, head injury causes a three- to sevenfold increase in the expression of both IL-1α and APP in the brain.[39] These data suggest that IL-1α may be more important in early phases of the progression of AD and could work as a risk factor for the disease.

Animal Models

Several different transgenic animal models for AD are currently available, and these models exhibit neuropathological patterns similar to those seen in human AD, including Aβ and tau pathology and brain inflammatory responses. A recent report by Schwab and colleagues, however, discussed that the activation pattern of microglia in a transgenic mouse model overexpressing APPswe is distinctly different from that observed in human AD brain.[40] The difference on the inflammatory responses observed in these mice may be due to mouse strain, transgene background, and other factors, thus more thorough investigation may be required. Transgenic mice overexpressing human APPswe show age-dependent increases in activated microglia that correlate well with increased formation of extraneuronal Aβ plaques.[27,41,42] These activated microglia are associated with plaques in the transgenic brain and show

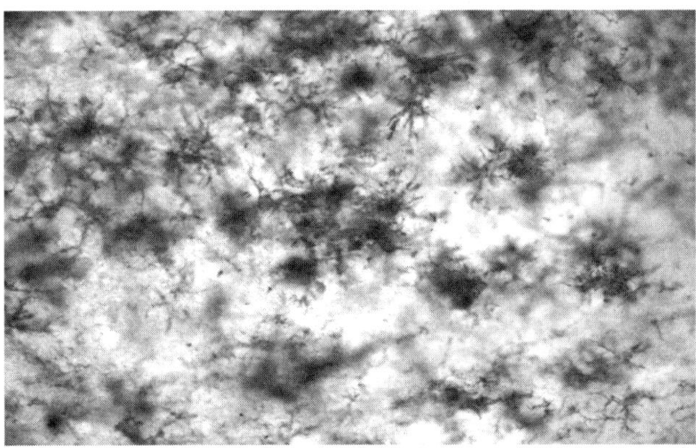

FIGURE 1. Colocalization of activated microglia with amyloid plaques in an animal model of AD. Double immunohistochemical staining of activated microglia (CD45 immunopositive) and amyloid plaques (6E10 immunopositive) in 24-month-old 3×Tg-AD mouse brain reveals that activated microglia (*black*) surround extraneuronal amyloid plaques (*light gray*) in the CA1 of the hippocampus.

some histological evidence of phagocytic activity.[43] In our laboratory, we have generated a triple transgenic mouse model of AD (3×Tg-AD) that develops both plaques and tangles in the brain in an age-dependent manner.[44] Using these mice, we have also found that CD45-immunopositive activated microglia colocalize around amyloid plaques (FIG. 1). Young 3×Tg-AD mice without plaques do not exhibit any activated microglia, but after extraneuronal plaques manifest in the brain, microglia are significantly activated and found closely associated with plaques (unpublished observation). These data suggest potential phagocytic activity of microglia on Aβ plaques in transgenic animal models although, as also described earlier, this activity is much limited.[45] More importantly, secretion of reactive molecules from microglia and astrocytes seems to occur earlier than the development of plaques in animal models. Elevated expression of certain cytokines including IL-6, IL-12, and IFN-γ, was detected prior to extraneuronal Aβ plaque formation in Tg2576 mice.[46,47] This is supported by the fact that ramified (resting) microglia are capable of producing more secretory molecules, and these physiological alterations may contribute to early cognitive impairments that appear before plaque development, as reported in probable AD patients.[48] Yet, it is unclear whether microglial activation and/or secreted cytokines further contribute to downstream pathogenic events in AD.

MOLECULAR LINK BETWEEN MICROGLIA AND TAU

Neurofibrillary tangles (NFTs) are mainly composed of hyperphosphorylated tau, and are found not only in the AD brain, but also in other neurodegenerative disorders including Pick's disease, corticobasal degeneration (CBD), progressive supranuclear palsy (PSP), and frontotemporal dementia with parkinsonism linked to chromosome 17 (FTDP-17).[49,50] The mechanism underlying tau hyperphosphorylation, and indeed whether all hyperphosphorylation events of tau are detrimental, and the effect of hyperphosphorylation on neuronal differentiation and death are all under investigation. As mentioned earlier, activation of microglia in AD brain has been studied and characterized, but it is not clear whether activated microglia affect plaque or tangle pathology. A recent study conducted by Ishizawa and Dickson may provide a specific link between microglia and NFTs. In this study, postmortem brain tissue from CBD and PSP were immunologically stained for activated microglia and NFTs. They found that there were more activated microglia in these brain tissues than in normal controls, and microglial burden correlated with tau burden in most of the pathologically afflicted areas.[51] Furthermore, NFTs are implicated in the loss of axonal integrity and connectivity between synapses.[52,53] Synaptic loss may contribute to the development of cognitive deficits and dementia in AD as well as other tauopathies.[54–56] Thus, studying the pathological link between microglia and NFTs and preventing NFT formation may spare neurons and slow the progression of dementia in these diseases.

Several kinases have been reported as possible candidates for tau phosphorylation: cyclin-dependent kinase 5 (cdk5), glycogen synthase kinase 3β (GSK-3β), and p38–mitogen-activated protein kinase (p38-MAPK). Each kinase has a unique activation process, but several lines of evidence suggest that microglia release cytokines that may initiate the activation of these kinases. Griffin and her colleagues recently demonstrated that the activation of microglia by secreted APP or lipopolysaccharide (LPS) results in the elevation of IL-1α, IL-1β, and TNFα, and subsequent tau hyperphosphorylation and neuronal loss.[57] In particular, IL-1–induced tau hyperphosphorylation is mediated by the activation of p38-MAPK, and the application of IL-1 receptor antagonist significantly reduces phosphorylated tau, activated p38-MAPK, and neuronal loss in rat primary cortical neurons. In an animal model of AD, chronic exposure to IL-1 causes hyperphosphorylation of tau through p38-MAPK activation.[58,59] Significant numbers of neurons that show colocalization of activated p38-MAPK and hyperphosphorylated tau (AT8-immunoreactivity) as well as IL-1–immunoreactive microglia are found in human AD brain,[58] implying a possible association between microglia and tau pathology. This p38-MAPK–mediated hyperphosphorylation of tau can also be observed in brains from Pick's disease, another major neurodegenerative disorder with tauopathy.[60] On the other hand, IL-6, another interleukin secreted from microglia and elevated in AD brain, has been shown to activate cdk5 by increasing levels of intracellular p35, an important cofactor of cdk5 and cause tau hyperphosphorylation in rat primary hippocampal neurons.[61] These results indicate that interleukins upregulate the activity of tau kinases and promote the development of NFTs.

On the other hand, inhibition of phosphatase activity could be another potential mechanism of tau hyperphosphorylation. Quinolinic acid, another molecule that is secreted from microglia, is a weak but selective *N*-methyl-D-aspartate (NMDA) receptor agonist[62] and may be implicated in the development of tau pathology in AD via excitotoxicity and inhibition of phosphatases. A recent *in vitro* study demonstrated that Aβ42 peptide significantly elevated the secretion of quinolinic acid by microglia,[63] indicating activation of the NMDA receptor and induction of excitotoxicity. Additionally, one subunit (NR3A) in the NMDA receptor has been shown to physically associate with phosphatase 2A (PP2A), contributing to its phosphatase activity. Once the NMDA receptor is stimulated, PP2A dissociates from the complex and reduces its activity.[64] This process is considered to be important for synaptic plasticity in neurons. In AD brain, however, abnormal stimulation of the NMDA receptor may occur locally in the vicinity of plaques by quinolinic acid. The resulting suppression of PP2A activity may lead to increased formation of hyperphosphorylated tau in neurons. Although the level of quinolinic acid in AD brains was found to be no different than that in age-matched control brains,[65,66] the mechanism involving phosphatase activity on tau via quinolinic acid or other inflammatory molecules must be investigated further. Based on these data, it is plausible that microglia activation may inadvertently lead to tau phosphorylation, providing a link between brain inflammation and NFT formation.

It remains to be resolved whether accumulation of hyperphosphorylated tau (or NFTs) eventually induces cognitive decline. In earlier studies, reduction of tau hyperphosphorylation by inhibiting cdk5 activity significantly rescues neurons from Aβ-induced toxicity.[67] This result correlates with the recent finding that cdk5 is involved in the apoptotic process[68] although there are opposing reports on this aspect.[69,70] Activation of cdk5 seems to occur in early stages of AD, and these neurons develop NFTs and undergo neurodegeneration.[71] More relevant evidence of hyperphosphorylated tau-induced neurodegeneration can be obtained from FTDP-17 studies. Mutations in the tau gene have been shown to cause FTDP-17,[72–74] and these discoveries shed light on the importance of tau in dementia and neurodegeneration, especially in light of the fact that FTDP-17 patients do not develop Aβ pathology.

If abnormal accumulation of hyperphosphorylated tau leads to neuronal loss, we may be able to attenuate or slow neurodegeneration by inhibiting chronic inflammatory responses in AD. In the last section of this review, we discuss possible therapeutic approaches of AD focusing on antioxidants and anti-inflammatory agents, and whether or not they have beneficial effects on AD.

POTENTIAL THERAPEUTIC APPROACHES TARGETING IMMUNE RESPONSES

Antioxidant Treatments

Oxidative stress is thought to play a critical role in the pathogenesis of AD and other dementias.[75,76] Microglia activated by Aβ have been reported to release various ROS and RNS.[77,78] These, in turn, may adversely affect neuronal viability and conceivably contribute to the clinical deterioration seen in AD. Thus, it is possible that antioxidant use may attenuate the neurodegenerative process induced by microglial-mediated ROS and RNS.

One of the most extensively studied antioxidants thus far is vitamin E. Several *in vitro* studies posit a neuroprotective role for vitamin E.[79,80] Further, *in vivo* studies using young Tg2576 mice maintained on a vitamin E–supplemented diet showed a decrease in Aβ40 and Aβ42 levels, suggesting that vitamin E may have a direct effect on attenuation of early AD pathology.[81] However, results of prospective studies and recent human clinical trials have questioned the efficacy of antioxidants in treatment or prevention of AD.[82–86]

The epidemiological studies of antioxidants in AD demonstrate this confusion. Two types of studies are apparent; those which assess dietary intake of antioxidants and those which analyze supplement use. Studies of dietary consumption have the advantage of being a rather stable assessment of long-term intake habits. In contrast, vitamin E and C supplements generally have considerably higher levels of antioxidants than those provided strictly by diet. However, plasma levels may be subjected to the vagaries of absorption and supplement use may not be as consistent as dietary intake over the period assessed. In either case, there are conflicting reports. The Rotterdam study, a large prospective study involving 5,395 participants with a 6-year followup, found a correlation between high dietary consumption of vitamin E or vitamin C and decreased risk for AD.[87] The Cache County study of 5,092 participants in Utah also found vitamin E and vitamin C supplements in combination were associated with a decreased incidence and prevalence of AD when assessed at a 3-year followup.[88] Findings from other groups support these positive results.[89,90] However, smaller studies failed to find any correlation between dietary or supplement intake of antioxidants and AD,[83,84] even when assessed as late as 30 years later for cumulative long-term effects.[82]

Although epidemiological studies have the advantage of investigating large cohorts, it is the clinical trial that provides a more rigorously controlled situation, defined subject population, and does not depend as heavily on patient dietary recall. Further, clinical trials allow direct assessment of therapeutic potential rather than a formulation of relative risk. Intriguingly, a randomized controlled trial of supplements as an actual therapy for 341 people diagnosed with moderately severe AD found significant delay in AD progression with vitamin E supplement use (progression defined as the time to death, institutionalization, progress to severe dementia, or loss of two-thirds of basic activities of daily living) over a 2-year period.[91] Notably, while behavioral deterioration was delayed, cognitive test scores did not improve.[91] These results are significant as the first randomized controlled trial showing a therapeutic benefit for vitamin E on actual AD patients.[91] A couple of other trials trying to assess the efficacy of donepezil versus vitamin E or donepezil/vitamin E combination treatments favor cholinesterase inhibition over vitamin E supplement treatment.[85,86] However, given the small size of these trials and the shorter durations, the results of Sano and colleagues seem to be more credible at this point.

The pathological effect of oxidative stress in AD has yet to be fully elucidated. Although microglia have been shown to increase the oxidative burden in affected brain regions, it is still not known whether this significantly contributes to neurodegeneration. An *in vitro* study suggests that the antioxidant vitamin E may exert beneficial effects in a manner entirely independent of its role as an antioxidant, likely, through its effects on specific cell signaling pathways in microglia. Studies by Li and colleagues demonstrate that pretreatment with vitamin E suppressed LPS-induced microglial activation and resulted in less neurotoxicity to PC12 cells.[80] Their data further suggest that activated microglia cause signaling through the NF-κB and p38-MAPK pathways, resulting in downstream inflammatory effects, including cytokine and nitric oxide release. Vitamin E seems to attenuate these signaling pathways and thus may downregulate a range of inflammatory factors in a role separate from, and possibly more wide-ranging than, its function as a free-radical scavenger.[80]

Thus, as a treatment for AD, vitamin E, and other antioxidants may suppress microglial activity and prevent subsequent neuronal death. Vitamin E has some promising support in prospective studies as well as a controlled trial. However, more studies, both clinical and research, are needed to assess true potential. Other antioxidants currently being tested for their efficacy against AD are estradiol-17B, tetra-hydracannabinol, aromatic amine/imines, TMP, and Cu/Zn chelators,[76] but results are still inconclusive. Antioxidants present something of a blanket approach to the problem; one that is diffuse and non-targeted in a system-wide downregulation of oxidative stress. Yet, given their usual lack of adverse side effects and affordability, they are promising candidates until more specifically targeted approaches can be developed.

Anti-inflammatory Treatments

If one takes the viewpoint that inflammation in the AD brain exacerbates the pathological processes, it follows that drugs that inhibit the inflammatory response may have therapeutic value.[92,93] Since Aβ can increase the inflammatory response through microglial activation, and the inflammatory response has been implicated in Aβ deposition, hindrance of inflammation could break this pathological cycle.[94] Indeed, in respect to microglial involvement in these processes, Mackenzie and colleagues examined postmortem brain tissue in non-demented elderly individuals with known use of non-steroidal anti-inflammatory drugs (NSAIDs) or no use and found that non-users had three times the number of activated microglia of NSAID users.[95] The authors interpret this finding as evidence that NSAID treatment in AD may exert its action through suppression of microglial activation.[95]

Given their history of common long-term use, efficacy in elderly patients, and well-characterized side-effect profile, NSAIDs hold promise of therapeutic potential. The main known target of NSAIDs is the cyclooxygenase (COX) enzymes. COX enzymes mediate the conversion of arachidonic acid to prostaglandins, crucial components of the inflammatory process. COX-2, the inducible isoform found in neurons and other cells, is found up-regulated in AD brain.[96] Human COX-2 overexpressing mice show an age-related cognitive decline, neuronal apoptosis, and astrocytic activation.[97] Mice with COX-2 overexpression in conjunction with the human APPswe and PS1 mutation show increased Aβ load and plaque formation.[98] Inhibition of COX-2 is thought to be neuroprotective in ischemic and excitotoxic injury.[99,100] In particular, there has been an impetus to develop drugs that selectively hinder COX-2 enzymes to circumvent the side effects of COX-1 inhibition, which include gastro-intestinal toxicity. Examples of COX-2 inhibitors include rofecoxib and celecoxib, which are the focus of several clinical trials. COX-1, the more constitutive isoform, is expressed in microglia, notably, in those found associated with neuritic plaques in AD.[101] Studies suggest that classical NSAIDs, such as ibuprofen and indomethacin, with their non-selective inhibition of COX enzymes, are capable of suppressing microglial prostaglandin production in inflammatory reactions and would thus be a more appropriate therapy.[102]

The epidemiological evidence in support of NSAID therapeutic efficacy seems particularly hopeful. More than 20 different studies show a decrease in frequency of AD in arthritic or other patients known to be treated with high levels of anti-inflammatory drugs.[6,103] The larger NSAID studies have been, on the whole, positive. For example, Stewart and colleagues assessed relative risk for AD in 1,686 partici-pants of the Baltimore Longitudinal Study of Aging over a 15-year period and found that NSAID use resulted in an overall relative risk of 0.74 compared to non-users.[104] In a later extensive study, in 't Veld and coworkers conducted a thorough examination of the pharmacy records of 6,989 participants in the Rotterdam cohort with a 6.8-year followup and found a clear-cut difference between increasing time on NSAIDs and decreasing risk for AD. This study found that NSAID use for a period of at least two years is capable of significantly decreasing AD risk.[105]

These promising studies are also supported by *in vivo* studies in transgenic animals. Several investigators have evaluated the efficacy of one of the most widely used NSAIDs, ibuprofen, in AD mouse models. Lim and colleagues found that 6 months of consumption of ibuprofen in chow of Tg2576 mice decreased amyloid plaque number, as well as lowered SDS-soluble and insoluble Aβ. Further, they found a decrease in activated microglia in ibuprofen-treated mice, as well as decreased inflammatory cytokine levels (IL-1β).[106] These results are further supported by Yan and colleagues whose treatment of Tg2576 mice for 4 months with ibuprofen resulted in a 63% reduction of SDS-soluble Aβ42 and a corresponding reduction in activated microglia compared to control animals.[107]

Further research performed by Weggen and colleagues have elaborated on these studies and made several important contributions.[108] The type of NSAID used is critical. Ibuprofen, indomethacin, and sulindac sulfide decreased Aβ42 levels preferentially, whereas other NSAIDs including aspirin (non-selective COX inhibitor), celecoxib (COX-2 inhibitor), and SC-560 (COX-1 inhibitor) did not lower either total Aβ levels or the Aβ42/40 ratio in cultured cells. They also found that ibuprofen administered to young Tg2576 mice in drinking water for 3 days resulted in a 39% decrease in Aβ42, but no change in Aβ40. They hypothesize that this change in Aβ42 is due to a shift in γ-secretase activity toward generation of Aβ1-38 species through a COX-independent mechanism.[108] In a more comprehensive study, Eriksen and colleagues screened 20 commonly used NSAIDs and found eight that were capable of lowering Aβ42 levels *in vivo*. Among these, they suggest that the COX-inactive R-enantiomer of flurbiprofen is the most suitable target for clinical trials due to its ability to lower Aβ42 as well as Aβ40, and as its method of action is through γ-secretase rather than COX. Consequently, it should not have the gastric and renal side effects often found in COX inhibitors. Notably, they find that neither naproxen nor aspirin has the capacity to lower Aβ42 *in vivo*.[94]

These reports could explain the results of clinical trials which have, on the whole, been discouraging. The one positive result came from a 6-month trial of indomethacin in patients with mild to moderate AD. The investigators found a 1.3% improvement in cognitive test scores of indomethacin-treated patients compared to a decline of 8.4% in controls.[109] However, the study started with only 44 patients and had a 21% drop-out rate from the treatment group, suggesting low tolerability of the treatment regime.[109] A second group investigated the effects of diclofenac, another non-selective COX inhibitor, in 41 mild-moderate AD patients over a 25-week period.[110] Misoprostol, a gastro-protective agent, was added in an attempt to reduce side effects, but the drop out rate from the trial was still 50%. Therefore, although there was a non-significant trend toward reduced deterioration in the treatment group, these results must be cautiously interpreted due to small sample size.[110] Further, clinical trials of COX-2 inhibitors celecoxib, nimesulide, and rofecoxib have also been resoundingly negative in reducing cognitive or behavioral deficits in AD patients. Each trial had more than 300 AD patients, who were tested for a year on a randomized, controlled paradigm.[111–113] Particularly disappointing was a recent clinical trial of both rofecoxib (COX-2 selective) and naproxen (non-selective) which had enrolled 351 patients and failed to show a slowing of cognitive decline after a year with either medication.[114] Lastly, a test of hydroxychloroquine, a medication used in malaria with some anti-inflammatory properties, also failed to ameliorate AD deficits.[115]

So, what explains the dichotomy in results derived from epidemiological observations versus clinical studies? One possibility is the fact that most epidemiological studies start with normal subjects and assess risk of developing disease and correlate with drug regimen, whereas past clinical trials have started with patients that already have a diagnosis of mild to moderate AD and determine if an improvement can be seen. Thus, there is a difference in the stage of the disease. It is wholly probably that at the stage studied in clinical trials, the disease is already so far advanced as to be irreversible by NSAIDs.[115,116] This makes sense if one thinks in terms of the pathology: if NSAIDs work by attenuating the inflammatory response, then removing the cause of the damage will not necessarily repair the damage already incurred. This may be resolved by early intervention trials currently in progress, which are studying the effects of COX-2 inhibitors on patients with mild cognitive impairment (MCI) or on cognitively normal elderly people.[117] Another possibility as suggested by the studies of Weggen and colleagues is that the choice of anti-inflammatory drug is crucial. If the efficacy of NSAIDs depends on their Aβ42 lowering ability or some other effect, not on their COX-inhibiting function, this may explain the negative result in trials of celecoxib, rofecoxib, and naproxen, but the positive findings with indomethacin and in epidemiological studies where ibuprofen was used. In either case, further clinical trials and research are necessary to explore fully the therapeutic potential of anti-inflammatory therapies.

Surprisingly, Jantzen and colleagues suggest that microglial activation may be beneficial from the results of their studies of a nitric oxide (NO)-releasing NSAID, NCX-2216.[118] This compound is a flurbiprofen derivative. Treating APPswe and PS1 overexpressing transgenic mice with NCX-2216 for five months resulted in a dramatic decrease in Aβ load (greater than corresponding treatment with ibuprofen or COX-2 inhibitor celecoxib and even greater than that found with Aβ vaccination). Unexpectedly, they also found increased microglial activation, leading them to hypothesize that these reduced Aβ levels resulted from phagocytic microglial clearance of Aβ.[118]

Immunotherapy

A possible therapeutic approach that has gained considerable attention in recent years involves harnessing the power of the immune system to fight AD. This has been carried out through active immunization against the synthetic Aβ peptide or its derivatives, or passive administration of antibody against Aβ. Dale Schenk and colleagues were the first to show that active immunization against Aβ42 decreases Aβ load and plaque development in the PDAPP mouse model of AD.[119] Interestingly, they also found a decrease in astrocytosis and microglial activation. The generation of anti-Aβ antibodies combined with the presence of Aβ-immunoreactive microglial in plaque regions led them to propose that clearance of Aβ may be through Fc receptor–mediated microglial phagocytosis of Aβ.[119] Microglial involvement in clearance of Aβ has been further supported by other studies.[120–122] However, other investigators believe that Aβ removal occurs through properties of the antibody itself;

that is, by inhibiting aggregation of Aβ[123] or by binding and withdrawing soluble Aβ to the peripheral system and thus reducing abundance in the brain.[124,125] Regardless of the mechanism, it is significant that not only has immunotherapy been confirmed to clear plaques in a variety of AD models, it has also been shown to slow cognitive deficits of AD in models.[126,127] These dramatic and indisputable findings lead many to believe that immunotherapy holds great potential as a treatment for AD.[128]

Given the positive finding for *in vitro* and *in vivo* work, immunotherapy moved quickly to human clinical trials. These trials, conducted by the pharmaceutical company Elan, used a synthetic Aβ42 peptide, AN-1792, and an adjuvant (QS21) for active immunization of patients with mild to moderate AD.[129] Although Phase I studies in smaller groups did not result in significant side effects, a large multicenter Phase IIA trial involving 375 patients had to be halted after less than a year in January 2002 due to the development of signs and symptoms of aseptic meningoencephalitis.[128] In all, 18 patients (approximately 6%), all from the treatment group, developed this adverse effect.[130]

Although there was disappointment about the outcome of the trials, the ongoing studies of the patients involved offer some intriguing results. Studies of immune serum from a Zurich cohort of 30 patients from the trial suggest high specificity of antibodies generated in that they react with aggregated Aβ in plaques, diffuse Aβ deposits, and vascular Aβ, but not with APP or soluble Aβ42.[131] Also, instances of meningoencephalitis did not correlate with the presence or levels of antibody titers to Aβ. These observations lead to the speculation that brain inflammation is due to a T-cell response in affected patients and not through cross-reactivity of antibodies generated.[131,132] Further, histological evidence from the brain of one patient who developed meningoencephalitis and later died demonstrated actual clearance of Aβ plaques from large areas of neocortex, as well as a lack of plaque-associated astrocytes and dystrophic neurites.[133] This strongly suggests that immunotherapy is capable of clearing plaques in humans. Exciting evidence that this therapy may also prevent symptomatic progression of AD was shown by further studies of Hoch and colleagues.[134] Following the same Zurich cohort of 30 patients they found that in the 20 patients who did develop antibodies to Aβ, there was a significant slowing of cognitive decline as well as a significant prevention in progression to severe dementia compared to the group who did not develop such antibodies.[134] Thus, immunotherapy may still hold potential promise, however, its methods must be refined before further trials are conducted.

In addition to its potential therapeutic value, immunotherapy has also been useful in extending our basic understanding of AD and the properties underlying development of pathology. Immunotherapy has also been instrumental for providing support for the amyloid cascade hypothesis, which states that Aβ aggregation is the trigger that initiates other pathological hallmarks of AD, such as the formation of neurofibrillary tangles and neuronal death.[135] The demonstration that plaque clearance in animal models leads to amelioration of memory deficits supports this idea. Further, our lab has shown that, in addition to the clearance of extracellular plaques, intracellular Aβ clearance also occurs, and that early tau pathology is reversed following immunotherapy with an antibody against Aβ.[136] The reduction of Aβ pathology precedes the reversal of tau pathology and further, Aβ pathology reemerges prior to tau pathology following a 30-day lapse in treatment. This provides support for the hypothesis that Aβ is an upstream of tau in the pathological timeline. Also from this work, it becomes apparent that only a subset of tau pathology is reversible by immuno-therapy; early tau pathology mislocalized to the somatodendritic compartment of neurons is reversible, but the later hyperphosphorylated tau aggregates do not clear. This suggests that there is a limit to the extent of disease modification that may be accomplished using immunotherapy, or possibly that a multitherapeutic approach (targeting both tau and Aβ lesions) may prove beneficial in treatment paradigms.[136]

CONCLUDING REMARKS

Existing reports from cell culture, transgenic animals, and human AD brain samples have revealed diverse effects of microglia on the disease progression. The activation of microglia appears to be triggered by formation of the extraneuronal Aβ plaques, and subsequent release of cytokines from activated microglia promotes the signaling pathways for tau hyperphosphorylation and formation of NFTs in neurons. Thus, microglia play a critical role in linking the two major hallmarks of AD pathol-ogy. Moreover, this series of molecular processes may eventually contribute to AD neurodegeneration. The inhibition of microglial activation may rescue neurons and slow the disease progression. For example, numerous studies have examined the effect of NSAIDs on AD. Both epidemiological studies and clinical trials show promising pharmacological effects of NSAIDs on AD patients, yet some controver-sial results still remain. Furthermore, the exact mechanism of how NSAIDs act in the brain and delay AD-related pathology and cognitive impairment is not known. Antioxidants and immunotherapies also seem to have some beneficial effects on delaying the progression of AD, but more studies are necessary to make a final con-clusion. Although we have presented current findings of the role of microglia and possible therapeutic approaches in AD, this field of study is still ongoing and more data will be necessary to discern whether microglia are the key pathological feature of AD and to ascertain the potential benefit of the use of NSAIDs, antioxidants, or immunotherapy for neuroprotection in AD.

ACKNOWLEDGMENTS

This work was supported by a grant from the Alzheimer's Association and by the National Institutes of Health (Grant Nos. AG17968 and AG0212982).

REFERENCES

1. HEBERT, L.E. *et al.* 2003. Alzheimer disease in the US population: prevalence estimates using the 2000 census. Arch. Neurol. **60:** 1119–1122.
2. MAIER-LORENTZ, M.M. 2000. Neurobiological bases for Alzheimer's disease. J. Neuro-sci. Nurs. **32:** 117–125.
3. SELKOE, D.J. & M.B. PODLISNY. 2002. Deciphering the genetic basis of Alzheimer's disease. Annu. Rev. Genomics Hum. Genet. **3:** 67–99.
4. SCHEUNER, D. *et al.* 1996. Secreted amyloid beta-protein similar to that in the senile plaques of Alzheimer's disease is increased in vivo by the presenilin 1 and 2 and APP mutations linked to familial Alzheimer's disease. Nat. Med. **2:** 864–780.

5. CORDER, E.H. *et al.* 1993. Gene dose of apolipoprotein E type 4 allele and the risk of Alzheimer's disease in late onset families. Science **261:** 921–923.
6. MCGEER, E.G. & P.L. MCGEER. 2003. Inflammatory processes in Alzheimer's disease. Prog. Neuropsychopharmacol. Biol. Psychiatry **27:** 741–749.
7. NELSON, P.T., L.A. SOMA & E. LAVI. 2002. Microglia in diseases of the central nervous system. Ann. Med. **34:** 491–500.
8. AKIYAMA, H. *et al.* 2000. Inflammation and Alzheimer's disease. Neurobiol. Aging **21:** 383–421.
9. DEL RIO HORTEGA, P. 1919. El 'tercer elemento' de los centros nerviosos. Poder fagocitario y movilidad de la microglia. Bol. Soc. Esp. Biol. Ano. **9:** 154–166.
10. KOUTSILIERI, E. *et al.* 2002. Degeneration of neuronal cells due to oxidative stress—microglial contribution. Parkinsonism Relat. Disord. **8:** 401–406.
11. MCGEER, P.L., S. ITAGAKI & E. G. MCGEER. 1988. Expression of the histocompatibility glycoprotein HLA-DR in neurological disease. Acta Neuropathol. (Berl.) **76:** 550–557.
12. ROGERS, J. & L.F. LUE. 2001. Microglial chemotaxis, activation, and phagocytosis of amyloid beta-peptide as linked phenomena in Alzheimer's disease. Neurochem. Int. **39:** 333–340.
13. WYSS-CORAY, T. & L. MUCKE. 2002. Inflammation in neurodegenerative disease—a double-edged sword. Neuron **35:** 419–432.
14. AKIYAMA, H. *et al.* 1996. Granules in glial cells of patients with Alzheimer's disease are immunopositive for C-terminal sequences of beta-amyloid protein. Neurosci. Lett. **206:** 169–172.
15. FUNATO, H. *et al.* 1998. Astrocytes containing amyloid beta-protein (Abeta)-positive granules are associated with Abeta40-positive diffuse plaques in the aged human brain. Am. J. Pathol. **152:** 983–992.
16. FRAUTSCHY, S.A., G.M. COLE & A. BAIRD. 1992. Phagocytosis and deposition of vascular beta-amyloid in rat brains injected with Alzheimer beta-amyloid. Am. J. Pathol. **140:** 1389–1399.
17. WELDON, D.T. *et al.* 1998. Fibrillar beta-amyloid induces microglial phagocytosis, expression of inducible nitric oxide synthase, and loss of a select population of neurons in the rat CNS in vivo. J. Neurosci. **18:** 2161–2173.
18. ARD, M.D. *et al.* 1996. Scavenging of Alzheimer's amyloid beta-protein by microglia in culture. J. Neurosci. Res. **43:** 190–202.
19. ROGERS, J. *et al.* 2002. Elucidating molecular mechanisms of Alzheimer's disease in culture models. *In* Neuroinflammation—From Bench to Bedside, pp. 25–44. Springer. Heidelberg.
20. AKIYAMA, H. & P.L. MCGEER. 2004. Specificity of mechanisms for plaque removal after A beta immunotherapy for Alzheimer disease. Nat. Med. **10:** 117–118 [author reply, pp. 118–119].
21. FRACKOWIAK, J. *et al.* 1992. Ultrastructure of the microglia that phagocytose amyloid and the microglia that produce beta-amyloid fibrils. Acta Neuropathol. (Berl.) **84:** 225–233.
22. WYSS-CORAY, T. *et al.* 2003. Adult mouse astrocytes degrade amyloid-beta in vitro and in situ. Nat. Med. **9:** 453–457.
23. ISHIZUKA, K. *et al.* 1997. Identification of monocyte chemoattractant protein-1 in senile plaques and reactive microglia of Alzheimer's disease. Psychiatry Clin. Neurosci. **51:** 135–138.
24. HOKE, A. *et al.* 1994. Regional differences in reactive gliosis induced by substrate-bound beta-amyloid. Exp. Neurol. **130:** 56–66.
25. SHAFFER, L.M. *et al.* 1995. Amyloid beta protein (A beta) removal by neuroglial cells in culture. Neurobiol. Aging **16:** 737–745.
26. WEGIEL, J. *et al.* 2000. Microglia cells are the driving force in fibrillar plaque formation, whereas astrocytes are a leading factor in plague degradation. Acta Neuropathol. (Berl.) **100:** 356–364.
27. STALDER, M. *et al.* 1999. Association of microglia with amyloid plaques in brains of APP23 transgenic mice. Am. J. Pathol. **154:** 1673–1684.
28. WEGIEL, J. & H.M. WISNIEWSKI. 1990. The complex of microglial cells and amyloid star in three-dimensional reconstruction. Acta Neuropathol. (Berl.) **81:** 116–124.

29. WEGIEL, J. *et al.* 2001. The role of microglial cells and astrocytes in fibrillar plaque evolution in transgenic APP(SW) mice. Neurobiol. Aging **22:** 49–61.
30. GRIFFIN, W.S. *et al.* 1989. Brain interleukin 1 and S-100 immunoreactivity are elevated in Down syndrome and Alzheimer disease. Proc. Natl. Acad. Sci. USA **86:** 7611–7615.
31. GRIFFIN, W.S. *et al.* 1998. Glial-neuronal interactions in Alzheimer's disease: the potential role of a 'cytokine cycle' in disease progression. Brain Pathol. **8:** 65–72.
32. DiPATRE, P.L. & B.B. GELMAN. 1997. Microglial cell activation in aging and Alzheimer disease: partial linkage with neurofibrillary tangle burden in the hippocampus. J. Neuropathol. Exp. Neurol. **56:** 143–149.
33. GRAMMAS, P. & R. OVASE. 2002. Cerebrovascular transforming growth factor-beta contributes to inflammation in the Alzheimer's disease brain. Am. J. Pathol. **160:** 1583–1587.
34. XIA, M.Q. *et al.* 1998. Immunohistochemical study of the beta-chemokine receptors CCR3 and CCR5 and their ligands in normal and Alzheimer's disease brains. Am. J. Pathol. **153:** 31–37.
35. HESSELGESSER, J. & R. HORUK. 1999. Chemokine and chemokine receptor expression in the central nervous system. J. Neurovirol. **5:** 13–26.
36. WALKER, D.G., S.U. KIM & P.L. MCGEER. 1995. Complement and cytokine gene expression in cultured microglial derived from postmortem human brains. J. Neurosci. Res. **40:** 478–493.
37. FIALA, M. *et al.* 1998. Amyloid-beta induces chemokine secretion and monocyte migration across a human blood–brain barrier model. Mol. Med. **4:** 480–489.
38. SHENG, J.G., R.E. MRAK & W.S. GRIFFIN. 1995. Microglial interleukin-1 alpha expression in brain regions in Alzheimer's disease: correlation with neuritic plaque distribution. Neuropathol. Appl. Neurobiol. **21:** 290–301.
39. GRIFFIN, W.S. *et al.* 1994. Microglial interleukin-1 alpha expression in human head injury: correlations with neuronal and neuritic beta-amyloid precursor protein expression. Neurosci. Lett. **176:** 133–136.
40. SCHWAB, C., M. HOSOKAWA & P.L. MCGEER. 2004. Transgenic mice overexpressing amyloid beta protein are an incomplete model of Alzheimer disease. Exp. Neurol. **188:** 52–64.
41. FRAUTSCHY, S.A. *et al.* 1998. Microglial response to amyloid plaques in APPsw transgenic mice. Am. J. Pathol. **152:** 307–317.
42. MASLIAH, E. *et al.* 1996. Comparison of neurodegenerative pathology in transgenic mice overexpressing V717F beta-amyloid precursor protein and Alzheimer's disease. J. Neurosci. **16:** 5795–5811.
43. SASAKI, A. *et al.* 2002. Amyloid cored plaques in Tg2576 transgenic mice are characterized by giant plaques, slightly activated microglia, and the lack of paired helical filament-typed, dystrophic neurites. Virchows Arch. **441:** 358–367.
44. ODDO, S. *et al.* 2003. Triple-transgenic model of Alzheimer's disease with plaques and tangles: intracellular Abeta and synaptic dysfunction. Neuron **39:** 409–421.
45. WISNIEWSKI, H.M., M. BARCIKOWSKA & E. KIDA. 1991. Phagocytosis of beta/A4 amyloid fibrils of the neuritic neocortical plaques. Acta Neuropathol. (Berl.) **81:** 588–590.
46. ABBAS, N. *et al.* 2002. Up-regulation of the inflammatory cytokines IFN-gamma and IL-12 and down-regulation of IL-4 in cerebral cortex regions of APP(SWE) transgenic mice. J. Neuroimmunol. **126:** 50–57.
47. TEHRANIAN, R. *et al.* 2001. Early induction of interleukin-6 mRNA in the hippocampus and cortex of APPsw transgenic mice Tg2576. Neurosci. Lett. **301:** 54–58.
48. CAGNIN, A. *et al.* 2001. In-vivo measurement of activated microglia in dementia. Lancet **358:** 461–467.
49. LEE, V.M., M. GOEDERT & J.Q. TROJANOWSKI. 2001. Neurodegenerative tauopathies. Annu. Rev. Neurosci. **24:** 1121–1159.
50. GOEDERT, M. 2004. Tau protein and neurodegeneration. Semin. Cell Dev. Biol. **15:** 45–49.
51. ISHIZAWA, K. & D.W. DICKSON. 2001. Microglial activation parallels system degeneration in progressive supranuclear palsy and corticobasal degeneration. J. Neuropathol. Exp. Neurol. **60:** 647–657.
52. IQBAL, K. & I. GRUNDKE-IQBAL. 2002. Neurofibrillary pathology leads to synaptic loss and not the other way around in Alzheimer disease. J. Alzheimers Dis. **4:** 235–238.

53. HALL, G.F. *et al.* 2000. Human tau filaments induce microtubule and synapse loss in an in vivo model of neurofibrillary degenerative disease. J. Cell Sci. **113:** 1373–1387.
54. TERRY, R.D. *et al.* 1991. Physical basis of cognitive alterations in Alzheimer's disease: synapse loss is the major correlate of cognitive impairment. Ann. Neurol. **30:** 572–580.
55. DeKOSKY, S.T. & S.W. SCHEFF. 1990. Synapse loss in frontal cortex biopsies in Alzheimer's disease: correlation with cognitive severity. Ann. Neurol. **27:** 457–464.
56. COLLINS, S.J. *et al.* 1995. Progressive supranuclear palsy: neuropathologically based diagnostic clinical criteria. J. Neurol. Neurosurg. Psychiatry **58:** 167–173.
57. LI, Y. *et al.* 2003. Interleukin-1 mediates pathological effects of microglia on tau phosphorylation and on synaptophysin synthesis in cortical neurons through a p38-MAPK pathway. J. Neurosci. **23:** 1605–1611.
58. SHENG, J.G. *et al.* 2001. Interleukin-1 promotion of MAPK-p38 overexpression in experimental animals and in Alzheimer's disease: potential significance for tau protein phosphorylation. Neurochem. Int. **39:** 341–348.
59. SHENG, J.G. *et al.* 2000. Interleukin-1 promotes expression and phosphorylation of neurofilament and tau proteins in vivo. Exp. Neurol. **163:** 388–391.
60. PUIG, B., F. VINALS & I. FERRER. 2004. Active stress kinase p38 enhances and perpetuates abnormal tau phosphorylation and deposition in Pick's disease. Acta Neuropathol. (Berl.) **107:** 185–189.
61. QUINTANILLA, R.A. *et al.* 2004. Interleukin-6 induces Alzheimer-type phosphorylation of tau protein by deregulating the cdk5/p35 pathway. Exp. Cell Res. **295:** 245–257.
62. STONE, T.W. 1993. Neuropharmacology of quinolinic and kynurenic acids. Pharmacol. Rev. **45:** 309–379.
63. GUILLEMIN, G.J. *et al.* 2003. A beta 1-42 induces production of quinolinic acid by human macrophages and microglia. Neuroreport **14:** 2311–2315.
64. CHAN, S.F. & N.J. SUCHER. 2001. An NMDA receptor signaling complex with protein phosphatase 2A. J. Neurosci. **21:** 7985–7992.
65. SOFIC, E. *et al.* 1989. Brain quinolinic acid in Alzheimer's dementia. Eur. Arch. Psychiatry Neurol. Sci. **239:** 177–119.
66. MORONI, F. *et al.* 1986. Senile dementia and Alzheimer's disease: lack of changes of the cortical content of quinolinic acid. Neurobiol. Aging **7:** 249–253.
67. ALVAREZ, A. *et al.* 1999. Inhibition of tau phosphorylating protein kinase cdk5 prevents beta-amyloid-induced neuronal death. FEBS Lett. **459:** 421–426.
68. WEISHAUPT, J.H. *et al.* 2003. Inhibition of CDK5 is protective in necrotic and apoptotic paradigms of neuronal cell death and prevents mitochondrial dysfunction. Mol. Cell. Neurosci. **24:** 489–502.
69. LI, B.S. *et al.* 2003. Cyclin-dependent kinase-5 is involved in neuregulin-dependent activation of phosphatidylinositol 3-kinase and Akt activity mediating neuronal survival. J. Biol. Chem. **278:** 35702–35709.
70. KEROKOSKI, P. *et al.* 2001. The levels of cdk5 and p35 proteins and tau phosphorylation are reduced during neuronal apoptosis. Biochem. Biophys. Res. Commun. **280:** 998–1002.
71. PEI, J.J. *et al.* 1998. Accumulation of cyclin-dependent kinase 5 (cdk5) in neurons with early stages of Alzheimer's disease neurofibrillary degeneration. Brain Res. **797:** 267–277.
72. SPILLANTINI, M.G. *et al.* 1998. Mutation in the tau gene in familial multiple system tauopathy with presenile dementia. Proc. Natl. Acad. Sci. USA **95:** 7737–7741.
73. HUTTON, M. *et al.* 1998. Association of missense and 5′-splice-site mutations in tau with the inherited dementia FTDP-17. Nature **393:** 702–705.
74. POORKAJ, P. *et al.* 1998. Tau is a candidate gene for chromosome 17 frontotemporal dementia. Ann. Neurol. **43:** 815–825.
75. BEHL, C. 1999. Vitamin E and other antioxidants in neuroprotection. Int. J. Vitam. Nutr. Res. **69:** 213–219.
76. BEHL, C. & B. MOOSMANN. 2002. Antioxidant neuroprotection in Alzheimer's disease as preventive and therapeutic approach. Free Radic. Biol. Med. **33:** 182–191.
77. MEDA, L. *et al.* 2002. Activation of microglial cells by β-amyloid protein and interferon-γ. Nature **374:** 647–650.
78. QIN, L. *et al.* 2002. Microglia enhance beta-amyloid peptide-induced toxicity in cortical and mesencephalic neurons by producing reactive oxygen species. J. Neurochem. **83:** 973–983.

79. HALKS-MILLER, M., M. HENDERSON & L.F. ENG. 1986. Alpha tocopherol decreases lipid peroxidation, neuronal necrosis, and reactive gliosis in reaggregate cultures of fetal rat brain. J. Neuropathol. Exp. Neurol. **45:** 471–484.
80. LI, Y. *et al.* 2001. Vitamin E suppression of microglial activation is neuroprotective. J. Neurosci. Res. **66:** 163–170.
81. SUNG, S. *et al.* 2004. Early vitamin E supplementation in young but not aged mice reduces Abeta levels and amyloid deposition in a transgenic model of Alzheimer's disease. FASEB J. **18:** 323–325.
82. LAURIN, D. *et al.* 2004. Midlife dietary intake of antioxidants and risk of late-life incident dementia: the Honolulu-Asia Aging Study. Am. J. Epidemiol. **159:** 959–967.
83. LUCHSINGER, J.A. *et al.* 2003. Antioxidant vitamin intake and risk of Alzheimer disease. Arch. Neurol. **60:** 203–208.
84. MASAKI, K.H. *et al.* 2000. Association of vitamin E and C supplement use with cognitive function and dementia in elderly men. Neurology **54:** 1265–1272.
85. ONOFRJ, M. *et al.* 2002. Donepezil versus vitamin E in Alzheimer's disease: Part 2: mild versus moderate-severe Alzheimer's disease. Clin. Neuropharmacol. **25:** 207–215.
86. SOBOW, T. & I. KLOSZEWSKA. 2003. Donepezil plus vitamin E as a treatment in Alzheimer disease. Alzheimer Dis. Assoc. Disord. **17:** 244.
87. ENGELHART, M.J. *et al.* 2002. Dietary intake of antioxidants and risk of Alzheimer disease. J. Am. Med. Assoc. **287:** 3223–3229.
88. ZANDI, P.P. *et al.* 2004. Reduced risk of Alzheimer disease in users of antioxidant vitamin supplements: the Cache County Study. Arch. Neurol. **61:** 82–88.
89. MORRIS, M.C. *et al.* 1998. Vitamin E and vitamin C supplement use and risk of incident Alzheimer disease. Alzheimer Dis. Assoc. Disord. **12:** 121–126.
90. MORRIS, M.C. *et al.* 2002. Dietary intake of antioxidant nutrients and the risk of incident Alzheimer disease in a biracial community study. J. Am. Med. Assoc. **287:** 3230–3237.
91. SANO, M. *et al.* 1997. A controlled trial of selegiline, alpha-tocopherol, or both as treatment for Alzheimer's disease. The Alzheimer's Disease Cooperative Study. N. Engl. J. Med. **336:** 1216–1222.
92. AISEN, P. S. 1997. Inflammation and Alzheimer's disease: mechanisms and therapeutic strategies. Gerontology **43:** 143–149.
93. MCGEER, P. L., M. SCHULZER & E. G. MCGEER. 1996. Arthritis and anti-inflammatory agents as possible protective factors for Alzheimer's disease: a review of 17 epidemiologic studies. Neurology **47:** 425–432.
94. ERIKSEN, J.L. *et al.* 2003. NSAIDs and enantiomers of flurbiprofen target gamma-secretase and lower Abeta 42 in vivo. J. Clin. Invest. **112:** 440–449.
95. MACKENZIE, I.R. & D.G. MUNOZ. 1998. Nonsteroidal anti-inflammatory drug use and Alzheimer-type pathology in aging. Neurology **50:** 986–990.
96. YASOJIMA, K. *et al.* 1999. Distribution of cyclooxygenase-1 and cyclooxygenase-2 mRNAs and proteins in human brain and peripheral organs. Brain Res. **830:** 226–236.
97. ANDREASSON, K.I. *et al.* 2001. Age-dependent cognitive deficits and neuronal apoptosis in cyclooxygenase-2 transgenic mice. J. Neurosci. **21:** 8198–8209.
98. XIANG, Z. *et al.* 2002. Cyclooxygenase-2 promotes amyloid plaque deposition in a mouse model of Alzheimer's disease neuropathology. Gene Expr. **10:** 271–278.
99. SALZBERG-BRENHOUSE, H.C. *et al.* 2003. Inhibitors of cyclooxygenase-2, but not cyclooxygenase-1 provide structural and functional protection against quinolinic acid-induced neurodegeneration. J. Pharmacol. Exp. Ther. **306:** 218–228.
100. NOGAWA, S. *et al.* 1997. Cyclo-oxygenase-2 gene expression in neurons contributes to ischemic brain damage. J. Neurosci. **17:** 2746–2755.
101. YERMAKOVA, A.V. *et al.* 1999. Cyclooxygenase-1 in human Alzheimer and control brain: quantitative analysis of expression by microglia and CA3 hippocampal neurons. J. Neuropathol. Exp. Neurol. **58:** 1135–1146.
102. HOOZEMANS, J.J. *et al.* 2003. Non-steroidal anti-inflammatory drugs and cyclooxygenase in Alzheimer's disease. Curr. Drug Targets **4:** 461–468.
103. ZANDI, P.P. *et al.* 2002. Reduced incidence of AD with NSAID but not H2 receptor antagonists: the Cache County Study. Neurology **59:** 880–886.
104. STEWART, W.F. *et al.* 1997. Risk of Alzheimer's disease and duration of NSAID use. Neurology **48:** 626–632.

105. IN T' VELD, B.A. *et al.* 2001. Nonsteroidal antiinflammatory drugs and the risk of Alzheimer's disease. N. Engl. J. Med. **345:** 1515–1521.
106. LIM, G.P. *et al.* 2000. Ibuprofen suppresses plaque pathology and inflammation in a mouse model for Alzheimer's disease. J. Neurosci. **20:** 5709–5714.
107. YAN, Q. *et al.* 2003. Anti-inflammatory drug therapy alters beta-amyloid processing and deposition in an animal model of Alzheimer's disease. J. Neurosci. **23:** 7504–7509.
108. WEGGEN, S. *et al.* 2001. A subset of NSAIDs lower amyloidogenic Abeta42 independently of cyclooxygenase activity. Nature **414:** 212–216.
109. ROGERS, J. *et al.* 1993. Clinical trial of indomethacin in Alzheimer's disease. Neurology **43:** 1609–1611.
110. SCHARF, S. *et al.* 1999. A double-blind, placebo-controlled trial of diclofenac/misoprostol in Alzheimer's disease. Neurology **53:** 197–201.
111. AISEN, P.S., J. SCHMEIDLER & G.M. PASINETTI. 2002. Randomized pilot study of nimesulide treatment in Alzheimer's disease. Neurology **58:** 1050–1054.
112. SAINATI, S. *et al.* 2000. Results of a double-blind, randomized, placebo-controlled study of celecoxib in the treatment of progression of Alzheimer's disease. Sixth International Stockholm/Springfield Symposium on Advances in Alzheimer Therapy, Stockholm, April, 180 (abstr.).
113. REINES, S.A. *et al.* 2004. Rofecoxib: no effect on Alzheimer's disease in a 1-year, randomized, blinded, controlled study. Neurology **62:** 66–71.
114. AISEN, P.S. *et al.* 2003. Effects of rofecoxib or naproxen vs. placebo on Alzheimer disease progression: a randomized controlled trial. J. Am. Med. Assoc. **289:** 2819–2826.
115. VAN GOOL, W.A. *et al.* 2001. Effect of hydroxychloroquine on progression of dementia in early Alzheimer's disease: an 18-month randomised, double-blind, placebo-controlled study. Lancet **358:** 455–460.
116. EIKELENBOOM, P. & W.A. VAN GOOL. 2004. Neuroinflammatory perspectives on the two faces of Alzheimer's disease. J. Neural Transm. **111:** 281–294.
117. AISEN, P.S. 2002. Evaluation of selective COX-2 inhibitors for the treatment of Alzheimer's disease. J. Pain Symptom Manage. **23:** S35–40.
118. JANTZEN, P.T. *et al.* 2002. Microglial activation and beta -amyloid deposit reduction caused by a nitric oxide-releasing nonsteroidal anti-inflammatory drug in amyloid precursor protein plus presenilin-1 transgenic mice. J. Neurosci. **22:** 2246–2254.
119. SCHENK, D. *et al.* 1999. Immunization with amyloid-beta attenuates Alzheimer-disease-like pathology in the PDAPP mouse. Nature **400:** 173–177.
120. WILCOCK, D.M. *et al.* 2004. Passive amyloid immunotherapy clears amyloid and transiently activates microglia in a transgenic mouse model of amyloid deposition. J. Neurosci. **24:** 6144–6151.
121. WILCOCK, D.M. *et al.* 2003. Intracranially administered anti-Abeta antibodies reduce beta-amyloid deposition by mechanisms both independent of and associated with microglial activation. J. Neurosci. **23:** 3745–3751.
122. BARD, F. *et al.* 2000. Peripherally administered antibodies against amyloid beta-peptide enter the central nervous system and reduce pathology in a mouse model of Alzheimer disease. Nat. Med. **6:** 916–919.
123. SOLOMON, B. *et al.* 1996. Monoclonal antibodies inhibit in vitro fibrillar aggregation of the Alzheimer beta-amyloid peptide. Proc. Natl. Acad. Sci. USA **93:** 452–455.
124. DEMATTOS, R.B. *et al.* 2002. Brain to plasma amyloid-beta efflux: a measure of brain amyloid burden in a mouse model of Alzheimer's disease. Science **295:** 2264–2267.
125. DEMATTOS, R.B. *et al.* 2001. Peripheral anti-A beta antibody alters CNS and plasma A beta clearance and decreases brain A beta burden in a mouse model of Alzheimer's disease. Proc. Natl. Acad. Sci. USA **98:** 8850–8855.
126. JANUS, C. *et al.* 2000. A beta peptide immunization reduces behavioural impairment and plaques in a model of Alzheimer's disease. Nature **408:** 979–982.
127. MORGAN, D. *et al.* 2000. A beta peptide vaccination prevents memory loss in an animal model of Alzheimer's disease. Nature **408:** 982–985.
128. SCHENK, D. 2002. Amyloid-beta immunotherapy for Alzheimer's disease: the end of the beginning. Nat. Rev. Neurosci. **3:** 824–828.
129. SENIOR, K. 2002. Dosing in phase II trial of Alzheimer's vaccine suspended. Lancet Neurol. **1:** 3.

130. ORGOGOZO, J.M. *et al.* 2003. Subacute meningoencephalitis in a subset of patients with AD after Abeta42 immunization. Neurology **61:** 46–54.

131. HOCK, C. *et al.* 2002. Generation of antibodies specific for beta-amyloid by vaccination of patients with Alzheimer disease. Nat. Med. **8:** 1270–1275.

132. WEINER, H.L. & D.J. SELKOE. 2002. Inflammation and therapeutic vaccination in CNS diseases. Nature **420:** 879–884.

133. NICOLL, J.A. *et al.* 2003. Neuropathology of human Alzheimer disease after immunization with amyloid-beta peptide: a case report. Nat. Med. **9:** 448–452.

134. HOCK, C. *et al.* 2003. Antibodies against beta-amyloid slow cognitive decline in Alzheimer's disease. Neuron **38:** 547–554.

135. HARDY, J. & D.J. SELKOE. 2002. The amyloid hypothesis of Alzheimer's disease: progress and problems on the road to therapeutics. Science **297:** 353–356.

136. ODDO, S. *et al.* 2004. Abeta immunotherapy leads to clearance of early, but not late, hyperphosphorylated tau aggregates via the proteasome. Neuron **43:** 321–332.

Inflammation and the Degenerative Diseases of Aging

PATRICK L. McGEER AND EDITH G. McGEER

Kinsmen Laboratory of Neurological Research, University of British Columbia, Vancouver, British Columbia, Canada

ABSTRACT: Chronic inflammation is associated with a broad spectrum of neurodegenerative diseases of aging. Included are such disorders as Alzheimer's disease (AD), Parkinson's disease (PD), amyotrophic lateral sclerosis, the Parkinson-dementia complex of Guam, all of the tauopathies, and age-related macular degeneration. Also included are such peripheral conditions as osteoarthritis, rheumatoid arthritis, atherosclerosis, and myocardial infarction. Inflammation is a two-edged sword. In acute situations, or at low levels, it deals with the abnormality and promotes healing. When chronically sustained at high levels, it can seriously damage viable host tissue. We describe this latter phenomenon as autotoxicity to distinguish it from autoimmunity. The latter involves a lymphocyte-directed attack against self proteins. Autotoxicity, on the other hand, is determined by the concentration and degree of activation of tissue-based monocytic phagocytes. Microglial cells are the brain representatives of the monocyte phagocytic system. Biochemically, the intensity of their activation is related to a spectrum of inflammatory mediators generated by a variety of local cells. The known spectrum includes, but is not limited to, prostaglandins, pentraxins, complement components, anaphylotoxins, cytokines, chemokines, proteases, protease inhibitors, adhesion molecules, and free radicals. This spectrum offers a huge variety of targets for new anti-inflammatory agents. It has been suggested, largely on the basis of transgenic mouse models, that stimulating inflammation rather than inhibiting it can be beneficial in such diseases as AD. If this were the case, administration of NSAIDs, or other anti-inflammatory drugs, would be expected to exacerbate conditions such as AD, PD, and atherosclerosis. However, epidemiological evidence overwhelmingly demonstrates that the reverse is true. This indicates that, at least in these diseases, the inflammation is harmful. So far, advantage has not been taken of opportunities indicated by these epidemiological studies to treat AD and PD with appropriate anti-inflammatory agents. Based on this evidence, classical NSAIDs are the most logical choice. Dosage, though, must be sufficient to combat the inflammation. Analysis of mRNA levels of inflammatory mediators indicates that the intensity of inflammation is considerably higher in AD hippocampus and in PD substantia nigra than in osteoarthritic joints. Thus, full therapeutic doses of NSAIDs, or combinations of anti-inflammatory agents, are needed to achieve the suggested neurological benefits.

Address for correspondence: Dr. Patrick L. McGeer, Kinsmen Laboratory of Neurological Research, University of British Columbia, 2255 Wesbrook Mall, Vancouver, British Columbia V6T 1Z3, Canada. Voice: 604-822-7380; fax: 604-822-7086.
mcgeerpl@interchange.ubc.ca

Ann. N.Y. Acad. Sci. 1035: 104–116 (2004). © 2004 New York Academy of Sciences.
doi: 10.1196/annals.1332.007

KEYWORDS: Alzheimer's disease; Parkinson's disease; amyotrophic lateral sclerosis; tauopathies; osteoarthritis; rheumatoid arthritis; atherosclerosis; myocardial infarction; NSAIDs

INTRODUCTION

Aging is associated with a greatly increased incidence of a number of degenerative conditions, including Alzheimer's disease (AD), Parkinson's disease (PD), amyotrophic lateral sclerosis (ALS), atherosclerosis, and myocardial infarction. All of these conditions are associated with a chronic inflammation which, while not causative, may greatly influence the pathogenesis. Accordingly, there may be potential for anti-inflammatory therapy. There have been several reviews recently published on inflammatory changes in AD,[1,2] PD,[3,4] and ALS.[5] In this paper, we only touch on some aspects that appear to offer therapeutic opportunities. Moreover, much of the emphasis will be on AD since research on inflammation has been particularly intensive in that condition.

The concept of inflammation, and particularly neuroinflammation, has undergone a major transformation in recent years. Classically, it had been equated with a prominent invasion of the brain by leukocytes.[6] Such an invasion occurs in all types of CNS infection—in presumed autoimmune diseases, such as multiple sclerosis, and in injuries or strokes where the blood-brain barrier is breached. However, this restricted view has failed to take into account landmark discoveries of the past that illustrated the local nature of inflammation. It was Metchnikoff[7] who first provided insight into this phenomenon. He impaled starfish larvae with rose thorns and noticed mesenchymal cells, which he named phagocytes, gathering around the site of injury. He concluded that inflammation was primarily a local phenomenon and that dolor, tumor, rubor, and calor, the cardinal inflammatory signs of Celsus, were a secondary reaction caused by exudation of serum elements into tissue. Del Rio Hortega[8] identified microglia as the phagocytes of brain and established that they were of mesenchymal origin. Van Furth[9] provided closure with his description of the monocyte phagocytic system. He showed that all tissue-based phagocytes were originally derived from monocytes and that they migrated into tissues to provide a first line of defense.

These concepts, particularly with regard to the origin and function of microglia, were regarded with considerable skepticism until recent years,[10] when more sophisticated molecular biological techniques became available. Now that the *in vivo* and *in vitro* properties of microglia have been more appropriately defined,[1,11] it is generally recognized that their activation signifies a primary inflammatory state and that leukocyte invasion, when it occurs, is a secondary phenomenon.

CELLULAR EVIDENCE

The key cellular event signaling the presence of neuroinflammation is the accumulation of reactive microglia in the degenerating areas. Clumps of activated microglia appear on the senile plaques in AD. Activated microglia are also evident in

TABLE 1. Some factors involved in microglia/macrophage activation[19]

	Classical	Alternative
Activating signals	IFN-γ, TNF	IL-4, glucocorticoids
Secretory products	TNF, IL-12, IL-1, IL-6	IL-1RA, IL-10
Biological markers	MHC class II, CD86, scavenger receptor, CD23	CD163, mannose receptor
Killer molecules	NO, O^{2-}	None
Chemokine production	IL-10, MIP-1α, MCP-1	AMAC-1

surrounding tissue.[12,13] Few, if any activated microglia, are seen in similar regions in control brains. Activated microglia are also seen in affected regions in PD[3] and ALS.[5] In gray matter, the cells become hypertrophied to form the classic morphology described by Hortega[8] and Penfield.[14] The cell body enlarges and the processes become thickened and retracted. In white matter, the cells may become engorged with myelin products, lose their processes, and become "fat granule cells," as originally described by Penfield. It is interesting that, years after the ingestion of MPTP, highly activated microglia are seen in the substantia nigra of both humans[15] and monkeys,[16] attesting to the chronicity of the inflammation. In a similar fashion, many activated macrophages are found in the arterial plaques of atherosclerosis[17] and in infarcted heart tissue years after an acute event.[18]

There is considerable debate as to whether activated microglia/macrophages are beneficial or harmful. There is much *in vitro* evidence that highly activated microglia/macrophages produce neurotoxic materials (see next section). However, they are also fundamentally beneficial because of their phagocytic potential and their ability to destroy invading pathogens. The problem lies in preventing them from destroying viable host tissue.

There is emerging evidence that macrophages may be activated to an anti-inflammatory state rather than the classical inflammatory state.[19] Stimulating such activation could be beneficial in chronic inflammatory states. Classical activation, which can be initiated by interferon-gamma (IFN-γ) and other factors such as lipopolysaccharide (LPS), results in a flooding of surrounding tissue with inflammatory mediators, oxidizing free radicals, pro-apoptotic factors, and matrix-degrading proteases (TABLE 1). The system is designed to dispatch foreign microbes but may result in considerable damage to viable host tissue.

Alternate activation may be initiated by interleukin-4 (IL-4) or glucocorticoids. The macrophage/microglia then secrete leukocyte-attracting chemokines, anti-inflammatory cytokines, and some extracellular matrix (ECM) components (TABLE 1). Factors secreted by alternatively activated macrophages/microglia promote cell proliferation, angiogenesis, and ECM reconstruction, thus promoting wound repair. Anti-inflammatory type activation may be distinguished by the upregulation of CD163. CD163 (M130) is a member of the scavenger receptor cysteine-rich (SRCR) superfamily, which is expressed by monocytes and macrophages. CD163 expression is suppressed by proinflammatory mediators like LPS, IFN-γ, and tumor necrosis factor-alpha (TNF-α), whereas IL-6 and the anti-inflammatory cytokine IL-10 strongly upregulate CD163 mRNA in monocytes and macrophages.[19]

A third type of activation has been reported to be initiated by ligation of Fcγ receptors (FcγRs), coupled with a macrophage stimulatory signal through any of the Toll-like receptors (TLRs), CD40, or CD44. This results in production of large amounts of IL-10. This can even occur in IFN-γ–primed macrophages, where the IL-12 production is cut off and IL-10 induced. However, the production of many of the other cytokines, such as TNF, IL-1, and IL-6 is unaffected.[19]

Much of the work on alternate forms of activation has been done on murine cells, which are easily followed because of their abundant production of NO following classical activation. It remains to be established whether similar alternative pathways can be induced in human macrophages/microglia.

Clearly it would be beneficial in AD and the other degenerative diseases characterized by chronic inflammation to switch from proinflammatory type macrophages to anti-inflammatory type. Whether this can be done while maintaining, or even stimulating phagocytosis, remains to be established. It is the phagocytic capacity that is counted upon to remove Aβ deposits following vaccination of amyloid precursor protein (APP) transgenic mouse models with Aβ. Whether proinflammatory microglia are harmful or beneficial may depend upon the degree of activation. Microglia in human AD are very highly activated, while those in the unvaccinated transgenic mice are less highly activated.[20]

BIOCHEMICAL EVIDENCE: OXIDATIVE STRESS, NEUROTOXINS, AND TYPES OF COMPOUNDS INVOLVED

Inflammation generates oxidative stress. It has long been suspected that oxidative stress contributes to neuronal death in diseases such as AD, PD, and ALS. The source of oxygen free radicals has usually been attributed to accidental leakage from the electron transport chain of mitochondria. However the most abundant source of oxygen free radicals in the central nervous system (CNS) is the respiratory burst system of activated microglia. When the system is turned on, large numbers of superoxide ions are generated on the microglial external membrane, from where they are released as a purposeful attack system.[21,22] Other, less abundant sources of free radicals are xanthine oxidase and nitric oxide synthase.

Evidence of free radical attack in AD cortex,[1,23,24] PD substantia nigra,[3] and ALS spinal cord[5] includes the presence of proteins that have been modified by glycation, the existence of low molecular weight compounds that have been oxidized and nitrated (such as 4-hydroxynonenal, malondialdehyde, 3-nitrotyrosine, 3-nitro-4-hydroxyphenylacetic acid, 5-nitrotocopherol, and 8-hydroxy-deoxyguanosin), and the identification of lipids that have been peroxidated. The nitrated products are mostly derived from peroxynitrite, a reaction product of nitric oxide and superoxide anions.

Activated microglia are also a source of neurotoxic materials other than free radicals. The damaging effects can be observed *in vivo*[25] as well as *in vitro*.[26,27] Glutamate has been identified as one potential neurotoxin released by activated microglia,[28] but there are others of low molecular weight that have not been identified. It seems probable that a combination of materials is responsible for the observed neurotoxic effects.[27]

The glial activation described should also be accompanied by numerous other inflammatory biochemical changes. Studies of AD tissue give some indication of the families of compounds whose production might be altered. These include complement proteins and complement inhibitors, pentraxins and other acute phase reactants, inflammatory cytokines, chemokines, anaphylotoxins, integrins, coagulation and fibrinolytic factors, prostaglandins, apolipoproteins and selective proteases, and protease inhibitors. Numerous reviews on the subject have appeared,[1,11,29] and the discussion here is limited to the complement proteins, pentraxins, and inflammatory cytokines because these appear to be major actors in the inflammatory phenomenon.

COMPLEMENT PROTEINS

A prominent part of the inflammatory reaction in these degenerative diseases is activation of the classical complement pathway. Complement is a sophisticated attack system designed to destroy invaders and to assist in the phagocytosis of waste materials. The complement system has components to carry out four major functions: recognition, opsonization, inflammatory stimulation through anaphylatoxins, and direct killing through the membrane attack complex (MAC). The classical pathway is activated by attachment of C1q to a target causing C1 dissociation. Amplification takes place through a cascade of proteases (C1r, C1s, C4, C2, C3) and the cleavage products C4d and C3d attach to exposed sites close to the C1q binding site. Covalent bonds are formed between exposed thiol esters on these cleavage fragments and hydroxyl or amino groups on the target tissue. This marks the target for opsonization since the attached complement fragments become ligands for complement receptors on phagocytes, which, in the case of brain, are microglia. If the complement system is fully activated, it proceeds to assemble the terminal components (C5b, C6, C7, C8, C9) into the lytic macromolecule C5b-9, known as the MAC. The MAC is intended to insert itself into foreign bacteria and viruses, but, if host cells are inadequately protected, it may damage them as well in a process called bystander lysis. Meanwhile, the small fragments C3a, C4a, and C5a, known as anaphylotoxins, stimulate inflammation. So the overall cascade identifies, opsonizes, and destroys its target, while dispatching messengers to seek help.

The tangles and plaques that are the hallmarks of AD are clearly marked with the activated complement fragments C4d and C3d.[1,29] They are not seen in control brain. Dystrophic neurites in AD brain are immunostained for the MAC,[29,30] indicating autolytic attack. Again such staining is not seen in control brains. The MAC has a very short half-life so that the abundant staining for the MAC in AD brain suggests such attack is responsible for much of the neurite loss in AD. Staining for the MAC is also seen in the substantia nigra in PD.[3]

How is complement activated in such cases? Traditional immunology would suggest antibody activity, but work on AD has demonstrated vigorous activation of complement in the absence of antibodies. A key finding regarding the mechanism of complement activation was that of Rogers and colleagues,[31] who demonstrated that amyloid protein (Aβ), when aggregated, was a strong complement activator. Thus, the senile plaques of AD have a unique activator of complement. In addition, the complement cascade can be activated by the pentraxins, amyloid P and C-reactive

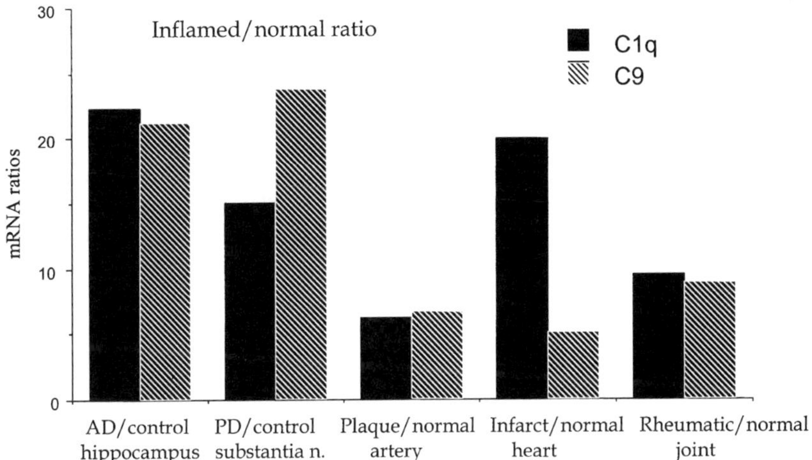

FIGURE 1. Ratio of mRNAs in inflamed and normal tissue for C1q and C9 in AD compared to normal hippocampus, PD compared to normal substantia nigra, atherosclerotic plaque compared to normal artery, infarcted heart compared to normal heart, and rheumatic joint compared to normal joint tissue. The rheumatic joint tissue was removed surgically because of intractable pain. (Data from Yasojima and colleagues[17,18,86] and unpublished data.)

protein, which are both upregulated in affected regions of AD brain.[32] Other molecules, as yet unidentified, may be responsible for the activation of the complement cascade in PD and ALS.

An estimate of the activity of the complement system in any tissue can be obtained by measurement of the relative mRNA levels. Fortunately, the coding regions of mRNAs appear to be surprisingly stable in postmortem tissue.[33] The mRNAs for complement proteins are sharply upregulated in affected regions of AD and PD brain, with the upregulation being greater than that seen in rheumatoid arthritis where active inflammation is established (FIG. 1). Thus it appears probable that, in these conditions, neurons are being progressively destroyed by complement self-attack. This we have termed autotoxicity.[29]

There are many steps in the complement cascade so that multiple opportunities exist for therapeutic intervention. The intervention, however, should not be of a nature that would seriously compromise the ability of the host to combat infection. One possibility that separates antibody activation of complement from that by Aβ or the pentraxins is the nature of C1q binding. Aβ, C-reactive protein (CRP), and amyloid P (AP) all activate the complement cascade by binding to the collagen tail of C1q, while antibodies bind to its globular head.[32] Thus, agents that block binding to the collagen tail of C1q might be effective therapeutic agents because they would not disturb antibody attack against an infectious agent.

Blocking formation of the MAC might be the most attractive method of limiting autotoxicity. Inhibiting this self attack could leave the more critical opsonization process undisturbed. Thus, high selectivity in inhibiting the damaging aspects of complement activation could be provided while the valuable function of phagocytosing debris could be preserved.

Examples of some inhibitors that block other steps in the complement cascade are the 13-residue cyclic peptide compstatin and the negatively charged sulfated glycosaminoglycan pentosan polysulfate (PPS). Compstatin binds to C3 and prevents its cleavage, thus inhibiting activation of both the classical and alternative complement pathways.[34] It has shown activity in a pig xenograft model.[35] PPS is an orally active, heparin-like compound that has been approved for the treatment of interstitial cystitis. It has been shown to prolong survival in a heterotopic rat cardiac transplant model[36] and to reduce myocardial infarct in a rabbit ischemia/reperfusion model.[37] Whether either would reach the brain *in vivo* is unknown, but these examples do demonstrate the possibility of designing synthetic complement inhibitors.

THE PENTRAXINS

The pentraxins may be important activators of the complement system in AD brain[38,39] since both are found extensively in affected regions. It had been generally believed for many years that CRP and AP were produced in the liver and carried in the circulation to other organs. The presence of AP in the brain in AD was even taken as an indication of leakage in the blood/brain barrier.[40] Application of molecular genetic techniques has made it possible to demonstrate that both CRP and AP, like the complement proteins, are produced locally in brain and that their production is sharply upregulated in areas damaged by AD.[41] Neurons are the most prominent generators of both. CRP is associated with damaged fibers within AD senile plaques, while AP is associated with the extracellular amyloid deposits.[42] Since they cannot activate the complement cascade unless appropriately bound, agents that block the binding of pentraxins to viable host tissue, or otherwise inhibit their ability to activate complement, might be of therapeutic benefit in reducing autotoxic attack in AD.

CYTOKINES

Cytokines are a heterogeneous group of small molecules that act in autocrine and paracrine fashion. They encompass several subfamilies that include interleukins (ILs), interferons (INFs), tumor necrosis factors (TNFs), growth factors, colony-stimulating factors, and chemokines. They have in common participation in inflammatory reactions. They typically act in combination so that attributing a specific set of *in vivo* properties to any given cytokine is difficult.

Only a few of the cytokines have been extensively studied in AD or PD. A finding of particular interest is that the risk of AD seems to be substantially influenced by several polymorphisms in the non-coding regions of these inflammatory genes.[43–54] The risk of PD is also reported to be influenced by a polymorphism in IL-1β.[55,56] The polymorphisms are in promoter and untranslated regions. Those alleles that favor increased expression of the inflammatory mediators are more frequent in AD and PD than in controls.

The polymorphisms reported to influence the risk for AD are fairly common ones in the general population, so there is a strong likelihood that any given individual will inherit one or more of the high risk alleles. The odds ratio for a single one of these polymorphisms is much lower than for polymorphisms in apolipoprotein E (apoE), where different forms of the protein are expressed. Inheritance of the apoE4 form substantially increases the risk of AD.[57] Moreover, the risk of AD in carriers of the apoE4 allele is substantially increased by carrying the high risk allele of TNFα.[50] It has also been reported that the odds ratio for contracting AD is greatly increased if an individual carries two of the high risk alleles for inflammatory cyto-kines.[54] For example, Nicoll and colleagues[51] found that simultaneous inheritance of the high risk alleles for IL-1α−889 and IL-1β+3953 increased the odds ratio for developing AD to 10.8. The overall chances of an individual developing AD might be profoundly affected by a "susceptibility profile" reflecting the combined influ-ence of inheriting multiple high risk alleles.[58] Identification of such profiles might in the future lead to strategies for therapeutic intervention in the very early stages of the disorder.

Each of the polymorphisms found to be a significant risk factor for AD has also been linked to at least one peripheral inflammatory condition. The implication is that an inflammatory stimulus is more likely to cause autotoxic damage at a vulnerable site in any one of numerous disorders in those individuals carrying genetic poly-morphisms that enhance inflammatory mediator expression.

The importance of TNFα as an inflammatory stimulus is emphasized by the widespread use in rheumatoid arthritis of TNFα blockers. Infliximab is an antibody to TNFα and etanercept is a TNF receptor–Fc fusion protein. Both types of TNFα inhibition induce a rapid improvement in multiple clinical measures of disease activity and patient functional status, as well as a beneficial effect on progression of joint damage as measured radiographically.[59,60] Infliximab has also been shown to be effective in Crohn's disease.[61]

Chemokines are a large subfamily of cytokines of relatively low molecular weight (8−14 kDa). So far, more than 50 members have been discovered, but their involvement in AD or other neuropathology has not been explored much. They may, however, have a significant influence on microglial activity. The cytokine fractalkine, and its receptor CX3CR-1, may prove to be particularly interesting. Fractalkine is produced by neurons and exists in a bound as well as a free state. When neurons are exposed to excitotoxic damage, fractalkine is cleaved prior to neuronal death.[62] An antibody to fractalkine markedly reduced the neurotoxic effects of microglia stimu-lated by lipopolysaccharide.[63] These data suggest that fractalkine might be a neuro-protective agent *in vivo*, being cleaved under neuronal stress and acting to reduce microglial activation. Agonists of CX3C-R1 might therefore be effective anti-inflammatory agents.

Clearly, research into defining the precise roles of chemokines in neuroinflamma-tion in general is a priority for the future.

POSSIBLE USE OF ANTI-INFLAMMATORY DRUGS
AS THERAPEUTIC AGENTS

The inflammatory reaction in these degenerative neurological disorders could be interpreted as representing nothing more than an epiphenomenon in which detritus, secondary to an unrelated degenerative phenomenon, is being scavenged. However, the inflammatory reaction in AD and PD is robust enough to favor the existence of a more aggressive process. In such a case, anti-inflammatory drugs might slow the disease progression.

There are now more than 20 published epidemiological studies that show that people known to be taking anti-inflammatory agents, or known to be suffering from conditions such as arthritis for which such agents are routinely used have a considerably reduced risk of developing AD.[64–68] Despite one negative report,[69] the evidence indicates that long term use of conventional NSAIDs reduces the risk by 60%[66] to 80%.[68] And one report[70] indicates that chronic use of NSAIDs reduces the risk of PD by 45%. Some anti-inflammatory drugs, such as selected NSAIDs and tetracyclines, are also reported to be protective in the 6-hydroxydopamine and MPTP models of PD.[3,4]

Can anti-inflammatory agents be used to treat these diseases? For this possibility to be realized, appropriate agents must be selected. They should act on targets based on correlations between epidemiology and molecular pathology. The need for such correlations is illustrated by failures in clinical trials in AD of prednisone, the COX-2 inhibitors celecoxib and nimesulide, and hydroxychloroquine.[71–74] These agents were known to be effective in treating arthritic conditions but there was little or no evidence that they would be useful in neuroinflammation. Steroids may be particularly bad because they themselves cause hippocampal damage.[75]

As far as selective COX-2 inhibitors are concerned, they have not been in use long enough for epidemiological data to accumulate, but immunohistochemical evidence was available that indicated they should fail. Unlike COX-1, COX-2 is highly expressed in normal pyramidal neurons, as well as in pyramidal neurons of AD cases.[76] Therefore, selective COX-2 inhibitors will primarily target pyramidal neurons rather than microglia. This, combined with evidence of exacerbation of neuronal death in some animal neurotoxicity models following COX-2 inhibition, suggests COX-2 inhibitors are an inappropriate choice.[77]

Hydroxychloroquine is not a general anti-inflammatory agent. Its mechanism of action in arthritis is uncertain. It is noteworthy, however, that while its main side effects are ototoxicity and retinal damage, some include neuronal damage.[78] Since there is no epidemiological or immunohistochemical evidence to support a role for hydroxychloroquine or other 4-aminoquinolines in neuroinflammation, the failure to be effective in AD is not surprising although disappointing.

The situation with respect to traditional NSAIDs is quite different. The epidemiological evidence in favor of their protective effect in AD is very strong. Moreover, one small, double-blind clinical trial of indomethacin, a COX-1 inhibitory NSAID, in established AD indicated arrest of progression.[79] Another NSAID trial, involving the mixed inhibitor diclofenac combined with misoprostyl, showed marginally less deterioration in drug compared with placebo patients, although the data fell short of statistical significance.[80] A significantly slower cognitive decline compared to placebo was also reported in a small group of Japanese cases treated with a combination of estrogen, vitamin E, and an NSAID.[81] In *in vitro* experiments, NSAIDs have been shown to reduce the neurotoxicity of activated microglia to cultured neuroblastoma cells.[82] Clearly, properly designed clinical trials of COX-1–inhibiting NSAIDs that reach the brain should be a high priority for AD. Relatively high doses may be required due to the strong inflammatory reaction present in established AD. Low dosage may have been the problem in the recent, failed trial with naproxen.[83] Gastrointestinal and other side effects are a problem with such agents, particularly at high doses, with chronic use and in the aged.[84] While such side effects are significant, they may be small in comparison with the inevitable progression and fatal outcome of AD with currently approved methods of treatment. It is possible that a new class of COX-1 inhibiting NSAIDs, based on introducing a nitrate ester moiety, may circumvent the side effect problem. These so-called NO-NSAIDs have greatly reduced gastrointestinal toxicity.[85]

Other types of anti-inflammatory agents may also be effective. The spectrum of inflammatory mediators upregulated in AD suggests many routes for future therapeutic intervention. It may be that multiple drug administration, targeted at different inflammatory mechanisms, will prove far more effective than utilization of any single agent. In many cases, the data suggest exploiting targets that so far have not been considered important in the immunological field.

ACKNOWLEDGMENTS

This work was supported by the Jack Brown and Family Alzheimer Disease Research Fund, the George Hodson estate, and grants from the Alzheimer Society of Canada/CIHR/Astra-Zeneca.

REFERENCES

1. NEUROINFLAMMATION WORKING GROUP. 2000. Inflammation and Alzheimer's disease. Neurobiol. Aging **21:** 383–421.
2. McGEER, E.G. & P.L. McGEER. 2003. Inflammatory processes in Alzheimer's disease. Progr. Neuro-Psychopharmacol. Biol. Psychiatry **27:** 741–749.
3. McGEER, P.L. & E.G. McGEER. 2004. Inflammation and neurodegeneration in Parkinson's disease. Parkinsonism Relat. Disord. **10:** S3–S7.
4. MADHAVI, T. *et al.* 2003. Minocycline and other tetracycline derivatives: a neuroprotective strategy in Parkinson's disease and Huntington's disease. Clin. Neuropharmacol. **26:** 18–23.
5. McGEER, P.L. & E.G. McGEER. 2002. Inflammatory processes in amyotrophic lateral sclerosis. Muscle Nerve **26:** 459–470.
6. HAYMAKER, W. & R.D. ADAMS, Eds. 1982. Histology and Histopathology of the Nervous System, pp. 1150–1173. Charles C. Thomas. Springfield, IL.
7. METCHNIKOFF, E. 1892. Lecons sur la pathologie comparée de l'inflammation. Masson. Paris.
8. DEL RIO HORTEGA, P. 1919. El 'tercer elemento' de los centros nerviosos. Poder fagocitario y movilidad de la microglia. Bol. Soc. Esp. Biol. Ano. **9:** 154–166.
9. VAN FURTH, R. 1982. Current view on the mononuclear phagocyte system. Immunobiology **161:** 178–185.
10. DAVIS, R.L. & D.M. ROBERTSON, Eds. 1991. Textbook of Neuropathology. Second edition, pp. 141–163. Williams & Wilkins. Baltimore.
11. McGEER, P.L. & E.G. McGEER. 1995. The inflammatory response system of brain: implications for therapy of Alzheimer and other neurodegenerative disease. Brain Res. Rev. **21:** 195–218.
12. LUBER-NAROD, J. & J. ROGERS. 1988. Immune system associated antigens expressed by cells of the human central nervous system. Neurosci. Lett. **94:** 265–273.
13. McGEER, P.L. *et al.* 1988. Expression of the histocompatibility glycoprotein HLA-DR in neurological disease. Acta Neuropathol. **76:** 550–557.

14. PENFIELD, W. 1925. Microglia and the process of phagocytosis in gliomas. Am. J. Pathol. **1:** 77–89.
15. LANGSTON, J.W. *et al.* 1999. Evidence of active nerve cell degeneration in the substantia nigra of humans years after 1-methyl-4-phenyl-1,2,3,6-tetrahydropyridine exposure. Ann. Neurol. **46:** 598–605.
16. McGEER, P.L. *et al.* 2003. Presence of reactive microglia in monkey substantia nigra years after 1-methyl-4-phenyl-1,2,3,4-tetrahydropyridine administration. Ann. Neurol. **54:** 599–604.
17. YASOJIMA, K. *et al.* 2001. Complement components, but not complement inhibitors, are upregulated in atherosclerotic plaques. Arterioscler. Thromb. Vasc. Biol. **21:** 1214–1219.
18. YASOJIMA, K. *et al.* 1998. Human heart generates complement proteins that are upregulated and activated after myocardial infarction. Circ. Res. **83:** 860–869.
19. MOSSER, D.M. 2003. The many faces of macrophage activation. J. Leukoc. Biol. **73:** 209–212.
20. SCHWAB, C. *et al.* 2004. Transgenic mice overexpressing amyloid beta-protein are an incomplete model of Alzheimer disease. Exp. Neurol. **188:** 52–64.
21. COLTON, C.A. & D.I. GILBERT. 1987. Production of superoxide anions by a CNS macrophage, the microglia. FEBS Lett. **223:** 284–288.
22. KLEGERIS, A. & P.L. McGEER. 1994. Rat brain microglia and peritoneal macrophages show similar responses to respiratory burst stimulants. J. Neuroimmunol. **53:** 83–90.
23. BUTTERFIELD, D.A. & J. KANSKI. 2001. Brain protein oxidation in age-related neurodegenerative disorders that are associated with aggregated proteins. Mech. Aging Dev. **122:** 945–962.
24. WILLIAMSON, K.S. *et al.* 2002. The nitration product 5-nitro-gamma-tocopherol is increased in the Alzheimer brain. Nitric Oxide **6:** 221–227.
25. BANATI, R.B. *et al.* 1993. Cytotoxicity of microglia. Glia **7:** 111–118.
26. GIULIAN, D. *et al.* 1996. Specific domains of β-amyloid from Alzheimer plaque elicit neuronal killing in human microglia. J. Neurosci. **16:** 6021–6037.
27. KLEGERIS, A. & P.L. McGEER. 2000. Interaction of various intrasignalling mechanisms involved in mononuclear phagocyte toxicity towards neuronal cells. J. Leukoc. Biol. **67:** 127–133.
28. KLEGERIS, A. *et al.* 1997. Regulation of glutamate in cultures of human monocytic THP-1 and astrocytoma U-373 MG cells. J. Neuroimmunol. **78:** 152–161.
29. McGEER, P.L. & E.G. McGEER. 2001. Inflammation, autotoxicity and Alzheimer disease. Neurobiol. Aging **22:** 799–809.
30. WEBSTER, S. *et al.* 1997, Molecular and cellular characterization of the membrane attack complex, C5b-9, in Alzheimer's disease. Neurobiol. Aging **18:** 415–421.
31. ROGERS, J. *et al.* 1992. Complement activation by β-amyloid in Alzheimer disease. Proc. Natl. Acad. Sci. USA **89:** 10016–10020.
32. McGEER, E.G. *et al.* 2001. The pentraxins: possible role in Alzheimer's disease and other innate inflammatory disorders. Neurobiol. Aging **22:** 843–848.
33. YASOJIMA, K. *et al.* 2001. High stability of mRNAs postmortem and protocols for their assessment by RT-PCR. Brain Res. Protocols **8:** 212–218.
34. FURLONG, S.T. *et al.* 2000. C3 activation is inhibited by analogs of compstatin but not by serine protease inhibitors or peptidyl alpha-ketoheterocycles. Immunopharmacology **48:** 199–212.
35. FIANE, A.E. *et al.* 1999. Compstatin, a peptide inhibitor of C3, prolongs survival of ex vivo perfused pig xenografts. Xenotransplantation **6:** 52–65.
36. SCHWARTZ, C.F. *et al.* 1999. Increased rat cardiac allograft survival by the glycosaminoglycan pentosan polysulfate. J. Surg. Res. **86:** 24–28.
37. TANHEHCO, E.J. *et al.* 1999. Reduction of myocardial infarct size after ischemia and reperfusion by the glycosaminoglycan pentosan polysulfate. J. Cardiovas. Pharm. **34:** 153–161.
38. JIANG, H. *et al.* 1992. Localization of sites through which C-reactive protein binds to and activates complement to residues 14-26 and 76-92 of the human C1q A chain. J. Exp. Med. **175:** 1373–1379.
39. HICKS, P.S. *et al.* 1992. Serum amyloid P component binds to histones and activates the classical complement pathway. J. Immunol. **149:** 3689–3694.

40. KALARIA, R.N. & I. GRAHOVAC. 1990. Serum amyloid P immunoreactivity in hippocampal tangles, plaques and vessels: implications for leakage across the blood-brain barrier in Alzheimer's disease. Brain Res. **516:** 349–353.
41. YASOJIMA, K. *et al.* 2000. Human neurons generate C-reactive protein and amyloid P: upregulation in Alzheimer's disease. Brain Res. **887:** 80–89.
42. AKIYAMA, H. *et al.* 1991. Association of amyloid P component with complement proteins in neurologically diseased tissue. Brain Res. **548:** 349–352.
43. BLACKER, D. *et al.* 1998. Alpha-2-macroglobulin is genetically associated with Alzheimer disease. Nature Genetics **19:** 357–360.
44. COLLINS, J.S. *et al.* 2000. Association of a haplotype for tumor necrosis factor in siblings with late-onset Alzheimer disease: the NIMH Alzheimer disease genetics initiative. Am. J. Med. Genet. **96:** 823–830.
45. DU, Y. *et al.* 2000. Association of an interleukin 1 alpha polymorphism with Alzheimer's disease. Neurology **55:** 480–483.
46. GRIMALDI, L.M. *et al.* 2000. Association of early-onset Alzheimer's disease with an interleukin-1a gene polymorphism. Ann. Neurol. **47:** 361–365.
47. KAMBOH, M.I. *et al.* 1997. Genetic effect of alpha-1-antichymotrypsin on the risk of Alzheimer disease. Genomics **40:** 382–384.
48. LICASTRO, F. *et al.* 2000. Polymorphisms of the IL-6 gene increase the risk for late onset Alzheimer's disease and affect IL-6 plasma levels. Neurobiol. Aging **21:** S38.
49. LICASTRO, F. *et al.* 2000. Gene polymorphism affecting α1-antichymotrypsin and interleukin-1 plasma levels increases Alzheimer's disease risk. Ann. Neurol. **48:** 388–391.
50. McCUSKER, S.M. 2001. Association between polymorphism in regulatory region of gene encoding tumour necrosis factor α and risk of Alzheimer's disease and vascular dementia: a case-control study. Lancet **357:** 436–439.
51. NICOLL, J.A.R. *et al.* 2000, Association of interleukin-1 gene polymorphisms with Alzheimer's disease. Ann. Neurol. **47:** 365–368.
52. PAPASSOTIROPOULOS, A. *et al.* 1999. A genetic variation of the inflammatory cytokine interleukin-6 delays the initial onset and reduces the risk for sporadic Alzheimer's disease. Ann. Neurol. **45:** 666–668.
53. REBECK, G.W. 2000. Confirmation of the genetic association of interleukin-1α with early onset sporadic Alzheimer's disease. Neurosci. Lett. **293:** 75–77.
54. HEDLEY, R. *et al.* 2002. Association of interleukin-1 polymorphisms with Alzheimer's disease in Australia. Ann. Neurol. **51:** 795-797.
55. SCHULTE, T. *et al.* 2000. Polymorphisms in the interleukin-1 alpha and beta genes and the risk for Parkinson's disease. Neurosci. Lett. **326:** 70–72.
56. McGEER, P.L. *et al.* 2000. Association of interleukin-1β polymorphism with idiopathic Parkinson's disease. Neurosci. Lett. **326:** 67–69.
57. STRITTMATTER, W.J. *et al.* 1993. Apolipoprotein E: high avidity binding to β-amyloid and increased frequency of type 4 allele in late-onset familial Alzheimer disease. Proc. Natl. Acad. Sci. USA **90:** 1977–1981.
58. McGEER, P.L. & E.G. McGEER. 2001. Polymorphisms in inflammatory genes enhance the risk of Alzheimer disease. Arch. Neurol. **58:** 1790-1792.
59. ALLDRED, A. 2001. Etanercept in rheumatoid arthritis. Exp. Opin. Pharmacother. **1:** 1137–1148.
60. HAMILTON, K. & E.W. CLAIR. 2000. Tumour necrosis factor-alpha blockade: a new era for the effective management of rheumatoid arthritis. Exp. Opin. Pharmacother. **1:** 1041–1052.
61. FEAGAN, B.G. *et al.* 2001. Infliximab for the treatment of Crohn's disease: efficacy, safety and pharmacoeconomics. Can. J. Clin. Pharmacol. **8:** 188–198.
62. CHAPMAN, G.A. *et al.* 2000. Fractalkine cleavage from neuronal membranes represents an acute event in the inflammatory response to excitotoxic brain damage. J. Neurosci. **20:** 2–6.
63. ZUJOVIC, V. *et al.* 2000. Fractalkine modulates TNF-alpha secretion and neurotoxicity induced by microglial activation. Glia **29:** 305–315.
64. BROE, G.A. *et al.* 2000. Anti-inflammatory drugs protect against Alzheimer disease at low doses. Arch. Neurol. **57:** 1586–1591.

65. McGeer, P.L. *et al.* 1996. Arthritis and antiinflammatory agents as possible protective factors for Alzheimer's disease: a review of 17 epidemiological studies. Neurology **147:** 425–432.
66. Szekely, C.A. *et al.* 2004. Nonsteroidal anti-inflammatory drugs for the prevention of Alzheimer's disease: a systematic review. Neuroepidemiology **23:** 159–169.
67. Stewart, W.F. *et al.* 1997. Risk of Alzheimer's disease and duration of NSAID use. Neurology **48:** 626–632.
68. Veld, B.A. *et al.* 2001 Non-steroidal antiinflammatory drug use and risk of Alzheimer's disease. New Engl. J. Med. **345:** 1515–1521.
69. Wolfson, C. *et al.* 2002. A case-control analysis of nonsteroidal anti-inflammatory drugs and Alzheimer's disease: are they protective? Neuroepidemiology **21:** 81–86.
70. Chen, H. *et al.* 2002. Nonsteroidal antiinflammatory drugs and the risk of Parkinson's disease. Movement Dis. **17:** S143–S144.
71. Aisen, P.S. *et al.* 2000. A randomized controlled trial of prednisone in Alzheimer's disease. Neurology **54:** 588–593.
72. Aisen. P.S., *et al.* 2002. Randomized pilot study of nimesulide in Alzheimer's disease. Neurology **58:** 1050–1054.
73. Sainali, S.M. *et al.* 2000. Results of a double-blind, placebo-controlled study of celecoxib for the progression of Alzheimer's disease. *In* Sixth International Stockholm-Springfield Symposium of Advances in Alzheimer Therapy, p. 180.
74. Van Gool, W.A. *et al.* 2001. Effect of hydroxychloroquine on progression of dementia in early Alzheimer's disease: an 18-month randomized, double-blind, placebo-controlled study. Lancet **358:** 455–460.
75. Hoschl, C. & T. Hajek. 2001. Hippocampal damage mediated by corticosteroids—a neuropsychiatric research challenge. Eur. Arch. Psychiatry & Clin. Neurosci. **251:** II81–I188.
76. Yasojima, K. *et al.* 1999. Distribution of cyclooxygenase-1 and cyclooxygenase-2 mRNAs and proteins in human brain and peripheral organs. Brain Res. **830:** 226–236.
77. McGeer, P.L. 2000. Cyclo-oxygenase-2 inhibitors.Drugs Aging **17:** 1–11.
78. Stein, M. *et al.* 2000. Hydroxychloroquine neuromyotoxicity. J. Rheumatol. **27:** 2927–2931.
79. Rogers, J. *et al.* 1993. Clinical trial of indomethacin in Alzheimer's disease. Neurology **43:** 1609–1611.
80. Scharf, S. *et al.* 1999. A double-blind, placebo-controlled trial of diclofenac misoprostol in Alzheimer's disease. Neurology **53:** 197–201.
81. Arai, H. *et al.* 2000. A new interventional strategy for Alzheimer's disease by Japanese herbal medicine. Jap. J. Ger. **37:** 212–215.
82. Klegeris, A. *et al.* 1999. Toxicity of human THP-1 monocytic cells towards neuron-like cells is reduced by non-steroidal anti-inflammatory drugs (NSAIDs). Neuropharmacology **38:** 1017-1025.
83. Aisen, P.S. *et al.* 2003. Effects of rofecoxib or naproxen vs. placebo on Alzheimer disease progression: a randomized controlled trial. J. Am. Med. Assoc. **289:** 2819–2826.
84. Capell, H.A. 2001. Disease modifying antirheumatic drugs: longterm safety issues. J. Rheumatol. (Suppl.) **62:** 10–15.
85. Wallace, J.L. *et al.* 1995. Nitric oxide-releasing NSAIDs: a novel class of GI-sparing anti-inflammatory drugs. Agents Actions (Suppl.) **46:** 121–129.
86. Yasojima, K. *et al.* 1999. Complement regulators C1 inhibitor and CD59 do not significantly inhibit complement activation in Alzheimer disease. Brain Res. **833:** 297–301.

Inflammation, Neurodegenerative Diseases, and Environmental Exposures

AREZOO CAMPBELL

Department of Community and Environmental Medicine, University of California, Irvine, Irvine, California 92697, USA

ABSTRACT: The etiology of neurodegenerative disorders is multifactorial and consists of an interaction between aging, environmental factors, and genetic predisposition. Neuronal cell loss in specific regions of the central nervous system and the resulting clinical symptoms are used to characterize different neurological syndromes. While the selectivity of neuronal cell death is not clearly understood, it is in part attributed to the physiological role and microenvironment of the impacted cells. In this review, innate immune responses in the central nervous system are described. Chronic upregulation of this pathway, orchestrated mainly by microglial cells, may jeopardize neuronal integrity through the prolonged production of toxic inflammatory mediators. Environmental exposures that further enhance the innate immune response may accelerate microglia-driven neurodegeneration. Environmental factors that can trigger inflammatory events in the central nervous system are lipopolysaccharide, aluminum, and particulate matter present in air pollution. These factors may enhance existing age-related inflammation in the central nervous system and thus accelerate neuronal toxicity.

KEYWORDS: neuroinflammation; neurodegenerative diseases; lipopolysaccharide; aluminum; particulate matter; air pollution

INTRODUCTION

Recent studies have shown that there is a strong link between inflammation and neurodegeneration. While this may in part be a consequence of the disease process, it is now clear that it can also directly contribute to formation of pathological lesions characteristic of neurological disorders. The purpose of this review is to describe the function of innate immune responses in the central nervous system (CNS) and to illustrate how chronic activation of this system may lead to neuronal cell loss. The focus will be on four neurological syndromes in which inflammatory events may play a role.

Multiple sclerosis is an autoimmune disorder in which cells attack myelin sheaths in both the peripheral and central nervous system leading to progressive loss in nerve conduction. Alzheimer's disease is characterized by gradual cell death in the hippo-

Address for correspondence: A. Campbell, Department of Community and Environmental Medicine, University of California, Irvine, Irvine, CA 92697-1825. Voice: 949-824-3439; fax: 949-824-2070.

aghadimi@uci.edu

Ann. N.Y. Acad. Sci. 1035: 117–132 (2004). © 2004 New York Academy of Sciences.
doi: 10.1196/annals.1332.008

campus and the frontal cortex, eventually leading to severe memory loss. In Parkinson's disease, there is extensive loss of dopaminergic neurons in the substantia nigra, which results in a unique movement disorder. Amyotrophic lateral sclerosis is a condition in which motor neurons are selectively destroyed, leading to paralysis and eventual death.

While familial forms of these diseases have been linked to mutations in specific genetic loci, a majority of cases are idiopathic. Thus environmental factors play a role in their pathogenesis. In the present review the potential role of three environmental factors, known to upregulate innate immune responses, will be evaluated. Lipopolysaccharide (LPS), a component of the cell wall of gram-negative bacteria, is a classical proinflammogen. Aluminum is a ubiquitous metal present in pharmaceutical agents, food, and drinking water. The potential adverse effect of this metal in the CNS is a controversial subject and under close scrutiny. Exposure to particulate matter present in air pollution is thought to be responsible for cardiovascular mortality. However, not much is known about the adverse effects in the CNS. Since the exposure is mainly through inhalation, there is a potential for compounds to enter the brain rapidly through the cribriform plate of the ethmoid bone, resulting in direct activation of innate immune responses in this organ. While acute activation of inflammatory events is a necessary component of the CNS defense against foreign antigens, unresolved stimulation and prolonged activation can lead to chronic inflammation which can eventually result in neuronal cell death.

INTERRELATIONSHIP BETWEEN INFLAMMATION, NEURODEGENERATION, AND ENVIRONMENTAL EXPOSURES

Innate Immune Response in the CNS

The immune system comprises a complex interrelated network of cellular, molecular, and chemical mediators that function to protect the body against environmental stress factors. These stressors can be as diverse as microorganisms (viral, bacterial, fungal agents), physical damage (burns, lacerations), or environmental toxins (snake venoms, nonessential metals, chemicals). The first line of defense is innate or natural immunity. The inflammatory component of this response is important in recruiting cells of the immune system to the compromised area. The mediators for this function are cytokines and chemokines. While the former orchestrate a specific response that is appropriate based on the type of foreign antigen that has penetrated the tissue, the latter factors are important in allowing cells of the immune system to reach the area under attack.

Although the brain has been considered immunologically privileged, it is now evident that innate immunity is present and plays an important role in defending this organ against foreign antigens and clearing debris resulting from normal age-related deterioration. Microglial cells, which can be activated to become phagocytic, are the main cellular component of innate immunity in the brain. Astrocytic cells are also important in that they provide a healthy microenvironment for neurons. They also contribute to the blood-brain barrier (BBB) by forming processes that surround the endothelial cells of the cerebral microvasculature (FIG. 1).

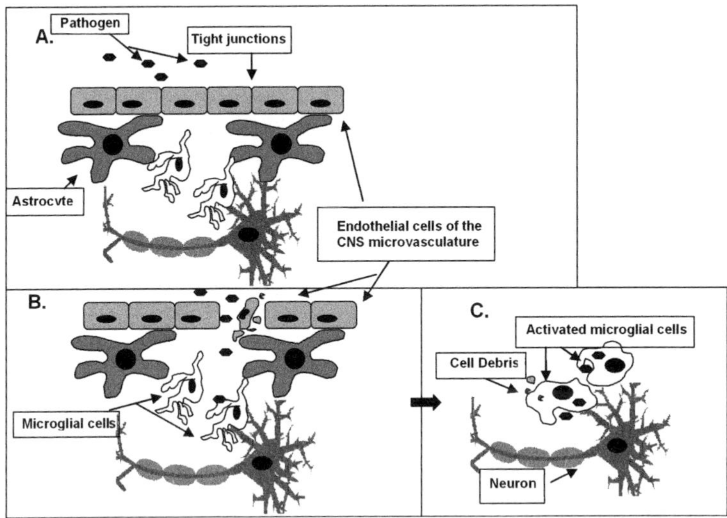

FIGURE 1. Innate immune responses in the CNS. (**A**) The CNS is protected from the entry of pathogens in the systemic circulation by the presence of the BBB, the main component of which is the tight junctions in between the endothelial cells comprising the cerebral microvasculature. (**B**) Deterioration of the BBB during the natural course of aging can leave areas of the CNS compromised. Pathogens can then enter the brain. The astrocytic cell processes that are another component of the BBB can function as a barrier. However, this may not always be sufficient. (**C**) Once pathogens have accessed the brain, microglial cells will be activated. The ramified morphological shape typical of quiescent microglia is changed to the amoeboid structure typical of activated phagocytic cells. These will clear both cellular debris and pathogens. Once this is accomplished, the inflammatory response subsides.

While the innate immune response had been considered to be non-specific, the identification of the evolutionarily well-conserved toll-like receptors (TLR) has revolutionized this idea. These are transmembrane receptors linked to signaling pathways that activate immune responses. To this date, ten different TLRs have been identified and they are shown to be specifically activated by unique structures present on pathogens known as pathogen-associated molecular patterns (PAMPs). Except for TLR 8 and TLR10, the ligand for all of these receptors has been identified.[1] For example, TLR9 selectively recognizes unmethylated CpG oligonucleotides, which are usually released by bacteria,[2] and the main ligand for TLR4 is LPS.[3] In the brain and spinal cord, expression of TLR in glial cells has been documented and this expression is increased during neuroinflammatory events.[4]

Stimulation of TLR leads to activation of NF-κB, a transcription factor involved in the innate immune response.[5–7] This promotes the expression of genes involved in inflammation, such as tumor necrosis factor–alpha (TNF-α), interleukin 1 (IL-1), inducible nitric oxide synthase (iNOS), and complement factors.[5] The importance of this protein in the CNS response to stress is evident in that activated forms of NF-κB are increased in a multitude of differing conditions, including experimental autoimmune encephalomyelitis,[8] prion disease,[9] and aluminum exposure.[10,11]

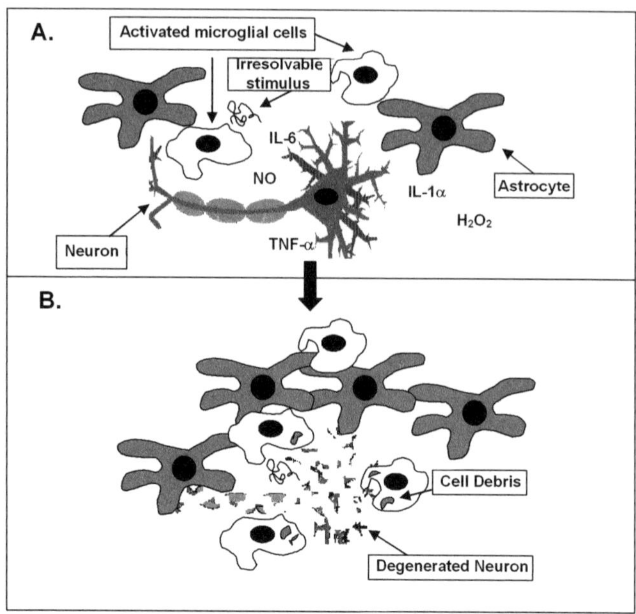

FIGURE 2. Consequences of chronic neuroinflammation. **(A)** If an inflammatory response is not resolved, prolonged stimulation of glial cells will lead to the production of proinflammatory cytokines (IL-6, TNF-α, IL-1α) and reactive oxygen species ($O_2^{\bullet-}$, NO, H_2O_2). **(B)** The glial response is incapable of resolving the stressor and prolonged production of deleterious factors will eventually lead to neuronal cell death.

The innate immune response in the CNS is necessary to resolve potential pathogenic conditions. It is usually short-lived and ensures that the stress factor is removed. Transient upregulation of inflammatory events in the brain is natural and does not lead to neuronal cell death.[12] This is because endogenous factors such as glucocorticoids moderate this response by inhibiting proinflammatory gene expression via negative feedback.[13] However, overactivation of innate immunity may lead to neurodegeneration (FIG. 2). Thus a three-day activation of microglial TLR9 by unmethylated CpG oligonucleotides led to a significant damage to neurites.[14]

Chronic Neuroinflammation in Neurodegenerative Diseases

As the brain ages, inflammatory events are upregulated.[15,16] It is possible that this is due to compromise of the BBB which may occur as a result of senescence, leading to activation and proliferation of both microglial and astrocytic cells. Cytokines, such as IL-1, IL-6, granulocyte-macrophage colony–stimulating factor (GM-CSF), and TNF-α, are synthesized. These are important for the recruitment of more microglia and macrophages to the site of infection or injury. These cells coordinate an immune response necessary for tissue regrowth and wound healing.[17] These mediators typically have a short half-life. However, irresolvable stimuli may cause chronic production of these cytokines leading to neuronal toxicity. Activated glial cells also produce reactive oxygen species (ROS). If the production of ROS is prolonged, the endogenous stores of antioxidants are exhausted and cell damage can ensue.[18]

During neuroinflammation, microglial cells produce chemokines to allow immune cells to infiltrate the CNS from the blood stream.[19] T cells, macrophages, and neutrophils can migrate into the brain by the process of diapedesis in which they squeeze between the endothelial cells of the microvasculature. This requires the interaction of adhesion molecules on both the vascular cells and leukocytes. Vascular cell adhesion molecule -1 (VCAM-1) has been shown to be important in facilitating the movement of immune cells into the brain during multiple sclerosis and experimental autoimmune encephalomyelitis (EAE), an animal model of multiple sclerosis.[20] The chemokine monocyte chemoattractant protein (MCP)-1, known as CCL2, has been implicated in the pathogenesis of EAE. Activated glial cells express mRNA for a type of CCL2 receptor known as L-CCR. During the early phases of EAE, expression of L-CCR is induced and correlated to the onset of the disease.[21] Another chemokine receptor (CXCR3) is upregulated on immune cells capable of migrating into the brain. This molecule appears to be a surface marker rather than a direct mediator of extravasation[22] and can be used in defining the subset of leukocytes capable of crossing the BBB during an inflammatory response.

Multiple Sclerosis

Multiple sclerosis (MS) is a chronic condition in which the immune system attacks the myelin sheaths surrounding neuronal axons. The site of the inflammatory damage is scarred, thus the name of the disease is derived from sclerosis meaning "scar" in Latin. Since these loci of injury can occur anywhere in the brain and spinal cord, the symptoms of the disease are usually diverse in different patients. These include fatigue, numbness, vision abnormalities, incontinence, muscle weakness, and paralysis. Patients diagnosed with MS fall into a spectrum ranging from benign, where individuals diagnosed may lead normal lives, to severe, where patients are progressively debilitated. The diagnosis is made after physical examination and neurological assessment. However, confirmation is by magnetic resonance imaging (MRI) where the demyelinated foci can be visualized.

Approximately 250,000 people in the United States are diagnosed with MS. There are more cases occurring in the northern compared to southern regions. Thus it is assumed that an environmental agent may be responsible for the onset and progression of the disease. Migration studies have provided evidence for this hypothesis in that people, who move from an area where the disease is more prevalent, to a region where the disease is rare, are at a lower risk for developing MS.[23] Furthermore, monozygotic twin studies show that genetic factors are only partial contributors, in that concordance rate is 30%.[24]

Bacterial or viral infections may be the environmental trigger of MS, but this is still uncertain.[25] Genetic predisposition also plays a role in MS and there is an association between the presence of certain major histocompatibility II (MHC-II) alleles and an increase in susceptibility to developing MS. However, individuals who carry these do not necessarily develop the disease.[24] Thus, the interaction between environmental exposures and genetic predisposition is important in the etiology of MS.[26]

MS is an autoimmune condition where foci of chronic inflammation lead to compromise of oligodendrocytes and destruction of the myelin sheath. This is followed by axonal damage and consequent neuronal degeneration.[27] Inflammation and neurodegeneration do not occur simultaneously and axonal damage and brain atrophy may follow months after an acute innate immune response.[28] Chronic exposure to ROS may account for this delay. Glutamate-mediated excitotoxicity can lead to oligodendrocyte death and both cyclooxygenase 2 (COX-2) and iNOS are found in close proximity of MS lesions.[29] A regimen consisting of anti-inflammatory and anti-excitatory factors can stop the pathogenesis in an EAE model.[30] However, cessation of treatment causes a relapse and thus chronic therapy is probably necessary to regulate the MS disease process.

Alzheimer's Disease

Alzheimer's disease is an untreatable, progressive disorder that destroys learning and memory. It is estimated that approximately four million people may now be suffering from the disease. The risk of developing AD increases with age. The two major hallmarks of Alzheimer's disease (AD) are neurofibrillary tangles (NFT) and senile plaques (SP). The former are composed of paired helical filaments (PHFs) made of hyperphosphorylated tau proteins and the latter are made of a core of aggregated amyloid-β (Aβ) peptides surrounded by reactive glia. Epidemiological studies show that familial forms of AD can be attributed to abnormalities in specific genes responsible for disease susceptibility. These findings have led to the development of transgenic animals over-expressing mutated forms of these genes.

The APP23 mouse expresses a mutant form of human amyloid precursor protein (APP). As they age, these animals develop amyloid plaques in the hippocampus and neocortex.[31] β-Site–APP cleaving enzyme (BACE) is involved in the processing of APP32 and overexpression of this protein leads to an increase in the formation of Aβ1-42 in APP23 mice.[33] Aged Aβ proteins cause an NF-κB–mediated increase in glial activation followed by induction of IL-6 and IL-1β mRNA[34] as well as iNOS gene expression.[35] Aβ activates astrocytes that produce chondroitin sulfate–containing proteoglycans (CSPG), which can then inhibit axonal growth.[36] There is regional variability in the ability of Aβ to activate astrocytes and only the hippocampal and cortical cells are able to deposit CSPG.[37] This may be one of the reasons why in AD, these areas show the most neurodegeneration.

Innate immune responses are clearly involved in Aβ-induced neuronal cell death. Exposure to the protein led to neuronal apoptosis and this required TNF type I receptors and NF-κB activation.[38] Furthermore, blocking the innate immune receptor CD14 significantly ameliorates microglial activation induced by Aβ.[39]

APP on monocytes has been shown to participate in a multisignaling complex, leading to activation of MAP kinase and subsequent production of TNF-α, COX-2, IL-1β, IL-8, and iNOS.[40] APP overexpressing mice have increased cytokine mRNA in the brain at 16 months, but not at 6 months.[41] In transgenic mice overexpressing both mutated APP and presenilin-1 protein, microglial activation is not observable until the animals are at least 12 months old. However, at earlier time points, aggregated amyloid deposits around dystrophic neurites and activated astrocytes are present.[42] It is possible that in the transgenic animal models of AD, inflammatory processes do not necessarily initiate the pathological lesions but may enhance the progression of the disease.

An increase in neuroinflammation is seen in AD patients. Levels of TNF-α in the cerebrospinal fluid of patients with "mild cognitive impairment" who after 9 months progressed to AD are significantly higher than controls.[43] The prevalence of AD in rheumatoid arthritis patients, who consume anti-inflammatory drugs over an extended period, is lower than in the normal population.[44] A review of 17 separate epidemiologic studies has confirmed that anti-inflammatory drugs may play a protective role.[45] Nonsteroidal anti-inflammatory drugs (NSAIDs) are able to suppress microglial activation and thus ameliorate inflammation associated with senile plaques.[46] Ibuprofen has been shown to decrease levels of iNOS mRNA in primary cell cultures[47] and dexamethasone reduces the release of IL-6 from human astrocytoma cells.[48]

Parkinson's Disease

While AD is the most prevalent neurological disorder in the aged population, PD is the second most common neurodegenerative disease. In the United States, approximately one million individuals have been diagnosed with the condition. Similar to AD, senescence is an important cofactor and the prevalence increases with age. The clinical symptoms of Parkinsonism are tremors, rigidity, and bradykinesia. Loss of dopaminergic neurons in the substantia nigra is the main pathological finding. Several genetic mutations have been associated with early-onset familial forms of the disease and these have shed some light on the potential mechanisms involved in the pathogenesis of PD.

Alpha synuclein (α-syn) is an evolutionarily well-conserved phosphoprotein expressed in the brain and believed to play an important role in synaptic plasticity.[49] Mutations in the α-syn gene, lead to aggregation of the protein and Lewy body formation.[50] In primary human embryonic cells derived from the mesencephalon, it has been demonstrated that dopaminergic neurons are selectively vulnerable to α-syn overexpression[51] and in a transgenic mouse expressing an α-syn mutation, the animals developed adult-onset disease which closely mimicked the symptoms of PD.[52] Mutations in the Parkinson gene are also associated with early onset PD. This gene is mainly expressed in the CNS and codes for a family of proteins involved in ubiquitination and proteosomal degradation.[53] Mutations in three other genes, DJ-1, ubiquitin carboxyl-terminal hydrolase-1 (UCHL1), and PTEN induced kinase 1 (PINK), have also been identified and these are respectively involved in oxidative stress response, ubiquitin proteosomal pathway, and mitochondrial kinase activity. These mutations imply that mitochondrial abnormalities, oxidative stress, and deregulation of protein degradation are common mechanisms in the disease process.[54]

Since the concordance rate of PD occurrence between monozygotic twins is low,[55] environmental factors play an important role in the etiology of late-onset PD. Possible environmental agents that may be contributing factors for the disease are pesticides, such as rotenone, LPS,[56] and a byproduct of synthetic heroin, 1-methyl-4-phenyl-1,2,3,6-tetrahydropyridine (MPTP). In these exposure settings, activation of microglia is found together with dopaminergic cell loss. In primary neuron-enriched or neuron-glia cultures derived from rat mesencephalon, rotenone-induced dopaminergic neurodegeneration was dependent on the presence of microglial cells. This was mediated by the production of superoxide from activated microglia.[57] The injection of LPS in the supranigral area of rat brains resulted in microglial and astroglial proliferation and these reactive glial cells were important mediators of the subsequent neuronal death.[58] Furthermore, inhibition of glial cell activation in the mouse brain decreased MPTP-induced neurotoxicity by blocking the formation of iNOS and interleukin 1β.[59]

Heightened innate immune responses are seen in the CNS of PD patients. There is an increase in the levels of proinflammatory cytokines in the CSF and nigrostriatal regions of PD brains.[60] Furthermore, extensive amounts of reactive microglia are found in the substantia nigra of PD patients.[61] These may chronically produce ROS, resulting in depletion of antioxidant stores that may jeopardize mitochondrial activity. Since aerobic respiration in mitochondria is responsible for most of the ROS produced in cells, abnormalities in these organelles may exacerbate oxidative stress. Thus, parallel to AD, NSAIDs and antioxidant therapy may benefit PD patients.

Amyotrophic Lateral Sclerosis (ALS)

ALS is a progressive neurodegenerative disease in which motor neurons in the brain and spinal cord are selectively destroyed. Worldwide, the number of cases is 1 to 2 per 100,000 individuals per year and a majority of these are idiopathic. The disease typically manifests itself during the mid-50s, although there are rare cases of early-onset ALS. The symptoms of the disease are muscle wasting and atrophy leading to eventual paralysis and death. Diagnosis is confirmed by an electromyogram, which measures the electrical activity of muscles.

Approximately 20% of familial ALS cases have been linked to a mutation in the copper-zinc superoxide dismutase (SOD1) gene. SOD is an enzyme involved in the conversion of superoxide to hydrogen peroxide. It is not known whether expression of SOD mutations in motor neurons can lead to their death.[62] While high levels of mutant protein accumulate in these cells, this does not lead to the pathological lesions found in motor neurons of ALS patients or transgenic animals carrying a SOD mutation. Thus, neuronal death may not be a consequence of non-functional SOD aggregation. However, the formation of advanced glycation end products is selectively increased in the astrocytes of both ALS patients with the SOD1 mutation and in the transgenic mice,[63] indicating that compromise of astrocytes might jeopardize neuronal integrity. Neurons themselves produce toxic reactive mediators that could lead to their death. Neuronal nitric oxide synthase increases steadily in spinal motor neurons of the SOD transgenic mice with disease progression. The subsequent increase in NO and thence peroxynitrite production, as well as the inability of the astrocytes to provide efficient protection, may contribute to the death of the motor neurons.[64]

There is an upregulation of innate immune responses in the CNS of ALS patients and the level of monocyte-chemoattractant protein (MCP-1) is increased in their cerebrospinal fluid but not their serum.[65] In transgenic mice overexpressing SOD1, levels of genes associated with inflammation and apoptosis are increased before symptoms of the disease and neuronal death is apparent.[66] While the SOD transgenic mice have a normal innate immune response after acute LPS treatment, chronic exposure to the endotoxin leads to accelerated motor neuron degeneration and a decrease in lifespan of these animals.[67] TNF-α, IL-12, and TLR-2 expression in microglial cells were associated with this neuronal cell loss. Thus the cell death that accompanies neurodegenerative disease and toxic insult is in part mediated by chronic glial activation. An inhibitor of microglial activation, minocycline, has been shown not only to delay the onset of ALS, but also to dose-dependently increase the survival of the SOD1 transgenic mice.[68]

ENVIRONMENTAL EXPOSURES CAN TRIGGER INFLAMMATORY EVENTS IN THE CNS

Lipopolysaccharide (LPS)

The TLR-4 pathway plays an integral role in the innate immune response to this endotoxin.[3] This receptor functions in conjunction with lipopolysaccharide binding protein (LBP) and CD14 to enable mitogen-activated protein kinases (MAPKs) to activate NF-κB.[69] Innate immune components necessary for a response to LPS are present in the CNS. In the brain, there is low-level constitutive expression of TLR4 mRNA, which is downregulated after peripheral LPS exposure.[70] In contrast, systemic LPS treatment increases CD14 expression, first in the circumventricular organs (CVO), which have an incomplete BBB, and then in the brain parenchyma.[71]

Microglial cells express TLR4 and through this pathway can secondarily cause LPS-induced toxicity in oligodendrocytes[72] and cortical neurons.[73] LPS-induced chronic inflammation in the rat brain causes astrogliosis and an increase in the levels of β-amyloid, IL-1, and TNF-α mRNA levels.[74] This is followed by impairment in spatial memory. In the dentate gyrus, neurogenesis plays an important role in hippocampal-dependent associative memory acquisition.[75] LPS-induced inflammation blocks neuronal generation[76] and this may play an important role in cognitive impairment. Thus, in animal models, inflammatory events are associated with symptoms similar to AD.

Inflammatory stimuli can also cause dopaminergic cell death, which is the main pathological finding in PD. In rats, LPS treatment led to microglial activation followed by selective loss of dopaminergic neurons.[77] Injection of LPS in the supranigral area of rat brains caused an increase in reactive glial cells expressing both increased iNOS immunoreactivity and 3-nitrotyrosine formation.[58] An important mediator of neuronal toxicity was iNOS since pretreatment of animals with an iNOS inhibitor substantially reduced the extent of cell death. LPS-induced toxicity in dopaminergic cells is not dependent on iNOS but rather the levels of TNF-α and IL-1β.[78] The effect of LPS in the brain is mainly mediated by TNF-α. Chronic infusion of rat brains with the cytokine produced the same neurotoxic effect as the endotoxin. Furthermore, blocking TNF-α with neutralizing antibody inhibited neuronal damage.[13] However, the TNF-α–mediated toxicity involved nitric oxide formation.

Aluminum

A relation between aluminum exposure and human health has been postulated. In several instances one can observe a direct causal role between exposure to the metal and abnormal neurological symptoms.[79–82] Epidemiological studies found a correlation between chronic exposure to aluminum in the drinking water and a higher incidence of AD.[83–85]

Aluminum modulates the levels of Aβ. Both *in vivo* and *in vitro* analysis show that aluminum does not affect the actual processing or expression of APP.[86] However, the metal causes aggregation of $A\beta$[87–89] and aluminum exacerbates oxidative stress, $A\beta$ deposition, and plaque formation in the brain of transgenic mice that over-express APP.[90] Both $A\beta$ and aluminum are able to stabilize the ferrous form of iron, which is involved in the promotion of the Fenton reaction[91] and thus the two compounds can potentiate ROS formation. aluminum also causes aggregation of tau protein to a product resistant to proteases and phosphatases.[92]

Aluminum enhances neuroinflammatory events in the brain. Intracerebroventricular injection of aluminum salts leads to activation of glial cells in the rat brain.[93] Aluminum caused an increase in TNFα production and NF-κB activation in a human glioblastoma cell line.[10] In mice treated for ten weeks with aluminum lactate in the drinking water, there was a dose-dependent increase in proinflammatory cytokines.[11] In these animals, the striatum had the highest number of astrocytes and activated microglia. The use of transgenic animal models of neurodegeneration will help to determine whether aluminum-induced inflammation plays a role in potentiating pathological lesions characteristic of neurological impairments.

Particulate Matter Present in Air Pollution

Epidemiological data show that particulate matter (PM) present in ambient air pollution may underlie increased morbidity and mortality rates related to pulmonary and cardiovascular systems.[94–96] However, few reports have looked at the potential adverse health effects of air pollution on the CNS. In one study, dogs living in a highly polluted region in Mexico City had an increase in brain inflammation compared to animals living in a less polluted area (Tlaxcala, Mexico). The brain tissue of animals from Mexico City had higher levels of NF-κB activation, iNOS production, and reactive astrocytes compared with the animals from Tlaxcala.[97] Levels of the immune-related transcription factor NF-κB as well as the principal proinflammatory cytokines IL-1α and TNF-α are increased in the brain of mice after exposure to concentrated particulate matter present in air pollution.[98] Since inflammatory events have been associated with neurodegenerative processes, it is possible that extended exposure to PM may aggravate the progression of these disorders. There is a correlation between MS relapse and the PM content of air.[99]

Since metals constitute a high proportion of fine particles that comprise PM, it is possible that metals may account for some of the responses following exposure. There is evidence of metal involvement in the pathology of neurodegenerative disorders. Abnormal metal interactions have been indicated in the pathogenesis of AD[100] and the levels of copper, zinc, and iron are increased in the rims of senile plaques.[101] Iron is also elevated in the brain of PD patients.[102] Airborne levels of these metals, as constituents of PM, are increased in air pollution.[98] These may directly reach the CNS through the olfactory pathway where cell processes of olfactory neurons enter the brain through the cribriform plate of the ethmoid bone. For inhaled manganese, the olfactory route has been shown to contribute significantly to the access of this metal into the brain.[103]

The extent to which PM exposure may have adverse neurological consequences is at present unknown. In parallel to effects of LPS and aluminum, chronic exposure to PM in polluted air may lead to exacerbation of inflammatory events associated with neurodegeneration. Since the etiology of a major fraction of neurodegenerative

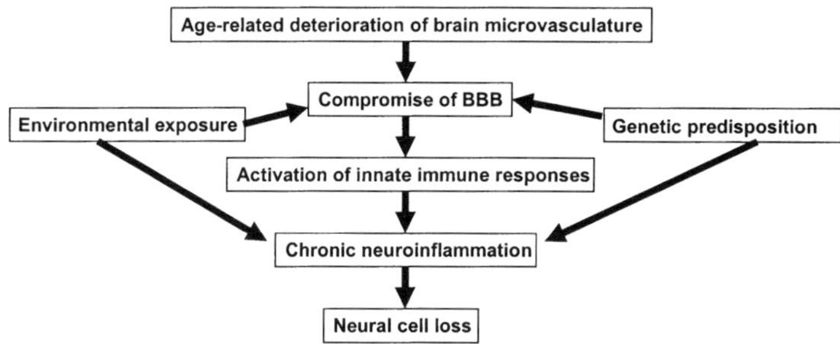

FIGURE 3. Interaction of aging, genetic predisposition, and environmental exposures in neurodegeneration. The process of senescence is not benign and eventually leads to compromise of the integrity of the BBB. This not only relies on the genetic profile of an individual, but also on environmental insults which may affect the BBB. Age-related damage to this structure will lead to initiation of innate immune responses, which if prolonged can lead to chronic neuroinflammation. The interaction between genetic and environmental factors can also determine the severity of this response, which can eventually lead to neuronal cell death.

cases is idiopathic, it is important to evaluate the potential role of environmental air pollution as another possible aggravating factor in these disorders.

SUMMARY

Controlled microglial activation may be advantageous to an aging brain. In APP and PS1 double-transgenic mice, intracranial injection of LPS in the hippocampus reduced Aβ levels.[104] Furthermore, two independent groups found that treatment with glial-derived neurotrophic factor (GDNF) has protective effects in an ALS transgenic mice model.[105,106] Limited and confined inflammation is appropriate and beneficial. However, irresolvable pathological lesions may lead to chronic activation of inflammatory events that can accentuate existing problems in the diseased brain.

Inflammatory events are likely to contribute to the pathogenesis of many disorders such as MS, AD, PD, and ALS. Environmental exposures appear to exacerbate the endogenous heightened CNS inflammation that is a result of normal aging and by doing so may accelerate neuronal cell loss (FIG. 3). Thus, anti-inflammatory intervention may slow down the progression of many different forms of neurodegenerative diseases.

ACKNOWLEDGMENTS

This study was supported in part by grants from the National Institutes of Health (Nos. ES 7992 and AG-16794).

REFERENCES

1. YAMAMOTO, M. *et al.* 2004. TIR domain-containing adaptors define the specificity of TLR signaling. Mol. Immunol. **40:** 861–868.
2. HEMMI, H. *et al.* 2000. A Toll-like receptor recognizes bacterial DNA. Nature **408:** 740–745.
3. POLTORAK, A. *et al.* 1998. Defective LPS signaling in C3H/HeJ and C57BL/10ScCr mice: mutations in Tlr4 gene. Science **282:** 2085–2088.
4. BSIBSI, M. *et al.* 2002. Broad expression of toll-like receptors in the human central nervous system. J. Neuropathol. Exp. Neurol. **61:** 1013–1021.
5. BAEUERLE, P.A. & T. HENKEL. 1994. Function and activation of NF-κB in the immune system. Annu. Rev. Immunol. **12:** 141–179.
6. MEDZHITOV, R. & C.A. JANEWAY. 1998. An ancient system of host defense. Curr. Opin. Immunol. **10:** 12–15.
7. HATADA, E.N. *et al.* 2000. NF-κB and the innate immune response. Curr. Opin. Immunol. **12:** 52–58.
8. KALTSCHMIDT, C. *et al.* 1994. Transcription factor NF-κB is activated in microglia during experimental autoimmune encephalomyelitis. J. Neuroimmunol. **55:** 99–106.
9. KIM, J. *et al.* 1999. Expression of cytokine genes and increased nuclear factor-kappa B activity in the brains of scrapie-infected mice. Mol. Brain Res. **73:** 17–27.
10. CAMPBELL, A. *et al.* 2002. Pro-inflammatory effects of aluminum in human glioblastoma cells. Brain Res. **933:** 60–65.
11. CAMPBELL, A. *et al.* 2004. Chronic exposure to aluminum in drinking water increases inflammatory parameters selectively in the brain. J. Neurosci. Res. **75:** 565–572.
12. RIVEST, S. 2003. Molecular insights on the cerebral innate immune system. Brain Behav. Immun. **17:** 13–19.
13. NADEAU, S. & S. RIVEST. 2003. Glucocorticoids play a fundamental role in protecting the brain during innate immune response. J. Neurosci. **23:** 5536–5544.
14. ILIEV, A.I. *et al.* 2004. Neuronal injury mediated via stimulation of microglial toll-like receptor-9 (TLR9) FASEB J. **18:** 412–414.
15. DAVID, J.P. *et al.* 1997. Glial reaction in the hippocampal formation is highly concentrated with aging in human brain. Neurosci. Lett. **235:** 53–56.
16. STREIT, W.J. *et al.* 1999. Reactive microgliosis. Prog. Neurobiol. **57:** 563–581.
17. FRANZEN, R. *et al.* 2004. Nervous system injury: focus on the inflammatory cytokine "granulocyte-macrophage colony stimulating factor". Neurosci. Lett. **361:** 76–78.
18. BONDY S.C. & A. CAMPBELL. 2002. Initiation of futile pathways common to many neurological diseases. *In* Neuroprotection. J. Marwah & E. Lo, Eds.: 299–309. Prominent Press. Scottsdale, AZ.
19. KIELIAN, T. 2004. Microglia and chemokines in infectious disease of the nervous system: views and reviews. Front. Biosci. **9:** 732–750.
20. GIMENEZ, M.A. *et al.* 2004. TNFR1-dependent VCAM-1 expression by astrocytes exposes the CNS to destructive inflammation. J. Neuroimmunol. **151:** 116–125.
21. BROUWER, N. *et al.* 2004. Induction of glial L-CCR mRNA expression in spinal cord and brain in experimental autoimmune encephalomyelitis. Glia **46:** 84–94.
22. CALLAHAN, M.K. *et al.* 2004. CXCR3 marks CD4+ memory T lymphocytes that are competent to migrate across the human brain microvascular endothelial cell layer. J. Neuroimmunol. **153:** 150–157.
23. GALE, C.R. & C.N. MARTYN. 1995. Migrant studies in multiple sclerosis. Prog. Neurobiol. **47:** 425–448.
24. HENSIEK, A.E. *et al.* 2003. Searching for needles in haystacks—the genetics of multiple sclerosis and other common neurological diseases. Brain Res. Bull. **61:** 229–234.
25. GRANIERI, E. *et al.* 2001. Multiple sclerosis: infectious hypothesis. Neurol. Sci. **22:** 179–185.
26. EBERS, G.C. & A.D. SADOVNICK. 1994. The role of genetic factors in multiple sclerosis susceptibility. J. Neuroimmunol. **54:** 1–17.
27. BRUCK, W. & C. STADELMANN. 2003. Inflammation and degeneration in multiple sclerosis. Neurol. Sci. **24:** S265–S267.

28. PAOLILLO, A. *et al.* 2004. The relationship between inflammation and atrophy in clinically isolated syndromes suggestive of multiple sclerosi: a monthly MRI study after triple dose gadolinium-DTPA. J. Neurol. **251:** 432–439.
29. ROSE, J.W. *et al.* 2004. Inflammatory cell expression of cyclooxygenase-2 in the multiple sclerosis lesion. J. Neuroimmunol. **149:** 40–49.
30. KANWAR, J.R. *et al.* 2004. Simultaneous neuroprotection and blockade of inflammation reverses autoimmune encephalomyelitis. Brain **127:** 1313–1331.
31. BONDOLFI, L. *et al.* 2002. Amyloid-associated neuron loss and gliogenesis in the neocortex of amyloid precursor protein transgenic mice. J. Neurosci. **22:** 515–522.
32. VASSAR, R. *et al.* 1999. Beta-secretase cleavage of Alzheimer's amyloid precursor protein by the transmembrane aspartic protease BACE. Science **286:** 735–741.
33. BODENDORF, U. *et al.* 2002. Expression of the human beta-secretase in the mouse brain increases the steady-state level of beta-amyloid. J. Neurochem. **80:** 799–806.
34. BALES, K.R. *et al.* 1998. The NF-κB/Rel family of proteins mediates Aβ-induced neurotoxicity and glial activation. Mol. Brain Res. **57:** 63–72.
35. AKAMA, K.T. *et al.* 1998. Amyloid β peptide stimulates nitric oxide production in astrocytes through an NF-κB-dependent mechanism. Proc. Natl. Acad. Sci. USA **95:** 5795–5800.
36. CANNING, D.R. *et al.* 1993. Beta-amyloid of Alzheimer's disease induces reactive gliosis that inhibits axonal outgrowth. Exp. Neurol. **124:** 289–298.
37. HOKE, A. *et al.* 1994. Regional differences in reactive gliosis induced by substrate-bound β-amyloid. Exp. Neurol. **130:** 56–66.
38. LI, R. *et al.* 2004. Tumor necrosis factor death receptor signaling cascade is required for amyloid-beta protein-induced neuron death. J. Neurosci. **24:** 1760–1771.
39. FASSBENDER, K. *et al.* 2004. The LPS receptor (CD14) links innate immunity with Alzheimer's disease. FASEB J. **18:** 203–205.
40. SONDAG, C.M. & C.K. COMBS. 2004. Amyloid precursor protein mediates proinflammatory activation of monocytic lineage cells. J. Biol. Chem. **279:** 14456–14463.
41. SLY, L.M. *et al.* 2001. Endogenous brain cytokine mRNA and inflammatory responses to lipopolysaccharide are elevated in the Tg2576 transgenic mouse model of Alzheimer's disease. Brain Res. Bull. **56:** 581–588.
42. GORDON, M.N. *et al.* 2002. Time course of the development of Alzheimer-like pathology in the double transgenic PS1+APP mouse. Exp. Neurol. **173:** 183–195.
43. TARKOWSKI, E. *et al.* 2003. Intrathecal inflammation precedes development of Alzheimer's disease. J. Neurol. Neurosurg. Psychiatry **74:** 1200–1205.
44. MCGEER, P.L. *et al.* 1990. Anti-inflammatory drugs and Alzheimer's disease. Lancet **42:** 447–449.
45. MCGEER, P.I. *et al.* 1996. Arthritis and anti-inflammatory agents as possible protective factors for Alzheimer's disease: a review of 17 epidemiologic studies. Neurology **47:** 425–432.
46. MACKENZIE, I.R.A. & D.G. MUNOZ. 1998. Nonsteroidal anti-inflammatory drug use and Alzheimer-type pathology in aging. Neurology **50:** 986–990.
47. STRATMAN, N.C. *et al.* 1997. Ibuprofen: effect on inducible nitric oxide synthase. Mol. Brain Res. **50:** 107–112.
48. BLOM, M.A.A. *et al.* 1997. NSAIDS inhibit the IL-1β-induced IL-6 release from human post-mortem astrocytes: the involvement of prostaglandin E_2. Brain Res. **777:** 210–218.
49. CLAYTON, D.F. & J.M. GEORGE. 1998. The synucleins: a family of proteins involved in synaptic function, plasticity, neurodegeneration and disease. Trends Neurosci. **21:** 249–254.
50. KAHLE, P.J. *et al.* 2000. Physiology and pathophysiology of alpha-synuclein: cell culture and transgenic animal models based on a Parkinson's disease-associated protein. Ann. N.Y. Acad. Sci. **920:** 33–41.
51. ZHOU, W. *et al.* 2002. Overexpression of human alpha-synuclein causes dopamine neuron death in primary human mesencephalic culture. Brain Res. **926:** 42–50.
52. LEE, M.K. *et al.* 2002. Human alpha-synuclein-harboring familial Parkinson's disease-linked Ala-53→Thr mutation causes neurodegeneration disease with alpha-synuclein aggregation in transgenic mice. Proc. Natl. Acad. Sci. USA **99:** 8968–8973.

53. NUSSBAUM, M.D. & C.E. ELLIS. 2003. Alzheimer's disease and Parkinson's disease. N. Engl. J. Med. **348:** 1356–1364.
54. GREENAMYRE, J.T. & T.G. HASTINGS. 2004. Parkinson's—divergent causes, convergent mechanisms. Science **304:** 1120–1122.
55. TANNER, C.M. *et al.* 1999. Parkinson disease in twins: an etiologic study. J. Am. Med. Assoc. **281:** 341–346.
56. LIU, B. *et al.* 2003. Parkinson's disease and exposure to infectious agents and pesticides and the occurrence of brain injuries: role of inflammation. Env. Health Perspect. **111:** 1065–1070.
57. GAO, H.M. *et al.* 2002. Distinct role for microglia in rotenone-induced degeneration of dopaminergic neurons. J. Neurosci. **22:** 782–790.
58. IRAVANI, M.M. *et al.* 2002. Involvement of inducible nitric oxide synthase in inflammation-induced dopaminergic neurodegeneration. Neuroscience **110:** 49–58.
59. WU, D.C. *et al.* 2002. Blockade of microglial activation is neuroprotective in the 1-methyl-4-phenyl-1,2,3,6-tetrahydropyridine mouse model of Parkinson disease. J. Neurosci. **22:** 1763–1771.
60. NAGATSU, T. *et al.* 2000. Changes in cytokines and neurotrophins in Parkinson's disease. J. Neural Transm. Suppl. **60:** 277–290.
61. MCGEER, P.L. *et al.* 1988. Reactive microglia are positive for HLA-DR in the substantia nigra of Parkinson's and Alzheimer's disease brains. Neurology **38:** 1285–1291.
62. LINO, M.M. *et al.* 2002. Accumulation of SOD1 mutants in postnatal motoneurons does not cause motoneuron pathology or motoneuron disease. J. Neurosci. **22:** 4825–4832.
63. SHIBATA, N. *et al.* 2002. Selective formation of certain advanced glycation end products in spinal cord astrocytes of humans and mice with superoxide dismutase-1 mutation. Acta Neuropathol. **104:** 171–178.
64. SASAKI, S. *et al.* 2002. Neuronal nitric oxide synthase (nNOS) immunoreactivity in the spinal cord of transgenic mice with G93A mutant SOD1 gene. Acta Neuropathol. **103:** 421–427.
65. WILMS, H. *et al.* 2003. Intrathecal synthesis of monocyte chemoattractant protein-1 (MCP-1) in amyotrophic lateral sclerosis: Further evidence for microglial activation in neurodegeneration. J. Neuroimmunol. **144:** 139–142.
66. YOSHIHARA, T. *et al.* 2002. Differential expression of inflammation- and apoptosis-related genes in spinal cords of mutant SOD1 transgenic mouse model of familial amyotrophic lateral sclerosis. J. Neurochem. **80:** 158–167.
67. NGUYEN, M.D. *et al.* 2004. Exacerbation of motor neuron disease by chronic stimulation of innate immunity in a mouse model of amyotrophic lateral sclerosis. J. Neurosci. **24:** 1340–1349.
68. VAN DEN BOSCH, L. 2002. Minocycline delays disease onset and mortality in a transgenic model of ALS. Neuroreport **13:** 1067–1070.
69. HOFFMAN, J.A. *et al.* 1999. Phylogenic perspectives in innate immunity. Science **284:** 1313–1318.
70. LAFLAMME, N. & S. RIVEST. 2001. Toll-like receptor **4:** the missing link of the cerebral innate immune response triggered by circulating gram-negative bacterial cell wall components. FASEB J. **15:** 155–163.
71. LACROIX, S. *et al.* 1998. The bacterial endotoxin lipopolysaccharide has the ability to target the brain in upregulating its membrane CD14 receptor within specific cellular populations. Brain Pathol. **8:** 625–640.
72. LEHNARDT, S. *et al.* 2002. The toll-like receptor TLR4 is necessary for lipopolysaccharide-induced oligodendrocyte injury in the CNS. J. Neurosci. **22:** 2478–2486.
73. LEHNARDT, S. *et al.* 2003. Activation of innate immunity in the CNS triggers neuro-degeneration through a Toll-like receptor 4-dependent pathway. Proc. Natl. Acad. Sci. USA **100:** 8514–8519.
74. HAUSS-WEGRZYNIAK, B. *et al.* 1998. Chronic neuroinflammation in rats reproduces components of the neurobiology of Alzheimer's disease. Brain Res. **780:** 294–303.
75. SHORS, T.J. *et al.* 2001. Neurogenesis in the adult is involved in the formation of trace memories. Nature **410:** 372–376.
76. MONJE, M.L. *et al.* 2003. Inflammatory blockade restores adult hippocampal neuro-genesis. Science **302:** 1760–1765.

77. GAO, H.M. *et al.* 2002. Microglial activation-mediated delayed and progressive degeneration of rat nigral dopaminergic neurons: relevance to Parkinson's disease. J. Neurochem. **81:** 1285–1297.
78. GAYLE, D.A. *et al.* 2002. Lipopolysaccharide (LPS)-induced dopamine cell loss in culture: roles of tumor necrosis factor-alpha, interleukin-1beta, and nitric oxide. Brain Res. Dev. Brain Res. **133:** 27–35.
79. ALFREY, A.C. *et al.* 1976. The dialysis encephalopathy syndrome: possible aluminum intoxication. N. Engl. J. Med. **294:** 184–188.
80. RIFAT, S.L. *et al.* 1990. Effect of exposure of miners to aluminum powder. Lancet **336:** 1162–1165.
81. BISHOP, N.J. *et al.* 1997. Aluminum neurotoxicity in preterm infants receiving intravenous-feeding solutions. N. Engl. J. Med. **336:** 1557–1561.
82. AUTHIER, F.J. *et al.* 2001. Central nervous system disease in patients with macrophagic myofascitis. Brain **124:** 974–983.
83. MCLACHLAN, D.R.C. *et al.* 1996. Risk for neuropathologically confirmed Alzheimer's disease and residual aluminum in municipal drinking water employing weighted residential histories. Neurology **46:** 401–405.
84. RONDEAU, V. *et al.* 2000. Relation between aluminum concentrations in drinking water and Alzheimer's disease: an 8-year follow-up study. Am. J. Epidemiol. **152:** 59–66.
85. FLATEN, T.P. 2001. Aluminium as a risk factor in Alzheimer's disease, with emphasis on drinking water. Brain Res. Bull. **55:** 187–196.
86. NEILL, D. *et al.* 1996. Effect of aluminum on expression and processing of amyloid precursor protein. J. Neurosci. Res. **46:** 395–403.
87. MANTYH, P.W. *et al.* 1993. Aluminum, iron and zinc ions promote aggregation of physiological concentrations of beta amyloid peptide. J. Neurochem. **61:** 1171–1174.
88. KAWAHARA, M. *et al.* 1994. Aluminum promotes the aggregation of Alzheimer's amyloid β-protein in vitro. Biochem. Biophys. Res. Comm. **198:** 531–535.
89. BONDY, S.C. & A. TRUONG. 1999. Potentiation of beta-folding of β-amyloid peptide 25-35 by aluminum salts. Neurosci. Lett. **267:** 25–28.
90. PRATICO, D. *et al.* 2002. Aluminum modulates brain amyloidosis through oxidative stress in APP transgenic mice. FASEB J. **16:** 1138–1140.
91. YANG, E.Y. *et al.* 1999. The stabilization of ferrous iron by a toxic β-amyloid fragment and by an aluminum salt. Brain Res. **839:** 221–226.
92. LI, W. *et al.* 1998. Phosphorylation sensitizes microtubule-associated protein τ to Al^{3+}-induced aggregation. Neurochem. Res. **23:** 1467– 1476.
93. PLATT, B. *et al.* 2001. Aluminum toxicity in the rat brain: histochemical and immunocytochemical evidence. Brain Res. Bull. **55:** 257–267.
94. DONALDSON, K. *et al.* 2001. Ambient particle inhalation and the cardiovascular system: potential mechanisms. Environ. Health Perspect. **109:** 523–527.
95. FRAMPTON, M.W. 2001. Systemic and cardiovascular effects of airway injury and inflammation: ultrafine particle exposure in humans. Environ. Health Perspect. **109:** 529–531.
96. POPE, C.A. *et al.* 2002. Lung cancer, cardiopulmonary mortality, and long-term exposure to fine particulate air pollution. J. Am. Med. Assoc. **287:** 1132–1141.
97. CALDERON-GARCIDUENAS, L. *et al.* 2002. Air pollution and brain damage. Toxicol. Pathol. **30:** 373–389.
98. CAMPBELL, A. *et al.* 2004. Particulate matter in polluted air increases inflammatory indices in the mouse brain. NeuroToxicology. In press.
99. OIKONEN, M. *et al.* 2003. Ambient air quality and occurrence of multiple sclerosis relapse. Neuroepidemiology **22:** 95–99.
100. BUSH A.I. 2003. The metallobiology of Alzheimer's disease. Trends Neurosci. **26:** 207–214.
101. LOVELL, M.A. *et al.* 1998. Copper, iron and zinc in Alzheimer's disease senile plaques. J. Neurol. Sci. **158:** 47–52.
102. HIRSCH, E.C. *et al.* 1991. Iron and aluminum increase in the substantia nigra of patients with Parkinson's disease: an X-ray microanalysis. J. Neurochem. **56:** 446–451.

103. BRENNEMAN, K.A *et al.* 2000. Direct olfactory transport of inhaled manganese (^{54}MnCl$_2$) to the rat brain: toxicokinetic investigations in a unilateral nasal occlusion model. Toxicol. Appl. Pharmacol. **169:** 238–248.
104. DICARLO, G. *et al.* 2001. Intrahippocampal LPS injections reduce Abeta load in APP+PS1 transgenic mice. Neurobiol. Aging **22:** 1007–1012.
105. MANABE, Y. *et al.* 2002. Adenovirus-mediated gene transfer of glial cell line-derived neurotrophic factor prevents motor neuron loss of transgenic model mice for amyotrophic lateral sclerosis. Apoptosis **7:** 329–334.
106. ACSADI, G. *et al.* 2002. Increased survival and function of SOD1 mice after glial cell-derived neurotrophic factor gene therapy. Hum. Gene Ther. **13:** 1047–1059.

Induction of Serine Racemase by Inflammatory Stimuli Is Dependent on AP-1

SHENGZHOU WU[a] AND STEVEN W. BARGER[a,b,c]

Departments of [a]Neurobiology and Developmental Sciences and [b]Geriatrics, University of Arkansas for Medical Sciences, Little Rock, Arkansas 72205, USA

[c]Geriatric Research Education and Clinical Center, Central Arkansas Veterans Healthcare System, Little Rock, Arkansas 72205, USA

ABSTRACT: Serine racemase (SRace) is an enzyme that catalyzes the conversion of L-serine to pyruvate or D-serine, an endogenous agonist for NMDA receptors. Our previous studies showed that inflammatory stimuli such as Aβ could elevate steady-state mRNA levels for SRace, perhaps leading to inappropriate glutamatergic stimulation under conditions of inflammation. We report here that a proinflammatory stimulus (lipopolysaccharide) elevated the activity of the human SRace promoter, as indicated by expression of a luciferase reporter system transfected into a microglial cell line. This effect corresponded to an elevation of SRace protein levels in microglia, as well. By contrast, dexamethasone inhibited the SRace promoter activity and led to an apparent suppression of SRace steady-state mRNA levels. A potential binding site for NFκB was explored, but this sequence played no significant role in SRace promoter activation. Instead, large deletions and site-directed mutagenesis indicated that a DNA element between −1382 and −1373 (relative to the start of translation) was responsible for the activation of the promoter by lipopolysaccharide. This region fits the consensus for an activator protein–1 binding site. Lipopolysaccharide induced an activity capable of binding this DNA element in electrophoretic mobility shift assays. Supershifts with antibodies against c-Fos and JunB identified these as the responsible proteins. An inhibitor of Jun N-terminal kinase blocked SRace promoter activation, further implicating activator protein–1. These data indicate that proinflammatory stimuli utilize a signal transduction pathway culminating in activator protein–1 activation to induce expression of serine racemase.

KEYWORDS: D-serine; dexamethasone; gene regulation; JNK; lipopolysaccharide; transcription

INTRODUCTION

Serine racemase (SRace) is a pyridoxal phosphate–dependent enzyme initially discovered in type I astrocytes ensheathing synapses.[1] Recently, we reported that SRace could be induced in microglia by the Alzheimer amyloid β-peptide (Aβ) and that several aspects of this effect could be duplicated by lipopolysaccharide (LPS).[2]

Address for correspondence: Dr. Steven W. Barger, Reynolds Center on Aging, 629 Jack Stephens Drive, #807, Little Rock, AR 72205. Voice: 501-526-5811; fax: 501-526-5830.
sbarger@uams.edu

Ann. N.Y. Acad. Sci. 1035: 133–146 (2004). © 2004 New York Academy of Sciences.
doi: 10.1196/annals.1332.009

We have also noted SRace expression in Schwann cells and fibroblasts derived from peripheral nerve.[3]

SRace synthesizes D-serine and pyruvate from L-serine.[4,5] D-Serine is a co-agonist of the NMDA class of glutamate neurotransmitter receptor, binding at a site traditionally known as the glycine site; depleting D-serine can block neurotransmission by the NMDA receptor.[4,6] Because the NMDA receptor is intimately associated with paradigms of synaptic plasticity, excitotoxicity, and pain, SRace and its product may play critical roles in these processes. Furthermore, elevation of their levels in microglia by proinflammatory stimuli indicates that they may be involved in the connections between neuroinflammation and excitotoxicity.[7–9] Along these lines, D-serine produced by an elevation of SRace appears to contribute to the neurotoxicity exhibited by Schwann cells[10] and Aβ- or LPS-treated microglia.[2]

Elevation of SRace by Aβ and LPS was associated with increases in the steady-state level of SRace mRNA. Incorporation of an upstream regulatory region of SRace into a reporter-gene construct conveyed responsiveness to Aβ and LPS.[2] Here we report that LPS elevated this apparent promoter activity in a manner dependent upon specific sequence elements. MatInspector screening of the upstream regulatory region of the human SRace gene showed several potential binding sites for known transcription factors, including an apparent NFκB site and five presumptive AP-1 *cis* elements, two of which are canonical. Through deletion and site-specific mutagenesis, evidence was acquired indicating that an activator protein–1 (AP-1) site localized between −1382 and −1373 bp (relative to the start of translation) was responsible for the induction by LPS. Furthermore, luciferase reporter assay and real-time PCR indicated that dexamethasone decreases expression of SRace.

MATERIALS AND METHODS

Materials

Cell culture media were purchased from Gibco, Invitrogen Corporation (Carlsbad, CA). High-fidelity PCR kit was from Roche Applied Science (Indianapolis, IN). The dual luciferase kit, pGL3-basic luciferase vectors, phRL-TK *Renilla* construct, Nco I, Xho I, and alkaline phosphatase were from Promega, Inc. (Madison, WI). γ-[^{32}P]ATP was from Amersham Biosciences, Inc. (Piscataway, NJ). Site-directed mutagenesis was performed with the QuickChange kit from Stratagene, Inc. (La Jolla, CA). Monoclonal mouse SRace antibody was from Becton-Dickinson/Transduction Laboratories (Mississauga, ON). The c-Jun, JunB, JunD, and pan-Fos antibodies used in supershifts were from Santa Cruz Biotechnology, Inc. (Santa Cruz, CA). Goat anti-mouse alkaline phosphatase–linked secondary antibody were from Vector, Inc. (Burlingame CA). RNA extraction materials (TriReagent) were from Molecular Research Center, Inc. (Cincinnati, OH). Cyber-green PCR master mixture and enzyme were from Applied Biosystems, Inc. (Foster City, CA).

Construction of Reporter Plasmids

Genomic DNA was extracted from the T98G astrocytoma cell line, and the region upstream from the SRace coding region (Entrez acc. no.: NM_021947) was amplified with a high-fidelity PCR kit from Roche Applied Science, producing an amplimer containing the sequence from -1508 (relative to the start codon) through -193 and having a HinD III site on either end. The amplimer was inserted into the HinD III site of pGL3-basic plasmid. After identifying a clone with the desired orientation, it was digested with Pfl MI and Nco I for the insertion of a second amplimer comprising nucleotides -268 through $+8$. (Forward primer: 5′-CAG TGC CAA CAG TGC CAA GAG A; reverse primer: 5′-GCA CCC ATG GTT CTG AAA CCC A) The reverse primer introduced a single mutation (*underlined*) adjacent to the "start" codon to create a Nco I site. After confirmation by sequencing, this construct was used as the template for amplification of four additional sequences, beginning at -1410, -638, -490, and -164, respectively. Forward primers were as follows: 5′-CCG CTC GAG ATT GAG AAT GCA GAA G (-1410 sequence); 5′-CCG CTC GAG ATT CAA GTA GCT TCA C (-638 sequence); 5′-CCG CTC GAG CGT GTC TAC TAA AAA T (-490 sequence); CCG CTC GAG GTC AAC TCT CTT TTA G (-164 sequence). Each forward primer included an Xho I restriction site (underlined). The reverse primer for all reactions was as follows: 5′-GCA CCC ATG GTT CTG AAA CCC A. This corresponds with a Nco I site in pGL3-basic, and the amplimers were inserted between this point and the Xho I site. The fidelity of each construct was confirmed by sequencing. Site-directed mutagenesis was performed to introduce a two-base change within the AP-1 consensus sequence running from -1382 to -1376 ($G_{-1381} \rightarrow A$, $A_{-1380} \rightarrow T$); the mutation was confirmed by restriction digest and sequencing.

Transient Transfections and Luciferase Assays

Microglial cell lines HAPI (courtesy of John Connor, Pennsylvania State University) and BV2 (courtesy of G.A. Weisman, University of Missouri) were grown in 24-well plates in minimal essential medium (MEM) (Invitrogen/Life Technol., Carlsbad, CA) supplemented to 10% with fetal bovine serum (FBS) until they had reached 90% confluency. The cells were then transfected using LipofectAMINE reagent in serum-free MEM. Each well received 0.3 µg of the respective serine-racemase/luciferase plasmid, 10 ng phRL-TK *Renilla* (Promega, Inc.; Madison, WI), and 0.69 µg inert DNA. The plasmid mixtures were incubated with LipofectAMINE at room temperature for 20 min, transferred to the cells for 3 h, and then washed away with MEM. When present, LPS was added immediately after this transfection period. Firefly and *Renilla* luciferase activities were measured 12 or 20 h later, using a dual-luciferase assay system (Promega) according to the manufacturer's instruction.

Electrophoretic Mobility Shift Assay

Nuclear extractions and binding reactions were performed essentially as described previously.[11] Aliquots of nuclear extracts were removed for protein quantification by BCA reaction (Pierce) so that the remainder of the sample could be frozen immediately and stored at $-80°C$ until use in binding reactions (performed within a week of extraction). For DNA-binding reactions, 3 µg of nuclear protein was diluted in binding buffer (10 mM Tris-HCl, 4% glycerol, 1 mM $MgCl_2$, 0.5 mM EDTA, 0.1% Nonidet P-40, 1 mM β-mercaptoethanol, 50 µg/mL poly[dI:dC]; pH 7.4). After a 15-min incubation on ice, a $[^{32}P]$-labeled oligonucleotide probe (30–50 fmol) was added, and the reaction was continued for another 20 min at room temperature. The probe was either a commercially available AP-1 probe (Promega) or a double-stranded oligonucleotide (Invitrogen/Life Technologies) corresponding to nucleotides −1387 to −1370 of the SRace sequence: 5′-GGC GCA GTG ACT CAC GCC (AP-1 site underlined). For competition assays, unlabeled oligonucleotide probe was added to the prebinding reaction at 10- or 30-fold molar excess over the amount of radiolabeled probe. For supershift analysis, antibodies to c-Jun, JunB, or the Fos family were added to the prebinding reaction. Protein-DNA complexes were resolved by nondenaturing polyacrylamide (6%) gel electrophoresis, buffered by 0.25× Tris-borate/EDTA (TBE). The gel was dried and exposed to X-ray film.

Western Blot Analysis

Immunoblotting was performed as described previously.[12] Equivalent amounts of protein (20 μg) were resolved by SDS-PAGE (12%), then electrophoretically transferred to nitrocellulose. A monoclonal antibody generated against SRace was applied at 1:500 for 2 h, followed by alkaline phosphatase-conjugated goat anti-mouse antibody; the blots were developed with BCIP/NBT.

Real-Time PCR

Real-time, reverse-transcriptase PCR was performed using an ABI 7700 Sequence Detection System (PE Applied-Biosystems) in the presence of SYBR-Green. Optimization of the real-time PCR reaction was performed according to the manufacturer's instructions. The PCR conditions were standard (SYBR-Green I core reagent protocol 4310521), and all reagents were from the SYBR-Green I core reagent kit, including AmpliTaq-GOLD polymerase (PE Applied-Biosystems), SYBR Green PCR Master Mix (P/N 4309155), and SYBR Green RT-PCR reagents kit (P/N 4310179). Primers were designed with the assistance of PE ExpressTM software (PE Applied-Biosystems) and spanned an intron-exon junction. The primers for mouse SRace were as follows: 5′-AGG CAG CAG AGA ACC ATG TGT (forward); 5′-CAA CAT TCA AGA CTC TAT CCA CCT CA (reverse). The amplicon for SRace was 90 bp and the predicted annealling temperature was 78°C. The following primers were used for GAPDH: 5′-TGT GTC CGT CGT GGA TCT GA (forward); 5′-CCT GCT TCA CCA CCT TCT TGA (reverse). Specificity was confirmed by dissociation curve and agarose gel analysis. To avoid genomic DNA contamination, RNA samples were treated with DNase I (Ambion). RT conditions were as follows: 10 min at 25°C, 30 min at 48°C, 5 min at 95°C. PCR was performed on 56 ng of the resulting cDNA. The PCR conditions were as follows: "hot start" at 50°C for 2 min and 95°C for 10 min, followed by 40 cycles of 95°C for 15 s and 60°C for 1 min.

RESULTS

LPS Induction of Serine Racemase

Our previous report demonstrated that amyloid β-peptide or LPS could increase the steady-state levels of SRace mRNA in microglia. To confirm that the LPS-evoked increase in mRNA translated into an elevation of protein, we performed Western blot analysis on cells of the N9 microglial line. Untreated cultures were maintained in parallel with cultures exposed to LPS (100 ng/mL) for 20 h, and pro-

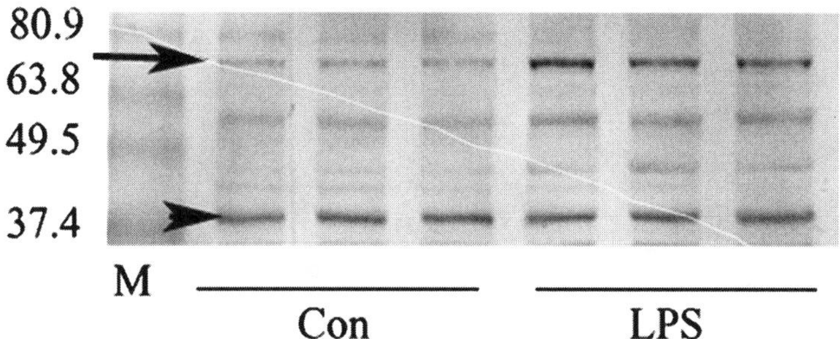

FIGURE 1. LPS elevates the levels of dimeric serine racemase. Triplicate cultures of the N9 mouse microglial cell line were incubated in the absence (Con) or presence (LPS) of 1 µg/mL LPS for 20 h. Cellular proteins were harvested and subjected to Western blot analysis with an antibody against SRace. The dimer (*arrow*) of SRace was elevated by LPS treatment while the monomer (*arrowhead*) appeared unchanged.

teins were isolated for immunoblotting. LPS treatment elevated the levels of a dimeric form of SRace protein (FIG. 1); identity was confirmed by a preabsorption control (as shown previously[2]).

LPS Activation of the Serine Racemase Promoter

Our previous demonstration that LPS elevates SRace mRNA[2] suggested that LPS might exert an influence on the gene's transcription. Approximately 1.5 kb of the sequence 5′ to the coding region of the human SRace gene was amplified by high-fidelity PCR and subcloned into a luciferase vector, creating pGL3/SRace (−1508). When transfected into HAPI cells, expression of firefly luciferase from this construct was induced by LPS (FIG. 2).

Analysis of the SRace sequence with MatInspector 2 revealed five potential AP-1 binding sites. AP-1 is composed of homodimers of c-Jun, JunB, JunD, or heterodimers of one of these proteins with a protein related to c-Fos. Phosphorylation of c-Jun by Jun N-terminal kinase (JNK) can activate AP-1 activity, and LPS is known to induce JNK activity in cells of the mononuclear phagocyte lineage. As an initial test of the role of this pathway in SRace induction, a JNK inhibitor was applied to luciferase assays of pGL3/SRace (−1508). HAPI cells were transfected and exposed to LPS in the absence or presence of SP600125 (15 µM). This JNK inhibitor completely abrogated transcriptional induction by LPS (FIG. 2).

Identification of a Functional AP-1 Binding Element
in the Serine Racemase Promoter

We sought to determine the relevant *cis* element(s) mediating activation of SRace transcription by LPS. As an initial step, deletions of the SRace construct were made, creating versions in which the 5′ ends of the SRace sequence were at −1410, −638, −490, or −164 from the start of translation. The parent construct contained five potential AP-1 binding sites, and each step to a smaller version removed a single AP-1

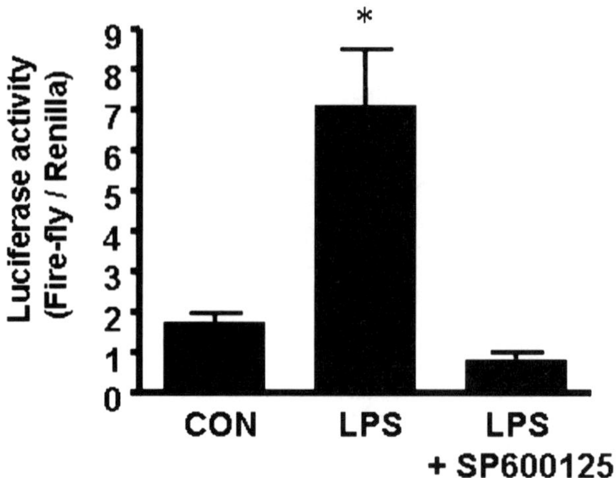

FIGURE 2. LPS elevates serine racemase promoter activity in a JNK kinase-dependent manner. Cultures of the HAPI cell line were transfected with pGL3/SRace (−1508) and phRL-TK. Cultures were either untreated (Con), treated with LPS (100 ng/mL) alone, or treated with LPS following a 1-h pretreatment with the JNK inhibitor SP600125 (15 μM). After 20 h, dual luciferase assays were performed. Values represent the mean (± SEM) of the firefly luciferase normalized to *Renilla* luciferase. Each experiment was performed in quadruplicate and the experiment was repeated three times (*P<.005 versus control).

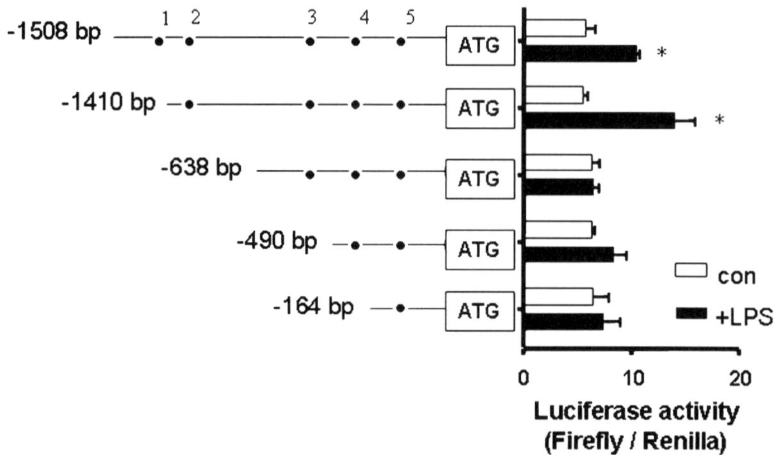

FIGURE 3. Responsiveness of SRace regulatory elements to LPS. Progressive 5′ deletion constructs of the SRace upstream region are depicted schematically; the enumerated *black dots* represent the AP-1 *cis* elements. Cultures of HAPI cells were transfected with each of the various constructs along with phRL-TK. Half the cultures of each set were then treated with LPS (300 ng/mL). After 12 h, dual luciferase assays were performed; values represent the mean (± SEM) of the firefly luciferase normalized to *Renilla* luciferase in quadruplicate cultures (*P<.005, LPS versus control for both the −1508 construct and the −1410 construct).

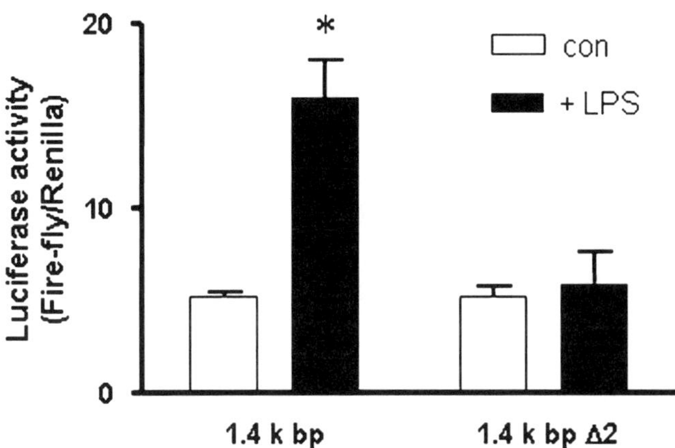

FIGURE 4. Requirement for AP-1 site at −1410 for induction by LPS. The second AP-1 site (−1382 to −1373) of the SRace upstream region was mutated from TGACTCA to TATCTCA within the context of pGL3/SRace. HAPI cells were transfected with this construct ("1.4 k bp Δ2") or the construct containing the wildtype sequence. Cultures were then treated with LPS (100 ng/mL) for 20 h. Values represent the mean (± SEM) of the firefly luciferase normalized to *Renilla* luciferase in quadruplicate cultures and the experiment was repeated three times (*P<.005, LPS versus control in construct of the wildtype sequence).

consensus sequence so that the shortest contained only one. These deletion constructs were transfected into HAPI cells that were subsequently incubated with or without LPS. The two longest constructs, pGL3/SRace (−1508) and pGL3/SRace (−1410), were inducible by LPS (see FIG. 3). However, removal of the 772 nucleotides between −1410 and −638 abolished responses to LPS. All the constructs smaller than pGL3/SRace (−1410) were unresponsive to LPS. Site-directed mutagenesis was utilized to confirm the role of the canonical AP-1 element at −1382. A 2-bp missense mutation ($G_{-1381} \rightarrow A$, $A_{-1380} \rightarrow T$) abolished inducibility by LPS (FIG. 4).

A sequence beginning at −124 showed similarity to a NFκB site, and NFκB plays an important role in many inflammation-related transcriptional inductions, including several of those evoked by LPS. The potential role of this sequence was assessed by testing a crude deletion of nucleotides −192 to −1 in the luciferase reporter vector (FIG. 5A). This construct responded to LPS equally as well as the full-length pGL3/SRace(-1508). We also tested the effect of cotransfecting pGL3/SRace (−1508) with an expression vector encoding RelA (a transactivating subunit of NFκB) or IκBα (the inhibitory regulator of NFκB) (FIG. 5B). RelA expression did not enhance expression from the full-length SRace reporter construct. Furthermore, expression of IκBα did not inhibit the stimulation of the reporter construct by LPS, as would be expected for a NFκB-dependent process.

LPS Induction of AP-1 DNA Binding to the Serine Racemase Sequence

As an additional test of the role of AP-1 in LPS-induced activation of the SRace promoter, we assayed DNA binding with EMSA. Initial experiments were performed with a commercial AP-1 consensus sequence as probe. Nuclear protein

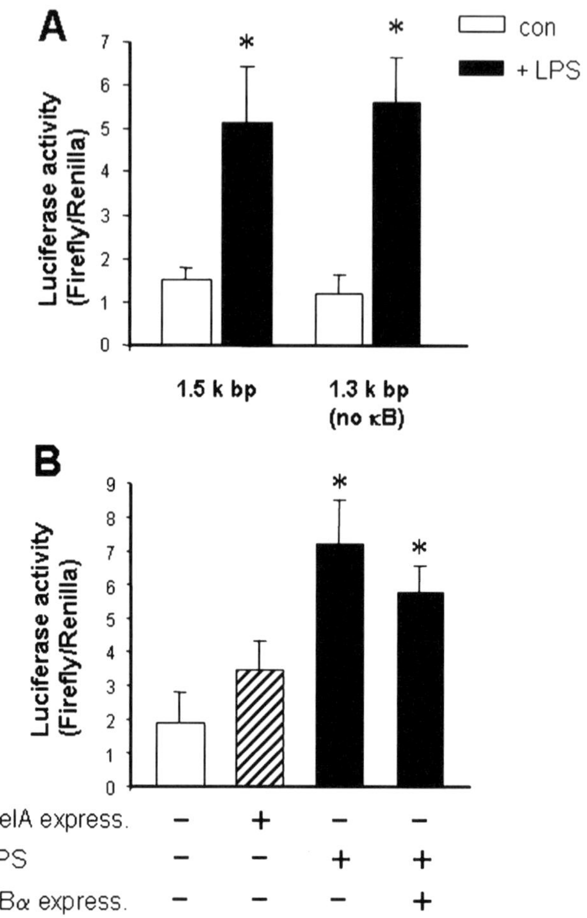

FIGURE 5. Lack of role for potential NFκB binding site. Cultures of the HAPI cell line were transfected with a pGL3/SRace and phRL-TK. Where indicated, cultures were treated with LPS (25 ng/mL). After 20 h, dual luciferase assays were performed. Values represent the mean (± SD) of the firefly luciferase normalized to *Renilla* luciferase. (*$P<.05$ versus no LPS). **(A)** The full-length reporter construct (1.5 kb) was compared to one in which nucleotides −192 to −1 were deleted (1.3 kb), removing the potential κB site. **(B)** The full-length reporter construct [pGL3/SRace(−1508)] was transfected alone or with expression vectors for either RelA or IκBα.

extracts from BV-2 mouse microglial cells treated with LPS showed an elevation in probe-binding activity compared to the untreated group (FIG. 6A). The binding ability was decreased by incubating the nuclear protein extract with an excess of un-labeled AP-1 probe before applying radiolabeled probe. To identify the proteins re-sponsible for this activity, antibodies against c-Fos, c-Jun, JunB, or JunD were added to the DNA-binding reaction to determine if they could diminish or further retard ("supershift") the LPS-induced protein/DNA complex. While c-Fos and JunB anti-

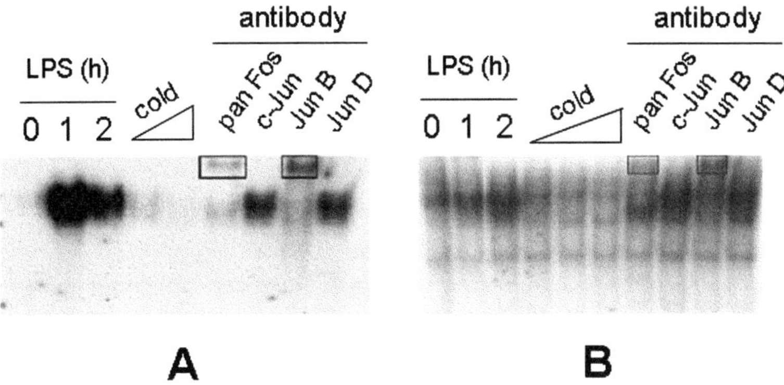

FIGURE 6. EMSA analysis of AP-1 DNA binding in response to LPS. **(A)** A canonical AP-1 *cis*-element was used as probe. BV-2 cells were treated with LPS (1 μg/mL) for 1 or 2 h and nuclear protein was extracted. LPS treatment increased a DNA-binding activity specific for the AP-1 *cis*-element, which was decreased by unlabeled AP-1 *cis*-element ("cold", 30× or 100× molar excess). Antibodies to c-Fos and JunB slowed the migration of protein-oligomer complex (*boxed*). **(B)** The sequence of the AP-1 *cis*-element from the SRace gene, including flanking sequences, was used as probe. HAPI cells were treated with LPS for 1 or 3 h. LPS treatment increased the nuclear protein binding to the oligomer, which was decreased by unlabeled oligomer ("cold", 10×, 30×, or 100× molar excess). Antibodies to c-Fos and JunB slowed the migration protein-oligomer migration (*boxed*).

bodies were effective in supershifting the complex, c-Jun and JunD antibodies were not. Because the AP-1 binding element in the SRace promoter has different flanking sequences compared to the commercial AP-1 consensus sequence, we also tested a probe sequence faithfully replicating the AP-1 element from the SRace promoter. And, in consideration of the possible different AP-1 components in different cell lines, we used nuclear protein extracts from HAPI cells. The results were very similar to the initial results: LPS induced a binding activity and antibody supershifts again implicated c-Fos and JunB as the primary components of the complex (FIG. 6B).

Dexamethasone Suppression of Serine Racemase Transcription

Dexamethasone is an anti-inflammatory steroid that antagonizes AP-1 or NFκB binding ability.[13–15] We tested the effects of dexamethasone on basal levels of SRace expression through analysis of quantitative, real-time RT-PCR. Dexamethasone caused an apparent decrease in SRace mRNA (FIG. 7A). This effect may result from diminished transcription rates, as dexamethasone also inhibited transcription from the SRace reporter construct as indicated by luciferase assays (FIG. 7B).

DISCUSSION

We have analyzed mechanisms controlling transcription from the human SRace gene. The enzyme it encodes catalyzes the synthesis of a biologically important

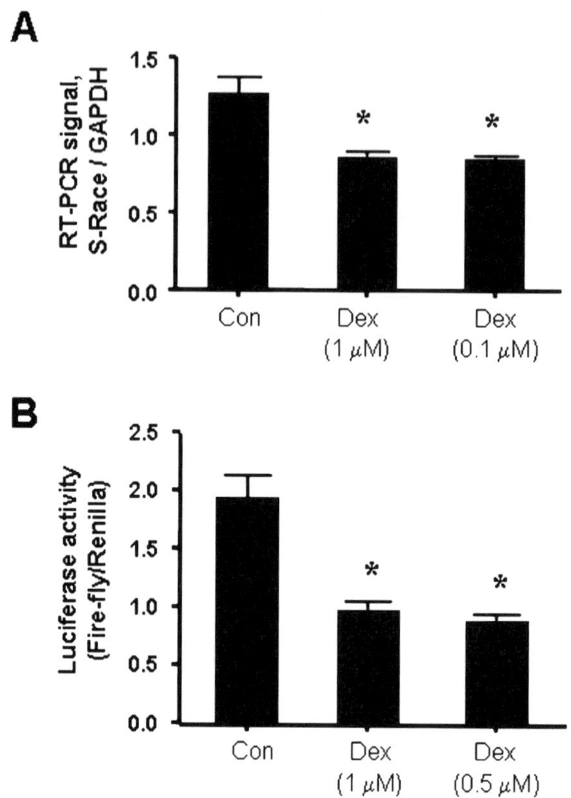

FIGURE 7. Dexamethasone suppresses SRace expression. **(A)** N9 microglial cells were treated with 100 nM or 1 μM dexamethasone for 20 h. RNA was extracted and quantified by real-time PCR. The control treatment included 0.1% ethanol as a vehicle control. The SRace signal was normalized to GAPDH. **(B)** HAPI cells and BV-2 cells were transfected with pGL3/SRace (−1508), along with phRL-TK. The cells were then treated with dexamethasone for 20 h. The firefly luciferase signal was normalized to *Renilla*. Control group received 0.1% ethanol as a vehicle control (*$P<$.005 between control and either dexamethasone treatment).

ligand of the NMDA receptor and is constitutively expressed in astrocytes and Schwann cells. The ability of proinflammatory stimuli to induce SRace expression in microglia has important implications for neurodegenerative consequences of microglial activation. Therefore, the information gleaned from the present body of work may be therapeutically useful toward attenuating the undesirable effects of neuroinflammation. We found that a proinflammatory stimulus, LPS, could elevate the steady-state level of dimeric SRace protein. This is consistent with our previous demonstration that LPS could elevate the level of SRace mRNA,[2] itself appearing to be a consequence of transcriptional induction through the AP-1 element we have identified here.

The elevation of an SRace protein dimer is consistent with the effect we previously reported for Aβ.[2] The dimeric form of SRace protein has been connected to the active state of the enzyme.[16] It is not clear what mechanisms control the dimerization process, but a recent report indicates that SRace interacts with protein kinase C. The resistance of the dimer to reducing agents and denaturing detergents in SDS-PAGE suggests a covalent bond distinct from disulfides, although there was also a noncovalent dimer apparent in the analysis by Cook and colleagues.[16] The possible role of chemical oxidation resulting from an oxidative burst is being investigated.

The human SRace gene is associated with cDNA sequences that indicate an unusually long first intron of more than 11.5 kb, all lying within the 5′ untranslated region. The rat gene is similar, with a 10.4-kb first intron; the mouse gene has an additional, untranslated exon within its analogous region. We have focused our initial analysis upon the first intron of the human gene, as it contains many sites that match the consensus sequences for binding by *trans*-acting factors. It is not uncommon for such intronic regions to contain important regulatory *cis* elements, including intronic AP-1 sites.[17-20] Although sequences 5′ to the start of transcription might be expected to participate in transcriptional regulation of SRace as well, this region apparently does not participate in responsiveness to proinflammatory stimuli. We placed approximately 1,500 bp of this region in a luciferase reporter construct and detected no induction by LPS (Wu and Barger, unpublished results). It remains to be seen whether or not that upstream region is responsible for other aspects of SRace expression, such as tissue-type or developmental specificity. Nevertheless, confidence in the promoter function of SRace intronic sequences is shored by the consistency between responses of the intronic reporter constructs and the endogenous gene's mRNA output, as both responded to LPS, Aβ, and dexamethasone.

There are five potential AP-1 binding elements in the first intron of human SRace, including two that are canonical. Our results show that at least one of these elements is functionally responsive to proinflammatory activation provided by LPS. It is not clear that the AP-1 site between −1382 and −1373 is solely responsible for control of the human SRace gene. Other investigators have documented cooperation between AP-1 complexes occupying adjacent sites.[21,22] Species conservation provides additional support for the role of AP-1; the mouse SRace sequence has four AP-1 consensus sites throughout the sequence upstream of the coding region, one at a relative position close to that of the functional site in the human sequence (−1719). The rat gene has six AP-1 consensus sites in its first intron, including one at −1348 and three others within 600 bp.

Antibody supershifts in our EMSA analysis indicated that the relevant AP-1 consists of a Fos protein and JunB. A JNK inhibitor completely inhibited the promoter induction by LPS. Together, these data suggest that JNK can phosphorylate JunB in HAPI cells or BV-2 cells, contributing to an active AP-1 complex. The JNK phosphorylation site in c-Jun (serines 63 and 73) or JunD is not conserved in JunB,[23,24] implying that JunB is not a good substrate for JNK. However, recent results demonstrate that JNK can indeed phosphorylate JunB, utilizing threonines 102 and 104.[22] Fos/Jun AP-1 heterodimers have higher affinity for DNA than that of homodimers of Jun family members.[25] The antibody utilized here cannot discriminate between several members of the Fos family, so it will be of interest to determine the JunB partner binding the SRace promoter element. Heterodimeric AP-1 activity is additionally regulated by phosphorylation of c-Fos by MAP kinases of the ERK family[26] and by induction of c-Fos expression.[27]

The precise composition of the AP-1 complex binding the SRace promoter could have additional implications for responses of the gene to other stimuli. Considerable data have shown that Aβ can activate JNK,[28,29] so it is likely that AP-1 is responsible for the induction of SRace by Aβ we reported previously.[2] That report also documented an elevation of steady-state mRNA for SRace by secreted amyloid precursor protein (sAPP). We have recently shown that JNK contributes to at least some aspects of the proinflammatory activation of microglia by sAPP.[30] Inhibitors of either JNK or p38-MAPK blocked the ability of sAPP to elevate the levels of inducible nitric oxide synthase and its nitrite indicator, but ERKs did not seem to be involved. Nevertheless, sAPP did activate ERKs; so their involvement in activation of AP-1 by sAPP to control genes other than inducible nitric oxide synthase is a viable possibility.

Our initial analysis of signals that might moderate SRace expression documented an ability of dexamethasone to inhibit the gene's expression. Dexamethasone is an anti-inflammatory drug that works largely through activation of glucocorticoid receptors to block NFκB binding.[31,32] Our present data concerning a potential NFκB site in the SRace promoter were negative, suggesting that NFκB activity is irrelevant to the actions of dexamethasone observed here. However, one mechanism by which glucocorticoid receptors block NFκB activity is through direct binding to NFκB, and a similar phenomenon appears to be relevant to AP-1.[13–15] The therapeutic potential of steroidal antiinflammatory drugs in neurological disorders is limited by the neurotoxic tendencies of glucocorticoids,[33] consistent with the disappointing results of a prednisone trial in Alzheimer's disease.[34] However, our studies with dexamethasone are part of a broader investigation of other steroids like estrogen and progesterone, for which regulatory elements appear to reside in the SRace gene. Together with attempts to regulate SRace enzyme activity and D-serine transport out of the cell, such manipulations of SRace comprise a rational approach to therapies for neurodegenerative forms of neuroinflammation.

ACKNOWLEDGMENTS

This work was supported by funds from the National Institutes of Health (R01AG17498, R01NS046439, R01HD037989, and P01AG12411). The authors thank Richard Jones for technical advice on real-time PCR.

REFERENCES

1. SCHELL, M.J., M.E. MOLLIVER & S.H. SNYDER. 1995. D-Serine, an endogenous synaptic modulator: localization to astrocytes and glutamate-stimulated release. Proc. Natl. Acad. Sci. USA **92:** 3948–3952.
2. WU, S.-Z. *et al.* 2004. Induction of serine racemase expression and D-serine release from microglia by amyloid β-peptide. J. Neuroinflammation **1:** 2–12.
3. WU, S., S.W. BARGER & T.J. SIMS. 2004. Schwann cell and epineural fibroblast expression of serine racemase. Brain Res. **1020:** 161–166.
4. MOTHET, J.P. *et al.* 2000. D-serine is an endogenous ligand for the glycine site of the N-methyl-D-aspartate receptor. Proc. Natl. Acad. Sci. USA **97:** 4926–4931.

5. DE MIRANDA, J. *et al.* 2002. Cofactors of serine racemase that physiologically stimulate the synthesis of the N-methyl-D-aspartate (NMDA) receptor coagonist D-serine. Proc. Natl. Acad. Sci. USA **99:** 14542–14547.

6. PANIZZUTTI, R. *et al.* 2001. A new strategy to decrease N-methyl-D-aspartate (NMDA) receptor coactivation: inhibition of D-serine synthesis by converting serine racemase into an eliminase. Proc. Natl. Acad. Sci. USA **98:** 5294–5299.

7. MASCARUCCI, P. *et al.* 1998. Glutamate release in the nucleus tractus solitarius induced by peripheral lipopolysaccharide and interleukin-1β. Neuroscience **86:** 1285-1290.

8. WILLARD, L.B. *et al.* 2000. The cytotoxicity of chronic neuroinflammation upon basal forebrain cholinergic neurons of rats can be attenuated by glutamatergic antagonism or cyclooxygenase-2 inhibition. Exp. Brain Res. **134:** 58–65.

9. BEZZI, P. *et al.* 2001. CXCR4-activated astrocyte glutamate release via TNFα: amplification by microglia triggers neurotoxicity. Nat. Neurosci. **4:** 702–710.

10. WU, S.-Z. *et al.* 2005. Schwann cells exhibit excitotoxicity consistent with release of NMDA receptor agonists. J. Neurosci. Res. In press.

11. MOERMAN, A.M. *et al.* 1999. Characterization of a neuronal κB-binding factor distinct from NF-κB. Brain Res. Mol. Brain Res. **67:** 303–315.

12. BARGER, S.W. & A.D. HARMON. 1997. Microglial activation by Alzheimer amyloid precursor protein and modulation by apolipoprotein E. Nature **388:** 878–881.

13. JONAT, C. *et al.* 1990. Antitumor promotion and antiinflammation: down-modulation of AP-1 (Fos/Jun) activity by glucocorticoid hormone. Cell **62:** 1189–1204.

14. SCHULE, R. *et al.* 1990. Functional antagonism between oncoprotein c-Jun and the glucocorticoid receptor. Cell **62:** 1217–1226.

15. YANG-YEN, H.F. *et al.* 1990. Transcriptional interference between c-Jun and the glucocorticoid receptor: mutual inhibition of DNA binding due to direct protein-protein interaction. Cell **62:** 1205–1215.

16. COOK, S.P. *et al.* 2002. Direct calcium binding results in activation of brain serine racemase. J. Biol. Chem. **277:** 27782–27792.

17. OSHIMA, R.G., L. ABRAMS & D. KULESH. 1990. Activation of an intron enhancer within the keratin 18 gene by expression of c-fos and c-jun in undifferentiated F9 embryonal carcinoma cells. Genes Dev. **4:** 835–848.

18. HENGERER, B. *et al.* 1990. Lesion-induced increase in nerve growth factor mRNA is mediated by c-fos. Proc Natl Acad Sci U S A. **87:** 3899–3903.

19. van DIJCK, P. *et al.* 1993. A Fos-Jun element in the first intron of an α-2 microglobulin gene. Mol. Cell Biochem. **125:** 127–136.

20. BERGERS, G. *et al.* 1995. Transcriptional activation of the fra-1 gene by AP-1 is mediated by regulatory sequences in the first intron. Mol. Cell Biol. **15:** 3748–3758.

21. CHIU, R., P. ANGEL & M. KARIN. 1989. Jun-B differs in its biological properties from, and is a negative regulator of, c-Jun. Cell **59:** 979–986.

22. LI, B. *et al.* 1999. Regulation of IL-4 expression by the transcription factor JunB during T helper cell differentiation. EMBO J. **18:** 420–432.

23. DERIJARD, B. *et al.* 1994. JNK1: a protein kinase stimulated by UV light and Ha-Ras that binds and phosphorylates the c-Jun activation domain. Cell **76:** 1025–1037.

24. KALLUNKI, T. *et al.* 1996. c-Jun can recruit JNK to phosphorylate dimerization partners via specific docking interactions. Cell **87:** 929–939.

25. HALAZONETIS, T.D. *et al.* 1988. c-Jun dimerizes with itself and with c-Fos, forming complexes of different DNA binding affinities. Cell **55:** 917–924.

26. MONJE, P., M.J. MARINISSEN & J.S. GUTKIND. 2003. Phosphorylation of the carboxyl-terminal transactivation domain of c-Fos by extracellular signal-regulated kinase mediates the transcriptional activation of AP-1 and cellular transformation induced by platelet-derived growth factor. Mol. Cell Biol. **23:** 7030–7043.

27. CHIU, R. *et al.* 1988. The c-Fos protein interacts with c-Jun/AP-1 to stimulate transcription of AP-1 responsive genes. Cell **54:** 541–552.

28. SHOJI, M. *et al.* 2000. JNK activation is associated with intracellular β-amyloid accumulation. Brain Res. Mol. Brain Res. **85:** 221–233.

29. JANG, J.H. & Y.J. SURH. 2002. β-Amyloid induces oxidative DNA damage and cell death through activation of c-Jun N terminal kinase. Ann. NY Acad. Sci. **973:** 228–236.

30. BODLES, A.M. & S.W. BARGER. 2004. Secreted β-amyloid precursor protein activates microglia via JNK and p38-MAPK. Neurobiol. Aging. In press.
31. SCHEINMAN, R.I. *et al.* 1995. Characterization of mechanisms involved in transrepression of NF-κB by activated glucocorticoid receptors. Mol. Cell Biol. **15:** 943–953.
32. AUPHAN, N. *et al.* 1995. Immunosuppression by glucocorticoids: inhibition of NF-κB activity through induction of IκB synthesis. Science **270:** 286–290.
33. SAPOLSKY, R.M. 1996. Stress, glucocorticoids, and damage to the nervous system: the current state of confusion. Stress **1:** 1–19.
34. AISEN, P.S. *et al.* 2000. A randomized controlled trial of prednisone in Alzheimer's disease. Alzheimer's Disease Cooperative Study. Neurology **54:** 588–593.

Neuroprotection from Complement-Mediated Inflammatory Damage

AMOD P. KULKARNI,[a] LAURIE A. KELLAWAY,[b] DEBOMOY K. LAHIRI,[c] AND GIRISH J. KOTWAL[a]

[a]*Division of Medical Virology,* [b]*Division of Neuroscience, University of Cape Town, Medical School, Observatory, Cape Town 7925, South Africa*

[c]*Department of Psychiatry, Indiana University School of Medicine, Indianapolis, Indiana 46202, USA*

ABSTRACT: Several neurodegenerative disorders, such as multiple sclerosis, Alzheimer's disease, and Parkinson's disease, are associated with inflammatory damage. The complex process of neuroinflammation involves various components of the immune system and the central nervous system. Particularly, brain astrocytes and microglial cells generate several inflammatory mediators like cytokines, leukotrienes, superoxide radicals, eicasonoids, and the components of the complement cascade. Complement plays an important role in the etiology of most of the neuroinflammatory disorders. To prevent long-term dysfunction inflammation in the central nervous system must be modulated with neuroprotective agents such as nonsteroidal anti-inflammatory drugs, steroids, phenolic thiazoles, nitrones, catechins, nitric oxide synthetase inhibitors, flavonoids, and phosphodiesterase inhibitors. Few drugs are found to be effective and their therapeutic benefit is hampered by side effects. Most of the neuroprotective agents are free radical scavengers and many inhibit only one or two aspects of inflammation. The complement inhibitory activity of most of these agents is either unknown or not established. Thus, there is doubt regarding their therapeutic value in most of the inflammatory disorders in which complement plays a major role. In this context the role of a multifunctional protein, vaccinia virus complement control protein (VCP), is quite significant as it may play a pivotal role in the treatment of several neuroinflammatory disorders. VCP is known to inhibit both complement pathways involved in inflammation. It is also known to inhibit cytokines and chemokines in inflammation. Our recent studies on rats demonstrate that VCP administration inhibits macrophage infiltration, reduces spinal cord destruction, and improves motor skills associated with spinal cord injury, establishing VCP as a strong candidate for neuroprotection. Thus, complement inhibitors such as VCP can serve as neuroprotective agents in inflammation associated with several neurodegenerative disorders.

KEYWORDS: aging; neurodegeneration; vaccinia viral complement control protein; neuroinflammation; complement regulatory agents; spinal cord injury

Address for correspondence: Girish J. Kotwal, Division of Medical Virology, Institute for Infectious Disease and Molecular Medicine (IIDMM), University of Cape Town Medical School, Anzio Road, Observatory, Cape Town 7925, South Africa. Voice: +(27)-(21)-406-6676; fax: +(27)-(21)-448-4110.

gjkotw01@yahoo.com

Ann. N.Y. Acad. Sci. 1035: 147–164 (2004). © 2004 New York Academy of Sciences.
doi: 10.1196/annals.1332.010

INTRODUCTION

Neuroinflammation is the most common phenomenon observed in the disorders of the central nervous system, namely, Alzheimer's disease (AD), Parkinson's disease (PD), brain trauma and spinal cord injury, Guillain-Barre syndrome, and multiple sclerosis (MS).[1–7] Most of the currently available agents provide only symptomatic relief and are not effective in the treatment of these disorders.[8,9] Overall complexity, involvement of several mediators of inflammation in the etiology, and identification of the key factor involved in the pathophysiology of such disorders are major challenges in designing an appropriate therapeutic regimen in the prevention and treatment of such disorders. Cells, such as brain microglial cells, monocytes, macrophages, and leukocytes, play a major role in neuroimmune activation and inflammation as evidenced from their presence in several neurodegenerative disorders, which in turn mediate their actions by expressing proinflammmatory mediators.[10,11]

Neurons, microglial cells, and oligodendrocytes are also involved in the production of complement components.[10–13] These cells express various receptors, through which activators like complement mediate their actions.[13–17] Apart from these receptor-mediated mechanisms, components like membrane attack complex (MAC) are involved in the direct actions of complement to mediate neurodegeneration. The interlinking of the components involved in the neuroinflammatory disorders marks the complexity of their interaction. Involvement of not only the cells of the central nervous system (CNS), but also migration of peripheral immune cells to the CNS adds to this complexity. Understanding the etiology of such disorders, the various factors involved therein, and their interrelationship with each other in mediating a particular disorder are all important to design an appropriate drug therapy. This report focuses on the components involved in the neuroinflammation, the impact of complement components as a key mediator in inflammation associated with CNS disorders via its direct and indirect actions, and the therapeutic strategies to be considered, with special emphasis on complement regulatory molecules.

CELLULAR COMPONENTS AND THEIR EXPRESSION PRODUCTS IN INFLAMMATION

The cellular components involved in the neuroinflammation and neuroimmune activation in the CNS are brain microglial cells, ependymal cells, macrophages, astrocytes, and mast cells. Microglial cells, which constitute around 10% of the CNS, are the first to respond to neuronal injury.[18] An altered chemical environment in the brain is a trigger for these cells to become activated. Microglial cells express receptors such as formyl peptide receptors (FPR), the macrophage scavenger receptors, and complement receptors after being activated. These cells are responsible for maintaining the normal biochemical homeostasis. This homeostatic regulatory function of the microglial cells is hampered in cases of injury or in inflammatory disorders of the brain leading to activation and upregulation of several neuroinflammatory mediators—cytokines, chemokines, reactive oxygen species, and adhesion molecules.[19,20] Glutamate released via protein kinase C, elevation of intracellular calcium levels mediated by complement anaphylatoxins, and activation of transcription factors are the consequences of microglial activation.[21,22] These cells, also described as brain macrophages, after being activated by inflammatory mediators migrate towards the target site.[23] Two types of chemotactic mediators operate by opsonin-dependent and -independent mechanisms. The opsonin-independent mechanisms include the formyl peptide receptor (FPR) and macrophage scavenger receptors expressed in disorders like AD.[24–26] Several chemokines like IL-8, macrophage inflammatory peptide–1α (MIP-1α), MIP-1β, and monocyte chemoattractant protein I (MCP–I) secreted by microglial cells mediate additional microglial recruitment to the target site. In case of opsonin-dependent mechanism, complement plays a major role as evidenced by its upregulation.

Phagocytosis mediated by microglial cells in the above manner or other mechanisms, such as free radical generation, is essential in the normal immune response against the inherent toxic proteins or proteins of foreign origin, but might prove detrimental in CNS disorders. These cells are also known to express cytokines, which play a dual role in the modulation of inflammation. Various cytokines modifying the inflammatory response are classified as growth factors, interleukins, interferons, and tumor necrosis factors. These cytokines play a dual role—neuroprotective as well as neurodegenerative.[19] Briefly, interferons and TNF-α are involved in the increase in the blood-brain barrier (BBB) permeability. TNF-γ causes macrophage activation and subsequent production of nitric oxide by macrophages and microglial cells, which is responsible for neurotoxic effects and favors permeability of BBB.[27] Production of glutamate and myelin removal by microglia also contribute to the damage to axons and oligodendrocytes. Apart from microglia, natural killer cells (NK), astrocytes, macrophages, oligodendrocytes, and epithelial cells play important roles in neuroinflammation. These cells release mediators like interferons and cytokines. As stated earlier, an underlying feature common to all these cells,[9] including neurons, is that they are capable of synthesizing most of the complement components. Thus, upregulation or overactivation of these cells may lead to an overproduction of the complement components.

Most of the cells are capable of producing complement regulatory molecules to protect themselves from the upregulated complement components. Neurons, however, express low levels of complement regulators and hence, are more susceptible to the attack by the upregulated components of the complement produced by various sources.[28] A net result of the direct and indirect actions mediated by the upregulated complement components is neuroinflammation and subsequent degeneration.[29] Attention must be focused on complement components while designing a therapeutic strategy against these disorders.

COMPLEMENT SYSTEM AND NEUROINFLAMMATION

The complement system consists of nearly 30 proteins involved in non-specific immune response and the role of various complement components in the pathophysiology of several disorders has been well studied in the past two decades. The complement system is activated in several disorders, particularly in response to foreign proteins, polysaccharides, cell surface components of microbial origin, or toxic proteins associated with the pathogenesis of several disorders. These foreign proteins activate the complement system by various pathways. The classical pathway of complement activation is found to be a major factor in the etiology of these disorders.[1,2,30–32] Recent evidence indicates the involvement of the alternate pathway of complement activation in the disorders of the central nervous system.[33] This emphasizes the importance of both pathways in the pathogenesis of neurodegenerative disorders. After being activated, these pathways lead to the generation of various complement components, which in broad terms can be classified as opsonins (C3b, iC3b, C4b etc.), anaphylatoxins (C3a, C4a and C5a), and MAC.[34]

These complement components are known to mediate different roles in the inflammatory and immune mechanisms.[35] The opsonins are involved in clearance function, anaphylatoxins are involved in the generation of inflammatory response, and MAC is involved in the inflammatory as well as cell-destructive mechanisms.[36] Anaphylatoxins mediate their individual *in vivo* actions through the various receptors present on the cells involved in the neuroimmune activation and neuro-inflammation. Although, the complement system is essential in the defense against pathogens, upregulated or improperly activated complement components lead to tissue destruction.[34]

CLASSICAL PATHWAY AND NEUROINFLAMMATION

Activation of a classical complement pathway through C1q component of the complement is evident in neurodegenerative disorders, such as AD.[1,37,38] Activated C1 cleaves both C4 and C2 to generate C4a and C2a fragments, which combine to form the classical pathway C3 convertase, involved in the cleavage of component C3 to form C3a and C3b. C3a is an anaphylatoxin and acts via various receptors present on the cellular surfaces. C3b combines with C4a and C2a to form C5 convertase, which leads to the formation of C5a and C5b. The former is an anaphylatoxin and the latter is involved in the production of terminal complement components, C6 to C9. C5b, with these terminal complement components, results in the formation of MAC.[39] The alternate pathway also results in the formation of complement anaphylatoxins and MAC, but activated through C3 component, requires factor B to form C3 convertase and C5 convertase.

Anaphylatoxins and Neuroinflammation

As noted previously, activation of complement by the major pathways involved in the neurodegeneration process results in the formation of anaphylatoxins. C3a and C5a are the potent anaphylatoxins. These are found to be associated with several neurodegenerative disorders. The role of anaphylatoxins in the inflammation is complex and not fully understood. Recent reports suggest that complement anaphylatoxins might play a neuroprotective role.[40,41] Anaphylatoxin 5a plays a neuroprotective role by mitogen-activated protein kinase inhibition of caspase 3.[42] Complement C3a is also found to have some neuroprotective role. Anaphylatoxin C5a is found to be beneficial in kainic acid toxicity and reduces the levels of glutamate, a neurotoxic agent found to be elevated in neurodegenerative disorders.[43] However, C3a does not protect against kainic toxicity though it has shown neuroprotective actions in NMDA-induced cell death.[44] The beneficial effects of complement anaphylatoxins must be balanced against their detrimental effects to understand the exact role played by these agents in neurodegeneration. Anaphylatoxins, which serve as potent signaling molecules in various proinflammatory reactions like smooth muscle contraction, granule secretion, and chemotaxis, increase vascular permeability by the cellular release of vasoactive peptides.[45–47] Activation of various myeloid and nonmyeloid cells involved in neuroimmune activation and inflammation takes place through the receptors present on their surfaces.[48]

After being activated, the immune complex mediates its action by different mechanisms, one of which is activation via complement anaphylatoxins. As noted earlier, the cells, which express receptors for C5a and C3a in CNS, include microglial cells, astrocytes, and endothelial cells. C5a and to a lesser extent C3a are potent chemoattractants. These recruit the polymorphonuclear cells from the periphery to the site of inflammation in the CNS.[1,7]

Anaphylatoxins and Microglial Cells

Microglial cells, which release nitric oxide, are the brain macrophages that mediate their actions by similar mechanisms.[49] Nitric oxide released by astrocytes and brain microglial cells combines with superoxide radicals resulting in peroxinitrite formation, which results in nitration of neuronal proteins and consequent degeneration.[50,51] Activated microglia generate free radicals, which are involved in neuronal cell death. Homooxygenase-1, a marker of oxidative stress, released by microglia can be correlated with neuronal death. Dying neurons may release free radicals and thereby activate microglial cells leading to further neurodegeneration.[52] Microglial cells are also shown to produce *in vitro* glutamate in cultured cells.[53] Although all these effects are beneficial initially, excessive activation by complement and other mediators is harmful.

Anaphylatoxins and Neutrophils

Neutrophils migrate from the periphery to the brain in neurodegenerative disorders or injury to brain. Complement component C5 is involved in the migration of neutrophils to the brain as evident from the study in AD.[1] These cells also express anaphylatoxin receptors for C3a and C5a.[54] Thus, complement anaphylatoxins play an important role in mediating the actions of neutrophils by recruiting them to the CNS. Nitric oxide synthetase released by neutrophils is responsible for neuronal damage.[55] These cells are responsible for BBB rupture and are involved in vasogenic edema.[56]

Anaphylatoxins and Endothelial Cells

Endothelial cells of the BBB are involved in inflammation. These cells are responsible for maintaining the integrity of the BBB by restricting the passage of molecules, cells, and fluid from the peripheral circulation to the brain. Anaphylatoxins, along with other mediators, are also involved in the rupture of the BBB by increasing the brain neutrophil count as discussed above. Endothelial cells also mediate their vasodilatory actions, neuronal damage, and alteration in the BBB permeability through NOS.[57]

Anaphylatoxins and Mast Cells

Anaphylatoxins are also involved in the activation and degranulation of mast cells. Previously, mast cells were considered to be restricted to the periphery, but recent reports suggest their presence in CNS disorders as well. It is also evident that complement anaphylotoxins play a role in their actions in such disorders.[58] These cells are found to be involved in the autoimmune and other chronic disorders of the CNS, where the activated immune complex plays an important role. C3a mediates mast cell degranulation via FcγRI.[59] Activated mast cells release cytokines, histamine and proteolytic enzymes. These are all vasoactive nociceptive agents and act as proinflammatory mediators in the inflammatory responses and allergic reactions.[60,61] IL-1, which is one of the major proinflammatory cytokines, results in the activation of various mediators like prostaglandin, leukotrienes, platelet activating factor, and nitric oxide. IL-1 is also involved in the expression of adhesion molecules by leukocytes and endothelial cells.[58]

Anaphylatoxins and Astrocytes

Another group of cells, activated by complement and involved in the CNS inflammatory process are the astrocytes. These cells play some protective role by expressing neurotrophic growth factor (NGF), cytokines, and antioxidant moieties (like glutathione) under normal conditions.

These cells have shown a specific increase in interleukin-6 (IL-6), after activation by complement, which may play a role in neuroprotection.[62,63] Complement anaphylotoxin C3a mediates excitotoxic neuronal death through astrocytes.[44] These cells also express chemokines and mediate migration of peripheral immune cells to the CNS, along with microglial cells, which are involved in the proinflammatory mediator nitric oxide.[64,65]

Membrane Attack Complex (MAC) in Neurodegeneration

The terminal complement components formed by the cleavage of C5 either by the classical or the alternate pathway result in the formation of MAC. The MAC formation is regulated by complement defense protein CD59, deficiency of which results in neurodegenerative diseases.[66] The neurotoxic effects of MAC on neuronal cells are time and concentration dependent. Mechanisms like free radical generation, cytokines, eicasonoids, and increased permeability to Na^+ and Ca^{2+} ions induced by MAC might be responsible for the observed effect.[67] Apart from their lytic properties, recent findings suggest that both cytolytically active and inactive forms of terminal complement complexes are involved in the accumulation of leukocytes into the cerebrospinal fluid and endothelial cell activation. At sublytic concentration, it not only protects host cells but also stimulates protein biosynthesis. The role of MAC, at sublytic and lytic concentration, is outlined by Wurzner.[68] This explains the concentration-dependent dual role of MAC. At lytic concentration, it acts as a neurodegenerative agent and at sublytic concentration it acts as a neuroprotective agent. Marked neurodegeneration in CNS disorders, even in the presence of the MAC, indicates the failure of regulation of MAC components and the need to restrict its activity to sublytic concentration by proper regulation of the pathways leading to

MAC formation. Thus, regulating the complement pathways leading to its generation can control formation of MAC.

ROLE OF COMPLEMENT IN NEURODEGENERATIVE DISORDERS

Alzheimer's Disease (AD)

The major hallmarks of AD are degeneration of basal forebrain cholinergic neurons, aggregation of Aβ and other proteins in these cholinergic target areas, and accumulation of hyperphosphorylated tau into neurofibrillary tangles.[69] AD may also result from the activation of the classical complement pathway by amyloid plaques. In addition, neurofibrillary tangles, associated tau, and other proteins are also involved in the activation of complement.[31,70] The complement opsonins and MAC are involved in the etiology of AD.[34,71] In AD, the complement system plays a dual role, and is explained by the yin and yang hypothesis.[36] Initially, the opsonin complements (i.e., iC3, C3b, etc.) play a beneficial role in the clearance of plaques, but in later stages of AD, particularly in sporadic AD, the upregulation of various inflammatory components (anaphylotoxins and MAC) results in neurodegeneration, which is associated with dementia.[37] Cyclooxygenase-I is involved in AD and is found to be associated with complement. The complement components are involved in the activation of cells of CNS and the migration of macrophage and leukocyte from periphery to CNS, thereby playing an important role in the pathogenesis. Now, there is evidence that the alternate pathway is activated in the frontal cortex of AD patients, where factor B is important.[72] In addition, cytokines, such as IL-1α and IL-1β, upregulate APP expression leading to Aβ depositions, which itself can trigger the cascade of inflammatory pathway.[73] Currently, there is an emphasis in research to understand the mechanism by which APP and cytokines interact with each other to develop novel drug targets for the treatment of AD.

Down Syndrome

Similar to AD, predominantly diffuse thioflavine-S–positive Aβ plaques in the frontal and entorrhinal cortex are involved in Down syndrome. These plaques activate the classical complement cascade by binding C1q component. This C1q component is associated with activated microglia as in AD.[74]

Multiple Sclerosis

Multiple sclerosis, in which there are multiple plaques of demyelination, affects individuals between 20 to 40 years of age. Complement plays a primary role in the etiology of this disease.[75] MAC formation is associated with demyelination of neurons in MS.[76] The inflammatory mediators involved in the MS are reactive oxygen species, complement, TNF-α, and antimyelin antibodies. The alternate pathway is activated in this disease, where factor B plays an essential role.[72]

Guillain-Barre Syndrome

This disease is typically an acute demyelinating neuropathy and has an anti-allergic basis. Of the two variants of the disease, complement plays a major role in demyelination of the dorsal root ganglion in acute inflammatory demyelinating polyneuropathy (AIDP). Complement C7 and the MAC (C5b–9) deposits formed on Schwann cell membranes are involved in the pathogenesis.[76,77]

Parkinson's Disease (PD)

PD is another disorder of the CNS associated with neuroinflammation. This disease involves chronic inflammation. Complement levels are found to be elevated in the substantia nigra, a part of the brain affected most in PD. Activation of microglia in the substantia nigra and other brain areas is also observed.[2,78]

Traumatic Brain Injury

Traumatic injury to the brain involves cellular components of inflammation like microglial cells and macrophages. Usually, there is a definite rupture of the BBB. Elevated levels of complement component C1q suggest the activation of complement cascade via the classical pathway. MAC is also involved in the etiology of this disorder.[79] MAC is also involved in evoking seizures. The components of MAC, when injected individually, evoke seizures and neurodegeneration by causing depolarization of the erythrocyte membrane.[80] Apart from these major disorders of the CNS, complement is found to play an important role in neurodegenerative disorder, like prion disease and Pick's disease.[81,82]

DUAL NATURE OF COMPLEMENT SYSTEM

From the above discussion, it is evident that the complement system plays a major role in the pathogenesis of several neuroinflammatory disorders. Although in most instances, the effects of complement system are detrimental, their beneficial roles, especially in glutamate and kainate toxicity should not be neglected.[43] The role played by the complement system along with other inflammatory mediators is outlined in FIGURE 1.

The role of complement in neurodegeneration is a double-edged sword.[28] This dual nature of the complement system suggests the necessity of thorough investigation of the roles played by various complement components. It can be concluded that the dual nature played by the complement system depends critically on the form of the disease and period of exposure to various complement components. In the normal immune response, in which an exposure to complement components is for a short period of time, the tissue repairing roles played by complement components are beneficial. However, chronic exposure results in their detrimental effects. An added complexity is that an acute exposure, as observed in accidental injury to the brain or spinal cord, is also destructive. The overall time and concentration-dependent actions of complement components can be diagrammatically represented by the minute, second, and hour hands of a clock (FIG. 2).

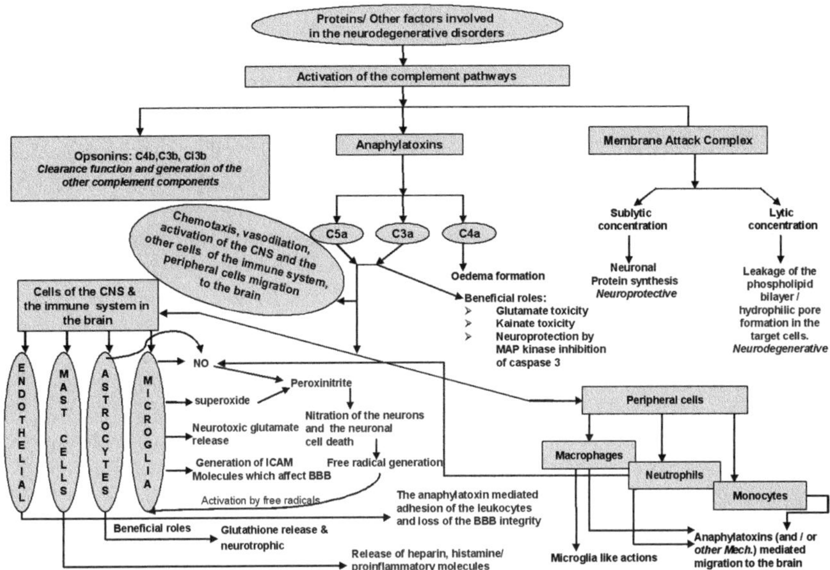

FIGURE 1. Diagrammatic representation of the overall neuroinflammatory process in CNS disorders and the role of complement components. This represents the overall picture of neuroinflammation in CNS disorders. The various immune cells involved in the inflammation, proinflammatory mediators, and the role of complement components by modulating cellular response and other mechanisms are shown.

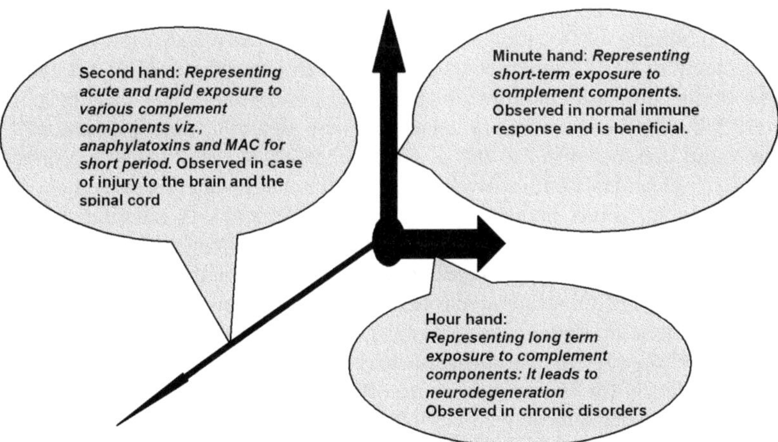

FIGURE 2. "Hands of a clock" representation of time-dependent actions mediated by various complement components in acute and chronic neurodegenerative disorders and in normal immune response.

THERAPEUTIC STRATEGY: SUCCESS AND LIMITATIONS

Current research from several laboratories suggests that inflammation is the primary consequence in the etiology of neurodegenerative disorders. Hence, it is no surprise that most of the agents used in the treatment of neurodegenerative disorders are anti-inflammatory molecules. Besides complement, other mediators involved in the neuroinflammation are free radicals, eicasonoids, nitric oxide, leukotrienes, cytokines, and cyclooxygenases.[83–85] The activated microglia, phagocytic, immune cells, or other cells of the CNS generate most of these proinflammatory molecules. As discussed earlier, apart from their direct actions, complement components play indirect roles in mediating the actions of the proinflammatory molecules, particularly those that are released or expressed by glial or other immune cells. It is evident from the fact that complement is involved in the activation and chemotaxis of glial and other cells involved in neuroimmune activation. In addition, some enzymes like cyclooxygenases are associated with the complement system or its receptors. However, no currently available agent in the market possesses direct complement inhibitory activity.[84] Anti-inflammatory drugs, which include nonsteroidal anti-inflammatory drugs (NSAIDs), indomethacin, and the other cyclooxygenase-1 (COX-1) inhibitors like rofecoxib, celecoxib, naproxen, and aspirin, are being tried and found to have some neuroprotective role, but at present no currently available agent offers significant neuroprotection in the neurodegenerative disorders.[8,9] These findings might lead one to question the significance of inflammation in neurodegenerative disorders. However, the reason for their failure can be attributed to their inability to directly inhibit the complement system. On the other hand, steroids like estrogens and progesterone have been tested for their neuroprotective roles.[87,88] Estrogen mediates its action by direct inhibition of microglial activation.[89] However, failure of prednisone and estrogen treatment in the controlled trial of AD patients raises serious questions regarding the therapeutic utility of these agents in allied disorders.[90,91]

Apart from steroids and NSAIDs, several agents are under development. Few of them mediate their actions through receptors (agonist/antagonists), nitric oxide synthesis inhibitors, or free radical scavengers.[92] Nitrones are also shown to have a neuroprotective role.[93] Cannabinoids acting via their own receptors, D3/D2 agonists in PD, serine protease inhibitors like FUT-175, phenolic thiazoles, phosphodiesterase inhibitors, and calcium channel blockers also offer neuroprotection.[94–98] These agents are shown in FIGURE 3. However, most of these agents are directed towards a single component involved in neuroinflammation and a few of them show some indirect or direct actions against the complement. As mentioned earlier, neurons are more prone to attack by the complement components, as they produce very low levels of complement regulatory proteins. Few agents like cannabinoids might play some neurodegenerative role apart from neuroprotecive roles.[99] Most of these agents show no direct activity against complement and they might not be of significant help in several neuroinflammatory disorders, where complement plays a major role. Hence, for effective neuroprotection, development of and/or search for the agents with complement regulatory activity as a major activity is a matter of urgency. Complement regulatory proteins offer hope in this context. This is evident from the recent findings that a complement regulatory protein, sCrry, plays an important role in the treatment of multiple sclerosis.[16] However, the same agent failed in the treatment of AD.[100] Attention to this contradiction should not be neglected.

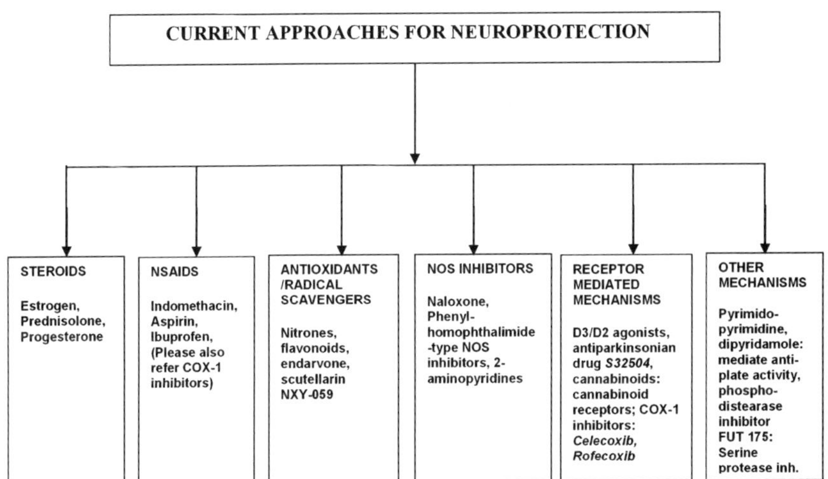

FIGURE 3. Current approaches for neuroprotection.

VACCINIA COMPLEMENT CONTROL PROTEIN: A NOVEL PROTEIN

Vaccinia complement control protein (VCP), a regulator of both complement pathways, has been found to be effective in treating spatial memory retention in a rodent model of AD. The possible involvement of different mechanisms in the neuroprotective roles of such agents must also be considered because complement inhibitor C1q-INH mediates its neuroprotective roles through mechanisms independent of C1q.[101] New complement inhibitors must be evaluated for their neuroprotective value in neuroinflammatory disorders.

Most of the times, the effects shown by small drug molecules are short lived. Frequent administration in chronic neurodegenerative disorders is associated with the adverse effects. Protein or other peptide molecules might be of great help in this context. Protein delivery to the brain or gene delivery to express the protein of therapeutic interest in the CNS to get expression over a prolonged period of time would be a better option in the treatment of neurodegenerative disorders, where long-term treatment is required.

VCP is a major protein secreted by vaccinia virus, and could be a drug of choice in the treatment of neurodegenerative disorders, where complement plays an important role. The role of VCP in various disorders is well documented in the recent review by Jha and Kotwal.[102] Briefly, it is a 26 kDa protein secreted by vaccinia virus that mimics the complement control proteins and chemokines of the host as an immune evasion strategy. It is composed of four complement control protein modules called sushi domains. Although it is more similar to the complement control protein C4b-BP structurally and to CR1 functionally, it also shares similarity to the other mammalian complement regulators like decay-accelerating factor (DAF), membrane cofactor protein (MCP), and factor H (fH).[103] VCP binds to C4b and regulates the classical complement pathway.[104] Through its ability to bind C3 and

C4 and ability as a cofactor of factor I to cleave C3b and C4b, it inhibits the classical complement pathway with greater potency than human C4b-BP.[105] VCP is also known to inhibit factor B–dependent complement-enhanced neutralization of antibody-sensitized virus, suggesting a regulatory role of this protein in the alternate complement pathway.[106] A possible mechanism involved might be an acceleration of the decay of the alternate pathway C3 convertase or through the cleavage of C3b into iC3b by acting as a cofactor for factor I.

Although, VCP regulates both pathways of complement activation, the concentration required to inhibit the alternate pathway is much higher than that for inhibiting the classical pathway. Regulation of these two pathways by VCP results in the inhibition of complement anaphylatoxins formation, which besides playing an important role in the neuroinflammatory disorders, also inhibits MAC. Apart from its complement regulatory activity, VCP has shown the ability to bind heparin and heparin-like molecules.[107] Heparin is a molecule released by the mast cells, which is found to be involved in the pathogenesis of CNS disorders. It may bind to other heparin-like molecules on the endothelial surface. Indeed, it is due to this property coupled with other roles that VCP is known to reduce the chemotactic migration of leukocytes. The heparin binding ability of VCP explains several physiologically interesting roles of VCP, for example, inhibition of complement-mediated killing of endothelial cells and blockade of interaction between (pig aortic) endothelial cells and neutrophils and natural killer cells thereby preventing cell death.[108]

All these actions mediated by VCP promote it as a potent anti-inflammatory agent. As illustrated, the anti-inflammatory activity of VCP involves multiple actions, complement inhibitory action being a major one. VCP inhibits more than one component involved in neuroinflammation and neuroimmune activation, its major action being complement control, which makes it a strong neuroprotective agent in the treatment of neurodegenerative disorders. Unlike several herbal ingredients, *in vitro* and *in vivo* activity of this protein in several neurodegenerative disorders is well established. sCrry, an inhibitor of the classical and the alternate pathways and effective in experimental allergic encephalomyelitis (EAE) in experimental animals, is found to be ineffective in treating AD.[100] Contrary to this, VCP is found to restore spatial memory deficit in Morris water maze model in rodents and might play an important role in dementia associated with AD.[1,109] Consequently, its role as a neuroprotective agent in animal models mimicking other neurodegenerative disorders involving head injury, traumatic brain injury, and spinal cord injury are well established.

Alzheimer's Disease

The pathogenic proteins in the etiology of AD, for example, tau protein and $A\beta$ derived from the amyloid precursor protein, are involved in the activation of the classical complement pathway. As mentioned earlier, the alternate pathway of activation is also involved in the pathogenesis of AD. VCP may play an important role in the prevention and treatment of dementia associated with AD.[1,109]

Traumatic Brain Injury

Traumatic brain injury involves complement and HSPG, a heparin conjugate. Traumatic brain injury inflammation is associated with cognitive dysfunction. VCP, with its ability to bind heparin like molecules and complement inhibitory activity, plays a beneficial role. Our study on rats using the lateral fluid percussion brain injury model showed that there was significant improvement in the cognitive function after the treatment with VCP.[110]

Hence, the use of novel strategies, such as the one used by poxviruses[111] and mediated by molecules like VCP with complement regulation as a key activity, might be a promising approach in the treatment of several neuroinflammatory disorders for which no suitable therapy is currently available. These compounds have an advantage of inhibiting a wide range of complement components involved in the neuroinflammation. However, it appears that inhibition of anaphylatoxins by the complement pathway regulators may actually play a devastating role in glutamate and kainate toxicity. Keeping the few controversies in mind, it may be concluded that regulators of both complement pathways can be effectively used in the treatment of neurodegenerative disorders.

OVERALL SUMMARY

Complement components serve as potent neuroinflammatory mediators in CNS disorders except for a very few beneficial roles in normal immune response or initial stage of disease. Complement components mediate their effects through direct actions or activation of cellular mechanisms involved in neuroinflammation. Failure of current neuroprotective agents can be attributed to their inability to direct inhibition of complement components.

VCP-like proteins (and/or genes expressing such proteins), which regulate both complement pathways, offer a promising approach in the treatment of neuroinflammation mediated by complement components in CNS disorders.

ACKNOWLEDGMENTS

The authors gratefully acknowledge the support of the Kentucky Spinal Cord and Head Injury Research Trust (KSCHIRT). G.J.K. is currently a Senior International Wellcome Trust Fellow for Biomedical Sciences in South Africa. A.P.K. is a recipient of the Poliomyelitis Research Foundation of South Africa Ph.D. Fellowship.

REFERENCES

1. DALY, J. & G.J. KOTWAL. 1998. Pro-inflammatory complement activation by the Aβ peptide of Alzheimer's disease is biologically significant and can be blocked by vaccinia virus complement control protein. Neurobiol. Aging **19:** 619–627.
2. McGEER, P.L. & E.G. McGEER. 2004. Inflammation and neurodegeneration in Parkinson's disease. Parkinson Rel. Disorders **10:** S3–S7.
3. EIKELENBOOM, P. *et al.* 2002. Neuroinflammation in Alzheimer's disease and prion disease. Glia. **40:** 232–239.
4. HUNOT, S. & E.C. HIRSCH. 2003. Neuroinflammatory processes in Parkinson's disease. Ann. Neurol. **53:** S49–S60.
5. BRADL, M. & R. HOHLFELD. 2003. Molecular pathogenesis of neuroinflammation. J. Neurol. Neurosurg. Psychiatry **74:** 1364–1370.

6. MULLER, H.D. *et al.* 2003. Inflammatory infiltrates in the spinal cord of patients with Guillain-Barre syndrome. Acta Neuropathol. **106:** 509–517.
7. REYNOLDS, D.N. *et al.* 2003. Vaccinia virus complement control protein reduces neutrophil infiltration following spinal cord injury. Ann. N.Y. Acad. Sci. **1010:** 534– 539.
8. AISEN, P.S. *et al.* 2003. Effects of rofecoxib or naproxen vs placebo on Alzheimer disease progression: a randomized controlled trial. J. Am. Med. Assoc. **289:** 2819–2826.
9. SCHARF, S. *et al.* 1999. A double-blind, placebo-controlled trial of diclofenac/misoprostol in Alzheimer's disease. Neurology **53:**197–201.
10. MCGEER, P.L. & E.G. MCGEER. 1998. Glial cell reactions in neurodegenerative diseases: pathophysiology and therapeutic interventions. Alzh. Dis. Assoc. Disord. **2:** S1–S6.
11. MCGEER, P.L. *et al.* 1993. Microglia in degenerative neurological disease. Glia **7:** 84–92.
12. SINGHRAO, S.K. *et al.* 1999. Increased complement biosynthesis by microglia and complement activation on neurons in Huntington's disease. Exp. Neurol. **159:** 362–376.
13. GASQUE, P., M. FONTAINE & B.P. MORGAN. 1995. Complement expression in human brain. Biosynthesis of terminal pathway components and regulators in human glial cells and cell lines. J. Immunol. **154:** 4726–4733.
14. NATAF, S. *et al.* 1999. Complement anaphylatoxin receptors on neurons: new tricks for old receptors? Trends Neurosci. **22:** 397–402.
15. NATAF, S. *et al.* 2001. Expression of the anaphylatoxin C5a receptor in the oligodendrocyte lineage. Brain Res. **894:** 321–326.
16. DAVOUST, N. *et al.* 1999. Central nervous system—targeted expression of the complement inhibitor sCrry prevents experimental allergic encephalomyelitis. **163:** 6551–6556.
17. O'BARR, S.A. *et al.* 2001. Neuronal expression of a functional receptor for the C5a complement activation fragment. J. Immunol. **166:** 4154–4162.
18. KREUTZBERG, G.W. 1996. Microglia: a sensor for pathological events in the CNS. Trends Neurosci. **19:** 312–318.
19. DELEO, J.A. & R.P. YEZIERSKI. 2001. The role of neuroinflammation and neuroimmune activation in persistent pain. Pain **90:** 1–6.
20. LIAO, S.L. *et al.* 2001. Association of immune responses and ischemic brain infarction in rat. Neuroreport. **12:** 1943–1947.
21. WERNER, P., D. PITT & C.S. RAINE. 2000. Glutamate excitotoxicity—a mechanism for axonal damage and oligodendrocyte death in multiple sclerosis? J. Neural Transm. Suppl. **60:** 375–385.
22. STEIN, V.M. *et al.* 2004. Microglial cell activation in demyelinating canine distemper lesions. J. Neuroimmunol. **153:** 122–131.
23. HICKEY, W.F. & H. KIMURA. 1988. Perivascular microglia are bone marrow derived and present antigen in vivo. Science **239:** 290–292.
24. TIFFANY, H.L. *et al.* 2001. Amyloid-beta induces chemotaxis and oxidant stress by acting at formylpeptide receptor 2, a G protein-coupled receptor expressed in phagocytes and brain. J. Biol. Chem. **276:** 23645–23652.
25. BELL, M.D. *et al.* 1994. Upregulation of the macrophage scavenger receptor in response to different forms of injury in the CNS. J. Neurocytol. **23:** 605–613.
26. CHRISTIE, R.H., M. FREEMAN & B.T. HYMAN. 1996. Expression of the macrophage scavenger receptor, a multifunctional lipoprotein receptor, in microglia associated with senile plaques in Alzheimer's disease. Am. J. Pathol. **148:** 399–403.
27. YANG, G.Y. *et al.* 1999. Tumor necrosis factor alpha expression produces increased blood-brain barrier permeability following temporary focal cerebral ischemia in mice. Mol. Brain. Res. **69:** 135–143.
28. SINGHRAO, S.K. *et al.* 2000. Spontaneous classical pathway activation and deficiency of membrane regulators render human neurons susceptible to complement lysis. Am. J. Pathol. **157:** 905–918.
29. GASQUE, P. *et al.* 2002. Roles of the complement system in human neurodegenerative disorders: pro-inflammatory and tissue remodelling activities. Mol. Neurobiol. **25:** 1–17.
30. FONSECA, M.I. *et al.* 2004. Absence of C1q leads to less neuropathology in transgenic mouse models of Alzheimer's disease. J. Neurosci. **24:** 6457–6465.
31. SHEN, Y. *et al.* 2001. Complement activation by neurofibrillary tangles in Alzheimer's disease. Neurosci. Lett. **305:** 165–168.

32. HEAD, E. *et al.* 2001. Complement association with neurons and β-amyloid deposition in the brains of aged individuals with Down syndrome. Neurobiol. Dis. **8:** 252–265.
33. HOLERS, V.M. & J.M. THURMAN. 2004. The alternative pathway of complement in disease: opportunities for therapeutic targeting. Mol. Immunol. **41:** 147–152.
34. VAN BEEK, J., K. ELWARD & P. GASQUE. 2003. Activation of complement in the central nervous system: roles in neurodegeneration and neuroprotection. Ann. N.Y. Acad. Sci. **992:** 56–71.
35. MORGAN, B.P. & P. GASQUE. 1996. Expression of complement in health and disease. Immunol. Today **17:** 461–465.
36. SHEN, Y. & S. MERI. 2003. Yin and Yang: Complement activation and regulation in Alzheimer's disease. Prog. Neurobiol. **70:** 463–472.
37. WEBSTER, S., C. GLABE & J. ROGERS. 1995. Multivalent binding of complement protein C1q to the amyloid beta-peptide (A beta) promotes the nucleation phase of A beta aggregation. Biochem. Biophys. Res. Commun. **217:** 869–875.
38. JOHNS, T.G. & C.C. BERNARD. 1997. Binding of complement component C1q to myelin oligodendrocyte glycoprotein: a novel mechanism for regulating CNS inflammation. Mol. Immunol. **34:** 33–38.
39. MULLER-EBERHARD, H.J. 1988. Molecular organisation and function of the complement system. Annu. Rev. Biochem. **57:** 321–327.
40. PASINETTI, G.M. *et al.* 1996. Hereditary deficiencies in complement C5 are associated with intensified neurodegenerative responses that implicate new roles for the C-system in neuronal and astrocytic functions. Neurobiol. Dis. **3:** 197–204.
41. MUKHERJEE, P. & G.M. PASINETTI. 2000. The role of complement anaphylatoxin C5a in neurodegeneration: implications in Alzheimer's disease. J. Neuroimmunol. **105:** 124–130.
42. MUKHERJEE, P. & G.M. PASINETTI. 2001. Complement anaphylatoxin C5a neuro-protects through mitogen-activated protein kinase-dependent inhibition of caspase 3. J. Neurochem. **77:** 43–49.
43. OSAKA, H. *et al.* 1999. The role of neuroinflammation and neuroimmune activation in persistent pain. Pain **90:** 1–6.
44. VAN BEEK, J. *et al.* 2001. Complement anaphylatoxin C3a is selectively protective against NMDA-induced neuronal cell death. Neuroreport **12:** 289–293.
45. GERARD, C. & N.P. GERARD. 1994. C5a anaphylatoxin and its seven transmembrane receptor. Annu. Rev. Immunol. **12:** 775–808.
46. DEL BALZO, U., M.J. POLLEY & R. LEVI. 1989. C3a-induced contraction of guinea pig ileum consists of two components: fast histamine-mediated and slow prostanoid-mediated. J. Pharmacol. Exp. Ther. **248:** 1003–1009.
47. KAWATSU, R. *et al.* 1996. Conformationally biased analogs of human C5a mediate changes in vascular permeability. Pharmacol Exp. Ther. **278:** 432–440.
48. GASQUE, P. *et al.* 1998. The receptor for complement anaphylatoxin c3a is expressed by myeloid cells and nonmyeloid cells in inflamed human central nervous system: analysis in multiple sclerosis and bacterial meningitis. J. Immunol. **160:** 3544–3554.
49. LIU, B. *et al.* 2002. Role of nitric oxide in inflammation-mediated neurodegeneration. Ann. N.Y. Acad. Sci. **962:** 318–331.
50. BROWN, G.C. & A. BAL-PRICE. 2003. Inflammatory neurodegeneration mediated by nitric oxide, glutamate, and mitochondria. Mol. Neurobiol. **27:** 325–355.
51. BAO, F. & D. LIU. 2002. Peroxynitrite generated in the rat spinal cord induces neuron death and neurological deficits. Neuroscience **115:** 839–849.
52. KE, Z.J. & GE. GIBSON. 2004. Selective response of various brain cell types during neurodegeneration induced by mild impairment of oxidative metabolism. Neurochem. Intl. **45:** 361–369.
53. NAKAMURA, Y. *et al.* 2003. Involvement of protein kinase C in glutamate release from cultured microglia. Brain Res. **962:** 122–128.
54. ZWIRNER, J. *et al.* 1999. Evaluation of C3a receptor expression on human leucocytes by the use of novel monoclonal antibodies. Immunology **97:** 166–172.
55. ACARIN, L. *et al.* 2002. Expression of inducible nitric oxide synthase and cyclooxygenase-2 after excitotoxic damage to the immature rat brain. J. Neurosci. Res. **68:** 745–754.

56. INGLIS, V.I. *et al.* 2004. Neutrophils both reduce and increase permeability in a cell culture model of the blood-brain barrier. Brain Res. **998:** 218–229.

57. TOGO, T., O. KATSUSE & E. ISEKI. 2004. Nitric oxide pathways in Alzheimer's disease and other neurodegenerative dementias. Neurol. Res. **26:** 563–566.

58. THEOHARIDES, T.C. & D.E. COCHRANE. 2004. Critical role of mast cells in inflammatory diseases and the effect of acute stress. J. Neuroimmunol. **146:** 1–12.

59. WOOLHISER, M.R. *et al.* 2004. Activation of human mast cells by aggregated IgG through FcγRI: additive effects of C3a. Clin. Immunol. **110:** 172–180.

60. WOOLLEY, D.E. & L.C. TETLOW. 2000. Mast cell activation and its relation to proinflammatory cytokine production in the rheumatoid lesion. Arth. Res. **2:** 65–74.

61. FERRER, M., K. NAKAZAWA & A.P. KAPLAN. 1999. Complement dependence of histamine release in chronic urticaria. J. Allergy Clin. Immunol. **104:** 169–172.

62. SAYAH, S. *et al.* 1999. Expression of cytokines by human astrocytomas following stimulation by C3a and C5a anaphylatoxins: specific increase in interleukin-6 mRNA expression. J. Neurochem. **72:** 2426–2436.

63. PENKOWA, M. *et al.* 2003. Astrocyte-targeted expression of interleukin-6 protects the central nervous system during neuroglial degeneration induced by 6-aminonicotinamide. J. Neurosci Res. **73:** 481–496.

64. HEALES, S.J. *et al.* 2004. Neurodegeneration or neuroprotection: the pivotal role of astrocytes. Neurochem. Res. **29:** 513–519.

65. WEISS, J.M. *et al.*1998. Astrocyte-derived monocyte-chemoattractant protein-1 directs the transmigration of leukocytes across a model of the human blood-brain barrier. J. Immunol. **161:** 6896–7903.

66. YANG, L.B. *et al.* 2000. Deficiency of complement defense protein CD59 may contribute to neurodegeneration in Alzheimer's disease. J. Neurosci. **20:** 7505–7509.

67. SHEN, Y. *et al.* 1997. Characterization of neuronal cell death induced by complement activation. Brain Res. Protocols **1:** 186–194.

68. WURZNER, R. 2003. Deficiencies of the complement MAC II gene cluster (C6, C7, C9): is subtotal C6 deficiency of particular evolutionary benefit? Clin. Exp. Immunol. **133:** 156–159.

69. LAHIRI, D.K. *et al.* 2003. A critical analysis of new molecular targets and strategies for drug developments in Alzheimer's disease. Curr. Drug Targets **4:** 97–112.

70. FONSECA, M.I. *et al.* 2004. Neuronal localization of C1q in preclinical Alzheimer's disease. Neurobiol Dis. **15:** 40–46.

71. MCGEER, E.G. & P.L. MCGEER. 2003. Inflammatory processes in Alzheimer's disease. Prog. Neuro-Psychopharmacol. Biol. Psychiat. **27:** 741–749.

72. STROHMEYER, R., Y. SHEN & J. ROGERS. 2000. Detection of complement alternative pathway mRNA and proteins in the Alzheimer's disease brain. Brain Res. Mol. Brain. Res. **81:** 7–18.

73. LAHIRI, D.K. *et al.* 2003. Role of cytokines in the gene expression of amyloid β-protein precursor: identification of a 5′-UTR-binding nuclear factor and its implications in Alzheimer's disease. J. Alz. Dis. **5:** 81–90.

74. HEAD, E. *et al.* 2001. Complement association with neurons and β-amyloid deposition in the brains of aged individuals with Down syndrome Neurobiol. Dis. **8:** 252–265.

75. SELLEBJERG, F. *et al.* 1998. Intrathecal activation of the complement system and disability in multiple sclerosis. J. Neurol. Sci. **157:** 168–174.

76. SANDERS, M.E. *et al.* 1986. Activated terminal complement in cerebrospinal fluid in Guillain-Barre syndrome and multiple sclerosis. J. Immunol. **136:** 4456–4459.

77. PUTZU, G.A. *et al.* 2000. Immunohistochemical localization of cytokines, C5b-9 and ICAM-1 in peripheral nerve of Guillain-Barre syndrome. J. Neurol. Sci. **174:** 16–21.

78. MCGEER, P.L., K. YASOJIMA & E.G. MCGEER. 2001. Inflammation in Parkinson's disease. Adv. Neurol. **86:** 83–89.

79. BELLANDER, B.M. *et al.* 2004. Activation of microglial cells and complement following traumatic injury in rat entorhinal-hippocampal slice cultures. J. Neurotrauma **21:** 605–615.

80. XIONG, Z. *et al.* 2003. Formation of complement membrane attack complex in mammalian cerebral cortex evokes seizures and neurodegeneration. J. Neurosci. **23:** 955–960.

81. KOVACS, G.G. *et al.* 2004. Complement activation in human prion disease. Neurobiol. Dis. **15:** 21–28.
82. SINGHRAO, S.K. *et al.* 1996. Role of complement in the aetiology of Pick's disease? J. Neuropathol. Exp. Neurol. **55:** 578–593.
83. LI, J. *et al.* 2003. Peroxynitrite induces apoptosis in canine cerebral vascular muscle cells: possible relation to neurodegenerative diseases and strokes. Neurosci. Lett. **350:** 173–177.
84. ROTILIO, G., K. AQUILANO & M.R. CIRIOLO. 2003. Interplay of Cu, Zn superoxide dismutase and nitric oxide synthase in neurodegenerative processes. IUBMB Life **55:** 629–634.
85. CONSILVIO, C. *et al.* 2004. Neuroinflammation, COX-2, and ALS—a dual role? Exp. Neurol. **187:** 1–10.
86. MAKRIDES, S.C. 1998. Therapeutic inhibition of the complement system. Pharmacol. Rev. **50:** 59–87.
87. HILTON, G.D. *et al.* 2004. Neuroprotective effects of estradiol in newborn female rat hippocampus. Brain Res. Dev. Brain Res. **150:** 191–198.
88. GONZALEZ DENISELLE, M.C. *et al.* 2002. Basis of progesterone protection in spinal cord neurodegeneration. J. Steroid Biochem. Mol. Biol. **83:** 199–209.
89. BRUCE-KELLER, A.J. *et al.* 2000. Antiinflammatory effects of estrogen on microglial activation. Endocrinology **141:** 3646–3656.
90. AISEN, P.S. *et al.* 2000. A randomized controlled trial of prednisone in Alzheimer's disease. Alzheimer's disease cooperative study. Neurology **54:** 588–593; Comment Neurology **55:** 1067.
91. REICHMAN, W.E. 2000. Alzheimer's disease: clinical treatment options. Am. J. Manag. Care **6:** S1125–S1132 [discussion: S1133–S1138].
92. KRISTIN, K.H. *et al.* 2003. The neuronal nitric oxide synthase inhibitor, TRIM, as a neuroprotective agent: effects in models of cerebral ischaemia using histological and magnetic resonance imaging techniques. Brain Res. **993:** 42–53.
93. FLOYD, R.A. 2002. Nitrones as neuroprotectants and antiaging drugs. Ann. N.Y. Acad. Sci. **959:** 321–329.
94. MIZUNO, T. *et al.* 2004. Neuroprotective role of phosphodiesterase inhibitor ibudilast on neuronal cell death induced by activated microglia. Neuropharmacology **46:** 404–411.
95. HARNETT, J.J. *et al.* 2004. Phenolic thiazoles as novel orally-active neuroprotective agents. Bioorganic Medicinal Chem. Lett. **14:** 157–160.
96. BLAKE, A.D. 2004. Dipyridamole is neuroprotective for cultured rat embryonic cortical neurons. Biochem.Biophys. Res. Commun. **314:** 501–504.
97. TOYODA, K. *et al.* 2004. Free radical scavenger, edaravone, in stroke with internal carotid artery occlusion. J. Neurol. Sci. **221:** 11–17.
98. KATSUMATA, T. *et al.* 2003. Neuroprotective effect of NS-7, a novel Na and Ca channel blocker, in a focal ischemic model in the rat. Brain Res. **969:** 168–174.
99. SARNE, Y. & O. KEREN. 2004. Are cannabinoid drugs neurotoxic or neuroprotective? Med. Hypotheses. **63:** 187–192.
100. WYSS-CORAY, T. *et al.* 2002. Prominent neurodegeneration and increased plaque formation in complement-inhibited Alzheimer's mice. **99:** 10837–10842.
101. DE SIMONI, M.G. *et al.* 2004. The powerful neuroprotective action of C1-inhibitor on brain ischemia-reperfusion injury does not require C1q. Am. J. Pathol. **164:** 1857–1863.
102. JHA, P. & G.J. KOTWAL. 2003. Vaccinia complement control protein: multi-functional protein and a potential wonder drug. J. Biosci. **28:** 265–271.
103. KOTWAL, G.J. & B. MOSS. 1988. Vaccinia virus encodes a secretory polypeptide structurally related to complement control proteins. Nature **335:** 176–178.
104. KOTWAL, G.J., S.N. ISSACS & R. MCKENZIE. 1990. Vaccinia virus major secretory protein inhibits the classical complement cascade. Science **250:** 827–830.
105. MCKENZIE, R. *et al.* 1992. Regulation of complement activity by vaccinia virus complement-control protein. J. Infect. Dis. **166:** 1245–1250.
106. SAHU, A. *et al.* 1998. Interaction of vaccinia virus complement control protein with human complement proteins: factor I-mediated degradation of C3b to iC3b1 inactivates the alternative complement pathway. J. Immunol. **160:** 5596–5604.

107. KEELING, K.L. *et al.* 2000. Local neutrophil influx following lateral fluid percussion brain injury in rats is associated with accumulation of complement activation fragments of the third component (C3) of the complement system. J. Neuroimmunol. **105:** 20–30.
108. AL-MOHANNA, F., R. PARHAR & G. J. KOTWAL. 2001. Vaccinia virus complement control protein is capable of protecting xenoendothelial cells from antibody binding and killing by human complement and cytotoxic cells. Transplantation **71:** 796–801.
109. KOTWAL, G.J., D.K. LAHIRI & R. HICKS. 2002. Potential intervention by vaccinia virus complement control protein of the signals contributing to the progression of central nervous system injury to Alzheimer's disease. Ann. N.Y. Acad. Sci. **973:** 317–322.
110. HICKS, R.H. *et al.* 2002. Vaccinia virus complement control protein enhances functional recovery after traumatic brain injury. J. Neurotrauma **19:** 705–714.
111. KOTWAL, G.J. 2000. Poxviral mimicry of complement and chemokine system components: what's the end game? Immunol. Today **21:** 242–248.

Vaccinia Virus Complement Control Protein Reduces Inflammation and Improves Spinal Cord Integrity Following Spinal Cord Injury

DAVID N. REYNOLDS,[a] SCOTT A. SMITH,[a] YI P. ZHANG,[b,c] QIU MENGSHENG,[c] DEBOMOY K. LAHIRI,[d] DANTE J. MORASSUTTI,[b] CHRISTOPHER B. SHIELDS,[b] AND GIRISH J. KOTWAL[a,e]

[a]*Department of Microbiology and Immunology, University of Louisville School of Medicine, Louisville, Kentucky 40202, USA*

[b]*Department of Neurological Surgery, University of Louisville School of Medicine, Louisville, Kentucky 40202, USA*

[c]*Department of Anatomical Sciences and Neurobiology, University of Louisville School of Medicine, Louisville, Kentucky 40202, USA*

[d]*Department of Psychiatry, Indiana University School of Medicine, Indianapolis, Indiana 46202, USA*

[e]*Division of Medical Virology, University of Cape Town, Medical School, Cape Town, South Africa*

ABSTRACT: Traumatic spinal cord injury (SCI) claims approximately 10,000 new victims each year in the United States alone. The injury usually strikes those under the age of 30 years, often leading to a lifetime of pain, suffering, and disability. Therapeutic agents targeting spinal cord injury are sorely lacking, and therefore our laboratory endeavored to evaluate the potential therapeutic benefits of immediate post-injury administration of the vaccinia virus complement control protein (VCP). VCP is a multifunctional anti-inflammatory protein that can inhibit both pathways of complement activation and bind heparin. Utilizing a common animal model of contusion SCI, motor function recovery tests, and immunochemical stains, we evaluated the effects of VCP injected into spinal cord tissue following injury. Results demonstrate that VCP administration inhibits macrophage infiltration, reduces spinal cord destruction, and improves hind-limb function, establishing VCP as a strong candidate for further investigation in the treatment of SCI.

KEYWORDS: spinal cord injury; vaccinia virus complement control protein; inflammation

Address for correspondence: Girish J. Kotwal, Division of Medical Virology, Institute for Infectious Disease and Molecular Medicine (IIDMM), University of Cape Town, Medical School, Anzio Road, Observatory, Cape Town, South Africa. Voice: +27-21-406-6676; fax: +27-21-448-4110.

gjkotw01@yahoo.com

Ann. N.Y. Acad. Sci. 1035: 165–178 (2004). © 2004 New York Academy of Sciences.
doi: 10.1196/annals.1332.011

INTRODUCTION

Every year in the United States, more than 10,000 people experience traumatic spinal cord injury (SCI), with an estimated total of 250,000 of those cases sufficiently severe to require wheelchair use.[1] A majority of SCI patients are injured while under the age of 30 years and will often experience a normal lifespan, leading to extremely high medical costs over the course of that lifetime.[2] It is important to realize that a seemingly minute degree of neuronal sparing or regeneration could result in a significantly improved quality of life, for voluntary muscle control can occur when only 5–10% of neurons remain intact through a lesioned segment of the spinal cord.

SCI is an extremely difficult condition to understand and manage in a clinical setting owing to the multitude of injury mechanisms involved in the injury. In addition to the primary injury, it is thought that a complex array of secondary-injury mechanisms account for the progression of damage from the central gray matter to the surrounding white matter that begins within minutes and persists long after the primary injury. After several days to weeks, the initial injury can expand in size, leading to a scar-encapsulated cavity many times the size of the original lesion.[3] The cavity is bounded by abnormally proliferating glial cells, primarily astrocytes, which form a physical barrier to any potential neuronal regeneration.[1] Suspected secondary-injury mechanisms include hemorrhage, ischemia–reperfusion, excitotoxicity, demyelination, and calcium-mediated injury. Disturbances in mitochondrial function, apoptosis and necrosis of neurons and oligodendrocytes, and inflammation have also been reported.[4] Clearly, a sound understanding of the secondary-injury mechanisms is critical to the development of effective pharmacologic therapies.

Currently, only one therapeutic agent, methylprednisolone (MP), is widely considered standard therapy after traumatic SCI. MP is a synthetic glucocorticosteroid that has been subjected to several large-scale human clinical trials and shown minor clinical benefits when administered within 48 h of SCI.[5] However, questions regarding MP's efficacy persist because of controversy surrounding study design and analysis/interpretation of data from clinical trials. Therefore, continued investigation and evaluation of potential therapeutic agents for traumatic SCI are paramount.[6,7]

Vaccinia virus complement control protein (VCP) is a secreted inflammation-modulatory protein possessed by the vaccinia virus, a member of the poxvirus family. VCP was identified in 1988 and found to inhibit the classical and alternative pathways of the complement cascade, a system of more than 30 proteins involved in the innate (nonspecific) immune response.[8,9] Because of the series of protein cleavages that occur when complement is activated, several potent inflammatory mediators, such as C3a, C4a, and C5a, are released. Experiments have shown that VCP possesses the ability to inhibit the complement cascade in the early stages of activation, thereby preventing release of inflammatory proteins and enabling the virus to "hide" from the host immune system.[10] Our lab has shown that VCP and its homologues in other poxviruses can significantly reduce the tissue damage caused by inflammatory responses *in vivo*,[11] and we recently discovered that VCP also possesses the ability to bind heparin and heparin-like molecules, possibly allowing prolonged tissue retention.[12,13] Because VCP is structurally similar to normal mammalian complement regulatory proteins, a host immune response against the protein is not mounted, making VCP an attractive potential anti-inflammatory therapy. Recently, the therapeutic ability of VCP was tested using a rat model of traumatic brain injury.[14]

Remarkably, VCP was able to reduce functional impairment, significantly improving spatial memory following brain injury.

MATERIALS AND METHODS

Production and Purification of VCP

VCP was produced by the *Pichia pastoris* yeast expression system (Invitrogen, Carlsbad, CA) described previously.[15,16] Purification of VCP was achieved through heparin HiTRAP (Pharmacia) column chromatography, with VCP elution attained with a gradient of NaCl (100 mM–1 M). VCP regularly eluted from the heparin column with the 400 mM fraction of NaCl. Presence of VCP was confirmed with SDS-PAGE and silver staining.

Spinal Cord Injury Model

All procedures involving experimental animals were performed according to the guidelines of the University of Louisville Institutional Animal Care and Use Committee. Impact injury was induced using a weight-drop device developed at New York University (the NYU impactor).[17,18] Adult Sprague-Dawley rats weighing between 200–250 g were anesthetized with pentobarbital (50 mg/kg, i.p.) and given prophylactic antibiotic injections (gentamicin sulfate, 15 mg/kg, s.c.) if survival times were planned to exceed 48 h. A laminectomy was performed at the T9-T10 level, and the spinous processes of T8 and T11 were rigidly clamped in a spinal frame in order to stabilize the spine. The exposed dorsal surface of the cord was then subjected to a mild impact injury in which a 10-g rod (2.5 mm in diameter) was dropped at a height of 12.5 mm and displaced the cord for duration of 23 ms, using an NYU Impactor. The mild (12.5 g/cm) severity of the impact was chosen because there is sufficient locomotor recovery to enable the rats to stand and walk for approximately 6 weeks post injury. The injury protocol used produces an anatomically consistent contusion lesion, which is reproducible between animals, and results in immediate and complete hind-limb paralysis, with partial recovery over the course of 5–6 weeks post injury.[19] The dura remained intact during injury induction. For animals not designated to receive post-injury intraparenchymal injections, their muscles were then sutured with No. 4-0 silk thread and their skin closed with clips. Animals designated to receive intraparenchymal injections were immediately subjected to the injection protocol described below, and their wounds closed with sutures and clips as described previously. Sham-operated control animals received T9-T10 laminectomy without weight-drop injury.

Following surgery, the animals were given 10 mL subcutaneous injections of 0.9% saline solution and placed on a heating pad (36.5–37.5°C) until recovery from anesthesia. The animals were then placed in their cages with easily accessible food and water and returned to the animal-holding facilities where they were maintained and monitored until the designated time of sacrifice. For animals that received contusion injury, their bladders were manually expressed twice daily until normal voiding was obtained (usually by 10–14 days).

Spinal Cord Intraparenchymal Injections

The Kentucky Spinal Cord Injury Research Center at the University of Louisville has developed an effective method of injecting small proteins into the rat spinal cord parenchyma.[20] Borosilicate pipettes (1.2 µm O.D.) were pulled on a Sutter Electrode Puller (P-87) and bevelled to 25 µm (WPI Beveller). The pipettes are premarked with 0.2–1.5 µL graduations and, with short pressure pulses (0.5–100 ms, 5–20 psi), the device is capable of delivering as little as 0.2 µL of solution with great accuracy. The pipettes were lowered into the spinal cord using a stereotaxic apparatus. Immediately prior to each injection, the dura was delicately opened and reflected with a 30-gauge needle in order to allow access for the injection pipette. All experimental animals designated to receive intraparenchymal injections were given two bilateral 5-µL injections, for a total of 10 µL per animal, of the desired solution at the visible T9 injury epicenter, or at the comparable site in uninjured control animals. The injection pipettes were placed 1.6 mm deep in the spinal cord tissue and 0.7 mm from the midline of the spinal cord. Immediately prior to injection, the pipettes were raised slightly (less than 1 mm) in order to provide a reservoir within the tissue in which the injected solution could pool. Each 5-µL injection was given gradually over a period of 5 min in order to avoid fluid pressure-induced tissue damage. Following injection, the muscles were sutured and the skin closed with clips. Control animals received injections of normal saline solution, while other animals received injections of VCP.

Rat Perfusions

After the appropriate recovery period, rats were deeply anesthetized via intra-peritoneal (i.p.) injections of 0.3–0.4 mL pentobarbital and placed securely on a dissecting rack. Using surgical scissors, the diaphragm was punctured and the heart exposed. A perfusion needle was then inserted through the left ventricle and left atrium, and into the ascending aorta. A small puncture was then made in the right atrium in order to allow blood and other fluids to drain. Next, 200–250 mL of 0.01 M phosphate-buffered saline (PBS) was pumped through the animals' circulatory system, followed by 400–500 mL of 4% paraformaldehyde (Sigma, St. Louis, MO) in 0.01 M PBS. The rats were then dissected and their spinal cord sections were removed using surgical scalpels and forceps, and placed in 4% paraformaldehyde overnight. The spinal cord sections were then cryoprotected by placing them in a solution of 25% sucrose in 0.01 M PBS and maintaining them at 4°C, until sectioning.

ED-1 Immunostaining

The spinal cord tissue was placed on a metal platform, embedded in TBS tissue-freezing medium (Triangle Biomedical Sciences, Durham, NC) in the desired orientation, and placed inside a Bright OTF Cryostat (Bright Instrument Co., Huntingdon, England) set at −20°C. The temperature of the tissue/tissue-freezing medium was allowed to equilibrate for a period of 30–45 min before sectioning. The section thickness was set to 20 µm and the tissue there cut in cross section or longitudinally. The tissue sections were immediately placed on Super frost/Plus microscope slides (Fisher) and stored at 4°C.

The mounted sections were washed three times in 0.01 M PBS in order to remove the freezing medium. Next, 200 µL of block solution (0.01 M PBS/0.3% Triton/10%

normal donkey serum) was added and allowed to incubate at room temperature for 1 h. A solution of mouse anti-ED-1 antibody (Serotec, Raleigh, NC) was then mixed with block solution at a dilution of 1 in 200 and 200 µL added to each slide. The slides were incubated overnight at room temperature and washed in PBS five times on day 2. A solution of donkey anti-mouse-(FITC) (Jackson Immuno Research Labs, West Grove, PA) was mixed with the block solution (without donkey serum) at a dilution of 1 in 100, and 1 in 200 µL was added to each slide. The slides were shaken gently in a dark at room for 2 h and washed in PBS three times. Slides were then dried, mounted with Gel/Mount (Biomeda, Foster City, CA), and stored in the dark at 4°C. Stained tissue was viewed with an Eclipse TE 300 (Nikon, Melville, NY) fluorescent microscope at magnifications of 40× or 100×. Images were captured with a SPOT TR Color camera (Diagnostic Instruments, San Diego, CA) and analyzed with SPOT Advanced software. Relative intensities of ED-1-stained tissue sections were measured as density values using the Alpha Imager 2000 software system.

Assessment of Locomotor Function

The 21-point Basso-Beattie-Bresnahan (BBB) open-field locomotor scale developed at the Ohio State University was used to evaluate functional recovery.[19] The BBB involves placing the rats in an empty plastic wading pool and assessing the hind-limb movements over a time period of 4 min. Three investigators observed the animals' movements independently, and a score for each animal was given based on the consensus of the investigators. Beginning 1 week post surgery, the animals were evaluated once per week for 6 weeks. The BBB scoring system evaluates all major motor groups of the hind limbs, bladder function, and ability to ambulate. The 21-point scale generally follows the progression of recovery, with a score of 21 representing the characteristics of a normal animal.

The grid-walking test assesses an animal's ability to walk over a plastic mesh (thickness of 0.5 mm) with diamond-shaped openings (4.5 × 5 cm) pulled over a square metal frame (46 inches square) for a period of 3 min. The grid surface was raised 12–24 inches in height in order to provide a lateral view of the hind limbs above and below the grid surface. The assessment was performed blind by two investigators, with each investigator observing only the right or left hind limb. The number of hind-limb footfalls through the mesh was recorded. Footfalls were counted only if the hind limb descended below the mesh to at least the hip (¾ of the limb). Multiple failed attempts to reposition the same limb at one particular location on the grid were not counted as additional footfall errors. Since animals with insufficient hind-limb recovery could not be used, the test was administered at 6 weeks post injury, a time point at which most of the injured animals were achieving a minimum score of 11 on the BBB scale. Statistical analysis was carried out using paired *t*-test.

RESULTS

Gross Appearance of Injured VCP-Treated Spinal Cords

Before the excision of the injured VCP-treated spinal cords, images of the exposed cords were captured with a 35-mm camera (FIG. 1). The pictures were taken after the skin, musculature, and appropriate vertebrae had been removed. The cords

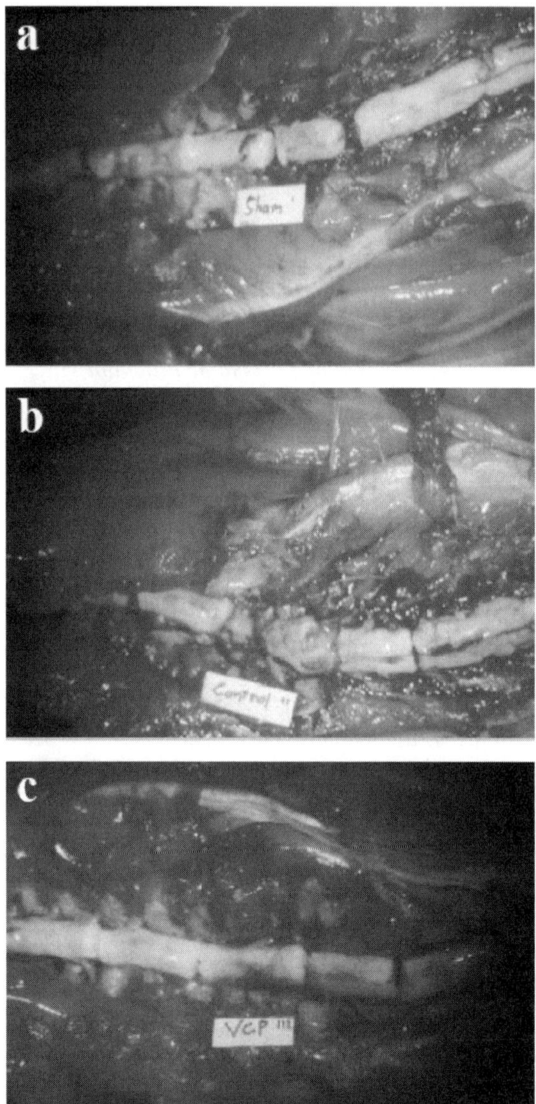

FIGURE 1. VCP reduces spinal cord destruction following contusion injury: (**a**) uninjured sham-VCP spinal cord after 24 h; (**b**) injured control spinal cord after 24 h; (**c**) injured-VCP spinal cord after 24 h. In each case, the spinal cords were cut into three sections (rostral, epicenter, and caudal).

were cut into three sections (rostral, epicenter, and caudal) with surgical scissors relative to the injury, but were not otherwise manipulated. The pictures were taken to provide a record of the gross appearance of spinal cord integrity prior to removal from the animal. The uninjured cord (sham) (FIG. 1A) received only an injection (~76 µg) of VCP. The integrity and appearance of the cord is very similar to that of a normal spinal cord. No bruising or discoloration is evident and, upon cutting of the cord, there was neither liquefaction nor subsequent leakage of spinal cord tissue. While the integrity of the sham-VCP cord was excellent (FIG. 1A), the injured control cord (FIG. 1B) was severely damaged. The epicenter section was bruised and discolored, with a significant degree of liquefaction and leakage upon cutting, resulting in loss of structural integrity. Similar characteristics were observed in the cord segments immediately rostral and caudal to the epicenter. Conversely, the injured VCP-treated cord (FIG. 1C) was similar in appearance to the uninjured cord. The injured VCP cord displayed only slight bruising, but no liquefaction nor leakage of cord contents upon cutting, enabling the structural integrity of the epicenter segment to remain intact (FIG. 1C).

Role of VCP in Altering Macrophage/Microglial Response after SCI

The role of VCP in altering the macrophage/microglial response following injury was assessed with the ED-1 antibody, which is specific for a lysosomal antigen in activated macrophages/microglial cells. Spinal cord tissue obtained from animals at three different time points (48 h, 7 days, and 14 days) was stained with ED-1 (FIG. 2). Initial results indicate that macrophage/microglial activation and/or influx is slightly reduced at the 48-h time point in injured-VCP animals when compared to injured-saline animals. After 7 days, there appears to be a substantial increase in macrophage/microglial influx in the injured-VCP tissue as compared to injured-saline tissue, with more intense staining in the central gray matter of the injured-VCP animals and more diffuse staining in the injured-saline animals (FIG. 2). After 14 days, the staining is much more intense in the injured-saline animals, with only a small area of positive staining in the dorsal funiculus of the injured-VCP animals. Uninjured animals show little to no positive ED-1 staining (FIG. 2).

Role of VCP in Altering Motor Function Recovery after SCI

The 21-point Basso-Beattie-Bresnahan (BBB) open-field locomotor scale and a grid-walking test were the methods used to evaluate locomotor function recovery following SCI. The BBB rates the ability of an animal to use its hind limbs during ambulation. A score of 21 would indicate a completely normal animal, while a score of 0 would indicate no observable hind-limb movement. BBB experiments involved sham-VCP ($n = 2$), saline-injured ($n = 5$), and injured-VCP animals ($n = 8$) (FIG. 3). VCP animals received 5 µL bilateral injections (4.80 µg/µL) for a total of 48 µg per animal. The hind limbs were rated separately once per week for 6 weeks following injury. The average scores for sham-VCP animals remained nearly normal during the 6-week study, with the left hind limb fluctuating between 19 and 20 (FIG. 3A), and the right hind limb between 18.5 and 20 (FIG. 3B). The average scores of the saline-injured animals were significantly worse, with the left hind limb scoring a 6.2 at week 1, a 12.8 at week 6, and achieving a maximum of 13 at week 5. The right hind

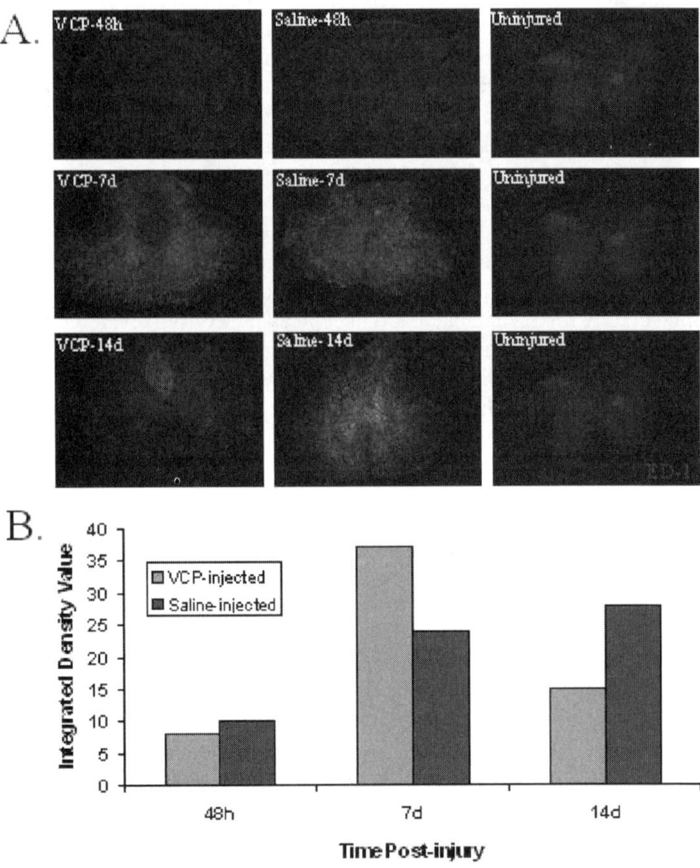

FIGURE 2. VCP alters the macrophage/microglial response following SCI: (**A**) summary of ED-1 staining of macrophages/microglial cells in uninjured control, injured-VCP, and injured-saline animals at 48 h, 7 days, and 14 days (40× objective); (**B**) comparison of relative intensities of ED-1 staining in VCP- and saline-treated injured animals as measured by density analysis.

limb scores reached an initial 7.8 at week 1, a final score of 13.2 at week 6, and a maximum score of 13.6 at weeks 4 and 5 (FIG. 3B). The average left hind limb scores of the injured-VCP animals at week 1 was 10.3 and ended with a maximum 14.9 at week 6 (FIG. 3A). The right hind limb scores began with a score of 10.9 at week 1 and rose to maximum of 15.5 by week 6. The scores for both hind limbs of the injured-VCP animals were substantially higher at week 1, but at each week thereafter the increases were not statistically significant, even though a trend of consistently higher scores for the injured-VCP animals is apparent.

Following the conclusion of the 6-week BBB study involving the animals mentioned above, the same animals were subjected to a grid-walking test as a further

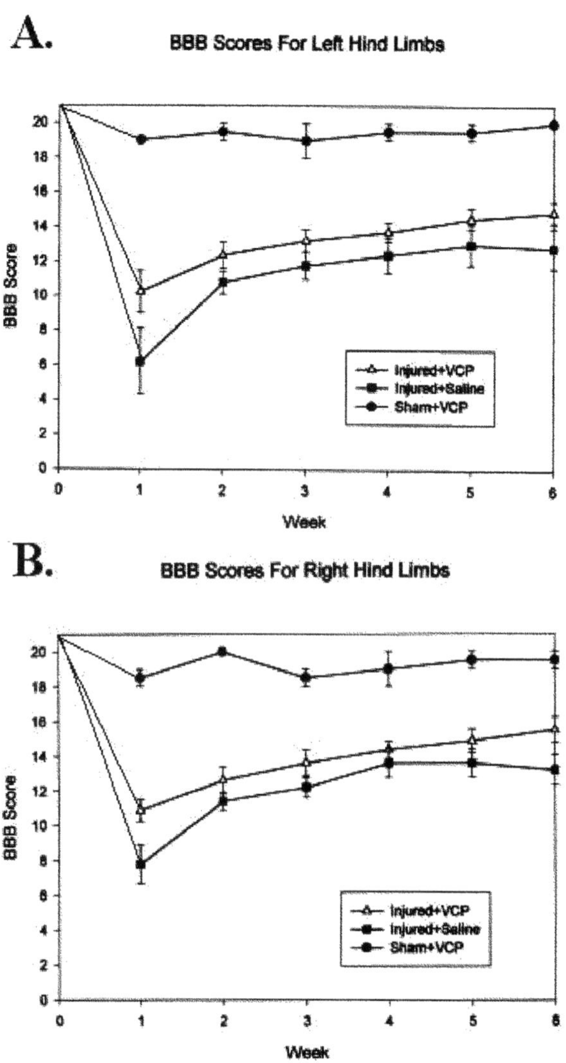

FIGURE 3. VCP increases motor function recovery after SCI as assessed by the Basso-Beattie-Bresnahan (BBB) open-field locomotor scale. Each VCP-treated animal received a total of 48 µg VCP in two bilateral injections. NYU impactor injuries were mild (12.5 g/cm) at T9 level. (**A**) BBB scores for left hind limbs of injured and control rats. (**B**) BBB scores for right hind limbs of injured and control rats.

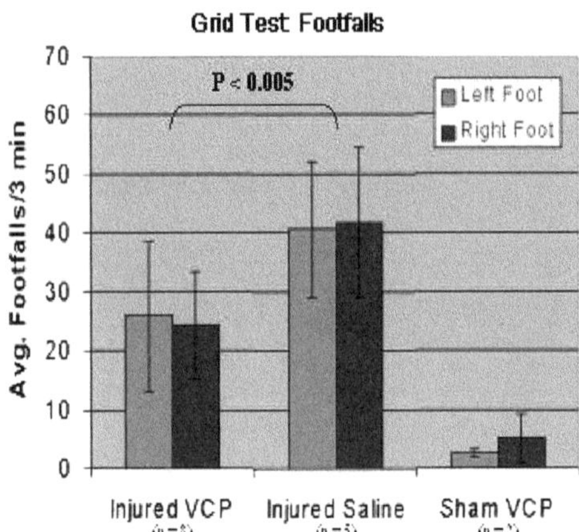

FIGURE 4. VCP increases motor function recovery after SCI as assessed by the grid-walking test. Grid-walking test results (right and left hind foot) for injured saline-injected, injured VCP-treated, and sham VCP-treated control animals 6 weeks after injury. Injured VCP-treated animals showed significantly fewer footfalls, combined right and left foot ($P < 0.005$), when compared to injured saline-injected animals.

measure of locomotor function recovery. The grid-walking test was administered only at week 6 and measured the number of times an animal's hind limbs slipped through (termed footfalls) a wire mesh during a 3-min period of ambulation. The sham-VCP animals averaged only 3.75 footfalls, while the saline-injured animals averaged 41.2 footfalls, and the injured-VCP animals averaged 25.1 footfalls (FIG. 4). The differences between saline-injured animals and the injured-VCP animals were statistically significant ($P < 0.005$) (FIG. 4).

DISCUSSION

The efforts invested in spinal cord injury (SCI) research have increased dramatically over the course of the past decade. Due to recent advancements in the understanding of SCI pathophysiologic mechanisms and renewed public interest, a great deal of attention has been channelled into research concerning spinal cord injury and potential therapeutic strategies. Until recently, SCI exploration languished mostly because of the complexity of the injury process after the initial physical trauma. It is now believed that multiple physiologic processes contribute to what has become known as the secondary-injury phase, which begins within minutes of primary injury and can persist for years. Hemorrhage, ischemia-reperfusion, excitotoxicity, demyelination, calcium mediated injury, disturbances in mitochondrial function, apoptosis and necrosis of neurons and oligodendrocytes, and inflammation are all mechanisms currently thought to be involved in the exacerbation of primary injury, although exactly how these events interact and which are most destructive are areas still subject to debate.[4]

Recent results of both myeloperoxidase (MPO) assays and H&E-stained section counts of spinal tissue have revealed that neutrophil infiltration into SCI lesion areas was reduced in animals that received VCP when compared to saline-injected controls.[21] Results demonstrated that animals receiving VCP exhibited MPO levels of roughly half those seen in injured control animals, indicating that neutrophil influx was substantially reduced. Histological staining and manual counting of neutrophils in injured spinal cord tissue corroborated MPO evidence. Previous studies have associated neutrophil influx inhibition with decreased tissue damage and improved functional recovery.[22–24] Activated neutrophils are postulated to significantly contribute to secondary injury on account of their release of proteases and oxygen radicals, which can be extremely harmful to local cells.

The gross appearances of the VCP-treated injured cords were quite revealing when compared to injured-control cords (saline-injected). While the sham-VCP cords closely resembled normal uninjured cords, the injured-control cords were extremely bruised and displayed a great deal of liquefaction of the inner contents and deformation upon cutting of the segments for removal (FIG. 1). The VCP-injured cords, however, did not resemble the injured-control cords, but rather displayed structural integrity more akin to that of the sham-VCP cords. Bruising was much less severe in the VCP-treated injured cords than in the injured-control cords, and the VCP-treated injured cords displayed much less liquefaction upon dissection. These results indicate that VCP administration may be able to limit lesion size and severity, leading to increased tissue sparing. Even a relatively small degree of neuronal sparing may have a significant effect upon improved functional recovery after SCI.

The macrophage/microglial cells most likely play a pivotal role in determining the outcome following SCI, although whether macrophage/microglial responses are beneficial, deleterious, or both, remains subject to debate. What is known, however, is that activated macrophages are first observed in injury epicenter areas within 12 h and peak within 14 to 21 days after injury.[24] Our experiments utilizing the ED-1 antibody, specific for a macrophage/microglial lysosomal antigen, indicate slightly reduced activation/influx in the epicenter of injured-VCP animals at the 48-h time point when compared to injured-saline animals. ED-1 staining after 7 days is substantially more intense in the injured-VCP cords, with staining more localized in the central gray matter when compared to the injured-saline tissue. Macrophage/microglial activation appears greater in injured-saline animals after 14 days than in injured-VCP animals. Previous studies have implicated macrophages' invading spinal cord tissue from the peripheral circulation as primary mediators of secondary injury, while assigning a more beneficial and potentially regenerative role to resident microglial cells. Unfortunately, it is impossible to differentiate between invading macrophages and resident microglia using the ED-1 antibody. In fact, short of depleting peripheral macrophages or creating chimeric animals, it can be virtually impossible to distinguish between the two cell-types of the same lineage. However, on the basis of our ED-1 results, it can be hypothesized that VCP, through its complement and chemotaxis-inhibition properties, is able to slightly reduce the influx of peripheral macrophages into injured epicenters within the first 48 h. However, the considerable increase in macrophage/microglial activation in VCP-treated animals at the 7-day time point and precipitous decrease at the 14-day time point in the same tissue is unexpected, but intriguing. Cord tissues of injured control animals receiving saline injection show a steady increase in macrophage/microglial activation throughout the 2-week time period, reflecting the typical situation in which influx and activation of such cells peak within a 2- to 3-week period.[25] While a clear explanation of the observed results is unavailable, it is possible that VCP, through its ability to inhibit peripheral macrophage chemotaxis, is able to promote early activation and expansion of resident microglial populations as a result of the dearth of peripheral macrophage infiltration. It is plausible that decreased early influx of peripheral macrophages, coupled with increased activation of resident microglia, could lead to less inflammatory damage to the cord and elevated capacity for regeneration on account of the putative beneficial activity of microglia.[26–29]

Behavioral tests suggest that VCP treatment promotes motor function recovery. The 21-point Basso-Beattie-Bresnahan (BBB) open-field locomotor scale is a commonly used test to analyze the recovery of hind-limb function over the course of several weeks after injury.[19] For our studies, animals were scored once per week for a total of 6 weeks. Injured-VCP animals demonstrated a substantially higher BBB score at week 1 for both hind limbs when compared to injured-saline animals. However, the gap between the two groups closed significantly after the first week, and while average scores for injured-VCP animals remained consistently higher than the injured-saline throughout the 6-week study, the discrepancies never approached the magnitude of that seen for week 1. While the difference in scores for injured-VCP versus injured-saline at week 1 were not statistically significant, the results indicate that VCP may be able to promote some degree of motor function recovery in the early stages of injury. Given that VCP injections were only given once immediately after the injury and not multiple times throughout the 6-week study, it is not surprising that the most substantial difference in scores was observed only within 1 week of injection.

The same animals subjected to the 6-week BBB study were also analyzed at week 6 with the grid-walking test, a less subjective analysis of hind-limb function.[30] It was found that injured-VCP animals committed significantly fewer footfalls per evaluation period than did the injured-saline animals. These results were statistically significant and demonstrated that the BBB test should not be the only motor function assessment used when dealing with spinal cord–injured animals. The BBB test relies on human graders to make subjective judgments concerning subtle but quick hind-limb movements of three different joints (hip, knee, and ankle). These rapid movements present a challenge to the observer to categorize in a short time. The grid-walking test requires human observers to simply record the number of times a single hind-limb is placed through the open squares of a grid apparatus, relying less upon subjective judgment. It was evident in our study that, even though there was no statistically significant difference between VCP-treated and untreated animals according to the BBB test at week 6, there was a clear motor function benefit displayed by VCP-treated animals when negotiating the grid test at the same time point. Thus, VCP appears to possess the ability to promote motor function recovery, and results would likely be more encouraging if multiple VCP injections were administered throughout the evaluation period. On the basis of these exciting results, it would be interesting to investigate whether a part of VCP is as effective as a full-length protein in terms of its functional effect in the model of spinal cord injury tested herein. This unique property of VCP is significant given that VCP has also been suggested to have a positive effect in CNS and other neurodegenerative disorders, such as Alzheimer's disease. Taken together, VCP establishes itself as a strong candidate for further investigation in the treatment of SCI.

In summary, VCP shows considerable promise as a potential therapeutic agent in the treatment of traumatic SCI. Its recently discovered ability to inhibit *in vitro* monocyte chemotaxis adds a new dimension to the anti-inflammatory properties of the viral protein. Given that many SCI studies have shown beneficial effects upon the inhibition of peripheral macrophage infiltration of the injured cord, VCP's chemotaxis-inhibitory properties, coupled with its capacity to inhibit complement, make further evaluation of VCP in SCI models quite necessary and potentially very valuable. This study has demonstrated that VCP is able to inhibit macrophage/microglial influx/activation in the early stages after SCI, while potentially elevating microglial activation within 1 week of injury. This inflammatory modulation may be directly related to improved motor function recovery observed via the grid-walking tests and BBB. In previous studies, VCP was also shown to inhibit neutrophil influx within 24 h of cord injury. However, it is unclear whether neutrophils actually play a major role in secondary damage, since the functional consequences of neutrophil activity still need further elucidation. While this study cannot present a cure for traumatic spinal cord injury, it does provide direction in the pursuit of a therapeutic agent that targets the inflammatory arm of secondary injury, which may eventually be administered synergistically with other therapeutic agents to significant clinical benefit.

ACKNOWLEDGMENTS

We would like to thank the Kentucky Spinal Cord Injury Research Center at the University of Louisville for the use of their facilities and Yingchun Han, Becky Gray, and Darlene Burke for their technical assistance. This work was supported by funding from the Kentucky Spinal Cord and Head Injury Research Trust (KSCHIRT) awarded to G.J.K., D.J.M., and C.B.S. G.J.K. is currently a senior Wellcome Trust International Fellow for Biomedical Science in South Africa.

REFERENCES

1. DUMONT, R.J., D.O. OKONKWO, S.VERMA, *et al.* 2001. Acute spinal cord injury, part I: pathophysiologic mechanisms. Clin. Neuropharmacol. **24:** 254–264.
2. ANDERSON, A.J. 2002. Mechanisms and pathways of inflammatory responses in CNS trauma: spinal cord injury. J. Spinal Cord Med. **25:** 70–79.
3. FITCH, M.T., C. DOLLER, C.K. COMBS, *et al.* 1999. Cellular and molecular mechanisms of glial scarring and progressive cavitation: in vivo and in vitro analysis of inflammation-induced secondary injury after CNS trauma. J. Neurosci. **19:** 8182–8198.
4. MCDONALD, J.W. 1999. Repairing the damaged spinal cord. Sci. Am. **281:** 64–73.
5. BRACKEN, M.B. 2001. Methylprednisolone and acute spinal cord injury: an update of the randomized evidence. Spine **26:** S47–S54.
6. HURLBERT, R.J. 2000. Methylprednisolone for acute spinal cord injury: an inappropriate standard of care. J. Neurosurg. **93:** 1–7.
7. HURLBERT, R.J. 2001. The role of steroids in acute spinal cord injury: an evidence-based analysis. Spine **26:** S39–S46.
8. KOTWAL, G.J. & B. MOSS. 1988. Vaccinia virus encodes a secretory polypeptide structurally related to complement control proteins. Nature **335:** 176–178.
9. KOTWAL, G.J., S.N. ISAACS, R. MCKENZIE, *et al.* 1990. Inhibition of the complement cascade by the major secretory protein of vaccinia virus. Science **250:** 827–830.
10. MCKENZIE, R., G.J. KOTWAL, B. MOSS, *et al.* 1992. Regulation of complement activity by vaccinia virus complement-control protein. J. Infect. Dis. **166:** 1245–1250.

11. KOTWAL, G.J., C.G. MILLER, D.E. JUSTUS. 1998. The inflammation modulatory protein (IMP) of cowpox virus drastically diminishes the tissue damage by down-regulating cellular infiltration resulting from complement activation. Mol. Cell Biochem. **185:** 39–46.

12. KOTWAL, G.J., D.N. REYNOLDS, K.L. KEELING, *et al.* 1998. Vaccinia virus complement control protein is a virokine with lysozyme-like heparin-binding activity: possible implications in prolonged evasion of host immune response. *In* Proceedings of the 10th International Congress of Immunology. G.P. Talwar & I. Nath, Eds.: 315–320. Monduzzi Editore Pub. Bologna, Italy.

13. REYNOLDS, D.N., K.L. KEELING, R. MOLESTINA, *et al.* 1999. Heparin binding activity of vaccinia virus protein confers additional properties of uptake by mast cells and attachment to endothelial cells. *In* Advances in Animal Virology. S. Jameel & J.D. Lambis, Eds.: 343–348. Oxford & IBH Pub. New York.

14. HICKS, R.H., K.L. KEELING, M.Y. YANG, *et al.* 2002. Vaccinia virus complement control protein enhances functional recovery after traumatic brain injury. J. Neurotrauma **19:** 705–714.

15. MURTHY, K.H., S.A. SMITH, V.K. GANESH, *et al.* 2001. Crystal structure of a complement control protein that regulates both pathways of complement activation and binds heparan sulfate proteoglycans. Cell **104:** 301–311.

16. SMITH, S.A., N.P. MULLIN, J. PARKINSON, *et al.* 2000. Conserved surface-exposed K/R-X-K/R motifs and net positive charge on poxvirus complement control proteins serve as putative heparin binding sites and contribute to inhibition of molecular interactions with human endothelial cells: a novel mechanism for evasion of host defense. J. Virol. **74:** 5659–5666.

17. GRUNER, J.A. 1992. A monitored contusion model of spinal cord injury in the rat. J. Neurotrauma **9:** 123–126.

18. BASSO, D.M., M.S. BEATTIE, J.C. BRESNAHAN. 1996. Graded histological and locomotor outcomes after spinal cord contusion using the NYU weight-drop device versus transection. Exp. Neurol. **139:** 244–256.

19. BASSO, D.M., M.S. BEATTIE, J.C. BRESNAHAN. 1995. A sensitive and reliable locomotor rating scale for open field testing in rats. J. Neurotrauma **12:** 1–21.

20. MAGNUSON, D.S., T.C. TRIDER, Y.P. ZHANG, *et al.* 1999. Comparing deficits following excitotoxic and contusion injuries in the thoracic and lumbar spinal cord of the adult rat. Exp. Neurol. **156:** 191–204.

21. REYNOLDS, D.N., S.A. SMITH, C.B. SHIELDS, *et al.* 2003. Vaccinia virus complement control protein reduces neutrophil infiltration following spinal cord injury. Ann. N.Y. Acad. Sci. **1010:** 534–539.

22. FAROOQUE, M., J. ISAKSSON, Y. OLSSON. 1999. Improved recovery after spinal cord trauma in ICAM-1 and P-selectin knockout mice. Neuroreport **10:** 131–134.

23. LACROIX, S., L. CHANG, S. ROSE-JOHN, *et al.* 2002. Delivery of hyper-interleukin-6 to the injured spinal cord increases neutrophil and macrophage infiltration and inhibits axonal growth. J. Comp. Neurol. **454:** 213–228.

24. LIU, Y., T. TACHIBANA, Y. DAI, *et al.* 2002. Heme oxygenase-1 expression after spinal cord injury: the induction in activated neutrophils. J. Neurotrauma **19:** 479–490.

25. POPOVICH, P.G., P. WEI, B.T. STOKES. 1997. Cellular inflammatory response after spinal cord injury in Sprague-Dawley and Lewis rats. J. Comp. Neurol. **377:** 443–464.

26. POPOVICH, P.G., Z. GUAN, P. WEI, *et al.* 1999. Depletion of hematogenous macrophages promotes partial hindlimb recovery and neuroanatomical repair after experimental spinal cord injury. Exp. Neurol. **158:** 351–365.

27. POPOVICH, P.G. & W.F. HICKEY. 2001. Bone marrow chimeric rats reveal the unique distribution of resident and recruited macrophages in the contused rat spinal cord. J. Neuropathol. Exp. Neurol. **60:** 676–685.

28. POPOVICH, P.G., Z. GUAN, V. MCGAUGHY, *et al.* 2002. The neuropathological and behavioral consequences of intraspinal microglial/macrophage activation. J. Neuropathol. Exp. Neurol. **61:** 623–633.

29. WATANABE, T., T. YAMAMOTO, Y. ABE, *et al.* 1999. Differential activation of microglia after experimental spinal cord injury. J. Neurotrauma **16:** 255–265.

30. BEHRMANN, D.L., J.C. BRESNAHAN, M.S. BEATTIE. 1994. Modeling of acute spinal cord injury in the rat: neuroprotection and enhanced recovery with methylprednisolone, U-74006F and YM-14673. Exp. Neurol. **126:** 61–75.

Melatonin Relieves the Neural Oxidative Burden that Contributes to Dementias

RUSSEL J. REITER, DUN-XIAN TAN, AND MIGUEL A. PAPPOLLA

Department of Cellular and Structural Biology, University of Texas Health Science Center, San Antonio, Texas 78229-3900, USA

ABSTRACT: This report summarizes some of the many publications that document the beneficial actions of melatonin within the central nervous system. Of particular interest are the multiple functions of melatonin and its metabolites as ubiquitously acting direct free radical scavengers and indirect antioxidants. The fact that melatonin and the metabolic progeny that are formed when it scavenges toxic reactants are all effective in neutralizing destructive molecules greatly increases the efficacy of melatonin as a protection against by-products of oxygen and nitrogen that normally mutilate essential molecules. Of the large number of situations in which oxidative stress may be the cause of disease processes or debilitating conditions, the current review examines melatonin's protection within the central nervous system, particularly in experimental ischemia/reperfusion (stroke) injury, Alzheimer's disease, and parkinsonism. In each of these conditions, melatonin has been found to provide significant neural protection against both the morphophysiological damage and the biobehavioral consequences of these infirmities. The report concludes with the suggestion that melatonin, alone or in combination with other antioxidants, be considered for routine usage to potentially combat some of the neural ravages of aging.

KEYWORDS: melatonin; free radicals; oxidative stress; ischemia/reperfusion; Alzheimer's disease; Parkinson's disease

INTRODUCTION

The functional repertoire of melatonin has expanded rapidly since the discovery that this endogenously produced indole is an uncommonly potent indirect antioxidant[1] and direct free radical scavenger.[2] These novel functions were discovered within essentially the last decade and, since then, the published literature defining and describing melatonin's efficacy in reducing oxidative damage has increased exponentially.[3–6] Melatonin has been tested under a remarkably large number of experimental situations in which free radical damage causes the accumulation of molecular debris and ultimately cellular loss in the brain. For example, melatonin's beneficial actions in the brain have been documented in models of stroke[7–9] and

Address for correspondence: Russel J. Reiter, Ph.D., Department of Cellular and Structural Biology, University of Texas Health Science Center, 7703 Floyd Curl Drive, MC 7762, San Antonio, TX 78229-3900. Voice: 210-567-3859; fax: 210-567-3805.
reiter@uthscsa.edu

Ann. N.Y. Acad. Sci. 1035: 179–196 (2004). © 2004 New York Academy of Sciences.
doi: 10.1196/annals.1332.012

Alzheimer's,[10–12] Parkinson's,[13–15] and Huntington's diseases.[15–17] Moreover, melatonin's protective actions in the central nervous system (CNS) have been confirmed in situations where neurons/glia are damaged owing to ionizing radiation,[18–20] diabetes,[21–23] toxins,[24] viral infections,[25] excitotoxicity,[26–28] metals,[29,30] seizures,[31] homocysteine,[32] aging,[33–35] etc.

The presumed reason that melatonin is effective in arresting molecular damage in these diverse situations relates to the fact that these conditions have a common pathophysiological denominator—namely, free radical damage. Because of its efficacy as a direct scavenger and indirect antioxidant, melatonin is capable of reducing the mutilation of essential molecules, thereby limiting the accumulation of molecular junk, preserving the functions of cells, and curtailing cellular death (and eventually organismal death) from apoptosis or necrosis.

The current review examines some of the many studies that have tested melatonin's ability and efficacy in limiting neuronal and glial injury, which results in situations where molecular oxygen (O_2) is converted to radicals and related reactants within cells. These reactants are usual progeny of O_2 under basal conditions, and their generation is exaggerated when organisms are exposed to toxins or subjected to disease processes as described above. This review only considers melatonin's protective actions in the CNS, although it is equally beneficial against oxidative stress in other organs.[36–39] Also, besides the free radical scavenging and antioxidative functions of melatonin, some of which are receptor-independent, additional receptor-mediated,[40] local functions of melatonin may contribute to its ability to limit cellular damage.[41–43]

MELATONIN AND ITS METABOLITES IN CELLS AND BODY FLUIDS

While achieving its high antioxidant capability, melatonin is in competition with a number of other direct free radical scavengers for this task. Considering melatonin's seemingly low intracellular concentrations compared with some other radical-detoxifying agents, it is sometimes difficult to reconcile its high efficacy in preventing the plundering of essential molecules by oxygen- and nitrogen-based reactants.

Relatively little, however, is known about the concentrations of melatonin in subcellular compartments and, likewise, rather limited information is available relating to the distribution and levels of other antioxidants within cells. It does seem certain, however, that melatonin concentrations are not in equilibrium in an organism or even within cells.[44] Typically, individuals make judgments concerning the concentrations of melatonin throughout the body based on the levels that are measured in the blood, which, even at their zenith at night, are in the low nanomolar range.[45] When other fluids have been examined, it has been commonplace to find that the concentrations of melatonin may exceed those in the blood by several orders of magnitude. Certainly in bile (of a number of mammalian species), melatonin levels are very greatly elevated over those in concurrent blood samples.[46] This is also true for some bone marrow cells.[47] Likewise, in the cerebrospinal fluid (CSF) of the third ventricle (of the sheep), the radioimmunoassayable values of melatonin far exceeded those in the blood, particularly at night when pineal melatonin synthesis and secretion are active.[48] In the fluid of the human graafian follicle as well, melatonin levels are greater than those in the blood.[49]

Within subcellular organelles, melatonin seems to be unequally dispersed. While one would predict that the concentrations of lipophilic melatonin would be highest in cell membranes, which are rich in fatty acids, this has never actually been determined. Preliminary estimates indicate that melatonin levels may be highest within the mitochondria[50] and the nucleus[51] of cells, but a limited number of tissues have been investigated in this regard. This conundrum will only be satisfied after more extensive and definitive studies are completed in reference to where and at what levels melatonin is present within cells. Of interest in this regard is that melatonin, functioning as an antioxidant, has been shown to protect membrane lipids,[52,53] cytosolic proteins,[54,55] and nuclear[56,57] and mitochondrial DNA,[14,58] from oxidative damage. This portends a wide intracellular distribution of this indole.

To assess the intracellular importance of the free radical–scavenging capability of the indole, the measurement of melatonin may, in a sense, be an inappropriate endpoint. When melatonin neutralizes certain reactive species, it is converted to metabolites that may be more efficient scavengers than melatonin itself. Thus, the products N^1-acetyl-N^2-formyl-5-methoxykynuramine (AFMK)[59–62] and N^1-acetyl-5-methoxykynuramine (AMK),[59] both of which are formed when melatonin interacts with oxygen-based reactants, are also potent radical scavengers.[63,64] Perhaps melatonin levels within cells are measurably low because the melatonin is quickly converted to its active metabolites, AFMK and AMK. The fact that AFMK and AMK are notable scavengers of radicals and/or their metabolites, the "effective concentration" of melatonin is magnified. At this point, however, the relative importance of melatonin versus its metabolites as scavengers are unknown, and certainly more information is required regarding subcellular levels and distribution of melatonin (and other scavengers) if we are to understand why melatonin is so effective in protecting against oxidative destruction.

A recent observation of Stefulj and colleagues[65] is germane to this discussion. While it has long been known that melatonin is not uniquely produced in the pineal gland,[66–68] its synthesis may be common to many cells. Using the reverse transcription–polymerase chain reaction (RT–PCR) method, this group determined the tissue-specific expression of mRNAs which encode the two enzymes (i.e., serotonin *N*-acetyltransferase [NAT] and hydroxyindole-*O*-methyltransferase [HIOMT]), which convert serotonin to melatonin. These investigators found these signals were present in the intestine, fundic stomach, testis, spinal cord, raphe nuclei of the brain stem, and striatum.[65] They surmised, consistent with the belief of other workers,[41,43] that melatonin, assuming it is indeed produced on-site, acts in a intracrine, autocrine, and/or paracrine manner. It would be especially important for its antioxidant protection if melatonin synthesis was inducible, particularly if the inducing process was increased free radical generation. Thus, intracellularly generated melatonin could then function in the scavenging of radicals and/or other toxicants in its cell of production or in adjacent cells. While there is no strong evidence to support such a series of events, the idea is introduced here because it is a testable hypothesis.

PROTECTIVE ACTIONS OF MELATONIN IN CELLS

The rate constant for the interaction of melatonin with the most damaging radical, that is, the hydroxyl radical (•OH), is similar to that of other •OH scavengers

TABLE 1. Calculated rate constants for the reaction of various free radical scavengers with the hydroxyl radical (•OH)

Reaction	Rate constant (M/s)
Ascorbyl + •OH	1.0×10^{10}
N-Acetylcysteine + •OH	1.4×10^{10}
Carnosine + •OH	2.5×10^{9}
β-Carotene + •OH	$<1.10 \times 10^{11}$
Desferroxamine + •OH	$6.6–7.1 \times 10^{9}$
Mannitol + •OH	1.7×10^{9}
Melatonin + •OH	$2.7–4.1 \times 10^{10}$
Reduced glutathione + •OH	8.8×10^{9}
Salicylic acid + •OH	$1.0–5.0 \times 10^{9}$
α-Tocopherol + •OH	1.0×10^{10}

NOTE: The •OH is highly reactive and damages any molecule in the immediate vicinity of where it is produced.

(TABLE 1). This being the case, melatonin has no advantage over other antioxidants in this regard. What seems to be frequently overlooked in terms of the efficacy of scavengers is their position relative to not only the site of free radical generation, but also where the scavenger is located in terms of the molecule it is destined to protect from a free radical. Since highly reactive oxygen- and nitrogen-based reactants travel very short distances (estimated to be a few angstroms or molecular diameters) before they destroy a bystander molecule, the scavenger, if it is to be protective, must be in the immediate vicinity of the radical product when it is generated. In this case, the damage that occurs is considered to be on-site and, likewise, the protection would be on-site. This phenomenon was emphasized by Borg,[69] who described what he referred to as the "reaction cage". The reaction cage is defined by the diameter of the area a toxic radical will travel before it mutilates a neighboring molecule. Borg[69] notes that, for a scavenger to be protective in this case, it must be within the "reaction cage" when the radical is generated.

Thus, the subcellular distribution of a scavenger is critical to its ability to protect against oxidative destruction. In this regard, the tocopherols (vitamin E) are excellent protectors against lipid peroxidation in membranes, since this is where they are located. Conversely, since hydrophilic ascorbic acid (vitamin C) is situated in the cytosol, it is particularly effective in limiting oxidative damage in this arena. The fact that melatonin reduces lipid damage within membranes,[52,53] protein carbonyls throughout the cell,[54,55] as well as mitochondrial[14,58] and nuclear DNA[56,57] damage suggests that this indole (or its metabolites) is in close proximity to each of these molecules. How this wide intracellular distribution is achieved is yet unknown.

The actions described above are presumably receptor-independent effects; the only requirement is for the scavenger to be in the right place at the right time. Additionally, melatonin's high efficacy in controlling the degree of oxidative damage may in part involve the interaction of the indole with identified membrane receptors.[40] Membrane receptors are known to mediate some of the actions of this ubiquitously acting agent. Whether membrane receptor–mediated actions account for the ability of this indole to lower oxidative damage has been only sparingly investigated, although it is known that these receptors are not required for the reduction of damage to mitochondrial DNA.[70] Also, how receptors for melatonin in other parts of the cell (e.g., in the nucleus) relate to the capability of melatonin as an antioxidant is not fully understood. The results published by Pablos and colleagues[71] indicate that nuclear receptors may be important in mediating some of the antioxidant actions of the indole. While for years the existence of nuclear melatonin receptors was questioned, recent evidence strongly supports their presence in at least some cells.[72,73]

Besides directly interacting with free radicals to neutralize them before they inflict damage, a major action of melatonin in limiting destruction of molecules by free radicals may be its ability to promote the activities of a number of metabolically essential antioxidative enzymes. These catalytic agents play an important role in antioxidative defense by metabolizing toxic reactants to less reactive or innocuous products. Examples of these enzymes include the superoxide dismutases (SODs), glutathione peroxidase (GPx), glutathione reductase (GRd), and catalase (CAT). They work in concert to initially metabolize $O_2^{\bullet-}$ (the SODs) to H_2O_2, which is subsequently converted to H_2O by GPx and CAT. In the process of metabolizing H_2O_2 to H_2O, GPx oxidizes reduced glutathione (GSH) to its disulfide form (GSSG); this latter product is recycled back to GSH by GRd and, in the process, utilizes NADPH. The effects of melatonin in promoting the activities of these essential antioxidative enzymes have been summarized in recent review articles, which should be consulted for specific details.[5,6]

MELATONIN PROTECTS AGAINST EXPERIMENTAL STROKE

Both physical and mental disabilities are common sequelae of the transitory interruption of the blood supply to a given area of the brain. These deficits are a consequence of the loss of neurons and glia resulting from the hypoxia/anoxia that accompanies the loss of the blood supply. Ironically, when blood flow is re-established to the afflicted area, the size of the lesion (i.e., the infarct) further increases in size, causing additional neurobehavioral deficits. Thus, both the ischemic episode as well as reperfusion (reoxygenation) contributes to the neural damage of stroke.

It is widely accepted that at least a portion of the molecular and cellular damage and loss that occur during neural ischemia/reperfusion (I/R) relates to the generation of biologically reactive oxygen- and nitrogen-based species during these processes. This being the case, antioxidants would be expected to provide protection against I/R injury if the agent gets into the CNS in sufficient quantities to scavenge a significant portion of the free radicals and related reactants generated during hypoxia and reflow. Melatonin, unlike some other antioxidants, readily crosses the blood–brain barrier[74] and, in many situations of neural damage, it has been shown to be beneficial.[75,76] Additionally, at least in sheep and likely in other vertebrates, melatonin from the pineal gland is released directly into the cerebrospinal fluid (CSF) of the third ventricle from where it has ready access to the brain.[77,78]

Although melatonin is only newly discovered to be a direct and indirect antioxidant, there are a rather extensive series of publications related to its beneficial actions in reducing the negative outcomes of an induced stroke in animals. Some of

TABLE 2. Some of the reports documenting the protective actions of melatonin against neural damage resulting from transitory ischemia and reperfusion

Species	Focal/global ischemia	Melatonin dose	Melatonin effects	Ref.
Rat	Focal (MCA occlusion)	4 mg/kg	↓ infarct volume	79
Rat	Focal (MCA occlusion)	10 mg/kg	↓ pyramidal neuron death	80
Rat	Focal (MCA occlusion)	10 mg/kg	↓ •OH radical generation	81
Rat	Focal (MCA occlusion)	10 mg/kg	↑ bcl-2 ↑ bcl-2 bax ratio ↓ apoptosis	82
Rat	Focal (MCA occlusion)	20 or 40 mg/kg	↓ infarct volume ↓ neurological deficits ↓ MDA ↑ GSH	83
Rat	Focal (MCA occlusion)	6 mg/kg	↓ cerebral edema ↓ infarct volume	84
Rat	Focal (MCA occlusion)	6 mg/kg	↓ cerebral edema ↓ striatal edema ↓ infarct volume	85
Mouse	Focal (MCA obstruction)	4 mg/kg (×2)	↑ neuronal survival ↓ cell injury ↓ TUNEL staining ↓ caspase 3	86
Rat	Focal (MCA occlusion)	1.5, 5, or 50 mg/kg	↓ neural nitric oxide	90
Fetal rat	Global (obstruction of utero-ovarian arteries)	10 mg/kg	↑ mitochondrial respiratory control index ↓ lipid peroxidation	9
Cat	Global (cardio-pulmonary arrest)	10 mg/kg/h for 6 h	↑ pyramidal neurons ↓ neurophysiological deficits	92

ABBREVIATIONS: GSH, reduced glutathione; MCA, middle cerebral artery; MDA, malondialdehyde.

these data are summarized in TABLE 2. The information in this table as well as several recent reviews[7,8,10] will provide the reader with the references necessary to examine melatonin's efficacy in protecting against I/R injury in depth. Additionally, the specifics of several more recent studies are summarized here.

Interestingly, the initial investigations designed to examine the relationship between melatonin and the severity of I/R injury took a somewhat unexpected approach. Rather than administering melatonin to possibly reduce lesion size after interruption and re-establishment of blood flow to the brain, Manev *et al.*[93] and Jou and colleagues[94] induced a relative melatonin deficiency in rats by surgically removing the pineal gland. Despite the fact that pinealectomy only removes one source of melatonin, after the middle cerebral artery (MCA) occlusion, the number of TUNEL-positive neurons (indicative of apoptosis), the frequency of dead cells (Nissl stain), the amount of damaged neural DNA, and the size of the infarct were all exaggerated compared to these parameters in nonpinealectomized control rats. The findings suggest that endogenously generated melatonin is important in maintaining the integrity of the CNS via its antioxidative actions. These results have been confirmed for other organs as well where loss of the pineal gland has been shown to accentuate the tissue destruction following a period of I/R. These findings also have important implications for aging since in animals, including humans,[95–97] melatonin levels dwindle to the point where they are equivalent to those following pinealectomy. Thus, the severity of neural damage after an I/R episode would be expected to be greater in an older individual relative to that in a younger person.

Not only is melatonin acutely beneficial in protecting against the neural damage associated with transient hypoxia and reoxygenation, but a recent report also claims that melatonin, given prophylactically, attenuates neural lesion size after I/R.[98] In this study, melatonin was given in the drinking water for 9 weeks prior to a 90-min MCA occlusion in rats. This advanced treatment with the indole led to a 30–35% reduction in infarct volume. Again, this has clear implications for the elderly where endogenous melatonin production is diminished. The routine use of melatonin by these individuals may be beneficial in reducing neural damage in the event of a stroke.

Clearly, a large number of studies have shown, in both focal and global ischemia models, that melatonin is highly protective against the brain damage that occurs during periods of relative ischemia and subsequent reperfusion. It seems important in light of these findings that melatonin's usage be considered in human stroke patients.

MELATONIN, NEURONAL APOPTOSIS, AND DEMENTIAS

Apoptosis, a form of programmed cell death, contributes to the pathological loss of neurons in a variety of neurodegenerative disorders.[99] The destruction of neurons in the aged contributes to a variety of dementias. Many of the neurodegenerative dementing illnesses have an overlapping component, that is, a reduction in the number of nerve cells subserving mental activity, emotional stability, motor control, etc. Prevention of the loss of brain cells during the later decades of life may help to preserve neurophysiology and neurobehavior and delay the onset or severity of several debilitating dementias, such as Alzheimer's disease (AD) or Parkinson's disease (PD). The goal of preserving neuronal function during aging is becoming increasingly important because of the prolonged life span of individuals in the present and subsequent generations. Without means to forestall these dementias, the number of the demented elderly will disproportionately increase, which will result in an overwhelming societal burden in terms of both the quality of care for these individuals and the financial resources available to provide proper treatment.

On the basis of the results of a wide variety of experiments in animals, melatonin seems to have considerable potential for reducing neuronal and glial loss and preserving function in models of both AD and PD. The cardinal signs of AD are well known, but nevertheless the condition is difficult to definitively diagnose. For example, there is no surefire diagnostic marker of this disease, and establishing guidelines for pinpointing the onset of cognitive decline in these patients is not without controversy. The major morphologic features of the brain in AD—that is, amyloid β peptide deposits (senile plaques) and neurofibrillary tangles (NFT)—are shared by other conditions. The major risk factors are a family history of the disease and the presence of the apoprotein E (Apo E) genotype.

One group of culpable agents that contributes to the destruction of neural tissue in AD is free radicals. Amyloid β (Aβ) peptide, the excessive neural deposition of which is a cardinal sign of AD, generates these oxidizing agents; in particular, Aβ1–42 is especially effective in producing radical species, and it is a major form of the Aβ family of peptides deposited in the AD brain.[100] Pappolla and coworkers[101,102] were the first to report that melatonin prevents cell death and oxidative damage in cultured neuroblastoma cells and primary neurons exposed to Aβ. In a subsequent study, this group also showed that melatonin strongly inhibited the spontaneous formation of β-sheets and β-amyloid fibrils.[103] The findings regarding the protective actions of melatonin against β-amyloid neurotoxicity have been repeatedly confirmed.[104–108] Furthermore, the deleterious neurobehavioral changes associated with the injection of Aβ25–35 directly into the hippocampus of rats have been shown to be reversed by melatonin treatment; these impairments following Aβ administration were evaluated using the Morris water maze.[109] Finally, it was recently shown that melatonin in the drinking water (2 mg/mL) partially reduced Aβ deposition in the brain of transgenic mice overexpressing human amyloid precursor protein (APP).[110] Also, the transgenic mice that received melatonin in the drinking water exhibited a reduced death rate relative to those not receiving the indolamine. Supplementing the diet with melatonin (rather than the drinking water) of mice also has been shown to limit the deposition of Aβ-peptide in the brain.[111]

Studies related to the use of melatonin as a treatment for human AD are limited. The reports have all been based on small, uncontrolled trials. While this shortcoming is significant, the positive effects of melatonin in relieving the behavioral signs of AD should stimulate additional investigations in this field.[112–115] In further support of this are the observations that individuals suffering with AD commonly have abnormally low endogenous melatonin levels, which may also exhibit aberrant rhythmicity.[116,117]

Basing our conclusion on the general consensus that AD is, in part, aggravated by free radical damage to the brain, we recently proposed a combination of antioxidants (i.e., melatonin plus vitamins C and E) as a potential prophylactic means to defer the onset and progression of this debilitating condition.[118]

As noted above, NFTs are also a major pathological component of the AD brain that contribute to the death of neurons. These complexes form in the parikarya and proximal dendrites of neurons and are most abundantly present in the hippocampus and cerebral cortex; they are made up of hyperphosphorylated microtubule-associated protein tau in the form of an insoluble polymer. The phosphorylation of tau is regulated by a host of protein phosphatases and protein kinases; protein kinase A (PKA) is particularly important in this regard.

Because of the association of NFTs with AD, Wang *et al.*[119] investigated the action of melatonin on tau phosphorylation. The injection of isoproterenol (ISO) directly and bilaterally into the hippocampus stimulated PKA activity and induced

NFT formation. When melatonin was given peripherally, PKA-induced phosphorylation of tau was reduced, as were the levels of lipid peroxidation products in the hippocampus. The implication is that melatonin may limit tau phosphorylation in the AD brain by suppressing both PKA activation and oxidative stress.

In a follow-up study, the same group[120] showed that prophylactic melatonin supplementation for 1 week before treatment with a melatonin synthesis–inhibiting drug arrested tau phosphorylation in the rat brain and reversed the memory impairments produced by a relative melatonin deficiency. The memory deficits were evaluated using the Morris water maze.

The cholinergic hypothesis of AD states that a deficiency in cholinergic neurotransmission may account for some of the cognitive impairment experienced by these patients. Mice transfected with the APP gene, which leads to the deposition of Aβ deposits in the CNS, exhibit a depressed choline acetyltransferase (ChAT) activity in the frontal cortex and hippocampus.[121] In this model of AD, melatonin supplementation re-established ChAT activity in the affected brain areas of transgenic mice, reduced DNA damage and neuronal apoptosis, and lessened the behavioral deficits.

As with AD, melatonin has been used in an attempt to abate neural damage in models of PD. A spurious compound (MPTP) formed as a result of an error in the synthesis of heroin roughly 20 years ago caused the users to develop precocious PD-like disease within a few weeks after its intake. The symptoms of this condition were similar to those of idiopathic PD, and the patients responded to levodopa treatment.[122] The toxic molecule was subsequently identified as N-methyl-4-phenyl-1,2,3,6-tetrahydropyridine (MPTP). After its uptake by glial cells in the substantia nigra, MPTP is converted to methyl-phenyl-pyridine$^+$ (MPP$^+$), which is released from glia and taken up by dopaminergic neurons of the pars compacta. MPP$^+$ eventually kills the neurons because of its toxic effects at the mitochondrial level and the generation of free radicals. When a large percentage of the dopamine neurons are destroyed, the symptoms of PD appear. While the circumstances under which MPTP was discovered are unfortunate, the use of the drug has provided an important model of PD in animals.

The MPTP model of PD has been used to examine the efficacy of melatonin to reduce the morphological damage and attenuate the seriousness of PD signs in animals. Also, melatonin was repeatedly found in cultured cells to stymie cellular damage when the cells were incubated in the presence of MPP$^+$ or other toxic agents. Mayo and coworkers[123] systematically investigated the potential beneficial actions of melatonin on PC12 cells exposed to a neural toxin—in this case, 6-hydroxy-dopamine (6-OHDA). They reported that melatonin prevented apoptosis induced by 6-OHDA, and the mechanisms of protection involved free radical scavenging, up-regulation of gene expression for several antioxidative enzymes, and an inhibition of cell proliferation in undifferentiated PC12 cells.[124] Additionally, melatonin overcame the necrotic changes experienced by neurons exposed to 6-OHDA.[125] The role of free radical quenching by melatonin as a mechanism of its protective actions in PC12 cells exposed to 6-OHDA has been confirmed by Park *et al.*[126]

As with 6-OHDA, exposure of cells to MPP$^+$ leads to death of a majority of the neurons within a relatively short interval. According to Lacovitti *et al.*[127] and Stull and colleagues,[128] incubating MPP$^+$-exposed neurons with melatonin allowed the cells to survive the toxin exposure. In these reports, the evidence is consistent with melatonin's antioxidative actions in providing the beneficial effects.

MPTP has also been administered to experimental animals to destroy the dopaminergic neurons of the substantia nigra and to inhibit tyrosine hydroxylase activity in both the striatum and the mesencephalon. The bulk of these studies,[10,15,118,126,129–131] but not all,[132,133] have shown that melatonin, given systemically, crosses the blood–brain barrier in sufficient quantities to limit oxidative stress and dopaminergic cell loss in animals treated with MPTP. Those studies that failed to confirm these observations were flawed, as pointed out by Tan *et al.*[118] and Yan.[134]

The most compelling documentation of the ability of melatonin to arrest the reduction in dopaminergic neuronal loss and loss of tyrosine hydroxylase activity comes from the work of Antolin and coworkers.[135] In this chronic study, mice were treated daily for 35 days with a low dose of MPTP with the intent of stimulating a gradual reduction of dopaminergic neurons from the substantial nigra; additionally, half of the animals were treated with melatonin. At the conclusion of the experiment, the mice given only MPTP had severely depleted tyrosine hydroxylase activity in both the striatum and substantia nigra and a marked reduction in the number of dopamine-containing neurons in the mesencephalon. Conversely, MPTP was ineffective in inducing either of these changes in mice cotreated with melatonin. This is the best evidence to date that melatonin, most likely because of its antioxidant and ancillary activities at the mitochondrial level,[14,136] is capable of arresting the destruction of dopaminergic neurons of the substantia nigra induced by a potent neurotoxin, MPTP. Given the drop in endogenous melatonin in aging humans, supplementation with melatonin may be useful in deferring the onset of PD.

In the majority of studies cited above, a reduction in neuronal apoptosis was a noteworthy feature when melatonin was given. A recent review summarizes the inhibitory effects of melatonin on apoptotic processes in normal cells.[137] Clearly, free radical damage to mitochondria can lead to apoptosis. Jou and colleagues[138] recently published an in-depth report on the mechanisms of inhibition of apoptosis by melatonin. Using a combination of time-lapse conventional, confocal, and multiphoton fluorescent imaging microscopy, they report that melatonin, because of its direct free radical scavenging activity at the mitochondrial level, prevents the initiation of the early apoptotic events, thereby reducing the subsequent changes that culminate in programmed cell death. In this scheme, melatonin prevented H_2O_2-induced mitochondrial calcium overload, mitochondrial potential depolarization, and the opening of the mitochondrial permeability transition (MPT) pore. These reductions were associated with a blockade of cytochrome *c* release from the mitochondria, no activation of caspase-3 activity, and reduced apoptotic fragmentation of nuclear DNA.[138] The results of this, and many other studies, document the preventive actions of melatonin on apoptosis in normal cells.

CONCLUSIONS

The information summarized in this report illustrates the high efficacy of melatonin in shielding essential macromolecules from rampaging free radicals and related reactants. Moreover, the results underscore the potential use of melatonin to forestall or treat degenerative neuronal conditions in humans that lead to dementia. The significance of deferring the debilitating neural diseases of the aged is of paramount importance, considering the rapidly aging population in the well-developed countries of the world.

Several features make melatonin of interest as a possible treatment for the conditions that cause feebleness in the elderly. Melatonin is an endogenously produced molecule which the body "recognizes", and it possesses the necessary molecular machinery to metabolize the indole. While melatonin is usually taken in doses that cause blood levels of exceed endogenous physiological concentrations, there are essentially no data that suggest this has serious sequelae. Melatonin has been regularly taken by many individuals for long periods of time (>10 years) with no reports of negative consequences. It is time, however, to conduct an epidemiological study on those individuals who regularly take melatonin (versus those who do not) for the purpose of evaluating its potential beneficial effects.

Another issue that is frequently raised is melatonin's potential interactions with prescription drugs that many elderly people take. Drugs are routinely examined for toxicity in animals and humans who have endogenous melatonin, so the drugs are normally tested in the presence of at least physiologic levels (if not pharmacologic concentrations) of melatonin, and drug interactions would be uncovered. Furthermore, prescription drugs typically have significant side effects (leading to their prescription drug status), and this toxicity is frequently abated by coadministration with melatonin with no impairment of drug efficacy.[139] Thus, the combination of melatonin and some prescription drugs may improve their benefits, reduce toxicity, and possibly allow for use of a higher dosage (with potential great efficacy) of the drug.

The seriously incapacitating nature of neurodegenerative diseases of aging in a progressively older population demands a revolutionary approach to the prevention or treatment of these conditions. The animal experiments to date suggest melatonin may have significant benefits in this arena. It is inexpensive, minimally toxic, and can be obtained in pure form. Either as a sole treatment, or in combination with other antioxidants as we recently suggested,[118] supplemental melatonin may improve the general health and reduce the drug-related expenses of the elderly. If melatonin were shown to have significant benefits in humans, as has been shown in animals, the cost advantage not only for the elderly individual but for the supporting governmental agencies could be tremendous.

REFERENCES

1. BARLOW-WALDEN, L.R., R.J. REITER, M. ABE, *et al.* 1995. Melatonin stimulates brain glutathione peroxidase activity. Neurochem. Int. **26:** 497–502.
2. TAN, D.X., L.D. CHEN, B. POEGGELER, *et al.* 1993. Melatonin: a potent endogenous hydroxyl radical scavenger. Endocrine J. **1:** 57–60.
3. REITER, R.J., D. ACUÑA-CASTROVIEJO, D.X. TAN, *et al.* 2001. Free radical mediated molecular damage: mechanisms of melatonin's protective actions in the central nervous system. Ann. N.Y. Acad. Sci. **939:** 200–215.
4. ALLEGRA, M., R.J. REITER, D.X. TAN, *et al.* 2003. The chemistry of melatonin's interaction with reactive species. J. Pineal Res. **34:** 1–10.
5. REITER, R.J., D.X. TAN, C. OSUNA, *et al.* 2000. Actions of melatonin in the reduction of oxidative stress. J. Biomed. Sci. **7:** 444–458.
6. RODRIGUEZ, C., J.C. MAYO, R.M. SAINZ, *et al.* 2004. Regulation of antioxidant enzymes: a significant role for melatonin. J. Pineal Res. **36:** 1–9.

7. REITER, R.J., R.M. SAINZ, S. LOPEZ-BURILLO, *et al.* 2004. Melatonin ameliorates neurological damage and neurophysiological deficits in experimental models of stroke. Ann. N.Y. Acad. Sci. **993:** 35–47.
8. CHEUNG, R.T.F. 2003. The utility of melatonin in reducing cerebral damage resulting from ischemia and reperfusion. J. Pineal Res. **34:** 153–160.
9. REITER, R.J., D.X. TAN, J. LEON, *et al.* 2004. When melatonin gets on your nerves: its beneficial actions in experimental models of stroke. Exp. Biol. Med. In press.
10. REITER, R.J. 1998. Oxidative damage in the central nervous system: protection by melatonin. Prog. Neurobiol. **56:** 359–384.
11. PAPPOLLA, M.A., Y.J. CHYAN, B. POEGGELER, *et al.* 2000. An assessment of the antioxidant and antiamyloidogenic properties of melatonin: implications for Alzheimer's disease. J. Neural Transm. **107:** 203–231.
12. PAPPOLLA, M.A., R.J. REITER, T.K. BRYANT-THOMAS, *et al.* 2003. Oxidative mediated neurodegeneration in Alzheimer's disease: melatonin and related antioxidants as neuroprotective agents. Curr. Med. Chem. **3:** 233–243.
13. MAYO, J.C., R.M. SAINZ, I. ANTOLIN, *et al.* 1999. Ultrastructural confirmation of neuronal protection by melatonin against the neurotoxin 6-hydroxydopamine in cell damage. Brain Res. **818:** 221–227.
14. ACUÑA-CASTROVIEJO, D., G. ESCAMES, A. CAROZO, *et al.* 2002. Melatonin: mitochondrial homeostasis and mitochondrial related diseases. Curr. Topics Med. Chem. **2:** 133–151.
15. REITER, R.J., J. CABRERA, R.M. SAINZ, *et al.* 2000. Melatonin as a pharmacological agent against neuronal loss in experimental models of Huntington's disease, Alzheimer's disease, and parkinsonism. Ann. N.Y. Acad. Sci. **890:** 471–485.
16. CABRERA, J., R.J. REITER, D.X. TAN, *et al.* 2000. Melatonin reduces oxidative neurotoxicity due to quinolinic acid: *in vitro* and *in vivo* findings. Neuropharmacology **39:** 507–514.
17. BEHAN, W.M., M. MCDONALD, L.G. DARLINGTON, *et al.* 1999. Oxidative stress as a mechanism for quinolinic acid-induced hippocampal damage: protection by melatonin and deprenyl. Br. J. Pharmacol. **128:** 1754–1760.
18. VIJAYALAXMI, E.R. THOMAS, R.J. REITER, *et al.* 2002. Melatonin: from basic research to cancer treatment clinics. J. Clin. Oncol. **20:** 2575–2601.
19. EROL, F.S., C. TOPSAKAL, M.F. OZUEREN, *et al.* 2003. Protective effect of melatonin and vitamin E in brain damage due to gamma radiation: an experimental study. Neurosurg. Dev. **27:** 65–69.
20. UNDEGER, U., B. GIRAY, A.F. ZORLU, *et al.* 2004. Protective effects of melatonin on the ionizing radiation induced DNA damage in the rat brain. Exp. Toxicol. Pathol. **55:** 379–384.
21. BAYDAS, G., R.J. REITER, A. YASAR, *et al.* 2003. Melatonin reduces glial reactivity in the hippocampus, cortex and cerebellum of streptozocin-induced diabetic rats. Free Rad. Biol. Med. **35:** 797–804.
22. BAYDAS, G., H. CANATAN & A. TURKOGLU. 2002. Comparative analysis of the protective effects of melatonin and vitamin E on streptozocin-induced diabetes mellitus. J. Pineal Res. **32:** 225–230.
23. COLANTUORI, A., B. LONGONI & P.L. MARCHIAFAVA. 2002. Retinal photoreceptors of Syrian hamsters undergo oxidative stress during streptozocin-induced diabetes. Diabetologia **45:** 121–124.
24. JUKNAT, A.A., M.L. KOTLER, A QUAGLINO, *et al.* 2004. Necrotic cell death by δ-aminolevulinic acid in mouse astrocytes: protective role of melatonin and other antioxidants. J. Pineal Res. **35:** 1–11.
25. BONILLA, E., N. VALERO, L. CHACIN-BONILLA, *et al.* 2004. Melatonin and viral infections. J. Pineal Res. **36:** 73–79.
26. TAN, D.X., L.C. MANCHESTER, R.J. REITER, *et al.* 1998. Melatonin protects hippocampal neurons in vivo against kainic acid-induced damage in mice. J. Neurosci. Res. **54:** 382–289.
27. CHUNG, S.Y., & S. H. HAN. 2003. Melatonin attenuates kainic acid-induced hippocampal neurodegeneration and oxidative stress through microglial inhibition. J. Pineal Res. 2003; **34:** 95–102.

28. ANANTH, G., P. GOPALAKRISHNAKONE & C. KAUR. 2003. Protective role of melatonin in domoic acid-induced neuronal damage in the hippocampus of adult rats. Hippocampus **13:** 375–387.

29. ESPARZA, J.J., M. GOMEZ, M. ROMEU, *et al.* 2003. Aluminum-induced pro-oxidant effects in rats: protective role of exogenous melatonin. J. Pineal Res. **35:** 32–39.

30. CHEN, K.B., A.M.Y. LIN & T.H. CHIU. 2003. Oxidative injury to the locus ceruleus of rat brain: neuroprotection by melatonin. J. Pineal Res. **35:** 109–117.

31. BIKJDAOUENE, L., G. ESCAMES, J. LEON, *et al.* 2003. Changes in brain amino acids and nitric oxide after melatonin administration in rats with pentylenetetrazole-induced seizures. J. Pineal Res. **35:** 54–60.

32. BAYDAS, G., S. KUTLU, M. NAZIROGLU, *et al.* 2003. Inhibitory effects of melatonin on neural lipid peroxidation induced by intracerebroventricular administered homocysteine. J. Pineal Res. **34:** 36–39.

33. REITER, R.J., D.X. TAN & S. BURKHARDT. 2002. Reactive oxygen and nitrogen species and cellular and organismal decline: amelioration with melatonin. Mech. Aging Dev. **123:** 1007–1019.

34. OKATANI, Y., A. WAKATSUKI, R.J. REITER, *et al.* 2002. Melatonin reduces oxidative damage to neural lipids and proteins in senescence-accelerated mouse. Neurobiol. Aging **23:** 639–644.

35. SHARMAN, E.H., K.G. SHARMAN, Y.W. GEE, *et al.* 2004. Age-related changes in murine CNS mRNA gene expression are modulated by dietary melatonin. J. Pineal Res. **36:** 165–170.

36. REITER, R.J. & D.X. TAN. 2003. Melatonin: a novel protective agent against oxidative injury of the ischemic/reperfused heart. Cardiovasc. Res. **58:** 10–19.

37. OHTA, Y., M. KONGO-NISHIMURA, T. MATSURA, *et al.* 2004. Melatonin prevents disruption of hepatic reactive oxygen species metabolism in rats treated with carbon tetrachloride. J. Pineal Res. **36:** 10–17.

38. YANUZ, M.N., A.A. YANUZ, C. ULKA, *et al.* 2003. Protective effect of melatonin against fractionated irradiation-induced epiphyseal injury in a weaning rat model. J. Pineal Res. **35:** 288–294.

39. PARLAKPINAR, H., M.K. OZER, E. SABINA, *et al.* 2003. Amikacin-induced acute renal injury in rats: protective role of melatonin. J. Pineal Res. **35:** 85–90.

40. BARRETT, P., S. CONWAY & P.J. MORGAN. 2003. Digging deep - structure-function relationships in the melatonin receptor family. J. Pineal Res. **35:** 221–230.

41. TAN, D.X., L.C. MANCHESTER, R. HARDELAND, *et al.* 2003. Melatonin: a hormone, a tissue factor, an autocoid, a paracoid and an antioxidant vitamin. J. Pineal Res. **34:** 75–78.

42. CABRERA, J., J. QUINTANA, R.J. REITER, *et al.* 2003. Melatonin prevents apoptosis and enhances HSP27 mRNA expression induced by heat shock in HL-60 cells: possible involvement of the MT2 receptor. J. Pineal Res. **35:** 231–238.

43. CARRILLO-VICO, A., J.R. CALVO, P. ABREU, *et al.* 2004. Evidence of melatonin synthesis by human lymphocytes and its physiological significance: possible role as an intracrine, autocrine, and/or paracrine substance. FASEB J. **18:** 537–539.

44. REITER, R.J. & D.X. TAN. 2003. What constitutes a physiological concentration of melatonin. J. Pineal Res. **34:** 79–80.

45. REITER, R.J. 1991. Pineal melatonin: cell biology of its synthesis and of its physiological interactions. Endocrine Dev. **12:** 151–180.

46. TAN, D.X., L.C. MANCHESTER, R.J. REITER, *et al.* 1999. High physiological levels of melatonin in the bile of mammals. Life Sci. **65:** 2523–2529.

47. TAN, D.X., L.C. MANCHESTER, R.J. REITER, *et al.* 1999. Identification of highly elevated melatonin in bone marrow: its origin and significance. Biochim. Biophys. Acta **1472:** 206–214.

48. SKINNER, D.C. & B. MALPAUX. 1999. High melatonin concentrations in third ventricular fluid are not due to Galen vein blood recirculating through the choroid plexus. Endocrinology **140:** 4399–4405.

49. BRZEZINSKI, A., M.M. SEIBEL & H.J. LYNCH, *et al.* 1987. Melatonin in human preovulatory follicular fluid. J. Clin. Endocrinol. Metab. **64:** 865–867.

50. MARTIN, M., M. MACIAS, G. ESCAMES, *et al.* 2000. Melatonin but not vitamins C and E maintains glutathione homeostasis in t-butyl hydroperoxide-induced mitochondrial oxidative stress. FASEB J. **14:** 1677–1679.
51. MENENDEZ-PELAEZ, A., B. POEGGELER, R.J. REITER, *et al.* 1993. Nuclear localization of melatonin in different mammalian tissues: immunocytochemical and radioimmuno-assay evidence. J. Cell. Biochem. **53:** 373–382.
52. REITER, R.J., D.X. TAN, S.J. KIM, *et al.* 1998. Melatonin as a pharmacological agent against oxidative damage to lipids and DNA. Proc. West. Pharmacol. Soc. **41:** 229–236.
53. SENER, G., K. PASKALOGLU, H. TOKLU, *et al.* 2004. Melatonin ameliorates chronic renal failure-induced oxidative organ damage. J. Pineal Res **36:** 232–241.
54. REITER, R.J., D.X. TAN, S.J. KIM, *et al.* 1999. Augmentation of indices of oxidative damage in life-long melatonin-deficient rats. Mech. Aging Dev. **110:** 157–173.
55. MAYO, J.C., D.X. TAN, R.M. SAINZ, *et al.* 2003. Oxidative damage to catalase induced by peroxyl radicals: functional protection by melatonin and other antioxidants. Free Rad. Res. **37:** 543–553.
56. REITER, R.J. 1999. Oxidative damage to nuclear DNA: amelioration by melatonin. Neuroendocrinol. Lett. **20:** 145–150.
57. ZAVODNIK, I.B., E.A. LAPSHINA, L.B. ZAVODNIK, *et al.* 2004. Hypochlorous acid–induced oxidative stress in Chinese hamster B14 cells: viability, DNA damage and protein. Mutat. Res. **559:** 39–48.
58. YAMAMOTO, H.A. & P.V. MOHANAN. 2003. Ganglioside GT1B and melatonin inhibit brain mitochondrial DNA damage and seizures induced by kainic acid. Brain Res. **964:** 100–106.
59. HIRATA, F., O. HAYAISHI, T. TOKUYAMA, *et al.* 1974. In vitro and in vivo formation of two new metabolites of melatonin. J. Biol. Chem. **249:** 1311–1313.
60. HARDELAND, R., R.J. REITER, B. POEGGELER, *et al.* 1993. The significance of the metabolism of the neurohormone melatonin: antioxidative protection and formation of bioactive substances. Neurosci. Biobehav. Dev. **17:** 347–357.
61. ROZOV, S.V., E.V. FILATOVA, A.A. ORLOV, *et al.* 2003. N^1-Acetyl-N^2-formyl-5-methoxy-kynuramine is a product of melatonin oxidation in rats. J. Pineal Res. **35:** 245–250.
62. DE ALMEIDA, E.A., G.R. MARTINEZ, C.F. KLETZKE, *et al.* 2003. Oxidation of melatonin by singlet molecular oxygen (O_2 (Δg)) produces N^1-acetyl-N^2-formyl-5-methoxy-kynuramine. J. Pineal Res. **35:** 131–137.
63. TAN, D.X., L.C. MANCHESTER, S. BURKHARDT, *et al.* 2001. N^1-Acetyl-N^2-formyl-5-methoxykynuramine, a biogenic amine and melatonin metabolite, functions as a potent scavenger. FASEB J. **15:** 2294–2296.
64. RESSMEYER, A.B., J.C. MAYO, V. ZELOSKO, *et al.* 2003. Antioxidant properties of the melatonin metabolite N^1-acetyl-5-methoxykynuramine (AMK): scavenging of free radicals and prevention of protein destruction. Redox Rept. **8:** 205-213.
65. STEFULJ, J., M. HÖRTNER, M. GHOSH, *et al.* 2001. Gene expression of the key enzymes of melatonin synthesis in extrapineal tissues of the rat. J. Pineal Res. **30:** 243–247.
66. ABE, M., M.T. ITOH, M. MIYATA, *et al.* 2000. Circadian rhythm of serotonin *N*-acetyltransferase activity in rat lens. Exp. Eye Res. **70:** 805–808.
67. LOPEZ-GONZALEZ, M.A., J.M. GUERRERO & F. DELGADO. 1997. Presence of the pineal hormone melatonin in the rat cochlea: its variations with lighting conditions. Neurosci. Lett. **238:** 81–83.
68. BUBENIK, G.A. 2002. Gastrointestinal melatonin: localization, function and clinical relevance. Dig. Res. Sci. **47:** 2336–2348.
69. BORG, D.C. 1995. Oxygen free radicals and tissue injury. *In* Oxygen Free Radicals and Tissue Damage. M. Tarr & F. Samson, Eds.: 12–53. Birkhaüser, Boston.
70. PAPPOLLA, M.A., Y.J. CHYAN, B. POEGGELER, *et al.* 1999. Alzheimer beta protein mediated oxidative damage of mitochondrial DNA: prevention by melatonin. J. Pineal Res. **27:** 226–229.
71. PABLOS, M.T., J.M. GUERRERO, G.G. ORTIZ, *et al.* 1997. Both melatonin and a protective nuclear melatonin receptor agonist CGP 52608 stimulate glutathione peroxidase and glutathione reductase activities in mouse brain in vivo. Neuroendocrinol. Lett. **78:** 49–58.

72. CARRILLO-VICO, A., A. GARCIA-PERGANEDA, L. NAJI, *et al.* 2003. Expression of membrane and nuclear melatonin receptor mRNA and protein in the mouse immune system. Cell. Mol. Life Sci. **60:** 2272–2278.
73. NAJI, L., A. CARRILLO-VICO, J.M. GUERRERO, *et al.* 2004. Expression of membrane and nuclear melatonin receptors in mouse peripheral organs. Life Sci. **74:** 2227–2236.
74. MENENDEZ-PELAEZ, A. & R.J. REITER. 1993. Distribution of melatonin in mammalian tissues: the relative importance of nuclear versus cytosolic localization. J. Pineal Res. **15:** 59–69.
75. REITER, R.J., J.J. GARCIA & J. PIE. 1998. Oxidative neurotoxicity in models of neurodegeneration: responses to melatonin. Restr. Neurol. Neurosci. **12:** 135–140.
76. REITER, R.J., D. ACUÑA-CASTROVIEJO, D.X. TAN, *et al.* 2001. Free radical mediated molecular damage: mechanisms of melatonin's protective actions in the central nervous system. Ann. N.Y. Acad. Sci. **939:** 200–215.
77. TRICOIRE, H., A. LOCATELLI, P. CHEMINEAU, *et al.* 2002. Melatonin enters the cerebrospinal fluid through the pineal recess. Endocrinology **143:** 84–90.
78. REITER, R.J. & D.X. TAN. 2002. Role of CSF in the transport of melatonin. J. Pineal Res. **3:** 61.
79. KILIC, E., Y.G. ÖZDEMIR, H. BOLAY, *et al.* 1999. Pinealectomy aggravates and melatonin administration attenuates brain damage in focal ischemia. J. Cerebr. Blood Flow Metab. **19:** 511–516.
80. CHO, S., T.H. JOH, H.H., BAIK, *et al.* 1997. Melatonin administration protects CA1 hippocampal neurons after ischemia in rats. Brain Res. **755:** 335–338.
81. LI, X.J., I.M. ZHANG, J. GU, *et al.* 1997. Melatonin decreases production of hydroxyl radical during ischemia reperfusion. Acta Pharmacol. Sinica **18:** 394–396.
82. LING, X., I.M. ZHANG, S.D. LU, *et al.* 1999. Protective effect of melatonin on injured cerebral neurons is associated with bcl-2 over expression. Acta Pharmacol. Sinica **20:** 409–414.
83. SINHA, K., M.N. DEGAONKAR, N.R. JAGANNATHAN, *et al.* 2001. Effect of melatonin on ischemia reperfusion injury induced by middle cerebral artery occlusion in rats. Eur. J. Pharmacol. **428:** 185–192.
84. KONDOH, T., H. UNEYAMA, H. NISHINO, *et al.* 2002. Melatonin reduces cerebral edema formation caused by transient forebrain ischemia in rats. Life Sci. **72:** 583–590.
85. TORII, K., H. UNEYAMA, H. NISHINO, *et al.* 2004. Melatonin suppresses cerebral edema caused by middle cerebral artery occlusion/reperfusion in rats assessed by magnetic resonance imaging. J. Pineal Res. **36:** 18–24.
86. KILIC, E., Ü. KILIC, B. YULUG, *et al.* 2004. Melatonin reduces disseminate neuronal death after mild focal ischemia in mice via inhibition of caspase-3 and is suitable as an add-on treatment to tissue-plasminogen activator. J. Pineal Res. **36:** 171–176.
87. CUZZOCREA, S., G. COSTANTINO, E. GITTO, *et al.* 2000. Protective effects of melatonin in ischemic brain injury. J. Pineal Res. **29:** 217–227.
88. GUERRERO, J.M., R.J. REITER, G.G. ORTIZ, *et al.* 1997. Melatonin prevents increases in neural nitric oxide and cyclic GMP production after transient brain ischemia and reperfusion in the Mongolian gerbil (*Meriones unguiculatus*). J. Pineal Res. **23:** 24–31.
89. PEI, Z., S.F. PANG & R.T.F. CHEUNG. 2002. Pretreatment with melatonin reduces volume of cerebral infarction in a rat middle cerebral artery occlusion stroke model. J. Pineal Res. **32:** 168–172.
90. PEI, Z., P.C.W. FUNG & R.T.F. CHEUNG. 2003. Melatonin reduces nitric oxide level during ischemia but not blood-brain barrier breakdown during reperfusion in rat middle cerebral artery occlusion stroke model. J. Pineal Res. **34:** 110–118.
91. WATANABE, K., A. WAKATSUKI, K. SHINOHARA, *et al.* 2005. Maternally administered melatonin protects against ischemia and reperfusion-induced oxidative mitochondrial damage in premature fetal rat brain. J. Pineal Res. In press.
92. LETECHIPIA-VALLEJO, G., I. GONZALEZ-BURGOS & M. CERVANTES. 2001. Neuroprotective effect of melatonin on brain damage induced by global cerebral ischemia in cats. Arch. Med. Res. **32:** 186–192.
93. MANEV, H., T. UZ, A. KHARLAMOV, *et al.* 1996. Increased brain damage after stroke or excitotoxic seizures in melatonin-deficit rats. FASEB J. **10:** 1546–1551.

94. Joo, J.Y., T. Uz & H. Manev. 1998. Opposite effects of pinealectomy and melatonin administration on brain damage following cerebral focal ischemia in rat. Restr. Neurol. Neurosci. **13:** 185–191.

95. Reiter, R.J. 1992. The aging pineal gland and its physiological consequences. BioEssays **14:** 169–175.

96. Reiter, R.J. 1995. The pineal gland and melatonin in relation to aging: a summary of the theories and of the data. Exp. Gerontol. **30:** 199–212.

97. Shene, D.J. & D.F. Swaab. 2003. Melatonin rhythmicity: effect of age and Alzheimer's disease. Exp. Gerontol. **38:** 199–206.

98. Kilic, E., Ü. Kilic, R.J. Reiter, et al. 2005. Prophylactic use of melatonin protects against focal cerebral ischemia in mice: role of endothelin correcting enzyme-1. J. Pineal Res. **37:** 247–251.

99. Thompson, C.B. 1995. Apoptosis in the pathogenesis and treatment of disease. Science **2671:** 1456–1462.

100. Butterfield, D.A. 2002. Amyloid β-peptide (1-42)-induced oxidative stress and neurotoxicity: implications for neurodegeneration in Alzheimer's disease brain. Free Radic. Res. **36:** 1307–1313.

101. Pappolla, M.A., M. Sos, R.A. Omar, et al. 1997. Melatonin prevents death of neuroblastoma cells exposed to the Alzheimer amyloid peptide. J. Neurosci. **17:** 1683–1690.

102. Pappolla, M.A., Y.J. Chyan, P. Bozner, et al. 1999. Dual anti-amyloidogenic and antioxidant properties of melatonin: a new therapy for Alzheimer's disease. *In* Advances in Alzheimer's Disease. K. Iqbal, J. Mortimer, B. Wimbled & H. Wisniewski, Eds: 661–669. Wiley, New York.

103. Pappolla, M.A., P. Bozner, C. Soto, et al. 1998. Inhibition of Alzheimer's β-fibrillogenesis melatonin. J. Biol. Chem. **273:** 7185–7188.

104. Shen, Y.X., S.Y. Yu, W. Wei, et al. 2002. Melatonin blocks rat hippocampal neuronal apoptosis induced by amyloid β-peptide 25-35. J. Pineal Res. **32:** 163–167.

105. Shen, Y.X., W. Wei & S.Y. Xu. 2002. Protective effects of melatonin on corticohippocampal neurotoxicity induced by amyloid β-peptide 25-35. Acta Pharmacol. Sinica **23:** 71–76.

106. Poeggeler, B., L. Miravalle, M.G. Zagarski, et al. 2001. Melatonin reverses the profibrillogenic activity of apolipoprotein E4 on the Alzheimer amyloid β-peptide. Biochemistry **40:** 14995–15001.

107. Olivieri, G., C. Hess, E. Savaskan, et al. 2001. Melatonin protects SHSY5Y neuroblastoma cells from cobalt-induced oxidative stress, neurotoxicity and increased β-amyloid secretion. J. Pineal Res. **31:** 320–325.

108. Shen, Y.X., S.Y. Xu, W. Wei, et al. 2002. The protective effects of melatonin from oxidative damage induced by amyloid β-peptide 25-35 in middle-aged rats. J. Pineal Res. **32:** 85–89.

109. Matsubara, E., T. Bryant-Thomas, J. Paebeco-Quinto, et al. 2003. Melatonin increases survival and inhibits oxidative and amyloid pathology in a transgenic model of Alzheimer's disease. J. Neurochem **85:** 1101–1108.

110. Lahiri, D.K., D. Chen, Y.W. Ge, et al. 2004. Dietary supplementation with melatonin reduces levels of amyloid beta-peptides in the murine cerebral cortex. J. Pineal Res. **36:** 224–231.

111. Brusco, L.I., M. Marques & D.P. Cardinali. 1998. Monozygotic twins with Alzheimer's disease treated with melatonin: case report. J. Pineal Res. **25:** 260–263.

112. Brusco, L.I., M. Marques & D.P. Cardinali. 1998. Melatonin treatment stabilizes chronobiologic and cognitive symptoms in Alzheimer's disease. Neuroendocrinol. Lett. **19:** 111–115.

113. Cohen-Mansfield, J., D. Garfinkel & S. Lipton. 2000. Melatonin for treatment of sundowning in elderly persons with dementia – a preliminary study. Arch. Gerontol. Geriatr. **31:** 65–76.

114. Asayama, K., H. Yamadera, T. Ito, et al. 2003. Double blind study of melatonin effects on the sleep-wake rhythm, cognitive and non-cognitive functions in Alzheimer type dementia. J. Nippon Med. Sch. **70:** 334–341.

115. Rebeck, G.W., J.S. Reiter, D.K. Strickland, et al. 1993. Apolipoprotein E in sporadic Alzheimer's disease allelic variation and receptor interactions. Neuron **11:** 575–580.

116. MISHIMA, K., T. TOZAWA, K. SATOH, *et al.* 1999. Melatonin secretion rhythm disorders in patients with senile dementia of Alzheimer's type with disturbed sleep-waking. Biol. Psychiatry **45:** 417–421.
117. ZHOU, J.N., R.Y. LIU, W. KAMPHORST, *et al.* 2003. Early neuropathological Alzheimer's changes in aged individuals are accompanied by decreased cerebrospinal fluid melatonin levels. J. Pineal Res. **35:** 125–130.
118. TAN, D.X., L.C. MANCHESTER, R. SAINZ, *et al.* 2003. Antioxidant strategies in protection against neurodegenerative disorders. Expert Opin. Ther. Patents **13:** 1513–1543.
119. WANG, D.L., Z.Q. LING, F.Y. CAO, *et al.* 2004. Melatonin attenuates isoproterenol-induced protein kinase A overactivation and tau hyperphosphorylation in rat brain. J. Pineal Res. **37:** 11–16.
120. ZHU, L.Q., S.H. WANG, Z.Q. LING, *et al.* 2004. Effect of inhibiting melatonin biosynthesis on spatial memory retention and tau phosphorylation in rat. J. Pineal Res. **37:** 71–77.
121. FENG, Z., Y. CHANG, Y. CHENG, *et al.* 2004. Melatonin alleviates behavioral deficits associated with apoptosis and cholinergic system dysfunction in the APP 695 transgenic mouse model of Alzheimer's disease. J. Pineal Res. **37:** 129–136.
122. LANGSTON, J.W., P. BALLARD, J.W. TETRUD, *et al.* 1983. Chronic Parkinsonism in humans due to product of meperidine-analog synthesis. Science **219:** 979–980.
123. MAYO, J.C., R.M. SAINZ, H. URIA, *et al.* 1998. Melatonin prevents apoptosis induced by 6-hydroxydopamine in neuronal cells: implications for Parkinson's disease. J. Pineal Res **24:** 179–192.
124. MAYO, J.C., R.M. SAINZ, H. URIA, *et al.* 1998. Inhibition of cell proliferation: a mechanism likely to mediate the prevention of neuronal cell death by melatonin. J. Pineal Res. **25:** 12–18.
125. MAYO, J.C., R.M. SAINZ, I. ANTOLIN, *et al.* 1999. Ultrastructural confirmation of neuronal protection by melatonin against the neurotoxin 6-hydroxydopamine cell damage. Brain Res. **818:** 221–227.
126. PARK, J.W., Y.C. YUON, O.S. KWON, *et al.* 2002. Protective effect of serotonin on 6-hydroxydopamine and dopamine-induced oxidative damage of brain mitochondria and synaptosomes and PC12 cells. Neurochem. Int. **40:** 223–233.
127. LACOVITTI, L., N.D. STULL & K. JOHNSTON. 1997. Melatonin rescues dopamine neurons from cell death in tissue culture models of oxidative stress. Brain Res **768:** 317–326.
128. STULL, N.D., D.P. POLAN & L. IACOVITTI. 2002. Antioxidant compounds protect dopamine neurons from death due to oxidative stress in vitro. Brain Res. **931:** 181–185.
129. ACUÑA-CASTROVIEJO, D., A. COTO-MONTES, M.G. MONTI, *et al.* 1997. Melatonin is protective against MPTP-induced striatal and hippocampal lesions. Life Sci. **60:** PL23–PL29.
130. TANG, Y.P., Y.L. MA, C.C. CHAO, *et al.* 1998. Enhanced glial cell line-derived neurotrophic factor mRNA expression upon deprenyl and melatonin treatments. J. Neurosci. Res. **53:** 593–604.
131. LI, X.J., J. GU, S.D. LU, *et al.* 2002. Melatonin attenuates MPTP-induced dopaminergic neuronal injury associated with scavenging the hydroxyl radical. J. Pineal Res. **32:** 47–52.
132. VAN DER SCHYF, C.J., K. CASTAGNOLI, S. PALMER, *et al.* 2000. Melatonin fails to protect against long term MPTP-induced dopamine depletion in mouse striatum. Neurotoxicol. Res. **1:** 261–269.
133. MORGAN, W.W. & J.F. NELSON. 2001. Chronic administration of pharmacological levels of melatonin does not ameliorate the MPTP-induced degeneration of the nigrostriatal pathway. Brain Res. **921:** 115–121.
134. YAN, M.T. 2002. Melatonin has antioxidant effects in the brain. J. Pineal Res. **33:** 125–126.
135. ANTOLIN, I., J.C. MAYO, R.M. SAINZ, *et al.* 2002. Protective effect of melatonin in a chronic experimental model of Parkinson's disease. Brain Res. **943:** 163–173.
136. LEON, J., D. ACUÑA-CASTROVIEJO, R.M. SAINZ, *et al.* 2004. Melatonin and mitochondrial function. Life Sci. **75:** 765–790.
137. SAINZ, R.M., J.C. MAYO, C. RODRIGUEZ, *et al.* 2003. Melatonin and cell death: differential actions on apoptosis in normal and cancer cells. Cell Mol. Life Sci. **60:** 1407–1426.

138. Jou, M.J., T.I. Peng, R.J. Reiter, *et al.* 2004. Visualization of the antioxidant effects of melatonin at the mitochondrial level during oxidative stress-induced apoptosis of rat brain astrocytes. J. Pineal Res. **37:** 55–70.
139. Reiter, R.J., D.X. Tan, R.M. Sainz, *et al.* 2002. Melatonin: reducing the toxicity and increasing the efficacy of drugs. J. Pharm. Pharmacol. **54:** 1299–1321.

Retardation of Brain Aging by Chronic Treatment with Melatonin

S. C. BONDY,[a] D. K. LAHIRI,[b] V. M. PERREAU,[c] K. Z. SHARMAN,[a]
A. CAMPBELL,[a] J. ZHOU,[d] AND E. H. SHARMAN[a]

[a]*Department of Community and Environmental Medicine, University of California,
Irvine, California 92697, USA*

[b]*Institute of Psychiatric Research, Indiana University School of Medicine,
Indianapolis, Indiana 46202, USA*

[c]*Institute for Brain Aging and Dementia, University of California,
Irvine, California 92697, USA*

[d]*Department of Molecular Biology and Biochemistry, University of California,
Irvine, California, 92697, USA*

ABSTRACT: Slowing the functional decline in the aging brain is not only relevant to nonpathological senescence but also to a broad range of neurodegenerative diseases. Although disorders such as Alzheimer's disease (AD) and Parkinson's disease (PD) are not found in the young adult, they gradually manifest with increasing age. AD, in particular, is an increasing major public health concern as the population ages; therapies that delay disease onset will markedly reduce overall disease prevalence. Aging of the brain has been repeatedly associated with cumulative oxidative damage to macromolecules and to abnormal levels of inflammatory activity. Melatonin has attained increasing prominence as a candidate for ameliorating these changes occurring during senescence. Recent research has focused on supplementation with dietary melatonin designed to elucidate the specific key intracellular targets of age-related inflammatory events, and the optimal means of affording protection of these targets. This report summarizes the progress made in this area.

KEYWORDS: brain aging; melatonin; antioxidants; neurodegenerative disease; inflammation

ADDRESSING THE PROBLEM OF NERVOUS SYSTEM DEFICITS IN THE AGING POPULATION

The median age of the United States population is rapidly increasing and accordingly there is an expectation of a corresponding increase in the incidence of many age-related syndromes. Aging is often associated with both memory and motor deficits that have their origin in the central nervous system (CNS). In addition to cognitive deficits, neurodegeneration contributes to many other ailments in the

Address for correspondence: S. C. Bondy, Ph.D., Department of Community and Environmental Medicine, University of California, Irvine, CA 92697-1825.
scbondy@uci.edu

Ann. N.Y. Acad. Sci. 1035: 197–215 (2004). © 2004 New York Academy of Sciences.
doi: 10.1196/annals.1332.013

elderly, such as injuries from falls that can be attributed to deficits in locomotor, postural, and balancing skills. The potential for large increases in the incidence of neurodegenerative disorders is especially pronounced as improved treatments and medical care have resulted in a declining cardiovascular death rate. The aging process is an essential factor in the progression of such diseases, which only gradually appear in the latter part of the life span. While the onset of neurological disease generally does not represent merely an acceleration of normal aging, it is often based on a platform of aging.

Application of appropriate dietary strategies could have an effect on a broad sector of the population. Dietary supplementation as a means of delaying age-related neural disorders is likely to have increased compliance compared to caloric restriction, which is known to retard aging processes.[1] Much research is focused on the elucidation of the specific key intracellular targets of age-related inflammatory and oxidative events and on identifying the optimal means of affording protection against them.

FACTORS ASSOCIATED WITH BRAIN AGING

Age-Related Changes in Cerebral Function Are in Part Attributable to Extended Exposure to Reactive Oxygen and Nitrogen Species

There is considerable evidence that age-related cellular changes in the CNS are in part attributable to an imbalance between pro-oxidant and antioxidant cerebral factors.[2,3] The brains of longer-lived animals tend to generate lower levels of free radicals and exhibit correspondingly lower activities of antioxidant enzymes.[4] Age-related changes in brain morphology include the appearance of lipofuscin bodies and other insoluble materials, such as amyloid plaques, that are resistant to normal intracellular catabolic processes. Amyloid deposits are considered to be one of the hallmarks of Alzheimer's disease (AD); however, these deposits are also found in the majority of apparently normal elderly individuals.[5] These inclusions are composed of proteinaceous and carbohydrate components. Their accretion is likely to adversely affect cellular function in a parallel manner to the more spectacular distortion of neuronal geometry seen in gangliosidoses.[6] The source of these gradually accumulating materials is from the formation of protein-carbohydrate complexes. Peptides within these complexes are cross-linked, and this is the basis of their resistance to ubiquitinylation and degradation by proteases. The presence of these irresolvable formations in the aging brain is proposed to constitute a focus for deleterious oxidative processes.[7] This hypothesis is supported by evidence of an association between oxidative events and the adverse consequences of aging. Treatment of aged gerbils with a free radical spin trapping agent, α-phenyl-N-*tert*-butyl nitrone, reverses age-related loss of memory skills, as evidenced by use of a radial arm maze test.[8] In a rapidly aging mouse line, such a spin trap can simultaneously reduce the extent of free radical-induced protein oxidation and improve cognition.[9] However, the evidence for a causal relation whereby such processes lead to impaired neurological or behavioral status is not definitive.

The Aging Brain Has a High Intrinsic Level of Inflammation Together with a Reduced Capacity to Respond to Exogenous Immune Stimuli

Several factors reflecting intrinsic immune status within the nervous system are chronically elevated with age in the absence of exogenous stimuli.[1,10–15] Heightened microglial activation in aged animals[16] may be due to a nonproductive response to endogenous factors which may elicit an aberrant reaction. Such intrinsic stress factors include aggregated amyloid peptide and other insoluble proteinaceous inclusions found in the aged brain.[17] The importance of microglia in promoting adverse inflammatory processes is illustrated by the finding that blockade of microglial activation is protective against MPTP toxicity to dopaminergic neurons.[18] Effective immune surveillance is, however, not elevated, but rather depressed in aged animals.[19] Thus, the responsiveness of the cortical immune system to a proinflammatory agent, lipopolysaccharide, is considerably decreased in the elderly mouse.[14] The deleterious effects of a prolonged and ineffective immune response is well illustrated in lung silicosis where the persistent presence of mineral particles leads to a futile phagocytic attack by alveolar macrophages on such irresolvable foci, which ultimately leads to severe pathological changes involving inflammatory cytokines.[20]

ATTENUATION OF INFLAMMATORY AND OXIDATIVE PROCESSES WITHIN THE AGING BRAIN BY MELATONIN TREATMENT

Many studies have reported that changes in both immune function and the presence of an imbalance between pro-oxidant and antioxidant factors occur with cerebral aging.[3,21–23] A relationship between oxidative stress and inflammatory events within nervous tissues has been described,[17,24] and both processes are likely to reflect parallel molecular changes. Recent therapeutic approaches to the most common disease associated with human brain aging, AD, have included both antioxidant and anti-inflammatory drugs. These directions are validated by epidemiological studies suggesting that the extended use of anti-inflammatory agents (e.g., by arthritis patients) reduces the risk of AD.[25] Other epidemiological data have proposed the utility of antioxidants in lowering the incidence of AD.[26] These findings may result from deceleration of changes occurring with normal brain aging rather than from a direct mitigation of AD-specific changes. The search for agents with properties that target the nervous system and restore a biochemical and behavioral profile more closely reflecting that found in younger animals may thus be of value in treatment of diseases such as AD.

The selection of appropriate agents, whose chronic use may optimally lead to beneficial changes within the CNS, poses some distinct problems. For example, global reduction of oxidative effects may impact negatively upon physiological events that rely on reactive oxygen species, such as the involvement of superoxide anion in the inflammatory response. Nitric oxide (NO) is a gaseous free radical that has the potential to cause substantial damage to cellular components; at the same time, it plays a beneficial role by modulating a number of signaling pathways critical to cellular and organismal health. NO can form the very potent oxidant, peroxynitrite; in addition, NO-generated protein nitrosylation is elevated with aging.[24,27] NO has a series of key functions relating to blood supply and neurotransmission. Thus, while inhibi-

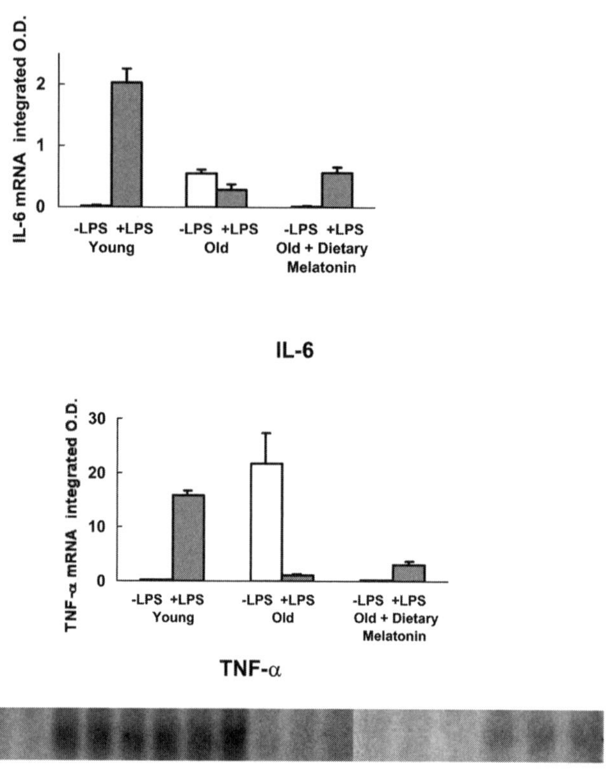

FIGURE 1. Levels of IL-6 and TNF-α mRNA in cerebral cortex of 5- and 26-month-old B6C3F1 mice. Some animals were challenged with an injection of lipopolysaccharide (LPS) 2 h before sacrifice. Two groups of older animals were fed a melatonin (MEL)–containing diet. Images of the Northern blots for TNF-α are also presented.

tion of the NO-producing enzyme, nitric oxide synthase, may protect against *acute* neurotoxic damage,[28] this would be an inappropriate long-term preventive strategy because of the potential for interfering with NO's beneficial endogenous signaling functions.

The evidence described here suggests that indices of immune activity of the aged cortex are less able to respond effectively to an acute inflammatory challenge. The potential ability of 8 weeks of dietary melatonin (200 ppm) to improve the capacity of the immune system to respond to the challenge was studied by focusing on the expression levels of mRNAs for two inflammatory cytokines, TNF-α and inter-leukin 6 (IL-6). In addition, the response of cortical cytokine mRNA levels to an inflammatory stimulus, lipopolysaccharide (LPS), was quantitated. Basal levels of mRNAs for inflammatory cytokines were markedly elevated in the cortex of aged

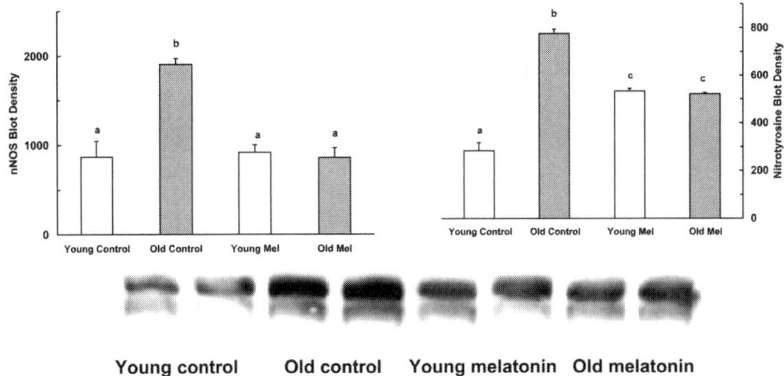

FIGURE 2. Densitometric quantitation of cortical nNOS protein and nitrotyrosine-residue-containing proteins. Values ± SE four replications of 4-month (young) and 27-month (old) B6C3F1 mice receiving control diet or melatonin supplementation. All groups bearing the same letter are statistically indistinguishable ($P<0.01$). Images of the Western blots for nNOS are also presented.

animals (FIG. 1), implying that the inflammatory response system of the aging brain is chronically activated.

This is in accord with a study reporting increased age-related basal expression of genes subserving inflammatory processes in the mouse hippocampus.[29] Expression of such genes is also elevated in hippocampus of the senescence accelerated mouse line.[30] However, cortical cytokine mRNA levels in the old mice did not increase in response to LPS challenge, as seen in young controls (FIG. 1). The high levels of constitutive gene expression of these inflammatory cytokines in the aged mice, prior to stimulation, may contribute to the diminished response to LPS challenge through a diminished signal/noise ratio. Melatonin treatment of 26-month-old mice reduced basal TNF-α and IL-6 cytokine mRNA to levels found in younger 4-month-old mice. This reduction was accompanied by restoration of the positive response to LPS challenge present in younger animals, but absent in untreated aged mice (FIG. 2).

These data in the CNS contrast strongly with parallel studies on five other organs (lung, heart, spleen, liver, and kidney) in the same animals. In all other organs tested and at both ages, basal mRNA levels of these cytokines were very low. In addition, a strong capacity to respond to LPS challenge was maintained, and the level of response was not greatly altered by melatonin supplementation.[14] This suggests that the inflammatory response system of the aging brain is distinctive in both the persistently high basal level of activation (perhaps by endogenous pathogenic signals) and its diminished capacity to respond to the challenge.

The restoration of CNS responses to LPS also parallels the enhancement of systemic immune function reported following melatonin administration.[19] Melatonin is able to attenuate the LPS-induced damage in nerve tissue.[31,32] In addition, melatonin has been reported to ameliorate behavioral indices of anxiety induced by LPS,[33] and to suppress beta-amyloid induced interleukin secretion.[34] Taken together, these findings suggest that, rather than being simply pro- or anti-inflammatory, melatonin may in fact act to optimize intrinsic immune responses.

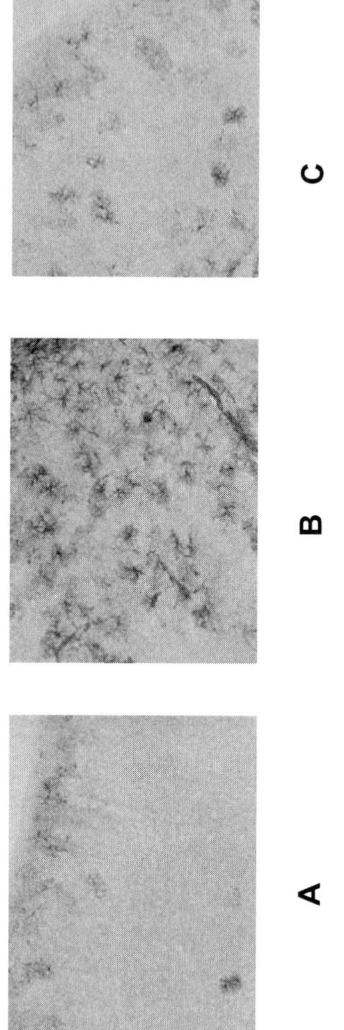

FIGURE 3. GFAP in sagittal sections of surface of murine mid-cortex: (A) 6-month-old mouse, (B) 27-month-old mouse, (C) 27-month-old mouse (B6C3F1) receiving 40 ppm melatonin in diet for the preceding 15 weeks. Magnification: 200×.

In agreement with the observation that mRNA levels of glial fibrillary acidic protein (GFAP) are increased in the aged brain,[15,35,36] immunohistochemical staining for GFAP revealed that both the number and soma size of activated astrocytes expressing this protein were increased in aged animals. This increase in number was largely reversed after aged mice received dietary melatonin for 8 weeks (FIG. 3). Thus, the potential value of melatonin in retardation of age-related oxidant and inflammatory events has a good experimental basis.[14,24,37,38]

REDUCTION OF AGE-RELATED MITOCHONDRIAL DAMAGE BY MELATONIN

The mitochondrion, by virtue of an intensely active respiratory chain and monoamine oxidase activity, is the major source of reactive oxidizing species. It also constitutes a major target of cumulative oxidative damage. Most of the reactive oxygen species produced intracellularly originate from leakage out of the respiratory chain. While electron transport is a very efficient process, it has been estimated that around 2% of oxygen utilized escapes complete reduction to water and can form transient reactive intermediates.[39] There is now an accumulation of evidence that the efficiency of mitochondrial respiration may diminish with age with a consequent increase in the production of superoxide and other oxidant species.[40,41] Mitochondrial respiratory function is compromised in aging human tissues; this can lead to oxidative stress and exhaustion of the endogenous antioxidant enzyme systems.[42] Furthermore, following chemical stress, mitochondria from aged mice are more prone to produce reactive oxygen species than those from young mice.[43] The impairment of mitochondrial function carries the hazard of oxidant-related damage, and the most proximal targets that are maximally at risk are likely to be molecules present within the mitochondrion.

Mitochondrial dysfunction has also been implicated in several common age-related neurodegenerative disorders including AD, Parkinson's disease (PD), Huntington's disease, and amyotropic lateral sclerosis.[44] Targets include mitochondrial membranes (which have an important inner and outer layered structure), mitochondrial proteins, and the mitochondrial DNA (mtDNA). Oxidative damage to mitochondrial proteins is suggested by the age-related decrease in cerebral levels of several enzyme components of the respiratory chain as well as by direct evidence of protein oxidation.[45,46] mtDNA is relatively unprotected in comparison to nuclear DNA, since it is located near the mitochondrial inner membrane where respiration occurs and it is not enclosed by basic histones; in addition, DNA repair enzymes are largely absent. Thus, the level of DNA damage in aging humans is 10-fold greater in the mitochondrion than in the nucleus.[47] In addition, the level of mitochondrial damage is 15-fold greater in people over 70 years of age compared to the younger population.[47] This is evidenced by the increased frequency of gene deletions and by a much higher level of 8-hydroxy-2-deoxyguanosine in mtDNA.[48,49] As a consequence, the mutation rate of mtDNA is increased many-fold in aged mice relative to young mice.[50] A high level of mutated mtDNA results in impaired mitochondrial respiration.[51] In addition, there is evidence that those mitochondria containing typical deletions, while less efficient in performing oxidative phosphorylation than normal mitochondria, are able to divide faster and appear to become more numerous in the CNS with age.[52,53] This raises the issue of such "malignant mitochondria" progressively replacing healthy mitochondria with increasing age. The utility of the mouse model to study this issue is in part due to the high metabolic rate of mice, which results in a much higher rate of mutagenesis of mtDNA compared to that in humans.[50] The action of melatonin on these parameters during mitochondrial aging is thus worthy of study. The potential of melatonin to retard aging processes may relate to its ability to improve mitochondrial function and to protect against oxidative and excitatory events.[51,52] Melatonin increases the activity of complexes II and IV within the brain while decreasing ROS levels.[41] Supercoiled (native) mtDNA in the brain can be partially converted into circular and linearized (denatured) forms following administration of ethanol, and this can be attenuated by concurrent treatment with melatonin.[54]

Melatonin has been found to be neuroprotective in a wide range of conditions including traumatic injury to the brain.[55,56] Melatonin treatment of rats during ischemia/reperfusion in the cerebral artery occlusion stroke model led to decreased cytochrome c release, apoptotic DNA fragmentation, loss of neurons, and infarct volume. These effects may be a consequence of melatonin's potent maintenance of mitochondrial inner membrane potential during oxygen and glucose deprivation of cultured striatal neurons.[57] Protection of mitochondrial integrity by the administration of exogenous melatonin has beneficial behavioral consequences most likely because of melatonin's antioxidant properties.[58]

CHANGES IN GENE EXPRESSION PRODUCED BY MELATONIN

An oligonucleotide microarray study on cortices from young and aged mice using an Affymetrix laser-activated fluorescence system revealed that dietary melatonin supplements changed the mRNA levels of many genes. In order to detect genes whose expression changed appreciably with senescence, a cutoff factor for a change in magnitude of expression of 1.7 or greater was used.[59] Only 107 of over 12,000 genes were altered to this extent. These results parallel those found using differential display analysis where only 1–2% of mRNAs were significantly altered with aging.[1,36,60] Many of the genes with the largest magnitude of age-associated increases were acute phase genes associated with short-term immune responses (TABLE 1).

Melatonin treatment of aged animals unequivocally brought about mRNA expression changes in a direction toward that found in younger mice. Such supplementation caused 89% of all genes whose expression altered by over 1.7-fold with age to be partially or completely restored to younger levels. These findings need to be consolidated by designing probe sets and making primers by RT-PCR to permit assay of mRNAs for genes whose age-related changes are completely reversed by melatonin. These include those for GFAP, Tom-40, and VHL (Von Hippel-Lindau). VHL is a signaling protein within the oxygen-sensing circuitry of the cell while Tom-40 is a mitochondrial outer membrane protein transporter. Age-related increases in the mRNA for glial fibrillary acidic protein, GFAP (a marker for astrogliosis), and for the apoptosis-signaling protein, Dedd (death effector domain-containing protein), were completely reversed by melatonin treatment.

A more recent microarray study with a different mouse strain (CB6F1) and the use of three animals per condition permitted a more rigorous statistical analysis of data. This study included testing of the effect of an LPS challenge and involved evaluation of over 40,000 genes.[61] While the variance between triplicate young animals was small, this increased markedly with aging (TABLE 2). Thus, the aging brain had a markedly increased divergence of gene expression so that differences in the profiles of mRNA isolated from individual senescent animals were greater than differ-

TABLE 1. Modulation of gene expression effected by melatonin treatment of 27-month-old B6C3F1 mice in comparison to expression profile of 4-month-old mice

UniGene cluster	GenBank no. and name	Function class	Fold-change OC vs. YC	OM vs. YC
Upregulated with age				
Mm.104747	M80423, X0065, M18237, IgM chain regions	Immunity	11.3	5.6
Mm.22339	AL843063	Unknown	4.9	2.3
Mm.22650	M64086	Immunity, acute phase	4.5	5.6
Mm.10160	AV355874	Unknown	3.8	2.0
Mm.9537	X81627, 24p3, lipocalin 2	Immunity, type 1 acute phase	3.5	1.4
Downregulated with age				
Mm.4137	M64278, chromogranin	Neurosecretory protein	−7.2	3.1
Mm.208443	AF0432049, Tom40	Mit. protein translocase	−4.5	2.3
Mm.5903	AB002136mGAA1	Glycosyl phosphatidyl-inositol transamidase	−4.1	2.2
Mm.213275	AA756275, T-cell delta chain precursor protein	Immune receptor	−3.4	0.2

TABLE 2. Number of genes and expressed sequence tags (ESTs) from melatonin-treated CB6F1 mice with greater variance than expected by assumption of random binomial distribution

Groups compared	Number of genes for which first group over second group variance is: Greater	Lesser	Identical	Random	Number of genes with variance not predicted by assumption of random value
Old control vs. young control	27,787 ± 339	17,247 ± 339	3	22,517	+5270 ± 479
Old melatonin vs. young control	20,894 ± 348	24,143 ± 348	5	22,516	−1627 ± 492
Old melatonin vs. old control	15,737 ± 333	29,297 ± 333	5	22,517	−6780 ± 471

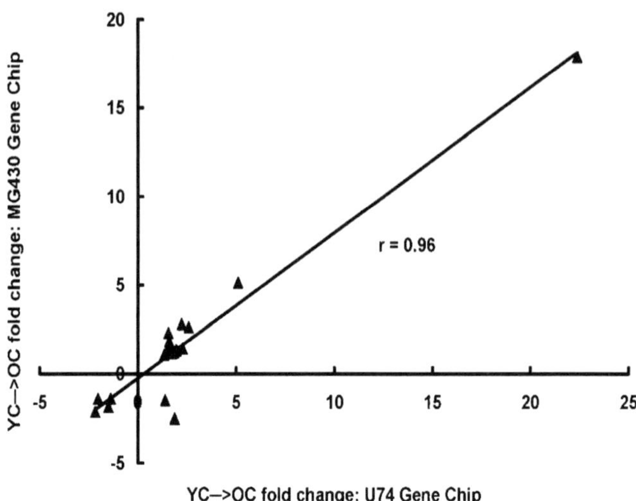

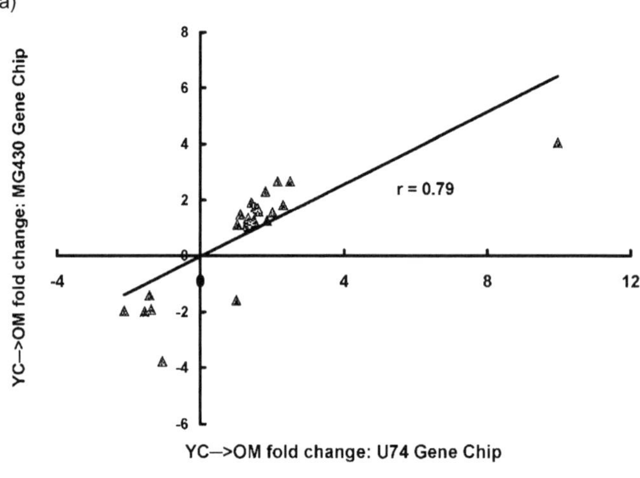

FIGURE 4. Expression correlation between two separate experiments involving use of B6C3F1 and CB6F1 strains of mouse and differing gene chips: **(a)** young/old groups versus **(b)** young compared to [old + melatonin] group. The U74Av2 Affymetrix gene chip was used with RNA prepared from B6C3F1 mice at 4 and 27 months. One set of aged mice received 200 ppm melatonin in the diet for the 6 weeks preceding death. The MG430 gene chip was used with RNA from CB6F1 mice at 4.5 and 26.5 months. One set of aged mice received 40 ppm melatonin in the diet for the 9.3 weeks preceding death. Correlations are for genes (a) changing markedly with aging or (b) where melatonin alters the aged mRNA profile toward one resembling a more youthful expression pattern.

ences found between younger animals. This age-associated genetic dispersion was arrested by melatonin treatment so that the gene expression of treated older animals had a variance even below that of the untreated young group of mice. The reduction of this dispersion of gene expression by melatonin treatment implies restoration of a more rigorous degree of genetic control in older animals.

Many of the results found for the prior gene analysis were replicated and, thus, validated in this second study, which used animals of a different strain and of a somewhat different age. The degree of correlation in age-related changes and responses to melatonin is shown in FIGURE 4. These parallels suggest that the findings are robust and may have extensive generality.

MECHANISM OF MELATONIN ACTION

Melatonin seems capable of modulating a number of changes in gene expression, some of which are associated with aging. The mechanisms through which these are affected may involve activation of transcription factors by way of specific receptors for melatonin.[62,63] Within the brain, there are three major classes of receptors for melatonin.[64] Two of these, ML1 and ML2, are within the plasma membrane coupled to G-proteins whose activation leads to the depression of cyclic AMP levels. However, the presence of melatonin-binding sites in the nucleus of many cell types suggests mechanisms of action other than through the G-protein coupled receptor.[65] The third class, M3, is a melatonin-regulated quinone reductase 2.[66] This antioxidant enzyme, which reduces quinone and blocks its redox cycling, is elevated in AD neurons exhibiting prominent tau immunostaining, and it is proposed to respond to excess oxidative events.[67]

The mechanism of action of melatonin is unlikely to be due to any direct antioxidant properties, as the normal brain concentration of melatonin is in the range of 4 to 5 pM,[68] while the less redox active 6-hydroxysulfate metabolite is constitutively present at 3–5 nM. In contrast, the levels of glutathione, a significant antioxidant, is around a millionfold greater in the CNS, generally being in the millimolar range. The evidence against melatonin being an important direct antioxidant is supported by the finding that it can actually promote ROS formation in an *in vitro* system. A biphasic potential for promotion of both pro- and antioxidant events by melatonin in *ex vivo* systems has been repeatedly described.[34,69,70] Nevertheless, melatonin as well as many of its catabolic products have antioxidant properties,[71] and this can contribute to the overall free-radical scavenging potential of this moiety. However, melatonin induces expression of antioxidant genes in the brain,[72] and selective derepression of redox-modulating factors most likely underlies its antioxidant potential.

THERAPEUTIC POTENTIAL OF MELATONIN IN NEURODEGENERATIVE DISEASE

There is extensive evidence for the potential utility of various agents in partially restoring both the biochemical and behavioral profile of older animals. Melatonin is an especially promising candidate in this regard for several reasons. It is a readily available and inexpensive chemical with almost no toxic potential. Melatonin does

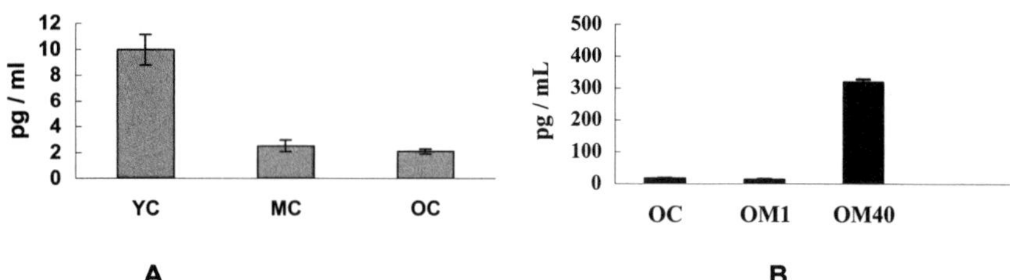

FIGURE 5. Serum concentration of melatonin in B6C3F1 mice—(**A**) concentration in untreated mice of various ages: YC = 6 months, MC = 12 months, OC = 27 months; (**B**) concentration in 27-month-old mice receiving 1 ppm (OM1) and 40 ppm (OM40) melatonin for 9 weeks. Control = OC.

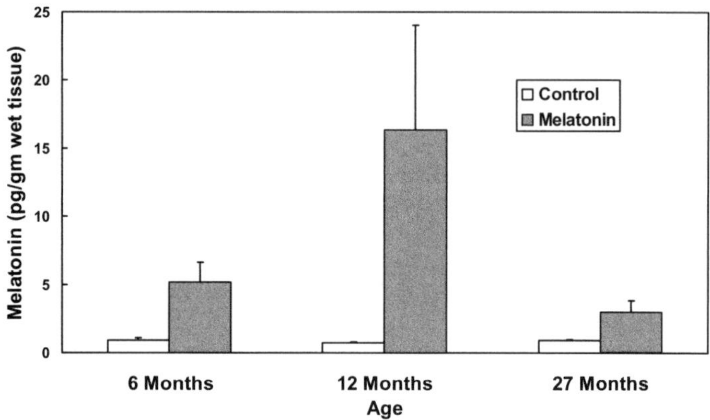

FIGURE 6. Cortical content of melatonin in B6C3F1 mice receiving 40 ppm melatonin for 9 weeks.

not act as a carcinogen or co-carcinogen. In fact, long-term supplementation lowers mammary tumor incidence from 63% to 23% in a cancer-prone mouse strain.[73] Finally, melatonin has been shown to increase both median and maximum life span of mice.[74] Thus, its widespread application to the aged sector of the population poses very little risk. Aged animals have significantly lower levels of circulating melatonin in comparison with levels in young or middle-aged mice[68] (FIG. 5). In addition, the diurnal fluxes of melatonin levels in plasma are not as pronounced in the aged.[75] Dietary melatonin administered for 8 weeks elevated serum levels of the neurohormone (FIG. 5). Melatonin is able to access the CNS through the blood–brain barrier. Following administration of melatonin, levels in the cerebral cortex of aged treated animals were also raised (FIG. 6). It may be significant that, in AD, the melatonin content of cerebrospinal fluid is even further reduced below the usual age related derepression.[76] Thus, deceleration of normal senescence using melatonin is likely to benefit the rate of progression of more specific neurodegenerative diseases such as AD and PD. Both normal aging and pathological processes may in part involve changes in identical loci. The identification and protection of such common targets will be valuable in the development of strategies designed to delay the manifestation of common neurodegenerative disorders. The slow progression of many neuro-degenerative disorders over a substantial portion of an individual's adult life span suggests that, in order to be effective, treatments, such as dietary supplementation, need to be maintained over many years.

Increased oxidative stress in the aged brain has been attributed to reduced efficiency of mitochondrial energy production.[77] Given the brain's high energy requirements, any decline in brain electron transport system enzyme activity could have a significant deleterious impact on the brain prior to an adverse effect on other organs with a lesser oxygen demand. While the ability of antioxidant nutrients to slow the decline in efficiency of mitochondrial energy processes has been extensively studied, the results have frequently been disappointing. Supplementation with α-tocopherol has been found to be ineffective in reducing ROS in the brain,[41] heart, or liver[78] of mice. With respect to the brain, this may be attributable to its poor penetrance. α-Tocopherol treatment of humans in the DATATOP study for mitigation of PD revealed that even after many months of treatment, cerebrospinal levels of this vitamin were not equilibrated with plasma levels and were still rising.[79] In contrast, as shown above, following its administration, levels of melatonin in the cerebral cortex of aged treated animals can be significantly raised.[68] These data reveal that dietary melatonin can both be absorbed in an intact unconjugated form into the bloodstream, and, importantly, can also pass across the blood–brain barrier resulting in increased levels in the CNS.

Using chronic administration of melatonin, good evidence has been found for the utility of melatonin in partially restoring the biochemical profile of older animals to that more closely resembling younger animals.[14,24,37,80] Pinealectomy, which removes the major source of melatonin synthesis within the brain, appears to accelerate the aging process.[81,82] Conversely, the thymic involution associated with aging can be arrested by pineal grafting or by administration of melatonin.[83] Aging may thus in part be a pineal-programmed event.[84] It is noteworthy that the overall appear-

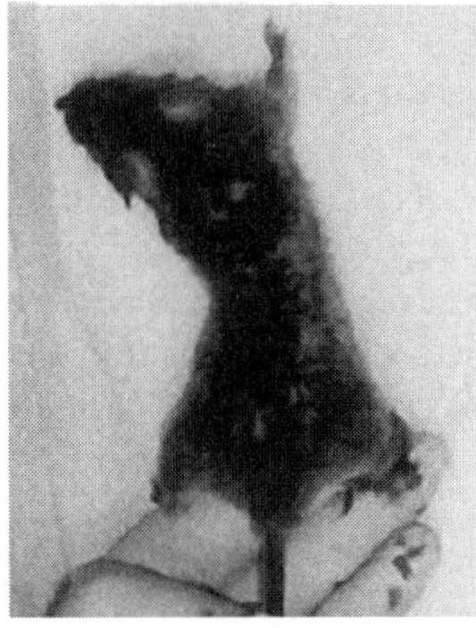
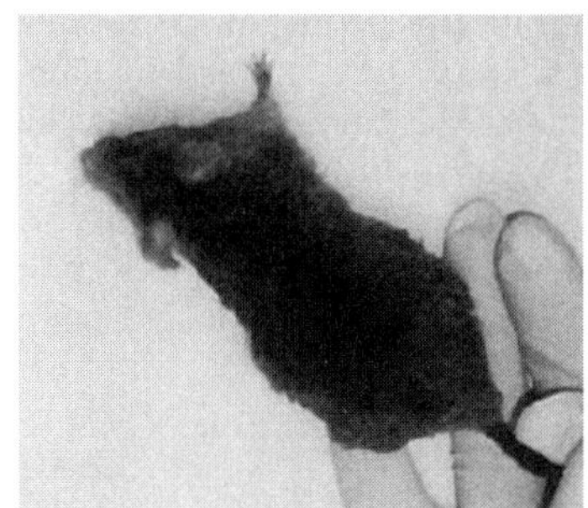

FIGURE 7. Appearance of 27-month-old CB6F1 mice. The treated animal received 40 ppm melatonin in the diet for 9.3 weeks.

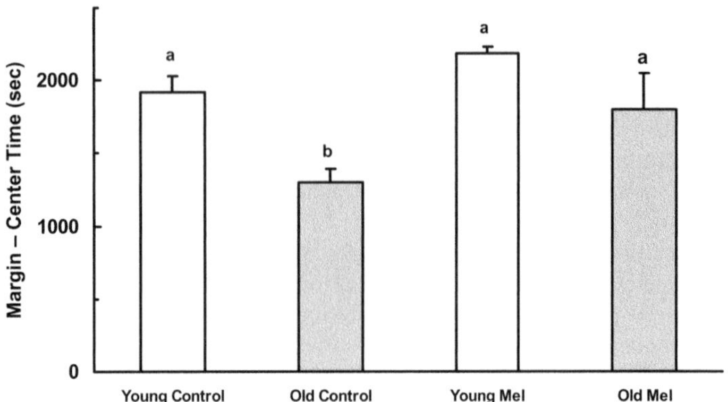

FIGURE 8. Time that B6C3F1 mice spent at test cage margin minus the time spent in the center of the area. Values represent time in seconds determined during a 1-h testing period and are mean ± SE of values derived from 5–7 animals. All groups bearing the same letter are statistically indistinguishable.

ance of aged animals chronically treated with melatonin is clearly superior to that of untreated mice in that the fur is less patchy and more glossy (FIG. 7).

The ultimate test of a therapeutic agent that is proposed to be of value in the retardation of brain aging involves demonstration of a beneficial behavioral effect. In untreated aged mice, there was a decreased proportion of time spent exploring cage margins relative to young mice.[24] This decreased exploratory activity was reversed in melatonin treated aged animals. Thus, restoration of a biochemical profile characterizing younger animals was paralleled by changes in behavioral indices so as to resemble those of younger animals. Exploratory behavior of younger animals treated with melatonin was entirely unaltered (FIG. 8).

The potential for delaying age related degenerative diseases in the CNS through the use of melatonin might be increased through its combination with other therapies. There is a rapidly expanding literature on the health benefits of exercise to healthy aging specifically relating to AD.[85,86] Exercise promotes neurogenesis and learning in the adult rodent brain[87] and ameliorates the antidepressant induction of BDNF expression in the hippocampus.[88] A recent study also suggests that exercise may prevent cognitive decline in humans.[89] There is an age-related decline in the amplitude of the circadian flux of melatonin levels,[76] and exercise enhances the diurnal expression levels of melatonin.[90] Thus, combining melatonin treatment together with exercise could provide more health benefits than either therapy alone.

CONCLUSIONS

The brain is distinct from other organs in that its aging is accompanied by a chronic enhancement of inflammatory markers in the absence of any external stimulus. Elevation of basal levels of inflammation can retard the response to exogenous inducers of inflammation, perhaps by leaving little room for maneuvering. Thus, reducing levels of inflammation in the aged may be an appropriate strategy in attempting to minimize age-associated CNS deficits. Rather than acting directly as an antioxidant, melatonin may alter gene expression by modulating the activity of a transcription factor. Elevation of basal levels can retard the response to exogenous inducers of inflammation, and this may be a relevant target in attempting to minimize age-associated CNS deficits. Supplementation of the diet with melatonin can retard the onset of, and even reverse, some of the biochemical and behavioral changes associated with aging and melatonin has been found to be neuroprotective in a wide range of conditions including traumatic injury to the brain.[55,56] Melatonin may alter gene expression rather than acting as a classical antioxidant. Since several neurological conditions are associated with a higher incidence of intrinsic inflammation, the capacity of melatonin to reduce basal levels of inflammation may be of value in retarding both normal brain aging and in slowing the progression of neurological disease. Aging is also characterized by dysregulation of immune responses to exogenous stimuli. This may in part account for the greater susceptibility to infection and higher incidence of cancer found in the aged. The ability of melatonin to arrest an attenuated immune response may prove beneficial in retarding deleterious trends associated with senescence.

ACKNOWLEDGMENTS

This work was supported in part by grants from the National Institutes of Health (ES 7992 and AG 16794).

REFERENCES

1. LEE, C.K., R. WEINDRUCH & T.A. PROLLA. 2000. Gene-expression profile of the ageing brain in mice. Nature Genet. **25:** 294–297.
2. LEBEL, C. & S.C. BONDY. 1992. Oxidative damage and cerebral aging. Prog. Neurobiol. **38:** 601–602.
3. CALABRESE, V. *et al.* 2000. NO synthase and NO-dependent signal pathways in brain aging and neurodegenerative disorders: the role of oxidant/antioxidant balance. Neurochem. Res. **25:** 1315–1341.
4. BARJA, G. *et al.* 1994. A decrease of free radical production near critical targets as a cause of maximum longevity in animals. Comp. Biochem. Physiol. Biochem. Mol. Biol. **108:** 501–512.
5. KNOPMAN, D.S. *et al.* 2003. Neuropathology of cognitively normal elderly. J. Neuropathol. Exp. Neurol. **62:** 1087–1095.
6. WALKLEY, S.U. 2003. Neurobiology and cellular pathogenesis of glycolipid storage diseases. Philos. Trans. R. Soc. Lond. B Biol. Sci. **358:** 893–904.
7. CAMPBELL, A. & S.C. BONDY. 2001. Particulates as contributory factors in neurodegenerative disease. *In* Inflammatory Events in Neurodegeneration. S.C. Bondy and A. Campbell, Eds.: 309–325. Prominent Press. Phoenix, AZ.
8. SACK, C.A. *et al.* 1996. Antioxidant treatment with phenyl-alpha-tert-butyl nitrone (PBN) improves the cognitive performance and survival of aging rats. Neurosci. Lett. **205:** 181–184.
9. BUTTERFIELD, D.A. *et al.* 1997. Oxidatively induced structural alteration of glutamine synthetase assessed by analysis of spin label incorporation kinetics: relevance to Alzheimer's disease. J. Neurochem. **68:** 2451–2457.
10. TERRAZZINO, S. *et al.* 1997. Interleukin-6, tumor necrosis factor and corticosterone induction by central lipopolysaccharide in aged rats. Life Sci. **61:** 695–701.

11. WEAVER, J.D. *et al.* 2002. Interleukin-6 and risk of cognitive decline: MacArthur studies of successful aging. Neurology **59:** 371–378.
12. BLALOCK, E.M. *et al.* 2003. Gene microarrays in hippocampal aging: statistical profiling identifies novel processes correlated with cognitive impairment. J. Neurosci. **23:** 3807–3819.
13. YU, W.H. *et al.* 2002. Phenotypic and functional changes in glial cells as a function of age. Neurobiol. Aging **23:** 105–115.
14. SHARMAN, E. *et al.* 2001. Reduced basal levels and enhanced LPS response of IL-6 mRNA in aged mice. J. Gerontol. **56B:** 520–523.
15. SHARMAN, E. *et al.* 2004. Age-related changes in murine CNS mRNA gene expression are modulated by dietary melatonin. J. Pineal Res. **36:** 165–170.
16. SLOANE, J.A. *et al.* 1999. Increased microglial activation and protein nitration in white matter of the aging monkey. Neurobiol. Aging **20:** 395–405.
17. BONDY, S.C. & A. CAMPBELL, Eds. 2001 Inflammatory Events in Neurodegeneration. Prominent Press. Phoenix, AZ.
18. WU, C. *et al.* 2002. Blockade of microglial activation is neuroprotective in the 1-methyl-4-phenyl-1,2,3,6-tetrahydropyridine mouse model of Parkinson disease. J. Neurosci. **22:** 1763–1771.
19. AKBULUT, K.G., B. GONUL & H. AKBULUT. 2001. The effects of melatonin on humoral immune responses of young and aged rats. Immunol. Invest. **30:** 17–20.
20. MOHR, C. *et al.* 1991. Systemic macrophage stimulation in rats with silicosis: enhanced release of tumor necrosis factor-alpha from alveolar and peritoneal macrophages. Am. J. Respir. Cell. Mol. Biol. **5:** 395–402.
21. HULL, M. *et al.* 1996. The participation of interleukin-6, a stress-inducible cytokine, in the pathogenesis of Alzheimer's disease. Behav. Brain Res. **78:** 37–41.
22. BONDY, S.C. 1998. Free radicals in neurodegenerative disease. *In* Advances in Neuro-degenerative Disorders, Vol. II. J. Marwah & H. Teitelbaum, Eds.: 1–21. Prominent Press. Phoenix, AZ.
23. SOHAL, R.S. 1998. Oxidative stress in senescent decline in brain function. *In* Advances in Neurodegenerative Disorders, Vol. II. J. Marwah & H. Teitelbaum, Eds.: 23–48. Prominent Press. Phoenix, AZ.
24. SHARMAN, E. *et al.* 2002. Reversal of biochemical and behavioral parameters of brain aging by melatonin and acetyl l-carnitine. Brain Res. **957:** 223–230.
25. BROE, G.A. *et al.* 2000. Anti-inflammatory drugs protect against Alzheimer disease at low doses. Arch. Neurol. **57:** 1586–1591.
26. PITCHUMONI, S.S. & P.M. DORAISWAMY. 1998. Current status of antioxidant therapy for Alzheimer's disease. J. Am. Geriatr. Soc. **46:** 1566–1572.
27. TOHGI, H. *et al.* 1999. Alterations of 3-nitrotyrosine concentration in the cerebrospinal fluid during aging and in patients with Alzheimer's disease. Neurosci. Lett. **269:** 52–54.
28. ITZHAK, Y. *et al.* 1998. The role of neuronal nitric oxide synthase in cocaine-induced conditioned place preference. Neuroreport **9:** 2485–2488.
29. TERAO, A. *et al.* 2002. Immune response gene expression increases in the aging murine hippocampus. J. Neuroimmunol. **132:** 99–112.
30. THA, K.K. *et al.* 2000. Changes in expressions of proinflammatory cytokines IL-1β, TNF-α and IL-6 in the brain of senescence accelerated mouse (SAM) P8. Brain Res. **885:** 25–31.
31. LEZOUALC'H, F., M. SPARAPANI & C. BEHL. 1998. N-acetyl-serotonin (normelatonin) and melatonin protect neurons against oxidative challenges and suppress the activity of the transcription factor NF-kappaB. J. Pineal Res. **124:** 168–178.
32. SEWERYNEK, E. *et al.* 1996. Lipopolysaccharide-induced DNA damage is greatly reduced in rats treated with the pineal hormone melatonin. Mol. Cell. Endocrinol. **117:** 183–188.
33. NAVA, F. & G. CARTA. 2001. Melatonin reduces anxiety induced by lipopolysaccharide in the rat. Neurosci. Lett. **307:** 57–60.
34. CLAPP-LILLY, K.L. *et al.* 2001. Melatonin reduces interleukin secretion in amyloid-beta stressed mouse brain slices. Chem. Biol. Interact. **134:** 101–107.
35. NICHOLS, N.R. *et al.* 1993. GFAP mRNA increases with age in rat and human brain. Neurobiol. Aging **14:** 421-429.

36. GOYNS, M.H. *et al.* 1998. Differential display analysis of gene expression indicates that age-related changes are restricted to a small cohort of genes. Mech. Ageing Dev. **101:** 73–90.
37. REITER, R.J. *et al.* 1998. Reactive oxygen intermediates, molecular damage, and aging. Relation to melatonin. Ann. N.Y. Acad. Sci. **854:** 410–424.
38. CUZZOCREA, S. *et al.* 2000. Protective effects of melatonin in ischemic brain injury. J. Pineal Res. **29:** 217–227.
39. BOVERIS, A. & B. CHANCE. 1973. The mitochondrial generation of hydrogen peroxide. General properties and effect of hyperbaric oxygen. Biochem. J. **134:** 707–716.
40. KU, H.H., U.T. BRUNK & R.S. SOHAL. 1993. Relationship between mitochondrial superoxide and hydrogen peroxide production and longevity of mammalian species. Free Radical Biol. Med. **15:** 621–627.
41. SHARMAN, E. & S.C. BONDY. 2001. Effects of dietary antioxidants and age on cortical electron transport chain activity. Neurobiol. Aging **22:** 629–634.
42. WEI, Y.H. *et al.* 2001. Oxidative stressing human aging and mitochondrial disease—consequences of defective mitochondrial respiration and impaired antioxidant enzyme system. Chin. J. Physiol. **44:** 1–11.
43. ALI, S.F. *et al.* 1994. MPTP-induced oxidative stress and neurotoxicity are age-dependent: evidence from measures of reactive oxygen species and striatal dopamine levels. Synapse **18:** 27–34.
44. BOWLING, A.C. & M.F. BEAL. 1995 Bioenergetic and oxidative stress in neurodegenerative diseases. Life Sci. **56:** 1151–1171.
45. BOWLING, A.C. *et al.* 1993. Age dependent impairment of mitochondrial function in primate brain. J. Neurochem. **60:** 1964–1967.
46. LENAZ, G.C. *et al.* 1997. Mitochondrial complex I defects in aging. Mol. Cell. Biochem. **174:** 329–333.
47. MECOCCI, P. *et al.* 1993. Oxidative damage to mitochondrial DNA shows marked age-dependent increases in human brain. Ann. Neurol. **34:** 609–616.
48. BROSSAS, J.Y. *et al.* 1994. Multiple deletions in mitochondrial DNA are present in senescent mouse brain. Biochem. Biophys. Res. Commun. **202:** 654–659.
49. MECOCCI, P. *et al.* 1997 Mitochondrial membrane fluidity and oxidative damage to mitochondrial DNA in aged and AD human brain. Mol. Chem. Neuropathol. **31:** 53–64.
50. WANG, E., A. WONG & G. CORTOPASSI. 1997. The rate of mitochondrial mutagenesis is faster in mice than humans. Mutat. Res. **377:** 157–166.
51. MARTIN, M. *et al.* 2002. Melatonin increases the activity of the oxidative phosphorylation enzymes and the production of ATP in rat brain and liver mitochondria. Int. J. Biochem. Cell. Biol. **34:** 348–347.
52. WALLACE, D.C. *et al.* 1995. Mitochondrial DNA mutations in human degenerative diseases and aging. Biochim. Biophys. Acta **1271:** 141–151.
53. BERTONI-FREDDARI, C. *et al.* 2004. Decay of mitochondrial metabolic competence in the aging cerebellum. Ann. N.Y. Acad. Sci. **1019:** 29–32.
54. MANSOURI, A. *et al.* 2001. Acute ethanol administration oxidatively damages and depletes mitochondrial DNA in mouse liver, brain, heart and skeletal muscles: protective effect of melatonin. J. Pharm. Exp. Therap. **298:** 737–743.
55. CIRAK, B. *et al.* 1999. Melatonin as a free radical scavenger in experimental head trauma. Pediatr. Neurosurg. **31:** 298–301.
56. BENI, S.M. *et al.* 2004. Melatonin-induced neuroprotection after closed head injury is associated with increased brain antioxidants and attenuated late-phase activation of NF-kappaB and AP-1. FASEB J. **18:** 149–151.
57. ANDRABI, S.A. *et al.* 2004. Direct inhibition of the mitochondrial permeability transition pore: a possible mechanism responsible for anti-apoptotic effects of melatonin. FASEB J. **18:** 869–871.
58. RAGHAVENDRA, V. & S.K. KULKARNI. 2001. Possible antioxidant mechanism in melatonin reversal of aging and chronic ethanol-induced amnesia in plus-maze and passive avoidance memory tasks. Free Radical Biol. Med. **30:** 595–602.
59. CAO, Z. *et al.* 2004. Detection of differentially expressed genes in healing mouse corneas, using cDNA microarrays. Invest. Ophthalmol. Vis. Sci. **43:** 2897–2904.

60. Jiang, C.H. *et al.* 2001. The effects of aging on gene expression in the hypothalamus and cortex of mice. Proc. Natl. Acad. Sci. USA **98:** 1930–1934.
61. Perreau, V.M. *et al.* 2004. Modulation of whole transcriptome mRNA expression patterns in murine CNS by age and dietary melatonin. In preparation.
62. New, D.C., S.T. Tsim & Y.H. Wong. 2003. G protein–linked effector and second messenger systems involved in melatonin signal transduction. Neurosignals **12:** 59–70.
63. Dubocovich, M.L. *et al.* 2003. Molecular pharmacology, regulation and function of mammalian melatonin receptors. Front. Biosci. **8:** 1093–1108.
64. Witt-Enderby, P.A. *et al.* 2003. Melatonin receptors and their regulation: biochemical and structural mechanisms. Life Sci. **72:** 2183–2198.
65. Filadelfi, A.M. & A.M. Castrucci. 1996. Comparative aspects of the pineal/melatonin system of poikilothermic vertebrates. J. Pineal Res. **20:** 175–186.
66. Nosjean, O. *et al.* 2000. Identification of the melatonin binding site MT3 as the quinone reductase 2. J. Biol. Chem. **275:** 31311–31317.
67. Wang, Y. *et al.* 2000. NAD(P)H:quinone oxidoreductase activity is increased in hippocampal pyramidal neurons of patients with Alzheimer's disease. Neurobiol. Aging **21:** 525–531.
68. Lahiri, D.K. *et al.* 2004. Age-related changes in serum melatonin in mice: higher levels of combined melatonin and 6-hydroxy melatonin sulfate in the cerebral cortex than in serum, heart, liver and kidney tissue. J. Pineal Res. **36:** 217–223.
69. Ianas, O., R. Olinescu & I. Badescu. 1991. Melatonin involvement in oxidative processes. Endocrinologie **29:** 147–153.
70. Bondy, S.C. *et al.* 2002. Dietary modulation of age-related changes in cerebral pro-oxidant status. Neurochem. Int. **40:** 123–130.
71. Tan, D.X. *et al.* 2000. Significance of melatonin in antioxidative defense: reactions and products. Biol. Signals Recep. **9:** 137–159.
72. Kotler, M. *et al.* 1998. Melatonin increases gene expression for antioxidant enzymes in rat brain cortex. J. Pineal Res. **24:** 83–9.
73. Subramanian, A. & L. Kothari. 1991. Melatonin, a suppressor of spontaneous murine mammary tumors. J. Pineal Res. **10:** 136–140.
74. Anisimov, V.N. *et al.* 2000. The effect of melatonin on the indices of biological age, on longevity and on the development of spontaneous tumors in mice. Vopr. Onkol. **46:** 311–319.
75. Magri, F.S. *et al.* 2004. Qualitative and quantitative changes of melatonin levels in physiological and pathological aging and in centenarians. J. Pineal Res. **36:** 256–261.
76. Liu, R.Y. *et al.* 1999. Decreased melatonin levels in postmortem cerebrospinal fluid in relation to aging, Alzheimer's disease, and apolipoprotein E-epsilon 4/4 genotype. J. Clin. Endocrinol. Metab. **84:** 323–327.
77. Liu, J. *et al.* 2002. Memory loss in old rats is associated with brain mitochondrial decay and RNA/DNA oxidation: Partial reversal by feeding acetyl-L-carnitine and/or R-alpha-lipoic acid. Proc. Natl. Acad. Sci. USA **99:** 2356–2361.
78. Sumien, N., M.J. Forster & R.S. Sohal. 2003. Supplementation with vitamin E fails to attenuate oxidative damage in aged mice. Exp. Gerontol. **38:** 699–704.
79. Vatassery, G.T., S. Fahn & M.A. Kuskowski. 1998. Alpha tocopherol in CSF of subjects taking high-dose vitamin E in the DATATOP study. Parkinson Study Group. Neurology **50:** 1900–1902.
80. Sharman, K.G., E. Sharman & S.C. Bondy. 2002. Dietary melatonin selectively reverses age-related changes in cortical basal cytokine mRNA levels, and their responses to an inflammatory stimulus. Neurobiol. Aging **23:** 633–638.
81. Payao, S.L. *et al.* 2001. Pinealectomy-associated decrease in ribosomal gene activity in rats. Biogerontology **2:** 105–108.
82. Reiter, R.J. *et al.* 1999. Augmentation of indices of oxidative damage in life-long melatonin-deficient rats. Mech. Ageing Dev. **110:** 157–173.
83. Provinciali, M. *et al.* 1996. Effect of melatonin and pineal grafting on thymocyte aopotosis in aging mice. Mech. Ageing Dev. **90:** 1–19.
84. Pierpaoli, W. 1998. Neuroimmunology of aging: a program in the pineal gland. Ann. N.Y. Acad. Sci. **840:** 491–497.

85. LARSON, E.B. & L. WANG. 2004. Exercise, aging, and Alzheimer disease. Alzheimer Dis. Assoc. Disord. **18:** 54–56.
86. TERI, L. *et al.* 2003. Exercise plus behavioral management in patients with Alzheimer disease: a randomized controlled trial. JAMA **290:** 2015–2022.
87. VAN PRAAG, H.B.R. *et al.* 1999. Running enhances neurogenesis, learning, and long-term potentiation in mice. Proc. Natl. Acad. Sci. USA **96:** 13427–13431.
88. RUSSO-NEUSTADT, A. *et al.* 1999. Exercise, antidepressant medications, and enhanced brain derived neurotrophic factor expression. Neuropsychopharmacology **21:** 679–682.
89. LYTLE, M.E. *et al.* 2004. Exercise level and cognitive decline: the Movies project. Alzheimer Dis. Assoc. Disord. **18:** 57–64.
90. BARGER, L.K. *et al.* 2004. Daily exercise facilitates phase delays of circadian melatonin rhythm in very dim light. Am. J. Physiol. Regul. Integr. Comp. Physiol. **286:** R1077–R1084.

Melatonin, Metals, and Gene Expression

Implications in Aging and Neurodegenerative Disorders

DEBOMOY K. LAHIRI,[a] DEMAO CHEN,[a] PREETI LAHIRI,[b] JACK T. ROGERS,[c] NIGEL H. GREIG,[d] AND STEPHEN BONDY[e]

[a]Department of Psychiatry, Institute of Psychiatric Research, Indiana University School of Medicine, Indianapolis, Indiana, USA

[b]Department of Chemistry, Women's College, Banaras Hindu University, Varanasi, India

[c]Harvard Medical School, Boston, Massachusetts, USA

[d]National Institute on Aging, National Institutes of Health, Baltimore, Maryland, USA

[e]Department of Community and Environmental Medicine, University of California, Irvine, California, USA

ABSTRACT: Melatonin is a hormone secreted by the pineal gland, mostly in the dark period of the light/dark cycle, with corresponding fluctuations reflected in the plasma melatonin levels. This hormone plays a critical role in the regulation of various neural and endocrine processes that are synchronized with daily change in photoperiod. Abnormal melatonin levels are associated with metabolic disturbances and other disorders. Melatonin potentially plays an important role in aging, prolongation of life span, and health in the aged individual. It may exert a beneficial action on neurodegenerative conditions in those with debilitating diseases. It interacts with metals and, in some cases, neutralizes their toxic effects. Levels of melatonin decrease with aging in mice. Its dietary supplementation has recently been shown to result in a significant rise in levels of endogenous melatonin in serum as well as all other tissue samples tested. The effects of dietary melatonin have been studied in the brain of mice with regard to nitric oxide synthase, synaptic proteins, and amyloid β peptides (Aβ), which are involved in amyloid deposition and plaque formation in Alzheimer's disease (AD). Melatonin supplementation has no significant effect on cerebral cortical levels of nitric oxide synthase or synaptic proteins, such as synaptophysin and SNAP-25. Notably, however, elevated brain melatonin levels resulted in a significant reduction in levels of toxic cortical Aβ of both 40- and 42-aminoacid forms. Taken together, these results suggest that dietary melatonin supplementation may slow the neurodegenerative changes associated with brain aging and that the depletion of melatonin in the brain of aging mice may, in part, account for this adverse change.

KEYWORDS: aging; amyloid; brain; diet; melatonin; mRNA; metals; mouse; synaptic protein

Address for correspondence: Debomoy K. Lahiri, Ph.D., Indiana University School of Medicine, 791 Union Drive, Indianapolis, IN 46202. Voice: 317-274–2706; fax: 317-274–1365.
dlahiri@iupui.edu

Ann. N.Y. Acad. Sci. 1035: 216–230 (2004). © 2004 New York Academy of Sciences.
doi: 10.1196/annals.1332.014

INTRODUCTION

The pineal gland secretes melatonin (*N*-acetyl-5-methoxy-tryptamine).[1] High-affinity binding sites specific for melatonin exist in human hypothalamus.[2] Its secretion is largely confined to the dark period of the light/dark cycle, and its diurnal fluctuation is reflected in the plasma levels of the hormone. Moreover, melatonin plays an important role in the regulation of various neural and endocrine processes that are synchronized with photoperiod changes.[3] Aberrant levels of melatonin are associated with metabolic disturbances and other disorders, such as sleep disorders, jet lag, depression, dementia, stress, schizophrenia, and anorexia nervosa, and some immunological disorders.[4] Melatonin can also be used as a pharmacological agent.[5] Currently, research is ongoing to understand the cellular, biochemical, and pathophysiological roles of melatonin in healthy adult and aging brains[3,4] as well as in disease. This review describes the effects of aging on melatonin levels, the physiological role of melatonin, and its interaction with different genes and metals.

MELATONIN IN AGING AND ALZHEIMER'S DISEASE

Melatonin potentially plays an important role in aging, in health in aged individuals, and in increasing the life span. Of particular relevance, melatonin may exert a beneficial action on neurodegenerative conditions in humans with debilitating diseases.[5] It mediates many of these functions through high-affinity, specific binding sites in the hypothalamus of humans and many other mammalian species.[3] A recent pilot study has determined that serum melatonin levels may decrease in AD patients.[6]

Current interest is high in studying age-associated biochemical changes and how these relate to brain function. Aging in animals results in a decline in several cellular functions, such as lysosomal enzyme activities,[7] mitochondrial respiration,[8] and rates of mitochondrial and nuclear DNA repair.[9] These reductions in cellular functions with aging correlate, to a degree, with the cognitive impairment observed in normal aging and other age-related conditions such as senile dementia, Alzheimer's disease (AD), and Parkinson's disease. Interestingly, functional deterioration runs parallel with age-related changes in gene expression profiles.[10,11] Therefore, it has been proposed that these biochemical changes may represent an "adaptive response" to the functional decline observed during the aging process. However, the role of melatonin in the biochemical changes characteristic of aging and age-related disorders, such as AD, is beginning to be understood.[3,12]

PROCEDURES TO SLOW AGE-RELATED COGNITIVE DECLINE: A ROLE FOR MELATONIN

Procedures to slow or reverse age-related cognitive decline are a current focus of considerable research. One approach involves the testing of exogenous agents or regimens to assess their ability to reverse age-induced changes in gene expression. This reversal has been somewhat successful in mice on a restricted-calorie diet.[13] A second approach is to identify potentially beneficial endogenous compounds, as exemplified by melatonin. We have studied the second approach to achieve a reversal of age-induced changes. Interest in melatonin and its implications in aging are based on the following important observations. The production of melatonin in the pineal gland declines progressively with age, and in elderly humans the amount of melatonin produced is much less than that of young individuals.[3] There are strong indications that melatonin can act as (i) a regulator of aging and senescence[14] and (ii) an intracellular scavenger of hydroxyl and peroxyl free radicals both *in vitro* and *in vivo*.[3] Cell culture experiments have established that melatonin prevents the death of neuroblastoma cells exposed to the Alzheimer amyloid beta-peptide (Aβ).[15] Thus, melatonin has a protective role for neurons and other cells. Recent results suggest that age-related changes in mRNA gene expression in the CNS of mice can be modulated by dietary melatonin.[14,16] Notably, a recent report is suggestive of age-reversion of gene expression levels in aged mice that were given diets supplemented with melatonin.[17]

MELATONIN AND METALS

A Neutralizing Effect of Melatonin on the Toxic Effect of Cobalt

Heavy metals have been implicated as potential causative agents of neurodegenerative diseases, such as AD. Cobalt, a positively charged transition metal, has been shown to be increased in AD brains as compared to controls. Recently, the effect of cobalt as an inducer of oxidative stress/cytotoxicity was studied. Olivieri *et al.*[18] have shown that cobalt is able to induce cytotoxicity and oxidative stress as measured by reduced MTT metabolism and reduced cellular glutathione, respectively. Notably, pretreatment of cells with melatonin prevented cytotoxicity and induction of oxidative stress. Cobalt treatment of the human neuroblastoma SHSY5Y cells increased the release of Aβ peptides compared with untreated controls (ratio of Aβ 40/42), but melatonin pretreatment reversed the deleterious actions of cobalt.[18] These results are of relevance as cobalt is an essential nutritional requirement for all animals; usually bound tightly to cobalamin (vitamin B12), its unbound form could lead to neurotoxicity.

Stable Complexes of Melatonin with Alkali Metals

Lack *et al.*[19] investigated the ability of serotonin and melatonin to bind metals that occur naturally in the brain by using an electrochemical technique called adsorptive cathodic stripping voltammetry (AdCSV). They reported that both serotonin and melatonin form stable complexes with lithium and potassium, with serotonin favoring lithium over potassium and melatonin favoring potassium over lithium. Coordination between either serotonin or melatonin and calcium was not favored. This binding and stable complex formation between both serotonin and melatonin with lithium, potassium, and sodium has biological importance.[19] As an example, the binding of serotonin to lithium may explain the therapeutic effects of lithium in the treatment of depression.

Melatonin and Aluminum

Using a novel model to represent the pathophysiology of AD, van Rensburg *et al.*[20] have shown that aluminum toxicity is exacerbated by hydrogen peroxide and attenuated by a fragment of Aβ and melatonin. These authors have further proposed that as melatonin is produced by the pineal gland only in the dark, the excess of electric light associated with developed countries may help explain why AD is more prevalent in these countries than in rural Africa. In addition, Lack *et al.*[19] showed that melatonin binds aluminum. Such a binding may shed light into the role of this element in the etiology of AD; however, the exact mechanism of this metal-melatonin interaction is presently unclear.

Melatonin and Zinc

A link between zinc and melatonin with a reconstitution of thymic functions has been recently reported in melatonin-treated old mice.[21] Notably, concomitant increments of the nocturnal peaks of zinc and melatonin, with synchronization of their circadian patterns, are achieved in old mice after melatonin treatment. *In vitro* experiments from old thymic explants suggest a direct action of zinc, rather than of melatonin, on thymulin production, which further suggests that the action of melatonin on the thymic efficiency is mediated by zinc bioavailability.[21] It has been suggested that the beneficial effect of the links between zinc and melatonin on thymic functions during the circadian cycle may be extended to prolong survival in aging, although zinc may play the predominant role in this particular system.

Several experiments indicate that melatonin can modulate zinc turnover: (i) both melatonin and zinc plasma levels decline with advancing age; and (ii) zinc supplementation in old mice is able to restore reduced immunological functions.[22] This has prompted investigations on the effect of chronic melatonin treatment and pineal grafts in old mice on age-related decline of thymic endocrine activity. Melatonin treatment or pineal grafts also restore a normalized zinc turnover in aged mice—specifically, a reduced zinc plasma level is restored to normal values. These findings support the idea that the effect of melatonin on thymic endocrine activity and peripheral immune functions may be mediated by the zinc pool.[22]

Melatonin and Iron

Limson *et al.*[23] used AdCSV to demonstrate that serotonin and melatonin complex with Fe^{3+} in the brain. Melatonin has also been shown to inhibit epileptic discharges in the brains of rats that had been injected with discharge-inducing levels of $FeCl_3$.[24] In addition, melatonin has been shown to suppress iron-induced lipid peroxidation and neurodegeneration in rat brain.[25] These and other neuroprotective activities against iron-induced damage may be mediated by the 6-hydroxymelatonin metabolite, as 6-hydroxymelatonin has been specifically shown to reduce Fe^{3+} to Fe^{2+} and to partially inhibit Fe^{2+} induction of lipid peroxidation in rat liver homogenates.[26] Of particular interest from a therapeutic standpoint, a systemic infusion of melatonin was shown to be effective in reducing iron-induced neuronal death in rat cerebral cortex while melatonin levels modified by light cycle were insufficient to reduce this damage.[27]

Melatonin and Copper

In addition to finding iron/melatonin complexes, Limson *et al.*[23] determined that melatonin forms complexes with copper in the brain. Melatonin has been shown to inhibit copper-mediated LDL oxidation in the serum of postmenopausal women[28] and to protect against copper-mediated free radical damage in rat liver homogenates.[29] Further evidence of complex interactions between copper and melatonin is a loss of circadian rhythm by fish that have undergone chronic subtoxic copper exposure (comparable to levels found in drinking water sources that have been treated by copper-based algicides).[30]

Melatonin and Calorie Restriction

Zanquetta *et al.*[31] recently measured insulin sensitivity and insulin-sensitive glucose transporter (GLUT4) expression protein levels in pinealectomized rats. They also determined the effects of melatonin and caloric restriction on the changes induced by pinealectomy.[31] Their results suggest that pinealectomy decreased insulin sensitivity and GLUT4 gene expression from a lack of melatonin. Caloric restriction improved insulin sensitivity in Pinx rats, and this was related to increased GLUT4 gene expression and insulin-induced GLUT4 translocation to the plasma membrane in white adipose tissue.[31]

Effect of Melatonin on Oxidative Stress Proteins and Its Role as Scavenger

In addition, melatonin has been reported to act as an intracellular scavenger of hydroxyl and peroxyl free radicals when administered at both physiological and pharmacological doses *in vitro* as well as *in vivo*.[3,32] Furthermore, melatonin has been shown to reverse the role of apolipoprotein E (ApoE) ε4 on the Aβ peptide.[33] Melatonin prevents the death of neuroblastoma cells exposed to Aβ,[15] and melatonin also promotes neuronal growth factor (NGF)–mediated neuronal differentiation in cell cultures.[34]

As far as antioxidant activity is concerned, melatonin, xanthurenic acid, resveratrol, epigallocatechin gallate (EGCG), vitamin C, and alpha-lipoic acid (LA) differentially reduce oxidative DNA damage induced by Fenton reagents as assessed in a study of their individual and synergistic actions.[35] The nucleic acid derivative, 8-hydroxydeoxyguanosine (8-OH-dG), is considered a biomarker of oxidative DNA damage. Among the antioxidants tested, melatonin was the most effective, and it proved capable of reversing the pro-oxidant effect of resveratrol and vitamin C. Interestingly, it had an antagonistic effect when used in combination with (−)-epigallocatechin-3-gallate (EGCG), and it exhibited synergism in combination with vitamin C and with LA.[35]

STUDIES OF MELATONIN IN THE HUMAN AND ANIMALS

Melatonin in Human Cerebrospinal Fluid

In the clinical setting, melatonin levels were decreased in postmortem cerebrospinal fluid with aging, AD, and *APOE*ε4/4 genotype.[12] These findings together with others suggest that reductions in brain melatonin, which occur during aging, may contribute to a proamyloidogenic microenvironment in the aging brain.

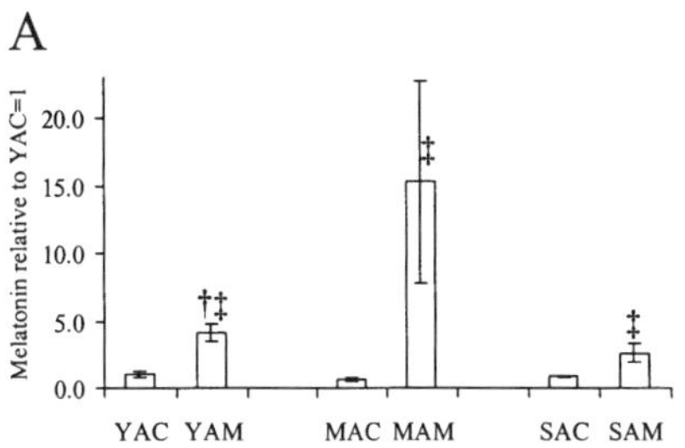
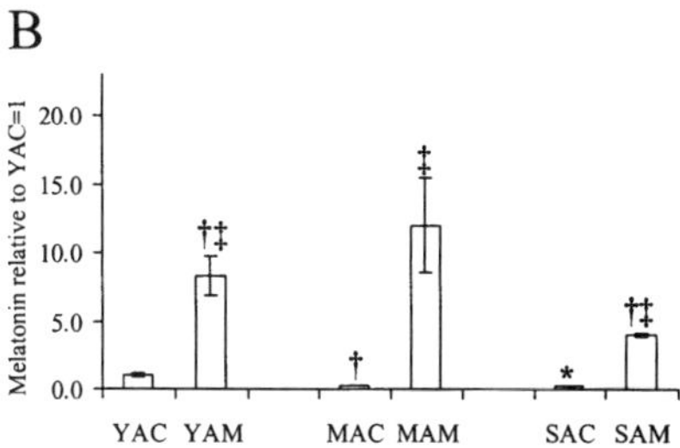

FIGURE 1. Relative levels of melatonin in serum and brain cortex samples from mice of different ages: young (12-month-old) and senescent, with or without dietary supplementation of melatonin. Three-letter abbreviations refer to mouse ages and treatments: YAC, young untreated; YAM, young melatonin-supplemented; MAC, middle-aged untreated; MAM, middle-aged melatonin-supplemented; SAC, senescent untreated; SAM, senescent melatonin supplemented. Melatonin was assayed using a sandwich ELISA and expressed relative to YAC mice, as indicated. Data were analyzed by multiple two-tailed t-test protected by the Bonferroni correction of $\alpha' = 1 - (1 - \alpha)^{1/k}$. *Indicates difference from YAC mice significant to $\alpha' < 0.05$. †Indicates difference from YAC mice significant to $\alpha' < 0.01$. ‡Indicates difference from unsupplemented mice of the same age group significant to $\alpha < 0.05$ in one-tailed t-test. (**A**) Cerebral cortex samples. (**B**) Serum samples.

Detection of Melatonin in Mouse Serum and the Brain

We recently reported the profile of endogenous melatonin in three age groups of mice and showed that melatonin levels decrease with age.[36] In addition, the effects of melatonin supplementation were tested on levels of endogenous melatonin and its sulfate derivative. In this particular study, levels of melatonin in young (6-month), middle-aged (12-month), and senescent (27-month) mice were compared before and after dietary melatonin supplementation.

Levels of Melatonin Decrease with Age

In serum, melatonin levels were highest in young mice, decreasing in 12- and 27-month-old animals. Serum melatonin level was reduced by ~70% in older animals as compared to the young. Interestingly, melatonin was detected in the cerebral cortex tissue. However, basal levels of melatonin are significantly lower in the cerebral cortex than in serum. Cortical levels were approximately 0.40 ± 0.07 pg per gram tissue from middle-aged control mice (FIG. 1A). The corresponding level in the serum was 20.1 ± 3.6 pg/g (FIG. 1).[37]

DIETARY SUPPLEMENTATION AS A MEANS OF RAISING MELATONIN

Effect of Dietary Supplementation on In Vivo Melatonin Levels

Hayter *et al.*[27] have reported that infusion of melatonin was more effective in inhibiting iron-induced oxidative damage than was light-cycle manipulation of melatonin. In treating humans, oral administration would be preferable to an injection, primarily for convenience and patient compliance. To determine possible efficacy of oral administration, Lahiri *et al.*[36] measured the effects of oral administration of melatonin to mice on plasma and cerebral cortex melatonin levels. Dietary melatonin (40 ppm) resulted in a significant increase in melatonin levels in all tissues of three ages of animals tested.[36]

Melatonin supplementation increased levels of melatonin in serum by approximately 50-fold in middle-aged and 20-fold in senescent mice. Interestingly, melatonin levels in all tissues studied (cerebral cortex, heart, liver, kidney, and serum) responded to dietary melatonin supplementation. Notably, this supplementation resulted in an increase in cerebral cortical levels in animals of all age groups tested. These increases were significant to $\alpha < 0.05$ by one-tailed t-test when comparing all untreated samples to treated samples of the same age group (FIG. 1A). The most dramatic mean effect of such supplementation was in middle-aged mice, which resulted in approximately 23-fold greater increases in endogenous melatonin levels in cerebral cortex. Melatonin supplementation increased brain levels from 0.40 ± 0.07 to 9.28 ± 4.52 pg/g tissue. Overall, the effect of dietary melatonin was greatest in the middle-aged group. Such supplementation caused a full compensation of the deficit in middle-aged mice with a net significant gain in melatonin levels. In addition, the oldest group's cerebral cortex melatonin was raised to a level not significantly different from those of young control mice.

Thus, endogenous melatonin, intrinsically present in the cerebral cortex and other tissues, can be increased by dietary melatonin supplementation. In addition, the amounts of melatonin sufficient to compensate for the loss because of aging can enter the brain, across the blood–brain and blood–CSF barriers, when exogenous melatonin is present in the diet.

Effect of Dietary Melatonin on In Vivo Melatonin Sulfate Levels

In the same animals, dietary melatonin resulted in a significant increase in 6-hydroxymelatonin sulfate levels in all tissues for all age groups of animals tested (data not shown). However, relative to the control mice, there was a smaller increase in 6-hydroxymelatonin sulfate levels in cerebral cortex than in serum with melatonin supplementation. Thus, the cerebral cortex had the highest levels of combined melatonin plus 6-hydroxymelatonin sulfate than other tissue tested in control mice, but not in melatonin-treated mice.

MELATONIN, AMYLOID, AND AD

Measuring Aβ and the β-Amyloid Precursor Protein (APP)

As mentioned in the previous section STUDIES OF MELATONIN IN THE HUMAN AND ANIMALS (see above), our results suggest that there was an age-dependent decline in melatonin levels, and since aging is a major risk factor for AD, the effects of melatonin supplementation were studied on levels of Aβ and the β-amyloid precursor protein from which it derives. AD is characterized by the presence of extracellular plaques and intracellular neurofibrillary tangles in the brain.[37] Extracellular plaques deposited in the brain consist of the 40–43 residue Aβ peptide, which is cleaved from the larger APP by secretase enzymes.[37] Recent research suggests that an increased release of the "longer form" of Aβ, Aβ42/43, which has a greater tendency to aggregate than does Aβ40, leads to abnormal deposition of Aβ and the associated neurotoxicity in AD. Therefore, it is important to assay Aβ40 and Aβ42 peptides in mouse brain and to investigate how their levels are affected by melatonin supplementation.

Briefly, we determined the effect of melatonin supplementation on neuronal proteins in cerebral cortical extracts. This included assaying levels of APP, Aβ, and synaptic proteins. A typical Western blot of cerebral cortical extracts revealed high molecular weight APP bands of 110–130 kDa (data not shown). The antibody used could detect all major alternatively spliced forms of APP as well as their posttranslationally modified derivatives.[38,39] The intensity of APP bands from different samples was compared after normalizing each APP band with the sample's corresponding β-actin band's density. This analysis demonstrated a small reduction (up to 16%) in APP levels in mouse cortex with melatonin addition. However, this was not statistically significant ($n = 6$).

Effect of Melatonin Supplementation on the Amyloid-β Proteins

Using two independent sensitive ELISAs, levels of major Aβ species Aβ40 (FIG. 2) and the more toxic form Aβ42 (FIG. 3) were measured separately.[39] Aβ40 concentrations of ~1000 pg/mg total protein were detected in middle-aged control mouse (MAC) cerebral cortical extracts. This was reduced approaching significance ($\alpha = 0.057$) after melatonin supplementation (MAM). Similarly, Aβ42 concentrations of ~750 pg/mg were detected in cortical extracts from the same mice (MAC). Levels of Aβ42 were significantly reduced in melatonin-supplemented mice (MAM). Overall, the effect of melatonin on Aβ42 was similar to that upon Aβ40 and was most pronounced in the middle-aged animals.

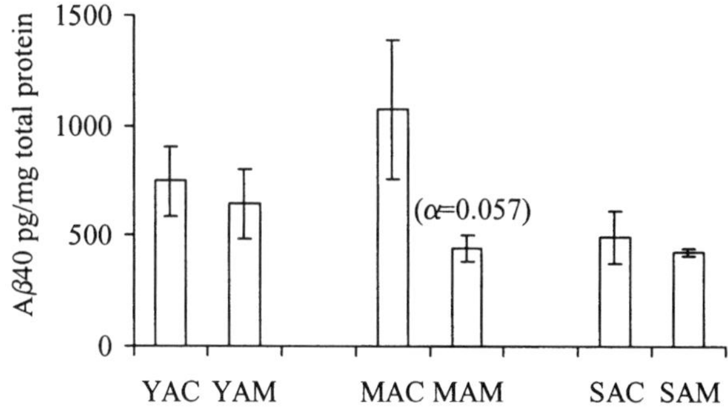

FIGURE 2. The effect of dietary melatonin on levels of Aβ40 in brain cortex tissue. Levels of Aβ40 were measured using a sandwich ELISA. Three-letter abbreviations refer to mouse ages and treatments: YAC, young untreated; YAM, young melatonin-supplemented; MAC, middle-aged untreated; MAM, middle-aged melatonin-supplemented; SAC, senescent untreated; SAM, senescent melatonin supplemented. Data were analyzed by one-tailed *t*-test, comparing each melatonin-supplemented population with the corresponding unsupplemented age-group population.

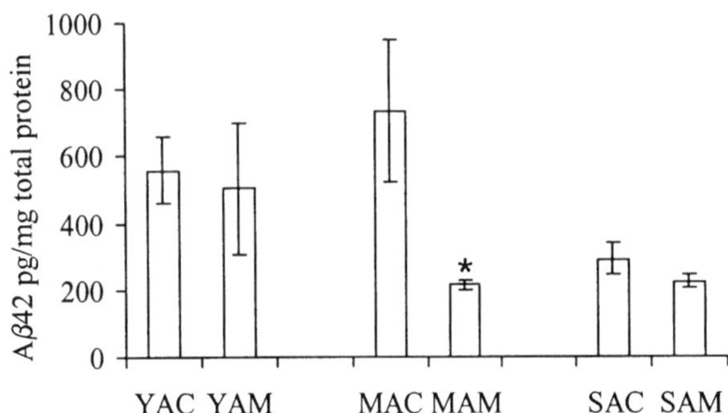

FIGURE 3. The effect of dietary melatonin on levels of Aβ42 in brain cortex tissue. Levels of Aβ42 were measured using a sandwich ELISA. Three-letter abbreviations refer to mouse ages and treatments: YAC, young untreated; YAM, young melatonin supplemented; MAC, middle-aged untreated; MAM, middle-aged melatonin supplemented; SAC, senescent untreated; SAM, senescent melatonin-supplemented. Data was analyzed by one-tailed t-test, comparing each melatonin-supplemented population with the corresponding unsupplemented age-group population. *α < 0.05.

Taken together, these results suggest that the addition of melatonin to the diet resulted in a significant increase in brain melatonin levels with a significant reduction in cortical Aβ levels. This effect of melatonin on Aβ had not previously been assessed or reported in an *in vivo* model of naive mice and is of significant biological relevance. Melatonin treatment in cell culture was previously shown to reduce levels of APP and Aβ,[40] which, for Aβ, is consistent with the present results in mouse brain. Thus, melatonin supplementation may retard age-related neurodegeneration by compensating for age-related depletion of melatonin in the brain.

Effect of Melatonin Supplementation on Synaptic Proteins

In Western blots of cerebral cortical extracts, a distinct band of synaptophysin protein at 38–40 kDa was detected. As in the case of APP, there was no statistically significant change in synaptophysin levels in cerebral cortex samples from middle-aged mice with melatonin supplementation. When levels of the 25-kDa synaptosomal-associated protein (SNAP-25) were measured in the same cerebral cortex samples, there was no statistically significant difference in levels of SNAP-25 as detected by Western blot. This is in contrast to another memory-enhancing drug, AIT-082.[41]

Effect of Melatonin on the Nitric Oxide Pathway

Since melatonin has been reported to act as an antioxidant,[3] the effect of dietary melatonin was tested on neuronal nitric oxide synthase, which is involved in nitric oxide generation. Levels of both neuronal (n)NOS and inducible (i)NOS were measured by Western blot in murine cerebral cortex samples. Although there was a trend towards a decrease in both NOS levels in the melatonin-supplemented mice, it was not statistically significant. Thus, the addition of exogenous melatonin *in vivo* had no significant effect on NOS enzymatic activity.[39]

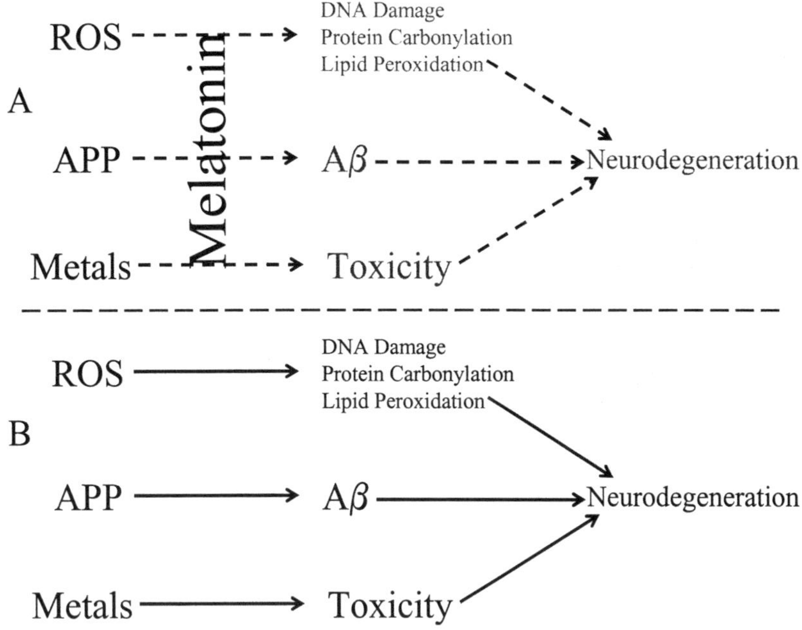

FIGURE 4. A proposed model showing the role of melatonin inhibition in AD. Postulated models showing the effect of **(A)** "melatonin sufficiency" and **(B)** "melatonin deficiency" on oxidative process and neurodegeneration. **(A)** Melatonin sufficiency. Melatonin serves to block a multitude of potentially pathogenic reactions (including oxidative DNA damage, protein carbonylation, and lipid peroxidation) by reactive oxidizing species of molecules, processing of APP into Aβ (at least in middle age, a period wherein it is presumed that the majority of the "molecular groundwork" for developing AD later in life begins), and metallotoxicity from a variety of metal ions. These inhibitions, in turn, result in reduced neurodegeneration. **(B)** Melatonin insufficiency. If melatonin levels fall below a critical level, lack of inhibition permits the activity of reactive oxidizing species, processing of APP into Aβ, and metallotoxicity, each and all of which lead to greater neurodegeneration.

MELATONIN AND AGE-DEPENDENT CHANGES

Changes in Brain Cellular Functions

Several studies suggest that there is an age-dependent decline in brain cellular functions and concomitant alteration in cerebral enzymatic activities linked to the mitochondria and the glutathione system.[42,43] Melatonin has also been suggested to be a pharmacologic agent to prevent neuronal loss in experimental models of neurodegenerative disorders such as AD.[5] To understand age-induced functional deterioration of the brain, several groups have investigated age-related changes in gene expression profile.[10,13,17,44] Several key genes involved in neuronal structure and signaling, such as synaptotagmin I and ApoE, are differentially expressed in the hypothalamus and cortex of aged animals.[44] Proteases that play essential roles in regulating neuropeptide metabolism, processing of APP, and neuronal apoptosis are upregulated in the aged brain; they may contribute significantly to brain aging.[44]

Changes in Age-Related Gene Expression

Sharman *et al.*[17] tested whether or not melatonin could reverse a wide variety of biochemical aspects of aging. An "aging paradigm" of normal mice with dietary supplementation of melatonin was used. Changes in levels of 12,423 genes were analyzed separately with respect to aging and with melatonin addition by gene array chip analyses. These results suggest that melatonin indeed can reverse age-related changes in levels of certain important genes.[17]

Changes in Signaling through G Protein–Coupled Receptors

Declines in melatonin levels associated with age should have consequences on cellular physiology. Our knowledge of melatonin's function has advanced considerably in the last few years through the cloning of the G protein–coupled seven-transmembrane domain melatonin receptors, MT1 and MT2, and the nuclear receptors associated with melatonin signaling, RZR/ROR and RZRβ.[3,45] Melatonin's effect on levels of gene expression has been a subject of intense research. A number of inflammatory and stress-related genes are activated following the binding of melatonin to nuclear receptor RZR/RORα.[45,46] Furthermore, melatonin treatment changes immune gene expression by modulation of glucocorticoid receptor activity.[45] The role of melatonin in regulating circadian and seasonal rhythms is presumably because of melatonin's binding to MT1 and MT2 receptors, which results in the sensitization of the ubiquitous-signaling enzyme, adenylate cyclase.[45] It is, therefore, apparent that an age-related decline in melatonin levels may be expected to induce concomitant changes in gene expression.

POTENTIAL NEUROLOGIC AND PHYSIOBIOCHEMICAL EFFECTS OF MELATONIN SUPPLEMENTATION

Effects of Melatonin Supplemention in Mice

A number of studies have investigated melatonin supplementation in mice and its effects on physio-biochemical processes. Melatonin reduces oxidative damage of neural lipids and proteins in the senescence-accelerated mouse.[47] In addition, it reduces memory changes and neural oxidative damage consequent to exposure of mice to D-galactose.[48] Acutely administered melatonin restores hepatic mitochondrial physiology in aged mice.[49] Notably, the administration of melatonin in drinking water promotes phase advance of the light-dark cycle in senescence-accelerated mice SAMR1 but not SAMP8 mice.[50] While a study reported that chronic dietary treatment with melatonin was not effective in reversing age-related deficits in psychomotor behavior,[51] another study of melatonin supplementation showed an improvement in the movement of aged C57BL/6 mice.[52]

Beneficial Effects of Melatonin in Both Animal and Human Settings

Beneficial effects of melatonin have been reported in both animal and human settings, which is consistent with our studies. Orally administered melatonin reduces oxidative stress and proinflammatory cytokines that are induced by Aβ in rat brain.[53] In a transgenic model of AD, melatonin increased survival and inhibits oxidative and amyloid pathology.[54] In human settings, interesting results were obtained in a recent case report of monozygotic twins with AD that were treated with melatonin.[55] Notably, one of the treated patients showed milder impairment of memory function, with substantial improvement of sleep quality and a reduction of "sundowning". In addition to these results, there is report of disturbed function of the pineal gland in familial amyloid polyneuropathy.[56]

Dietary Compensation of Melatonin for the Decline during Aging and Other Disorders

Taken together, all these results lead to a working model to explain the effect of melatonin on oxidative process and neurodegeneration (FIG. 4). This model/ hypothesis is based on our work as well as several other reports.[5,12,17,35,57] In the melatonin sufficiency model, as exemplified by the youthful state, endogenous melatonin provides greater overall antioxidant and antifibrillogenic activity, resulting in inhibition of the formation of amyloid plaque from Aβ peptides. Also, it inhibits oligomeric Aβ (Aβ*) from contributing to other reactive oxygen species and neurotoxicity. This results in low levels of DNA damage, protein carbonylation, and lipid peroxidation.

In the melatonin-deficiency model, as exemplified by aging or AD, the brain has significantly lower endogenous melatonin. In this case, Aβ peptides are free to associate into amyloid plaque and contribute to greater reactive oxidative species (ROS) activity. With aging and AD, there is excessive ROS, ROS-mediated oxidative damage, and toxic Aβ generation, which results in DNA damage, protein carbonylation, lipid peroxidation, and cell death. This may in part be affected by reduced levels of melatonin. Interestingly, dietary supplementation of melatonin restores, in whole or in part, brain melatonin levels to those of the healthy young brain state. Thus, in the youthful state, the proper balance of ROS and Aβ production is maintained so that excessive ROS/Aβ-mediated ill effects are held in check. This more-youthful profile may be restored by exogenous melatonin treatment of senescent animals.

SUMMARY

Overall, our results suggest that dietary melatonin supplementation in mice reduced total levels of Aβ proteins in cerebral cortex. In addition, other studies have shown that dietary melatonin supplementation is followed by extensive age reversion in gene expression profiles. Supplementation with melatonin could lead to neuroprotection of aged neurons, prevent the accumulation of fibrillogenic Aβ, and inhibit the cascade of neurodegenerative events in the senescent brain. Our finding of lowered cortical Aβ levels following dietary melatonin supplementation and the discovery by Sharman *et al.*[17] of apparent age reversion in gene expression following such supplementation may have implications in the prevention of age-related disorders exemplified by AD. Since an elevated brain melatonin level resulted in a concomitant decrease in cortical Aβ levels, melatonin addition may restore the neuroprotection that is lost because of a depletion of melatonin in the aged brain. We have found that exogenous melatonin can, indeed, elevate its levels within the CNS. Thus, the reported effects of melatonin on levels of certain genes and proteins are a direct consequence of melatonin supplementation, and further inquiry into potential relevance to human aging is likely to be rewarding, particularly in light of the fact that melatonin represents such a well-tolerated, inexpensive, and readily available agent.

ACKNOWLEDGMENTS

This work was supported in part by grants from the National Institutes of Health: AG 18379, AG 18884 AG 16794, and ES 7992. We sincerely thank the support from Yuan-Wen Ge and Bryan Maloney.

REFERENCES

1. AXELROD, J. 1974. The pineal gland: a neurochemical transducer. Science **184:** 1341–1348.
2. MASANA, M.I., P.A. WITT-ENDERBY & M. L. DUBOCOVICH. 2003. Melatonin differentially modulates the expression and function of the hMT1 and hMT2 melatonin receptors upon prolonged withdrawal. Biochem. Pharmacol. **65:** 731–739.
3. REITER, R.J. 1992. The ageing pineal gland and its physiological consequences. Bioessays **14:** 169–175.
4. BUIJS, R.M., C.G. VAN EDEN, V.D. GONCHARUK, et al. 2003. The biological clock tunes the organs of the body: timing by hormones and the autonomic nervous system. J. Endocrinol. **177:** 17–26.
5. REITER, R.J., J. CABRERA, R.M. SAINZ, et al. 1999. Melatonin as a pharmacological agent against neuronal loss in experimental models of Huntington's disease, Alzheimer's disease and parkinsonism. Ann. N.Y. Acad Sci. **890:** 471–485.
6. OZCANKAYA, R. & N. DELIBAS. 2002. Malondialdehyde, superoxide dismutase, melatonin, iron, copper, and zinc blood concentrations in patients with Alzheimer disease: cross-sectional study. Croat. Med. J. **43:** 28–32.
7. NAKAMURA, Y., M. TAKEDA, H. SUZUKI, et al. 1989. Age-dependent change in activities of lysosomal enzymes in rat brain. Mech. Ageing Dev. **50:** 215–225.
8. WEI, Y.H., C.Y. LU, H.C. LEE, et al. 1998. Oxidative damage and mutation to mitochondrial DNA and age-dependent decline of mitochondrial respiratory function. Ann. N.Y. Acad. Sci. **854:** 155–170.
9. STEVNSNER, T., T. THORSLUND, N.C. DE SOUZA-PINTO, et al. 2002. Mitochondrial repair of 8-oxoguanine and changes with aging. Exp. Gerontol. **37:** 1189–96.
10. LEE, C.K., R. WEINDRUCH & T.A. PROLLA. 2000. Gene-expression profile of the ageing brain in mice. Nat. Genet. **25:** 294–297.
11. CAO, S.X., J.M. DHAHBI, P.L. MOTE, et al. 2001. Genomic profiling of short- and long-term caloric restriction effects in the liver of aging mice. Proc. Natl. Acad. Sci. USA **98:** 10630–10635.
12. LIU, R.Y., J.N. ZHOU, J. VAN HEERIKHUIZE, et al. 1999. Decreased melatonin levels in postmortem cerebrospinal fluid in relation to aging, Alzheimer's disease, and apolipoprotein E-epsilon 4/4 genotype. J. Clin. Endocrinol. Metab. **84:** 323–327.
13. LEE, C.K., R.G. KLOPP, R. WEINDRUCH, et al. 1999. Gene expression profile of aging and its retardation by caloric restriction. Science **285:** 1390–1393.
14. BONDY, S.C., Y.E. YANG, T.J. WALSH, et al. 2002. Dietary modulation of age-related changes in cerebral pro-oxidant status. Neurochem. Int. **40:** 123–130.
15. PAPPOLLA, M.A., M. SOS, et al. 1997. Melatonin prevents death of neuroblastoma cells exposed to the Alzheimer amyloid peptide. J. Neurosci. **17:** 1683–1690.

16. SHARMAN, K.G., E.H. SHARMAN, E. YANG, *et al.* 2002. Dietary melatonin selectively reverses age-related changes in cortical cytokine mRNA levels, and their responses to an inflammatory stimulus. Neurobiol. Aging. **23:** 633–638.
17. SHARMAN, E.H., K.G. SHARMAN, Y.W. GE, *et al.* 2004. Age-related changes in murine CNS mRNA gene expression are modulated by dietary melatonin. J. Pineal. Res. **36:** 165–170.
18. OLIVIERI, G., C. HESS, E. SAVASKAN, *et al.* 2001. Melatonin protects SHSY5Y neuroblastoma cells from cobalt-induced oxidative stress, neurotoxicity and increased beta-amyloid secretion. J. Pineal Res. **31:** 320–325.
19. LACK, B., S. DAYA & T. NYOKONG. 2001. Interaction of serotonin and melatonin with sodium, potassium, calcium, lithium and aluminium. J. Pineal Res. **31:** 102–108.
20. VAN RENSBURG, S.J., W.M. DANIELS, F.C. POTOCNIK, *et al.* 1997. A new model for the pathophysiology of Alzheimer's disease. Aluminium toxicity is exacerbated by hydrogen peroxide and attenuated by an amyloid protein fragment and melatonin. S. Afr. Med. J. **87:** 1111–1115.
21. MOCCHEGIANI, E., L. SANTARELLI, A. TIBALDI, *et al.* 1998. Presence of links between zinc and melatonin during the circadian cycle in old mice: effects on thymic endocrine activity and on the survival. J. Neuroimmunol. **86:** 111–122.
22. MOCCHEGIANI, E., D. BULIAN, L. SANTARELLI, *et al.* 1994. The immuno-reconstituting effect of melatonin or pineal grafting and its relation to zinc pool in aging mice. J. Neuroimmunol. **53:** 189–201.
23. LIMSON, J., T. NYOKONG & S. DAYA. 1998. The interaction of melatonin and its precursors with aluminium, cadmium, copper, iron, lead, and zinc: an adsorptive voltammetric study. J. Pineal Res. **24:** 15–21.
24. KABUTO, H., I. YOKOI & N. OGAWA. 1998. Melatonin inhibits iron-induced epileptic discharges in rats by suppressing peroxidation. Epilepsia **39:** 237–243.
25. LIN, A.M. & L.T. HO. 2000. Melatonin suppresses iron-induced neurodegeneration in rat brain. Free Radical Biol. Med. **28:** 904–911.
26. MAHARAJ, D.S., J.L. LIMSON & S. DAYA. 2003. 6-Hydroxymelatonin converts Fe (III) to Fe (II) and reduces iron-induced lipid peroxidation. Life Sci. **72:** 1367–1375.
27. HAYTER, C.L., G.M. BISHOP & S.R. ROBINSON. 2004. Pharmacological but not physiological concentrations of melatonin reduce iron-induced neuronal death in rat cerebral cortex. Neurosci. Lett. **362:** 182–184.
28. WAKATSUKI, A., Y. OKATANI, N. IKENOUE, *et al.* 2000. Melatonin inhibits oxidative modification of low-density lipoprotein particles in normolipidemic post-menopausal women. J. Pineal Res. **28:** 136–142.
29. PARMAR, P., J. LIMSON, T. NYOKONG, *et al.* 2002. Melatonin protects against copper-mediated free radical damage. J. Pineal Res. **32:** 237–242.
30. HANDY, R.D. 2003. Chronic effects of copper exposure versus endocrine toxicity: two sides of the same toxicological process? Comp. Biochem. Physiol. A. Mol. Integr. Physiol. **135:** 25–38.
31. ZANQUETTA, M.M., P.M. SERAPHIM, D.H. SUMIDA, *et al.* 2003. Calorie restriction reduces pinealectomy–induced insulin resistance by improving GLUT4 gene expression and its translocation to the plasma membrane. J. Pineal Res. **35:** 141–148.
32. PARLAKPINAR, H., E. SAHNA, M.K. OZER, *et al.* 2002. Physiological and pharmacological concentrations of melatonin protect against cisplatin-induced acute renal injury. J. Pineal Res. **33:** 161–166.
33. POEGGELER, B., L. MIRAVALLE, M.G. ZAGORSKI, *et al.* 2001. Melatonin reverses the profibrillogenic activity of apolipoprotein E4 on the Alzheimer amyloid Abeta peptide. Biochemistry (Mosc.) **40:** 14995–5001.
34. SONG, W. & D.K. LAHIRI. 1997. Melatonin alters the metabolism of the beta-amyloid precursor protein in the neuroendocrine cell line PC12. J. Mol. Neurosci. **9:** 75–92.
35. LOPEZ-BURILLO, S., D.X. TAN, J.C. MAYO, *et al.* 2003. Melatonin, xanthurenic acid, resveratrol, EGCG, vitamin C and alpha–lipoic acid differentially reduce oxidative DNA damage induced by Fenton reagents: a study of their individual and synergistic actions. J. Pineal Res. **34:** 269–277.
36. LAHIRI, D.K., Y.W. GE, E.H. SHARMAN, *et al.* 2004. Age-related changes in serum melatonin in mice: higher levels of combined melatonin and 6–hydroxymelatonin

sulfate in the cerebral cortex than serum, heart, liver and kidney tissues. J. Pineal Res. **36:** 217–223.

37. LAHIRI, D.K., M.R. FARLOW, K. SAMBAMURTI, *et al.* 2003. A critical analysis of new molecular targets and strategies for drug developments in Alzheimer's disease. Curr. Drug Targets **4:** 97–112.

38. LAHIRI, D.K., M.R. FARLOW & K. SAMBAMURTI. 1998. The secretion of amyloid beta-peptides is inhibited in the tacrine-treated human neuroblastoma cells. Brain Res. Mol. Brain Res. **62:** 131–140.

39. LAHIRI, D.K., D. CHEN, Y.W. GE, *et al.* 2004. Dietary supplementation with melatonin reduces levels of amyloid beta-peptides in the murine cerebral cortex. J. Pineal Res. **36:** 224–231.

40. LAHIRI, D.K. 1999. Melatonin affects the metabolism of the beta-amyloid precursor protein in different cell types. J. Pineal Res. **26:** 137–146.

41. LAHIRI, D.K., Y.W. GE & M.R. FARLOW. 2000. Effect of a memory-enhancing drug, AIT-082, on the level of synaptophysin. Ann. N.Y. Acad. Sci. **903:** 387–393.

42. BENZI, G. & A. MORETTI. 1995. Age- and peroxidative stress-related modifications of the cerebral enzymatic activities linked to mitochondria and the glutathione system. Free Radical Biol. Med. **19:** 77–101.

43. LOVELL, M.A., C. XIE & W.R. MARKESBERY. 2000. Decreased base excision repair and increased helicase activity in Alzheimer's disease brain. Brain Res. **855:** 116–123.

44. JIANG, C.H., J.Z. TSIEN, P.G. SCHULTZ, *et al.* 2001. The effects of aging on gene expression in the hypothalamus and cortex of mice. Proc. Natl. Acad. Sci. USA **98:** 1930–1934.

45. PERSENGIEV, S.P. 1999. Multiple domains of melatonin receptor are involved in the regulation of glucocorticoid receptor-induced gene expression. J. Steroid. Biochem. Mol. Biol. **68:** 181–187.

46. VON GALL, C., J.H. STEHLE & D.R. WEAVER. 2002. Mammalian melatonin receptors: molecular biology and signal transduction. Cell Tissue Res. **309:** 151–162.

47. OKATANI, Y., A. WAKATSUKI, R.J. REITER, *et al.* 2002. Melatonin reduces oxidative damage of neural lipids and proteins in senescence-accelerated mouse. Neurobiol. Aging. **23:** 639–644.

48. SHEN, Y.X., S.Y. XU, W. WEI, *et al.* 2002. Melatonin reduces memory changes and neural oxidative damage in mice treated with D-galactose. J. Pineal Res. **32:** 173–178.

49. OKATANI, Y., A. WAKATSUKI, R.J. REITER, *et al.* 2003. Acutely administered melatonin restores hepatic mitochondrial physiology in old mice. Int. J. Biochem. Cell. Biol. **35:** 367–375.

50. ASAI, M., M. IKEDA, M. AKIYAMA, *et al.* 2000. Administration of melatonin in drinking water promotes the phase advance of light-dark cycle in senescence-accelerated mice, SAMR1 but not SAMP8. Brain Res. **876:** 220–224.

51. SHUKITT-HALE, B., D.E. SMITH, M. MEYDANI, *et al.* 1999. The effects of dietary antioxidants on psychomotor performance in aged mice. Exp. Gerontol. **34:** 797–808.

52. ARAGHI-NIKNAM, M., L. LANE & R.R. WATSON. 1999. Modification of physical movement in old C57BL/6 mice by DHEA and melatonin supplementation. Proc. Soc. Exp. Biol. Med. **221:** 193–197.

53. ROSALES-CORRAL, S., D. X. TAN, R. J. REITER, *et al.* 2003. Orally administered melatonin reduces oxidative stress and proinflammatory cytokines induced by amyloid-beta peptide in rat brain: a comparative, in vivo study versus vitamin C and E. J. Pineal Res. **35:** 80–84.

54. MATSUBARA, E., T. BRYANT-THOMAS, J. PACHECO QUINTO, *et al.* 2003. Melatonin increases survival and inhibits oxidative and amyloid pathology in a transgenic model of Alzheimer's disease. J. Neurochem. **85:** 1101–1108.

55. BRUSCO, L.I., M. MARQUEZ & D.P. CARDINALI. 1998. Monozygotic twins with Alzheimer's disease treated with melatonin: Case report. J. Pineal. Res. **25:** 260–263.

56. HIGA, S., T. SUZUKI, S. SAKODA, *et al.* 1987. Disturbed function of the pineal gland in familial amyloid polyneuropathy. J. Neural. Transm. **69:** 97–103.

57. LAHIRI, D.K. & C. GHOSH. 1999. Interactions between melatonin, reactive oxygen species, and nitric oxide. Ann. N.Y. Acad. Sci. **893:** 325–330.

The Degeneration of Dopamine Neurons in Parkinson's Disease

Insights from Embryology and Evolution of the Mesostriatocortical System

PHILIPPE VERNIER,[a] FREDERIC MORET,[a] SOPHIE CALLIER,[a] MARINA SNAPYAN,[a] CHRISTOPHE WERSINGER,[b] AND ANITA SIDHU[b]

[a]*Development, Evolution, Plasticity of the Nervous System, Institute of Neurobiology A. Fessard, CNRS, 91198 Gif-sur-Yvette, France*

[b]*Department of Pediatrics, Georgetown University, Washington, District of Columbia 20007, USA*

ABSTRACT: Parkinson's disease (PD) is, to a large extent, specific to the human species. Most symptoms are the consequence of the preferential degeneration of the dopamine-synthesizing cells of the mesostriatal–mesocortical neuronal pathway. Reasons for that can be traced back to the evolutionary mechanisms that shaped the dopamine neurons in humans. In vertebrates, dopamine-containing neurons and nuclei do not exhibit homogenous phenotypes. In this respect, mesencephalic dopamine neurons of the substantia nigra and ventral tegmental area are characterized by a molecular combination (tyrosine hydroxylase, aromatic amino acid decarboxylase, monoamine oxidase, vesicular monoamine transporter, dopamine transporter—to name a few), which is not found in other dopamine-containing neurons of the vertebrate brain. In addition, the size of these mesencephalic DA nuclei is tremendously expanded in humans as compared to other vertebrates. Differentiation of the mesencephalic neurons during development depends on genetic mechanisms, which also differ from those of other dopamine nuclei. In contrast, pathophysiological approaches to PD have highlighted the role of ubiquitously expressed molecules such as α-synuclein, parkin, and microtubule-associated proteins. We propose that the peculiar phenotype of the dopamine mesencephalic neurons, which has been selected during vertebrate evolution and reshaped in the human lineage, has also rendered these neurons particularly prone to oxidative stress, and thus, to the fairly specific neurodegeneration of PD. Numerous evidence has been accumulated to demonstrate that perturbed regulation of DAT-dependent dopamine uptake, DAT-dependent accumulation of toxins, dysregulation of TH activity as well as high sensitivity of DA mesencephalic neurons to oxidants are key components of the neurodegeneration process of PD. This view points to the contribution of nonspecific mechanisms (α-synuclein aggregation) in a highly specific cellular environment (the dopamine mesencephalic neurons) and provides a robust framework to develop novel and rational therapeutic schemes in PD.

Address for correspondence: Dr. Philippe Vernier, Development, Evolution, Plasticity of the Nervous System, UPR2197, Institute of Neurobiology A. Fessard, CNRS, 91198 Gif-sur-Yvette, France. Voice: +33-169-823-430; fax: +33-169-823-447.

vernier@iaf.cnrs-gif.fr

Ann. N.Y. Acad. Sci. 1035: 231–249 (2004). © 2004 New York Academy of Sciences.

doi: 10.1196/annals.1332.015

KEYWORDS: Parkinson's disease (PD); development; dopamine transporter; dopamine receptors; α-synuclein; neuroprotection

INTRODUCTION

Parkinson's disease (PD) is a neurodegenerative disorder primarily affecting the elderly. It is characterized by a progressive impairment of automatic aspects of behaviors leading to hypokinesia, sensory neglect, and rigidity. Numerous works performed in the mid-60s and 70s have established that the most severe symptoms of PD are the consequence of the degeneration of the dopamine-synthesizing cells of the mesostriatal–mesocortical neuronal pathway.[1] Degeneration of these anatomical systems causes dopamine depletion in the basal ganglia and prefrontal cortex. The absence of dopamine impairs elicitation of automatic behaviors and responses to novelty, which are clinically reflected in akinesia and apathy. The first symptoms occur when degeneration of dopamine neurons is already severe, rendering vital substitution therapy. Since dopamine is acting essentially as a modulatory, slow-acting neurotransmitter in the brain areas, substitutive therapy based on the oral intake of L-dopa, the metabolic precursor of dopamine, has proven to be very efficient for parkinsonian symptoms, at least at the first clinical stages.[2] From a pathophysiological point of view, the occurrence of abnormal protein aggregates, known as Lewy bodies, not only in the substantia nigra, but also in many other brain structures, has been considered as a key diagnostic element in post-mortem studies.[1,3] The mechanistic link between protein aggregation and the predominant degeneration of dopamine neurons of the substantia nigra is now one of the gold standards of the search for the initial causes of parkinsonian neurodegeneration.[4]

A Human Disease in Search of Its Roots

PD, like many other neurodegenerative diseases, is, to a large extent, specific to the human species. This remark suggests the existence of human-specific features that may provide the dopamine-synthesizing cells located in the mesencephalon (substantia nigra and ventral tegmental area) with unusual susceptibility to neurodegeneration. The question of human-specific neurodegeneration has been a matter of debate for a long time. It is as if the existence of exquisite cognitive functions, which depend on the tremendous increase of brain size in human as compared to other mammals, including primates, has an intrinsic weakness, an Achilles' heel. In other words, this would mean that, during the evolution of Hominid ancestors, the selection of genetic mechanisms allowing the development of a very large and efficient cognitive brain has been flawed by the occurrence of large-scale neural degeneration and cell death later in life of human beings. It has been stressed that neurodegenerative diseases and other diseases of old age are certainly a consequence of the way of life and the better access to medical care in developed countries that allows people to live much longer than in the recent past.[5] However, even as it is trivial to say that the number of neurodegenerative diseases is increasing as the population is getting older, it is essential to realize that diseases of the elderly population are the consequences of biological processes, which, to be fully understood, need to be examined from an evolutionary angle.[6]

To put it succinctly, an animal with PD or Alzheimer's disease will not survive in the wild for long. Thus, no selective pressure could have been applied to our ancestors to provide them with strong resistance to neurodegeneration. Moreover, natural selection acts on genetic and phenotypic characters that increase individual reproductive efficiency and fitness. Humans, as all the other mammals, reproduce rather early in life, whereas neurodegenerative diseases occur later, when the reproductive capabilities have decreased or disappeared. Thus, no mechanisms capable of overcoming neural degeneration could have been selected during animal evolution since this will not provide a better fitness to individuals having this aptitude.

Contrary to what is often believed, the evolution of species and the process of natural selection do not often lead to optimal character in every aspect of animal physiology. In addition, what has been selected upon specific functional constraints may not be so beneficial several thousands of years later, when the species do not live in the same environment. As a matter of fact, many human diseases are very often the consequence, the outcome of an evolutionary process of character selection, which was made for another purpose and in another context than the one in which humans are living today. For example, the capability to store energy in fat tissues, or the response to dangerous situations, was highly beneficial at a time when access to food was rare or irregular, and when enemies or predators were everywhere. These wonderful faculties, in the meantime, have rendered contemporary humans vulnerable to such pathological conditions as obesity, atherosclerosis, diabetes, or stress-related diseases, as soon as food was abundant and rich and stressful situations were of an entirely different nature.[7]

In a similar respect, there are ample reasons to believe that PD is strongly favored by some of the molecular and cellular characteristics of the dopamine systems, which have been otherwise selected for the advantages they confer on human behavior, when our hominoid ancestors began to become human about 5 million years ago. Thus, some of the reasons for the existence of PD can be traced back to the developmental and evolutionary mechanisms that shaped the dopamine neuronal systems of the human brain.

In this paper, we shall first examine one of the current and prominent hypotheses of the pathophysiology of PD by discussing both the cellular mechanisms that have been recently put forward and the pathological processes that take place during the course of the disease. Then we shall discuss, from an evolutionary perspective, how different the phenotypes of dopamine-containing neurons are from one brain area to another and, similarly, how different the genetic mechanisms are that determine those phenotypes. Our current knowledge of the differentiation of dopamine systems has indeed direct implications in the pathophysiology of PD. On the basis of a comparative approach in vertebrates and chordate animals, we will provide an overview of the general organization of the dopamine systems in the brain and how they could contribute to parkinsonian syndromes.

ELEMENTS OF THE PATHOPHYSIOLOGY OF PD

The seminal and compelling work of Hornykiewicz and colleagues[8] has established that the loss of dopamine in the substantia nigra of parkinsonian patients was fundamental to the neuropathology of the disease. Although degeneration of the substantia nigra has been recognized for almost a century,[9] its place in the pathophysiology of the disease began to be understood only when the anatomy of basal ganglia and dopamine systems was unraveled. Then the efficacy of L-dopa in relieving motor deficits associated with PD set the central place of dopamine systems in the pathological process, opening the way to thousands of studies published since then.[10] Our purpose here is different. We would like to simply emphasize that several lines of research, including biochemistry of the molecular components of the dopamine systems, comparative anatomy, and embryology of dopamine systems, have provided many elements for a revisited view of the disease and possible significant therapeutic implications.

The Pathological Process of PD

The analysis of the neuropathology of PD has revealed that the neurodegeneration process does not reach only the dopamine cells of the mesencephalon (substantia nigra and ventral tegmental area). Recent studies by Braak and others,[11] who carefully studied the time course of the pathological process, showed that the neurodegeneration reaches the dorsal motor nuclei of the hypoglossus and vagus nerves, the giganto-cellular and dorsal part of the raphe nuclei as well as the anterior olfactory nucleus and olfactory bulb, before it extends to the mesencephalic areas. It also progressively extends to other neuronal cell groups, synthesizing serotonin in the raphe nuclei or norepinephrine in the isthmic nuclei (locus coeruleus/sub coeruleus) and dorsal nucleus of the vagus nerve.[11] In a later phase only, neurodegeneration reaches the dopaminergic areas of the mesencephalon (substantia nigra and ventral tegmental area). Thus, PD is not solely a disease of dopamine systems, and, more importantly, it involves many anatomical structures before the substantia nigra and ventral tegmental area begin to degenerate.

Pathophysiological Hypotheses of PD

Studies of parkinsonian neurodegeneration have made significant progress these last 20 years This is primarily owing to better understanding of the mechanisms of action of toxins, such as 6-hydroxydopamine, 1-methyl-4-phenyl-1,2,3,6-tetrahydropyridine (MPTP), rotenone or others.[12] Two major features emerged from these studies, namely the importance of oxidative stress in the neurodegenerative process and the crucial role of the DAT present at the plasma membrane of the mesencephalic dopamine cells, since most of these toxins (with the notable exception of rotenone) enter into the neurons through the DAT.[13,14] In addition, the identification of mutations in rare familial forms of the diseases has also shed a new light on the pathological process of PD (FIG. 1). Indeed, studies have recognized mutations in gene-encoding proteins, such as α-synuclein (a synaptic protein), parkin (an E3 ligase transferring ubiquitin onto proteins targeted for proteasome degradation), or UCH-L1 (ubiquitin carboxy-terminal hydrolase L1, another component of the ubiquitination pathway).[14,15] These genetic findings led to a better understanding of the contribution of the aggregation of fibrillar proteins, such as phosphorylated tau, neurofilaments, and other cytoskeletal proteins, which form the Lewy bodies, another factor long recognized as a key feature of the neuropathology of PD.[16] These findings are also interesting because, as stated above, the degenerative process extends

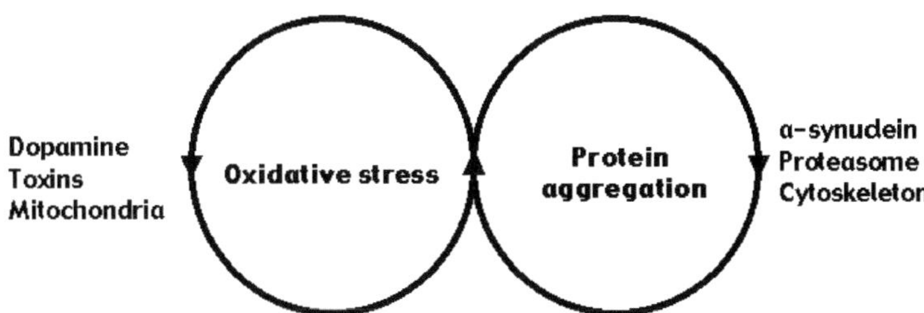

FIGURE 1. The degeneration of neurons in Parkinson's disease associates two interconnected processes: (1) Oxidative stress, which can be promoted by dopamine itself or other oxidant products; by toxins such as MPTP, which blocks the complex I of mitochondria; or by other kinds of mitochondrial insults. (2) Aggregation of proteins, such as α-synuclein or microtubule-associated proteins, favored by decreased chaperone and proteasome activities. The two processes are also able to reinforce each other by creating a self-sustained and deleterious mechanism of cellular degeneration.

far beyond the dopamine neurons of the substantia nigra and VTA in PD patients, and these proteins are ubiquitously expressed in the brain.

Although the degeneration of dopaminergic neurons neither recapitulates nor even corresponds to the first lesions occurring in the course of PD, it established and experimentally supported the concept that dopaminergic degeneration gives its specificity to PD, and that the key symptoms of the disease are the consequence of the dopamine loss. In this respect, the implication of perturbed dopamine metabolism in eliciting oxidative stress has been recognized to be instrumental in promoting the peculiar dopaminergic degeneration seen in PD.[17] A convergent set of evidence points to a link between protein aggregation and the formation of Lewy neurites and Lewy bodies in neurons, and the regulation of dopaminergic metabolism.[18] This link is particularly tight in the diencephalo-mesencephalic neurons in human. In this respect, the role played by α-synuclein seems to be specifically important. This protein is one of the most abundant components of the Lewy bodies, and mutations of α-synuclein (substitutions A30P and A53T) are associated with familial forms of PD. In a normal situation, the presence of α-synuclein as a soluble or lipid-bound structure in dopamine-synthesizing neurons tends to limit the amount of dopamine at nerve terminals.[14] This is because of three basic mechanisms. The first one is to decrease the activity of TH,[19] the second is to increase the number of synaptic vesicles, including those containing VMAT2,[20,21] and the third one is to dampen the uptake of released dopamine by DAT at nerve terminals.[22]

In pathological states, when its amount increases in neurons as well as upon the occurrence of oxidative stress, nucleation of α-synuclein aggregation may occur under the form of protofibrils.[17] This triggers more complete and severe aggregation into Lewy bodies. Although the precise mechanisms of protofibril formation are not known, the aggregation process seems to be similar to that occurring for prion-like or amyloid proteins.[23] This may account also for what is now known as generic synucleopathies, including several forms of dementia and PD.[24] Nevertheless, special features relate α-synuclein to the pathophysiology of PD, and the severe degeneration of the substantia nigra. Indeed, the formation of protofibrils tends to reduce the availability of the physiological form of α-synuclein and increase the toxic potential of dopamine at nerve terminals. Since, in the meantime, free radicals and oxidized dopamine and catecholamines structurally related to dopamine accelerate and stabilize the formation of α-synuclein protofibrils, a vicious circle of protein aggregation and dysregulation of dopamine metabolism is established[18] (FIG. 1). Indeed, the diminished availability of free α-synuclein will impair storage of dopamine by decreasing the number of synaptic vesicles and the amount of the transporter VMAT2. It will also stimulate dopamine synthesis by TH and increase the activity of DAT-processes that all contribute to increasing the levels of free intracellular dopamine. We have suggested that this self-sustained process could contribute significantly to the degeneration of the dopamine-synthesizing neurons of the mesencephalon in human PD.[14]

In this paper, we would like to propose that the highly peculiar phenotype of the dopamine mesencephalic neurons, which has been selected during vertebrate evolution and reshaped in the human lineage to efficiently regulate striatal and cortical functions in this species, has also rendered dopamine neurons more prone to oxidative stress. Indeed, dopamine-synthesizing neurons of the substantia nigra and VTA exhibit a peculiar arrangement of molecules related to dopamine metabolism and function (not found in other neurons), which may provide interesting clues to the pathophysiological process leading to neurodegeneration in PD. For example, the lower amount of α-synuclein immunoreactivity described in the substantia nigra, compared to other brain areas, suggests that nigral dopaminergic neurons may be particularly vulnerable to a pathological increase in α-synuclein protein levels.[14] Similarly, DAT-dependent accumulation of toxins, dysregulation of TH activity, and high sensitivity of dopamine mesencephalic neurons to oxidants are important aspects to better understand the neurodegeneration of substantia nigra and VTA. Several studies have shown that the expression of DAT confers the selectivity of the neurotoxin MPTP toward substantia nigra since the active metabolite of MPTP, MPP$^+$, enters the dopaminergic neuron through DAT in an energy-dependent manner. Once in the cell, MPP$^+$ inhibits complex I of the mitochondrial respiratory chain, releasing cytochrome *c*, which accelerates aggregation of α-synuclein and ultimately affects the properties of α-synuclein.[4] This view, which points to the contribution of nonspecific mechanisms (α-synuclein aggregation for example) in a highly specific cellular environment (the dopamine mesencephalic neurons), provides a robust framework for a more accurate understanding of both the physiology and the pathology of dopamine neurotransmission (FIG. 1). Since it considers molecular components, such as TH, DAT, VMAT2, dopamine receptors, and α-synuclein, as key players in the chain of events leading to PD protein, it also allows for developing novel and rational therapeutic schemes in PD.

ORGANIZATION OF DOPAMINE SYSTEMS IN THE CENTRAL NERVOUS SYSTEM OF HUMAN AND OTHER VERTEBRATES

Comparing dopaminergic systems among the various groups of vertebrate species provides invaluable information on the fundamental organization and function of these systems in the vertebrate phylum. As far as humans are concerned, it allows us to better determine what is common to human and many other vertebrate species, and what makes humans specific. A comparative approach is also required to adequately apply to human advances made in animals of experimental interest (rat, mouse, and zebrafish, for example), showing, in terms of physiology or physiopathology, what can be extrapolated from one species to another and what cannot be.

How to Compare Dopamine Systems in Vertebrates?

A large amount of data have now been accumulated about the anatomy and physiology of dopamine systems in all the main groups of vertebrates. Studies of the anatomy of dopamine and other catecholamine systems generally use the nomenclature of letters and numbers elaborated by Hökfelt and colleagues[25] for the rat brain, the cell group being labeled from A1 to A17. The application of this rat nomenclature to other species has been often difficult, but it was a good starting point for comparison between species. More recently, the comparison has highly benefited from the recognition of the fundamental segments that patterned the neural tube during embryogenesis according to the expression of developmental genes and anatomical cues.[26–28] Since most of the defined segments of the developing and adult brain and spinal cord contain dopamine neurons, comparison between species can easily be interpreted in terms of gain-or-loss of expression in a given territory.

Compiled data, thoroughly reviewed by Smeets and Reiner[29] and Smeets and Gonzalez,[30] led to two major conclusions. Firstly, a majority of the identified dopamine-containing cell groups are found in similar areas, in the different groups of vertebrates analyzed so far. These groups are, for example, dopamine neurons of the retina and the olfactory bulb, those of the hypothalamus, of the substantia nigra, and its homologue in nonmammalian species, the posterior tuberculum, and finally the dopamine neurons of the area postrema, of the nucleus of the tractus solitarius, and of the spinal cord. It is relevant to mention here that most, if not all, the dopamine groups found to exist in the human brain are also present in most of the other vertebrate species. As a consequence, many extrapolations can be made, in terms of physiology and anatomy, from "model" vertebrates such as mouse, rat, or zebrafish, to human. Secondly, significant differences also exist between vertebrate species. Examples are the dopamine-accumulating cells of the paraventricular organ, which does not exist in mammals, or, to a lesser extent, the dopamine neurons of the ventral thalamus and pretectum—this latter group not existing in adult mammals. The comparative analysis also led to the recognition that if many catecholaminergic structures are common to all vertebrates, they often display tremendous differences in size (the number of neurons in the different nuclei relative to the brain size) and in the number and topographic details of their projections.

The Case of the Mesencephalic Dopaminergic Neurons

Mesencephalic dopaminergic neurons correspond to the areas A8, A9, A10 of the Hökfelt nomenclature for rodents. Although these divisions are difficult to apply to the human, the A8-A9 groups correspond, overall, to the substantia nigra pars compacta. The A10 group comprises neurons of the ventral tegmental area (VTA), the Edinger-Westfal nucleus, interfascicular nucleus as well as neurons located in the dorsal raphe and supramamillary nucleus. Until recently, several investigators doubted that teleost fish, or even amphibians, have an equivalent of the human substantia nigra and ventral tegmental area. This issue is now resolved by the demonstration that homologues of these neurons are located in a posterior diencephalic position in fish[31,2] and that humans have also a diencephalic component of the substantia nigra.[33]

Comparison of the human substantia nigra and VTA with those of other mammals or vertebrates reveals a tremendous increase in the number of dopamine neurons. Whereas lizards (*Gekko*) have about 2000 neurons and turtles (*Pseudemys*) about 5500, rats have 45,000 dopamine neurons, *Macaca* 165,000, and humans 590,000 in the first four decades of their life. This very large number of dopamine neurons in humans is significant since, in the meantime, the brain size is only two to three times bigger in human than in *Macaca*, in close correlation with the body weight of the animal. This peculiarity is even more astonishing since a single dopamine neuron of the substantia nigra or VTA sends many collaterals with a very large arborization to several areas of the forebrain.[34] The projections of these neurons are essentially similar among the different vertebrate species. A general feature is that they abundantly innervate the striatal areas and, more scarcely, pallial (cortical) areas, underlining their role in the control of incentive and sensorimotor behaviors. Details of these connections are well described only in mammals and especially in the human.[30]

In humans, the substantia nigra has been divided into a ventral tier and a dorsal tier based on calbindin and TH immunoreactivity and on their projections on the telencephalon. The ventral tier (caudal, lateral and ventral) of the substantia nigra is

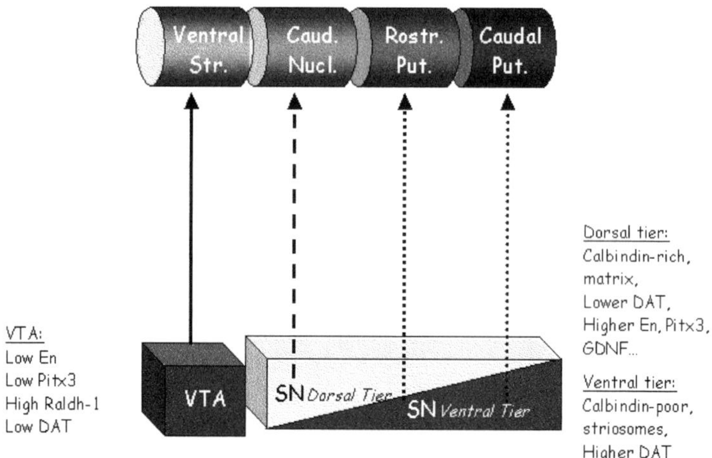

FIGURE 2. Schematic representation of anatomical relationships of the "mesencephalic" dopamine neurons of substantia nigra (SN) and ventral tegmental area (VTA) with their subpallial targets. In primates and humans, substantia nigra is divided into a ventral tier and a dorsal tier based on its differential content of molecular markers (calbindin and DAT, for example) and projections to the striatum. The ventral tier projects to the striosomes whereas the dorsal tier projects to the striatal matrix, and the VTA to the ventral striatum. This delineation reflects specificities in the genetic networks that operate to specify the phenotype of these neurons, which, in turn, is reflected in their differential susceptibility to neurodegeneration in Parkinson's disease. The more caudal part of the ventral tier of the substantia nigra degenerates before the more rostral and dorsal parts.[58]

poorly immunoreactive for calbindin. It projects mainly to the striosomes, or patches of the striatum, and to the caudal putamen (involved in sensorimotor control). The dorsal tier (rostral and dorsal) is calbindin-rich. It projects primarily to the striatal matrix and mainly to the rostral putamen and caudate nucleus (involved in more complex associative behaviors). The VTA projects mainly to the ventral striatum, including the olfactory bulb (FIG. 2). Topographically organized projections from these "mesencephalic" areas also exist on the prefrontal cortex, the pallidum, the subthalamic nucleus, and superior colliculus. Taken together, the anatomical organization of the diencephalo-mesencephalic dopamine neurons, the striking increase in the number of these neurons, and their cellular shape, provide important information in the context of the pathophysiology of PD. In a similar perspective, the biochemical characteristics of these neurons need to be fully taken into account. This issue is more complicated than may appear at first glance and needs to be addressed in some detail.

THE "DOPAMINERGIC PHENOTYPE" CORRESPONDS TO VERY DIFFERENT SITUATIONS IN THE CNS OF VERTEBRATES

A survey of the phenotypic characteristics of dopamine-containing neurons in all the main groups of vertebrate revealed that they exhibit all but a homogenous phenotype. In fact, the "dopaminergic phenotype" is somewhat hard to precisely define. Obviously, a dopaminergic neuron should at least contain dopamine. However, dopamine neurons are also characterized by a collection of molecules involved in dopamine neurotransmission and metabolism, namely synthesizing enzymes (such as tyrosine hydroxylase [TH], and aromatic amino acid decarboxylase [AADC]), degradation enzymes (such as monoamine oxidase), membrane and vesicular transporter (such as, dopamine transporter [DAT] and vesicular monamine transporter [VMAT2]), and membrane receptors (such as D_2 dopamine receptors). By definition, dopamine neurons should not contain dopamine-β-hydroxylase (DBH) or phenyl-ethyl-*N*-methyl transferase—the two enzymes required to make noradrenaline and adrenaline, respectively (TABLE 1).

Tyrosine Hydroxylase and Dopamine

The conspicuous presence of TH-positive, but dopamine-negative cells at several places in the CNS of many vertebrate species questions the validity of stating that TH-positive and DBH-negative cells equal dopaminergic neurons. These neurons have no detectable labeling for AADC, and it is very probable that these TH-positive/dopamine-negative cells are L-dopa–synthesizing neurons. Such cells are the magnocellular neurons of the supraoptic and the paraventricular nuclei of the hypothalamus, or some neurons of the olfactory bulb, for example. In another respect, it has been consistently reported that in lampreys, ray-finned fish, and amphibians, cells containing dopamine, but which were immunonegative for TH, were located around the ventricles in hypothalamic diencephalon (paraventricular organ).[29] These cells are likely to accumulate dopamine from the cerebrospinal fluid with which they are in direct contact and have been shown to accumulate several different monoamines (TABLE 1).

TABLE 1. Variable "dopamine phenotype"

TH⁺, AADC⁻, DAT⁺, VMAT2⁻	TH⁺, AADC⁻, DAT⁻, VMAT2⁺	TH⁻, AADC⁺, DAT⁻, VMAT2⁺	TH⁻, AADC⁻, DAT⁻, VMAT2⁺	TH⁺, AADC⁺, DAT⁺, VMAT2⁺
DA–	DA–	DA+	DA+	DA+
L-DOPA?	L-DOPA cells?	Dopamine-synthesizing cells after L-DOPA uptake? (*D-type neurons*)	Dopamine-accumulating cells	Dopamine-synthesizing cells
Olfactory bulb (internal granular layer)	Arcuate nucleus	Several hypothalamic nuclei	Paraventricular organ	Substantia nigra/ VTA/posterior tuberculum

NOTE: This table summarizes the presence of the different molecular components of the so-called "dopaminergic phenotype" in different neuronal nuclei in the vertebrate brain. It highlights the fact that dopamine-containing neurons are highly heterogeneous, providing them with a differential sensitivity to the pathophysiological process of PD. It also shows that the substantia nigra is indeed a very peculiar case of dopaminergic neurons since it is almost the only structure in the brain that simultaneously and abundantly expresses the full complement of the molecules known to play a role in dopamine metabolism and activity. This peculiarity certainly contributes to the specific and severe degeneration that strikes dopamine and other catecholamine neurons in PD.

The Dopamine Transporter

The use of dopamine transporter as a dopaminergic marker is also questionable since, again, not all the dopamine-containing cells express it, and it may also be present in cells that do not contain dopamine. DAT is found in abundance in the substantia nigra and VTA in mammals as well as in the homologous structure in teleost fish, the posterior tuberculum. It is also found, but at much lower levels, in the neurons of the internal granular layer, and glomerular layer of the olfactory bulb, in the inner nuclear layer of the retina,[6,35] and in the dorsomedial part of the arcuate nucleus of the hypothalamus (A12d[37]). These DAT-immunoreactive neurons also contain dopamine and AADC, which is not the case for the ventromedial neurons since these neurons are likely to produce L-dopa only (A12v[37]). Still, in the hypothalamus, neurons from the anterior paraventricular nuclei possess TH, dopamine, and DAT together, as do neurons from the zona incerta (A13). However, many other dopamine-containing neurons of the hypothalamus are not immunoreactive for DAT, in agreement with the very low density of DAT ligand binding sites observed in these areas[36,38] (TABLE 1).

Interestingly, there is some heterogeneity in the mesencephalic neurons labeled simultaneously with DAT and TH. Whereas TH and DAT immunoreactivities are strong in the substantia nigra pars compacta, the medial VTA exhibits a lower DAT labeling relative to TH. Conversely, in the superficial layers of the rat cingulate cortex, DAT immunolabeling is clearly stronger than that of TH. There is also an obvious heterogenity of DAT labeling in the basal ganglia, DAT being enriched in patches or striosomes of the dorsal and ventral striatum.[36]

The Vesicular Monamine Transporter

The presence of the vesicular monamine transporter (VMAT2) is also not universal to the catecholaminergic neurons of the brain. Indeed, VMAT2 is not found in the olfactory bulb or in the supraoptic nucleus of the hypothalamus. In the brainstem, VMAT2 is not present in the area postrema nor in the nucleus of the tractus solitarius.[39] This observation is of high interest for the pathophysiology of PD since some of the neurons that do not express VMAT2 are among the first to degenerate in the course of the disease.

To summarize, the so-called "dopamine phenotype" indeed corresponds to very different situations in the CNS of vertebrates and is clearly a strikingly versatile phenotype (TABLE 1). Different types of cells contain different sets of the molecular components required for the cells to make, store, and release dopamine. In this respect, the diencephalo-mesencephalic dopamine neurons of the substantia nigra and VTA exhibit the most complete phenotype that one can envisage since they contain TH, AADC, monoamine oxidase, VMAT2, DAT, and even the D_2 receptors—a molecular combination that is highly specific for this category of neurons.

DIFFERENT GENETIC NETWORKS PROMOTE THE DIFFERENTIATION OF DOPAMINE CELLS IN THE BRAIN

The conservation of the general anatomical organization of dopamine systems in vertebrates argues for the existence of ancient genetic mechanisms of specification, which has probably been set up as soon as vertebrates emerged more than 550 million years ago. However, as discussed above, the dopaminergic nuclei distributed along the dorso-ventral and antero-posterior axis of the encephalon are clearly heterogeneous, both from the anatomical and biochemical point of view. Not only are they located at different segmental position, but they also send projections to different brain areas, forming distinct functional systems. Not only is each group of dopamine neuron heterogeneous in the type of cells that constitute it, but dopamine-containing neurons also have a different complement of the molecules involved in dopamine synthesis, storage, re-uptake, and other related functions. A direct consequence of these considerations is that several different mechanisms of neuronal differentiation may operate during embryonic development and adulthood to determine and maintain this versatile phenotype. A number of genes have been implicated in the differentiation of dopamine-containing cells in the central nervous system of vertebrates. The topic has been extensively reviewed recently,[40–42] but little attention has been paid to how the differentiation mechanisms relate to the astonishing phenotypic diversity of dopaminergic neurons.

Signals Involved in Dopaminergic Differentiation

The determination of the dopaminergic phenotype requires the action of extracellular signals emitted in the vicinity of the neural plate soon after neurulation takes place. Little is known about the nature of these signals and signaling structures for most of the dopaminergic nuclei in the brain. One exception is the mesencephalic dopamine cell group, for which a strong emphasis has been given to the role of two systems of extracellular signals, sonic hedgehog (Shh) and fibroblast growth factor 8 (FGF8).[43,44] Shh is secreted by the floor plate, establishing a ventro-dorsal gradient of the morphogen, whereas FGF8 is produced orthogonally by the organizing center of the midbrain–hindbrain boundary, forming a postero-anterior gradient.[45] It is indeed striking that the most important dopamine-synthesizing areas in mammals (substantia nigra and VTA) are located at the intersection of the two structures that produce the highest amount of the two morphogens in the brain. The hypothesis for a major role of these signals was supported by "gain-of-function" and "loss-of-function" experiments carried out both *in vivo* and *in vitro*. Overexpression, or ectopic expression, of Shh and FGF8 was able to induce a dopaminergic phenotype in neurons similar to that of mesencephalic dopamine neurons.[40]

However, this hypothesis does not take into account the differentiation of many other dopaminergic cell groups, which clearly do not depend on this orthogonal array of signals. This is, for example, the case of the dopamine neurons of the ventral thalamus, which are determined by nonconvergent signaling pathways involving *Pax6* and *Lhx1* on the one hand and *Dlx1/2* and *Islet1* on the other.[46] In addition, in many groups of vertebrates other than mammals such as teleost fish or amphibians, the nucleus homologous to mammalian substantia nigra is not located in the mesencephalon just upstream of the midbrain–hindbrain boundary. Instead, dopaminergic neurons are located far upstream at the posterior edge of the diencephalon, a region named the posterior tuberculum.[29,47] Some inconsistencies also exist in the mammalian literature. Authors have reported that the first dopaminergic cells of the "mesencephalic" group arise at a very ventral position: at the edge of the neuro-epithelium along the mesencephalic flexure. However, this description is not precise enough to specify whether this neuronal population is truly mesencephalic or posterior diencephalic. In contrast, Verney and Puelles have shown that, even in human, the first contingent of TH-expressing cells appears at the diencephalon–mesencephalon border very much like in the other nonmammalian species.[48] Thus, the precise topological assignment of the primordium of the substantia nigra and VTA to either a diencephalic or mesencephalic position requires further work and particularly cell-fate studies.

Nevertheless, the morphogenetic factors Shh and FGF8 produced near the isthmus cannot be the sole determinant of dopaminergic phenotype in these areas. Indeed, analysis of zebrafish mutants has demonstrated that Nodal (a growth factor of the TGFβ superfamily) and its signaling pathway (in particular the gene $FoxH_1/Fast1$), but not Shh, is strictly required for the induction of the dopaminergic phenotype of the homologue of substantia nigra.[49] Nodal is expressed before and is required to induce Shh in the floor plate. It may well be that Nodal is the key determinant of the dopaminergic cells in the anterior portion of the substantia nigra—that is, the group of dopamine neurons located in the posterior diencephalon at its border with mesencephalon. Then it is possible that the truly mesencephalic component of the substantia nigra and VTA indeed requires Shh to be differentiated. The mesencephalic extension of the main dopaminergic neuronal group of the brain could have been acquired secondarily during vertebrate evolution, accompanying the concomitant enlargement of the basal ganglia and cortical areas, the main target areas of the diencephalo-mesencephalic dopaminergic nuclei. These observations are relevant to the pathophysiology of PD since the posterior component of substantia nigra degenerates before and more strongly than the anterior most part[1] (FIG. 2).

Genes Involved in Dopaminergic Differentiation

In addition to these signaling pathways, several intrinsic regulatory genes have also been implicated in inducing the dopaminergic phenotype. Again, the substantia nigra has been the topic of the vast majority of the investigations. The best-known factor of dopaminergic differentiation is *Nurr1*, an orphan nuclear receptor, the knock-out of which completely abolishes the expression of TH in the substantia nigra, but not in any other dopaminergic cell groups.[50] The presence of Nurr1 is essential for the expression of the whole phenotype of these dopaminergic neurons, including the expression of c-Ret, a receptor for growth factors such as GDNF. It does not seem that the lack of growth factor receptors is responsible for the disappearance of the dopaminergic phenotype. Rather, Nurr1 exerts a direct action on the TH promoter as well as on the genes of several other major determinants of the dopamine phenotype. Recent data from Perlman's group have suggested that Nurr1 may act as a regulator of cell cycle exit for the progenitors of dopaminergic neurons of the diencephalo-mesencephalic group in conjunction with p57-KIP, another regulator of the cell cycle, and independently of the cyclin pathway.[51] It is thus possible that Nurr1 is making a link between the exit of the cell cycle and the start of the dopaminergic differentiation.

Other important factors contribute to determining the dopaminergic phenotype of the substantia nigra and VTA, namely, the LIM-homeodomain gene (*Lmx-1b*), the genes *Engrailed1* and *2* (*En1*, *En2*), and the paired-box gene (*Pitx-3/Ptx-3*). The *Lmx-1b* gene is initially expressed in the dorsal neural tube and at the midbrain–hindbrain boundary and, later, more ventrally, in the presumptive diencephalo-mesencephalic dopaminergic neurons. Its expression precedes those of *Pitx-3* and *TH*. Invalidation of *Lmx-1b* abolishes the expression of *Pitx-3*, but not that of *Nurr1*. In these *Lmx-1b*-knock-out mice, TH begins to be normally expressed, but it is not maintained after birth. In agreement with these results, the mouse mutant *aphakia* (*Ak*), which lacks the *Pitx-3* gene, displays an early expression of TH in the diencephalo-mesencephalic, which disappears at later stages.[42] The *Pitx-3* gene seems to be strictly and uniquely expressed in TH-positive neurons, although the target genes of *Pitx-3* are not known. In particular, the expression of other components of the dopaminergic phenotype (VMAT2, AADC, DAT) is not affected in the *Ak* mutant. It is interesting to notice that neuronal projection on the caudate-putamen is lost in these mice but not that of the nucleus accumbens, which appears hyperactive. These data strongly suggest that *Nurr1*, on the one hand, and *Lmx-1b* and *Pitx-3*, on the other, belong to independent pathways that differentially contribute to the differentiation (*Nurr1*) and maintenance (*Lmx-1b* and *Pitx-3*) of the expression of TH and probably of the other molecular components of the dopaminergic phenotype in these neurons, such as DAT and VMAT2.

Interestingly enough, in the double-knock out mice for the Engrailed genes (*En1*$^{-/-}$, *En2*$^{-/-}$), TH expression is also lost soon after birth, and these mice are also completely devoid of α-synuclein, the protein mutated in rare forms of familial PD.[52] Thus, the Engrailed genes, in addition to being important survival factors for the dopaminergic neurons of the diencephalo-mesencephalic area, make a link between the presence of α-synuclein and the existence of a peculiar arrangement of molecules defining the dopaminergic phenotype of substantia nigra and VTA. Another interesting observation in the context of PD pathophysiology is that in the $En1^{-/-}$, $En2^{+/-}$ heterozygous mice, the terminal field of TH-positive cells is abolished in the caudate-putamen but not in the nucleus accumbens.[53] This indicates that the presence of Engrailed factors in the dopaminergic neurons of the diencephalo-mesencephalic area is more important for neurons of the dorsal tier of the substantia nigra than for the neurons of the ventral tier and of the VTA. This situation is very similar to that observed in the *Ak*-mutant lacking Pitx3, but the functional relevance of this observation is not known yet (FIG. 2).

Although no good evidence has been shown implicating the retinoic acid signaling pathway in dopaminergic differentiation, class 1-retinaldehyde deshydrogenase is abundantly present in a subset of the neurons of substantia nigra and VTA. Interestingly, the retinaldehyde deshydrogenase-containing terminals of these neurons are present at the highest density in the anterior and dorsal part of the caudate-putamen and nucleus accumbens in the rat. These regions are the last to degenerate in toxic models of PD as well as in the human disease itself. Retinoic acid has a major effect on the neuronal differentiation along the antero-posterior axis of the neural tube, but its precise role in dopamine neuron differentiation is not known. *Nurr1* has been shown to form heterodimers with retinoic acid receptors of the RXR family, but it is not clear whether such an interaction may interfere with retinoic acid signaling or not. In this respect, the only demonstrated effect of retinoic acid and its receptor in the substantia nigra and VTA concerns the expression of the dopamine D_2 receptor.[54] It is thus possible that retinoic acid may, in combination with *Nurr1*, contribute both to the setup of the expression of the molecular components of the mesencephalo-diencephalic dopamine neurons and the establishment of connections and synaptogenesis.

Other Factors

Besides these important factors of dopaminergic differentiation, a very large number of growth factors, or neurotrophic factors, have been implicated in aspects of differentiation of dopaminergic neurons *in vitro*. These include BMP-like factors, interleukins (IL-1 and IL-11), FGFα, TGFα, PACAP, neurotrophins (such as BDNF, NGF, NT3, NT4, and NT4-5), and a stromal factor of unknown nature.[55] The most compelling data concern glial cell line–derived neurotrophic factor (GDNF), which acts as a key survival factor for the diencephalo-mesencephalic dopamine neurons.[56] In addition, the GDNF receptor c-RET is specifically expressed in these dopaminergic neurons under the control of the same factors as TH. GDNF has been used with some success as a therapeutic agent in animal models as well as in clinical trials in humans, and it may represent one of the significant hopes in the treatment of nigral neurodegeneration in PD. Another interesting case of secreted factors are the members of the Wnt family since Wnt1 and Wnt3a are found at a high level in the mesencephalic area just in front of the midbrain–hindbrain boundary, whereas Wnt5a expression is restricted to the ventral portion of this area. It is likely that Wnt signals, by controlling the complex balance between proliferation and exit of the cell cycle in the neuronal precursors of the midbrain, play a role similar to that of *Nurr1* in the differentiation of dopamine cells. It has been shown that Wnt5a is able to stimulate the expression of Pitx3 and c-RET in *Nurr1*-positive neurons.[57]

To conclude here, although more and more features of the differentiation of dopamine neurons become deciphered, a lot remains to be done to understand how differentiation mechanisms differ from one cell group to another. However, it is already very clear that the action of genes, such as *Pitx3* and *En*, are fully relevant to the pathophysiology of PD (FIG. 2).

THE RELEVANCE OF DIFFERENTIATION AND ORGANIZATION OF DOPAMINE SYSTEMS TO THE PATHOPHYSIOLOGY AND TREATMENT OF PD

Taken together, the various observations that have been accumulated on mechanisms of differentiation and the molecular organization of dopamine systems bring a renewed view of the pathophysiology of PD. We prioritize the idea of a direct influence of the dopamine phenotype on the rather specific degeneration of dopamine neurons and its gradual progression during the course of the disease. We also think that multiple factors are able to trigger a neurodegenerative process with the typical characteristics of PD, which depends on the mutual reinforcement of two basic processes, protein aggregation and oxidative stress, as stated in the earlier section ELEMENTS OF THE PATHOPHYSIOLOGY OF PD and FIGURE 1.

Basically, the formation of protein aggregates, such as Lewy bodies, is a nonspecific mechanism. It depends on a phenomenon of nucleation of proteins prone to forming protofibrils (such as α-synuclein) or small aggregates (such as the β-amyloid component of APP or phosphorylated tau). Protein aggregation is essentially a self-sustained process favored by different conditions, such as increased protein concentration, decrease of protein degradation (especially by the proteasome system), specific mutations of the aggregating proteins, increased concentrations of metals, decreased activity of chaperones, or strong oxidative conditions (such as oxidative stress).[23,13] Oxidative stress can also be triggered by several means, including impairment of mitochondrial metabolism, production of oxidative radicals, or reactive oxygen species of different sources.[14]

Here, dopamine and molecules related to dopamine metabolism come into play. Dopamine itself is a highly oxidable compound that rapidly forms reactive oxygen species. Thus, increased activity of TH and AADC (the biosynthetic enzymes), increased activity of DAT (the membrane transporter taking up dopamine from the extracellular space), or decreased activity of VMAT2 (the vesicular transporter that safely accumulates dopamine into presynaptic vesicles) will all favor the cytoplasmic accumulation of free dopamine and its oxidated derivatives. We have already underlined the crucial role played by α-synuclein in this respect since its aggregation is precisely favored under these conditions. Thus, a dangerous connection exists between oxidative stress and protein aggregation as well as between dopamine metabolism and α-synuclein. The time course and detailed anatomy of neuronal lesions in PD clearly reflects this pathological condition.

Chemical Neuroanatomy of Parkinsonian Degeneration

It is striking to observe that the neurons that begin to degenerate first are those neurons expressing a high amount of DAT and/or low amount of VMAT2, as is the case in the olfactory bulb, for example. Neurons of the olfactory bulb are also among the very first to exhibit Lewy neurites or Lewy bodies. In the substantia nigra, posterolateral neurons are those reached more extensively by neural degeneration, and they express the highest amount of DAT transcripts and proteins. It should be emphasized that these statements are mainly conjectural at this point since little attention has been paid to the correlation between the presence of specific components, such as the vesicular transporter VMAT2 or the DAT, and the time of occurrence and severity of the disease. A piece of evidence is brought by the effect of toxins such as MPTP, which promotes the degeneration of the dopaminergic neurons of the mesencephalon and enters into the neurons through the DAT.[12] In agreement with this hypothesis, the expression of DAT reflects the sensitivity of these neurons to the toxins and the intensity of the neurodegeneration (FIG. 2). The caudo-medial regions of the substantia nigra degenerate first and most intensively in animal models of PD as well as in the human disease. It is possible that a similar phenomenon may account for the early and severe degeneration of the locus coeruleus—the noradrenergic nuclei of the isthmus that express high amounts of the norepinephrine transporter—a membrane transporter functionally closely related to DAT.

The neurons of the substantia nigra and VTA are particularly numerous in humans, and they concentrate a high amount of the molecular components that contribute to the exquisitely complex and precise mechanisms of synthesis, storage, release, and extracellular action of dopamine. This specific phenotype, which renders the neurons sensitive to dopamine-induced oxidative stress and neurodegeneration, is the consequence of peculiar developmental mechanisms. We have shown that neurons expressing *Pitx3* and *En1/2* are also the first to degenerate in the course of PD. In contrast, anterior neurons, phylogenetically the most conserved and ontogenetically appearing first, also express a high amount of class 1-retinaldehyde deshydrogenase and degenerate last.

Many aspects of this hypothesis have clear clinical therapeutic implications. Looking for nonmotor symptoms, such as smell impairment or subtle neurovegetative symptoms, which correspond to the earliest stages of PD, will allow an earlier diagnosis of PD and permit the use of treatments able to slow down the neurodegenerative process.[11] The effectiveness of compounds able to reduce oxidative stress and local inflammation should be thoroughly tested. Screening for new drugs able to activate genes such as *Pitx3* or *En1/2*, or even *Nurr1* needs to be more systematically undertaken. Cell therapy with neurotrophic factors, such as GDNF, is already under investigation. Pharmacological compounds that decrease aberrant or excessive dopamine uptake through DAT or increase dopamine storage into synaptic vesicles could be highly beneficial to the substitutive treatment of PD.

To conclude, we would like to advance the idea that the general molecular organization of dopamine and other catecholamine systems and their tremendous increased size in humans pave the way for the occurrence of a "specific" degeneration process, namely PD. The role of dopamine is modulatory in essence. It affects sensory information (in the retina, olfactory bulb, and some nuclei of sensory cranial nerves in the hindbrain), hypothalamic control of endocrine, reproductive, and vegetative functions, sensorimotor programming in the subpallial areas, emotions, and motivation and memory in the pallial-cortical areas. The quantitative modifications undergone by the dopaminergic neurons of the diencephalo-mesencephalic region and their neuronal projections reflects the concomitant tremendous enlargement of pallial-cortical regions, which are extremely specialized and compartmentalized in mammals and human as compared to amphibians and fish, for example. To accommodate such huge changes in the way sensory perception and motor action are elaborated, regulatory pathways such as the dopamine systems need to be adapted. The natural history of dopamine systems in vertebrates sheds a bright light on the physiology of dopamine systems in humans. It reveals its heritage of fundamental necessity for motivational behavior, for example, but also its genetic weakness, which may have favored susceptibility to oxidative stress and neurodegenerative diseases.

ACKNOWLEDGMENTS

This work was supported by grants from the CNRS, University Paris-sud, and the National Institutes of Health [NS-34914, NS-45326, and NS041555].

REFERENCES

1. FEARNLEY, J.M. & A. LEES. 1991. Ageing and Parkinson's disease: substantia nigra regional selectivity. Brain **114**: 2283–2301.
2. COTZIAS, G.C., M.H. VAN WOERT & L.M. SCHIFFER. 1967. Aromatic amino acids and modification of parkinsonism. N. Engl. J. Med. **276**: 374–379.
3. PRZEDBORSKI, S., V. KOSTIC, N. GILADI, *et al.* 2003. Dopaminergic systems in Parkinson's disease, in dopamine receptors and transporters. A. Sidhu, M. Laruelle & P. Vernier, Eds.: 363–402. Marcel Dekker. New York.
4. DAUER, W. & S. PRZEDBORSKI. 2003. Parkinson's disease: mechanisms and models. Neuron **39**: 889–909.
5. WICK, G., P. BERGER, P. JANSEN-DURR, *et al.* 2003. A Darwinian-evolutionary concept of age-related diseases. Exp. Gerontol. **38**: 13–25.
6. ROSE, M., L. MUELLER & A. LONG. 2002. Pharmacology, genomics, and the evolutionary biology of ageing. Free Radical Res. **36**: 1293–1297.
7. STEARNS, S. & D. EBERT. 2001. Evolution in health and disease: work in progress. Q. Rev. Biol. **76**: 417–432.
8. EHRINGER, H. & O. HORNYKIEWICZ. 1960. Verteilung von noradrenalin und dopamine 3-hydroxy-tyramin in Gehirn des Menschen und ihr Verhalten by Erkrankungen des Extrapyramidalen systems. Klin. Wschr. **38**: 1236–1239.
9. FOIX, M. 1921. Les lésions anatomiques de la Maladie de Parkinson. Rev. Neurol. **28**: 593–600.
10. SAMII, A., J.G. NUTT & B.R. RANSOM. 2004. Parkinson's disease. Lancet **363**: 1783–1793.
11. BRAAK, H., K. DEL TREDICI, U. RÜB, *et al.* 2003. Staging of brain pathology associated to sporadic Parkinson's disease. Neurobiol. Aging **24**: 197–211.
12. HIRSCH, E.C., G. HOGLINGER, E. ROUSSELET, *et al.* 2003 Animal models of Parkinson's disease in rodents induced by toxins: an update. J. Neural Trans. suppl. **65**: 89–100.
13. DAWSON, T. M., & V.L. DAWSON. 2003 Molecular pathways of neurodegeneration in Parkinson's disease. Science **302**: 819–822.
14. SIDHU, A., C. WERSINGER & P. VERNIER. 2004 Does α-synuclein modulate dopaminergic synaptic content and tone at the synapse? FASEB J. **18**: 637–647.
15. GIASSON, B.I. & V.M. LEE. 2003. Are ubiquitination pathways central to Parkinson's disease? Cell **114**: 1–8.

16. BABA, M., S. NAKAJO, P.H. TU, *et al.* 1998. Aggregation of alpha-synuclein in Lewy bodies of sporadic Parkinson's disease and dementia with Lewy bodies. Am. J. Pathol. **152:** 879–884.

17. CONWAY, K.A., J.C. ROCHET, R.M. BIEGANSKI, *et al.* 2001. Kinetic stabilization of the alpha-synuclein protofibril by a dopamine-alpha-synuclein adduct. Science **294:** 1346–1349.

18. SIDHU, A., C. WERSINGER & P. VERNIER. 2004 Alpha-synuclein regulation of the dopaminergic transporter: a possible role in the pathogenesis of Parkinson's disease. FEBS Lett. **265:** 1–5.

19. PEREZ, R.G., J.C. WAYMIRE, E. LIN, *et al.* 2002. A role for alpha-synuclein in the regulation of dopamine biosynthesis. J. Neurosci. **22:** 3090–3099.

20. LOTHARIUS, J., S. BARG, P. WIEKOP, *et al.* 2002 Effect of mutant alpha-synuclein on dopamine homeostasis in a new human mesencephalic cell line. J. Biol. Hematol. **277:** 38884–38894.

21. LOTHARIUS, J. & P. BRUNDIN. 2002. Pathogenesis of Parkinson's disease: dopamine, vesicles and alpha-synuclein. Nat. Rev. Neurosci. **3:** 932–942 .

22. WERSINGER, C., D. PROU, P. VERNIER, *et al.* 2003. Mutations in the lipid-binding domain of alpha-synuclein confer overlapping, yet distinct, functional properties in the regulation of dopamine transporter activity. Mol. Cell Neurosci. **24:** 91–105.

23. EL-AGNAF, O.M. & G.B. IRVINE. 2002 Aggregation and neurotoxicity of alpha-synuclein and related peptides. Biochem. Soc. Trans. **30:** 559–565.

24. LUCKING, C.B. & A. BRICE. 2000 Alpha-synuclein and Parkinson's disease. Cell. Mol. Life Sci. **57:** 1894–1908.

25. HÖKFELT, T., R. MARTENSSON, A. BJÖRKLUND, *et al.* 1984 Distributional maps of tyrosine hydroxylase-immunoreactive neurons in the rat brain. *In* Handbook of Chemical Neuroanatomy. T. Hökfelt, Ed.: 277–386. Elsevier. Amsterdam.

26. PUELLES, L. & J.L. RUBENSTEIN. 1993. Expression patterns of homeobox and other putative regulatory genes in the embryonic mouse forebrain suggest a neuromeric organization. Trends Neurosci. **16:** 472–479.

27. PUELLES, L. & J. RUBENSTEIN. 2003. Forebrain gene expression domains and the evolving prosomeric model. Trends Neurosci. **26:** 469–476.

28. WULLIMANN, M.L. & L. PUELLES. 1999 Postembryonic neural proliferation in the zebrafish forebrainand its relationships to prosomeric domains. Anat. Embryol. **201:** 329–348.

29. SMEETS, WJ. & A. REINER. 1994. Phylogeny and development of catecholamine systems in the CNS of vertebrates. Cambridge University Press. London.

30. SMEETS, W.J. & A. GONZALEZ. 2000. Catecholamine systems in the brain of vertebrates: new perspectives through a comparative approach. Brain Res. Rev. **33:** 308–379.

31. KAPSIMALI, M., F. BOURRAT & P. VERNIER. 2001 Distribution of the orphan nuclear receptor nurr1 in medaka *Oryzias latipes*: cues to the definition of homologous territories in the vertebrate brain. J. Comp. Neurol. **431:** 276–292.

32. RINK, E. & M.L. WULLIMANN. 2002. Connections of the ventral telencephalon and tyrosine hydroxylase distribution in the zebrafish brain *Danio rerio* lead to identification of an ascending dopaminergic system in a teleost. Brain Res. Bull. **57:** 385–387.

33. PUELLES, L. & C. VERNEY. 1998. Early neuromeric distribution of tyrosine-hydroxylase-immunoreactive neurons in human embryos. J. Comp. Neurol. **394:** 283–308.

34. PRENSA, L. & A. PARENT. 2001 The nigrostriatal pathway in the rat: a single-axon study of the relationship between dorsal and ventral tier nigral neurons and the striosome/matrix striatal compartments. J. Neurosci. **21:** 7247–7260.

35. CERRUTI, C., D. WALTHER, M. KUHAR, *et al.* 1993. Dopamine transporter mRNA expression is intense in rat midbrain neurons and modest outside midbrain. Brain Res. Mol. Brain Res. **18:** 181–186.

36. CILIAX, B.J., C. HEILMAN, L.L. DEMCHYSHYN, *et al.*. 1995 The dopamine transporter: immunochemical characterization and localization in brain. J. Neurosci. **15:** 1714–1723.

37. MEISTER, B. & R. ELDE. 1993. Dopamine transporter mRNA in neurons of the rat hypothalamus. Neuroendocrinology **58:** 388–395.

38. CILIAX, B.J., G.W. DRASH, J.K. STALEY, *et al.* 1999. Immunocytochemical localization of the dopamine transporter in human brain. J. Comp. Neurol. **409:** 38–56.

39. WEIHE, E. & L. EIDEN. 2000. Chemical neuroanatomy of the vesicular amine transporters. FASEB J. **14:** 2435–2449.

40. LIN, J.C. & A. ROSENTHAL. 2003. Molecular mechanisms controlling the development of dopaminergic neurons. Cell Dev. Biol. **14:** 175–180.

41. RIDDLE, R. & J. POLLOCK. 2003. Making connections: the development of mesencephalic dopaminergic neurons. Brain Res. Dev. Brain Res. **147:** 3–21 .

42. SMIDT, M., S. SMITS & J. BURBACH. 2003. Molecular mechanisms underlying midbrain dopamine neuron development and function. Eur. J. Pharmacol. **480:** 75–88.

43. HYNES, M., J.A. PORTER, C. CHIANG, *et al.* 1995 Induction of midbrain dopaminergic neurons by Sonic hedgehog. Neuron **15:** 35–44.

44. KIM, J., J. AUERBACH, J. RODRIGUEZ-GOMEZ, *et al.* 2002 Dopamine neurons derived from embryonic stem cells function in an animal model of Parkinson's disease. Nature **418:** 50–56.

45. WURST, W. & L. BALLY-CUIF. 2001 Neural plate patterning: upstream and downstream of the isthmic organizer. Nat. Rev. Neurosci **2:** 99–108.

46. ANDREWS, G., K. YUN, J.L. RUBENSTEIN, *et al.* 2003. Dlx transcription factors regulate differentiation of dopaminergic neurons of the ventral thalamus. Mol. Cell Neurosci. **23:** 107–120.

47. RINK, E. & M. WULLIMANN. 2002. Development of the catecholaminergic system in the early zebrafish brain: an immunohistochemical study. Brain Res. Dev. Brain Res. **137:** 89–100.

48. VERNEY, C. & L. PUELLES. 2001. Structures of longitudinal brain zones that originate the substantia nigra and ventral tegmental area in human embryos, as revealed by cytoarchitecture, and tyrosine hydroxylase, calbindin, calretinin and GABA immunoreaction. J. Comp. Neurol. **429:** 22–44.

49. HOLZSCHUH, J., G. HAUPTMANN & W. DRIEVER. 2003. Genetic analysis of the roles of Hh, FGF8, and nodal signaling during catecholaminergic system development in the zebrafish brain. J. Neurosci. **23:** 5507–5519.

50. ZETTERSTROM, R.H., L. SOLOMIN, L. JANSSON, *et al.* 1997. Dopamine neuron agenesis in Nurr1-deficient mice. Science **276:** 248–250.

51. JOSEPH, B., A. WALLEN-MACKENZIE, G. BENOIT, *et al.* 2003. p57Kip2 cooperates with Nurr1 in developing dopamine cells. Proc. Natl. Acad. Sci. USA **100:** 15619–15624.

52. ABELIOVICH, A., Y. SCHMITZ, I. FARINAS, *et al.* 2000. Mice lacking alpha-synuclein display functional deficits in the nigrostriatal dopamine system. Neuron **25:** 239–252.

53. SIMON, H., H. SAUERESSIG, W. WURST, *et al.* 2001. Fate of midbrain dopamine neurons controlled by the Engrailed genes. J. Neurosci. **21:** 3126–3134.

54. VALDENAIRE, O., P. VERNIER, M. MAUS, *et al.* 1994. Transcription of the rat dopamine-D2-receptor gene from two promoters. Eur. J. Biochem. **220:** 577–584.

55. KAWASAKI, H., H. SUEMORI, K. MIZUSEKI, *et al.* 2002. Generation of dopaminergic neurons and pigmented epithelia from primate ES cells by stromal cell-derived inducing activity. Proc. Natl. Acad. Sci. USA **99:** 1580–1585.

56. MOORE, M.W., R.D. KLEIN, I. FARINAS, *et al.* 1996. Renal and neural abnormalities in mice lacking GDNF. Nature **382:** 76–79.

57. CASTELO-BRANCO, G., J. WAGNER, F. RODRIGUEZ, *et al.* 2003. Differential regulation of midbrain dopaminergic neuron development by Wnt-1, Wnt-3a, and Wnt-5a. Proc. Natl. Acad. Sci. USA **100:** 12747–12752.

58. DAMIER, P., E. HIRSCH, Y. AGID, *et al.* 1999. The substantia nigra of the human brain. II. Patterns of loss of loss of dopamine-containing neurons. I. Parkinson's disease. Brain **122:** 1437–1448.

The Role of α-Synuclein in Both Neuroprotection and Neurodegeneration

ANITA SIDHU,[a] CHRISTOPHE WERSINGER,[a] CHARBEL E-H. MOUSSA,[a] AND PHILIPPE VERNIER[b]

[a]*Department of Pediatrics, Georgetown University, Washington, District of Columbia 20007, USA*

[b]*Institut de Neurobiologie Alfred FESSARD, CNRS, 91198 Gif-sur-Yvette Cedex, France*

ABSTRACT: Although α-synuclein is a central player in the pathophysiology of the dopaminergic neurodegeneration that occurs in Parkinson's disease (PD), emerging results suggest that the fundamental property of the wild-type form of this protein may be one of neuroprotection, as it can inhibit apoptosis in response to various pro-apoptotic stimuli. Such properties may be lost by its familial PD-linked mutations upon alterations in its expression levels or clearance (overexpression of the gene, reduced protein degradation) or following exposure to certain neurotoxins. Moreover, converging observations suggest that a primary function for α-synuclein in dopaminergic neurons may be the regulation of dopamine content and tone at the synapse. In this paper, we review how, indeed, α-synuclein regulates both the synthesis of dopamine, its storage into vesicles, its release in the synapse, and its re-uptake into the dopaminergic neurons. We also show how disruption of these events, and of the neuroprotective effects of α-synuclein, can initiate the observed neurotoxicity of α-synuclein in dopaminergic neurons and the genesis of the degenerative processes associated with PD.

KEYWORDS: dopamine transporter; α-synuclein; Parkinson's disease; MPTP; neurodegeneration; neuroprotection; apoptosis

INTRODUCTION

α-Synuclein (Syn) is a synaptic protein of still unknown function that is a major component of Lewy bodies (LBs)—neuronal cytoplasmic inclusions of aggregated proteins that are characteristic hallmarks of idiopathic and familial forms of Parkinson's disease (PD).[1–3] Syn aggregates are, however, not at all specific for PD since they are also found in the neuronal and glial cytoplasmic inclusions of multiple system atrophy and in the LBs of variants of Alzheimer's disease, Down syndrome with Alzheimer's disease, and in other neurodegenerative diseases collectively known as synucleinopathies.[2–4] Two substitution mutations in the gene encoding wild-type (*wt*) Syn, alanine[30]-proline (A30P) and alanine[53]-threonine (A53T), are

Address for correspondence: Dr. Anita Sidhu, Head, Laboratory of Molecular Neurochemistry, The Research Building, Room W222, 3970 Reservoir Road, NW, Washington, D.C. 20007. Voice: 202-687-0282; fax: 202-687-0279.
sidhua@georgetown.edu

Ann. N.Y. Acad. Sci. 1035: 250–270 (2004). © 2004 New York Academy of Sciences.
doi: 10.1196/annals.1332.016

associated with familial, autosomal-dominant forms of PD,[5,6] but these mutations are not found in idiopathic PD[7] or other forms of inherited PD.[8]

Extensive evidence from the literature shows that Syn is neurotoxic and that it is, somehow, implicated in the pathophysiology of PD.[1] Syn neuropathy is associated with its oligomerization into soluble protofibrils, which are believed to be the most toxic Syn species, followed by the coalescence of these oligomeric forms into insoluble fibrils composed of β-sheets, which are also neurotoxic, and amyloid-like filaments prior to their aggregation into insoluble fibrillar structures and inclusions, which then accumulate as LBs.[1,2,9–12] Several experimental conditions—including overexpression of the protein, presence of the A30P or A53T mutations, exposure to neurotoxins and oxidative factors, alterations in posttranslational modifications (such as phosphorylation or transglutamination), altered degradation of the protein through dysfunctions of the ubiquitin/proteasome pathway, or a crowded milieu— induce or accelerate Syn aggregation, both *in vivo* and *in vitro* through procedures that remain poorly understood.[1,2,9–12] However, many studies in the literature that we review in this paper have also found a neuroprotective effect for Syn since it was found to inhibit apoptosis induced by a wide variety of apoptotic stimuli or to modulate the expression levels or activity of proteins implicated in the induction or control of apoptosis. It is conceivable that neuroprotection may be a putative physiological function for this protein that may be lost either by the familial PD-linked mutants, or after exposure to certain neurotoxins, or after an overexpression of the protein.

Whereas PD is characterized by the preferential degeneration of dopamine-producing neurons of the substantia nigra pars compacta (*SNpc*), Syn is ubiquitously expressed at high levels in virtually all regions of the brain, where it is believed to account for up to 0.1% of total brain proteins.[3,13] Such a wide immunoreactivity in the brain renders it unlikely that high expression levels of Syn are the sole criteria to cause protofibril and/or LB formation and/or subsequent neuronal death both in PD and in other synucleinopathies. Moreover, the *SNpc* dopaminergic neurons that preferentially degenerate in PD express considerably less Syn compared to other areas of the brain[14] under nonpathologic conditions, whereas other brain regions expressing higher levels of Syn are relatively spared in PD. Increasingly then, the specific vulnerability of the *SNpc* neurons to degenerate in PD may be linked to some other additional factors—the prime candidate being dysfunctions in dopamine handling inside these neurons.[15,16] Indeed, metabolism of free intracellular dopamine by monoamine oxidases produces H_2O_2 while its spontaneous autoxidation at normal intracellular pH—that is, out of the acidic storage vesicles—produces toxic and reactive dopamine-quinones, superoxide free radicals, and H_2O_2.[15–17] Oxidized dopamine has been shown to give rise to dopamine-Syn adducts, which stabilize the formation of Syn protofibrils,[9] the most toxic form of Syn,[18] by inhibiting the conversion of soluble protofibrils into insoluble fibrils *in vitro*.[9] Moreover, after modifications of Syn by reactive oxygen- and reactive nitrogen species generated upon free intracellular dopamine autoxidation and/or metabolism, the neuroprotective and anti-apoptotic effects of Syn may be lost. Therefore, alterations in intraneuronal dopamine homeostasis may lead to a sustained oxidative stress that could potentiate or initiate Syn neuropathy in the *SNpc*.[15–17]

Interestingly, results obtained by our groups[15,16] and others[17,19,20] show there is even a closer relationship between Syn and dopamine whereby this protein probably participates in regulating the biosynthesis, the storage into vesicles, the release into the synapse after neuronal stimulation, and the re-uptake of this neurotransmitter in dopaminergic neurons. In essence, Syn may be an adaptor protein or a chaperone, regulating nearly every step of the bio-cycle of dopamine in *SNpc* neurons (FIG. 1), but in particular the function of the dopamine transporter (DAT), which is the key molecule dictating dopaminergic content and synaptic tone of dopamine.[15,16] Once aggregation of the protein is initiated, the bioavailability of the physiological form of Syn is substantially diminished such that normal physiological functions regulated by this protein may be severely compromised, which, in turn, could further exacerbate the initial cellular insult, since Syn may then play a central role both as a mediator and facilitator of the dopaminergic neurotoxicity that occurs in PD.[15,16,19] Thus, a loss-of-function phenomenon for Syn needs also to be taken into account in the pathophysiology of PD—at least in as much as a gain of toxic function because of protein aggregates.

STRUCTURAL AND FUNCTIONAL CHARACTERISTICS OF α-SYNUCLEIN

Human Syn is a 140-amino-acid acidic protein of ~19 kDa originally isolated both from amyloid plaques of Alzheimer's disease brains as a protein called the precursor of the non-Aβ-amyloid component (or NAC) of plaques and from cholinergic vesicle preparations isolated from the electric organ of the ray *Torpedo californica*.[3,13,15] Syn is highly enriched in presynaptic terminals, where its immunoreactivity appears equally distributed between cytosolic and membrane fractions and where it is in close proximity to, but loosely associated with, synaptic vesicles.[17,20–22] It is widely expressed in various brain regions[3,13]—including the neocortex, hippocampus, dentate gyrus, olfactory bulb, thalamus, and cerebellum[21]—and also in the amygdala and nucleus accumbens.[14] Somata of dopamine neurons of the *SNpc* contain lower levels of Syn, which, in turn, may be accumulated inside the terminals of the corresponding projections in the striatum.[14,23]

Structurally (FIG. 1), the protein is composed of three modular protein domains:[3,13,24] a highly conserved amino terminal lipid binding α-helix (residues 1–61); a variable internal hydrophobic NAC domain (residues 61–95) that makes up the highly amyloidogenic part of the molecule and is the building block of Syn aggregates[11,25] with critical residues for the aggregation, or fibrillization, of the protein seen in LBs inside the "GAV motif" (residues 66–74)[26] ; and a variable carboxyl terminal acidic tail (residues 95–140) composed primarily of glutamate and aspartate residues that appears critical for the chaperone-like activity of Syn[24] and contains several consensus phosphorylation sites for protein tyrosine kinases and serine/threonine kinases.[3] Over half of the molecule (amino acids 7–87) is composed of seven imperfect repeat sequences of 11 amino acids, each with the core consensus sequence motif KTKEGV.[3,13,24] Although the function of these repeats is still unknown, the structure of Syn allows the molecule to exhibit different conformations depending on its interacting environment,[24] such as natively unfolded in solution,[3] an α-helical conformation upon binding to lipid vesicles,[27] or β-pleated sheets in its aggregated form,[11] suggesting highly dynamic structural changes depending upon the local cellular milieu. According to recent nuclear magnetic resonance studies,

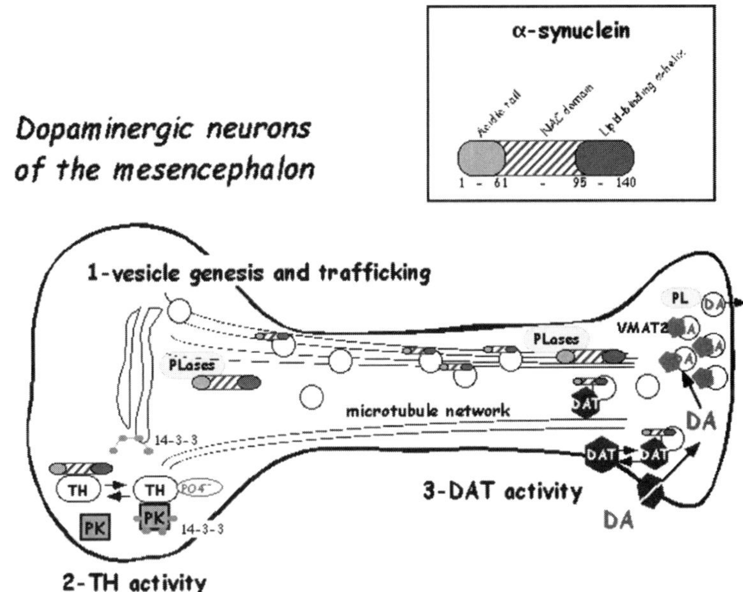

FIGURE 1. Schematic representation of the sites of action of α-synuclein on various components of the dopamine metabolic pathway in mesencephalic neurons. The three main parts of the Syn structure are schematically represented to highlight the multiple interactions discussed in the text: (1) In normal situations, or when synaptic plasticity needs to be increased, Syn contributes to the formation of synaptic vesicles, both by inhibiting phospholipase D activity (Plases) and by its lipid-binding properties. At the synaptic terminals, vesicles bearing the vesicular transporter, VMAT2, quickly and efficiently accumulate dopamine. (2) Syn modulates the activity of tyrosine hydroxylase (TH), the limiting enzyme of catecholamine biosynthesis, by preventing interactions with kinases (PK). In contrast, 14-3-3 proteins favor TH activity by enhancing TH phosphorylation by calmodulin kinases or ERKs. (3) The shuttling of dopamine transporter (DAT) to and away from the plasma membrane is also modified by the action of Syn, thereby changing the efficiency of dopamine uptake at the nerve terminals.

the lipid binding domain is composed of two α-helices that are interrupted by a short break when bound to phospholipids vesicles or synthetic membranes.[28] An *O*-glycosylated 22-kDa form of Syn is a specific substrate for the E3 ubiquitine ligase activity of parkin, which accumulates in autosomal recessive PD and leads to juvenile onset of the disease.[29]

Although the function(s) of Syn is still unknown, several lines of evidence suggest that it may be a chaperone protein, closely related to the function of 14-3-3 chaperone molecules, with whom it shares considerable sequence homology,[30] thus displaying pleiotropic effects in cells. Moreover, Syn may be involved in many molecular interactions, especially inside presynaptic terminals, which permits the protein to be implicated in the physiological maintenance of synaptic homeostasis and plasticity—a physiological function that may be altered in pathological conditions such as PD or other synucleinopathies.[15,17,19] Some of the physiological processes modulated by Syn may be quite general, such as synaptic vesicle formation,[17,20] neuronal development/synaptic plasticity,[15,31] regenerative sprouting of damaged axons,[32] or axonal transport[15,33], whereas others may be restricted to a given neuronal phenotype. In particular, Syn may be instrumental in the physiological maintenance of dopamine homeostasis and dopamine synaptic tone in dopaminergic neurons of the *SNpc* (FIG. 1), as already extensively reviewed by our groups[15,16] and others.[17,19,20] Data obtained by our groups show that one of the main consequences of the presence of Syn in dopaminergic nerve terminals is the modulatory effect it exerts on the trafficking and, thereby, on the activity of the dopamine transporter (DAT) of the plasma membrane of *SNpc* dopaminergic neurons.[15,16] Syn is also a possible transcriptional regulator of the expression of certain genes. Indeed, Syn was shown to decrease the expression of genes (such as the immediate early genes *c*-fos, and zif-68) modulated by the ERK (extracellular signal-regulated kinase) signaling pathway by decreasing the amount of phosphorylated ERK1/2[34] and thereby decreasing the phosphorylation of the transcription factor Elk-1 and its translocation to the nucleus, which normally mediates the transcription of ERK-dependent genes.[35] In addition, microarrays and quantitative RT-PCR in neuroblastoma cell lines transfected with either the *wt*, A30P, or A53T variants of Syn showed significant alterations in the expression of members of diverse groups of genes—such as stress response, transcription regulators, apoptosis-inducing molecules, transcription factors, and membrane-bound proteins[36]—and of the orphan nuclear receptor Nurr1, a transcription factor involved in the differentiation and maturation of catecholaminergic neurons.[36,37] There was also a coordinated downregulation by *wt* Syn, but not the A30P or A53T mutants, of various dopamine synthesis genes (see below) probably linked to the reduced expression of Nurr1.[36] Moreover, 51 signature transcripts, including lipid, energy, and membrane transport mRNAs, are tightly associated with Syn transgenic expression in *Drosophila*.[38]

GENERAL FUNCTIONS OF α-SYNUCLEIN

Is Wild-Type α-Synuclein Neuroprotective?

Some results in the literature are in accordance with a physiological role for Syn in neuroprotection and/or as an anti-apoptotic molecule for physiological concentrations of *wt* Syn, which may be partly lost by the two mutants, A30P and A53T, or after an overexpression of *wt* synuclein, or after exposure to certain neurotoxins. Hence, physiological concentrations of the *wt*, but not the A53T, variant of Syn reduce the activity and expression of pro-apoptotic proteins (caspase 3, p53) in neuronal TSM1 cells exposed to various apoptotic stimuli [staurosporine, etoposide, and ceramide C(2)]—the presence of 6-OHDA totally abolishing this anti-apoptotic effect of *wt* Syn.[39,40] Physiological concentrations of *wt* Syn, but not its A30P or A53T variants, were found to protect either cortical and hippocampal neurons, human pheochromocytoma PC12 cells differentiated into catecholaminergic cells, NT-2/D1 and SK-N-MC neuroblastoma cells, and the catecholaminergic human neuroblastoma SH-SY5Y cell line against the neurotoxicity induced by serum deprivation, H_2O_2-induced oxidative stress, and glutamate-induced excitotoxicity.[39,41–43] This anti-apoptotic effect of *wt* Syn seems to be mediated by a stimulation of the PI3/Akt signaling pathway,[42] followed by an increase in the expression levels of the anti-apoptotic protein Bcl-2,[42] and an inhibition of the activity of pro-apoptotic proteins. (There was increased phosphorylation of caspase-9, which inactivates this pro-apoptotic protein; there was also increased phosphorylation of the pro-apoptotic protein Bad, thereby decreasing its inhibitory interaction with the anti-apoptotic protein Bcl-xL and promoting Bcl-xL–dependent cell survival.)[39,41–43] *wt* Syn, but not its A30P or A53T variants, attenuated after serum deprivation the decreases of intracellular levels of reduced glutathione.[41] Similarly, a neuronal cell line stably expressing Syn was protected against H_2O_2-induced oxidative stress via an inactivation of the pro-apoptotic JNK signaling pathway secondary to an increased expression and activity of the JNK-interacting protein, JIP-1β/islet-brain (IB)1, the scaffold protein of the JNK pathway.[43] Moreover, Syn and JIP-1β/IB1 are colocalized in the axon growth cones of this neuronal cell line, suggesting that these two proteins are putative binding partners.[43] Similarly, the neurotoxicity of paraquat, a PD-linked neurotoxin, against *SNpc* dopaminergic neurons was strongly reduced in transgenic mice over-expressing either the *wt* or the A53T variant of Syn, compared to their control littermates, via an increase in the expression levels of the chaperone protein HSP-70 in the transgenic mice.[44] Recently, Jensen *et al.*[45] have shown that *wt* Syn, but not its A30P or A53T mutants, can protect nondifferentiated central nervous system dopaminergic cells from the neurotoxicity induced by either MPP^+ or rotenone—inhibitors of mitochondrial complex I that have been linked to the development of PD-like syndromes—or by 3-nitropropionic acid—an inhibitor of mitochondrial complex II.[45] Protection from MPP^+ was directly correlated with the preservation of mitochondrial function—that is, blockage of the MPP^+-induced decreases in mitochondrial dehydrogenase activity and loss of ATP levels by utilizing ketosis.[45] *wt* Syn-mediated neuroprotection and blockage of MPP^+-induced alterations in energy were not found in dibutyryl-cAMP-differentiated dopaminergic neuronal cells, suggesting that *wt* Syn may be neuroprotective or neurotoxic, depending on the levels of differentiation of the cells/neurons and/or that the normal physiological function of *wt* Syn may change during development.[45] Another possible explanation would be that the prevention of mitochondrial dysfunction in MPP^+-induced apoptosis by *wt* Syn might be lost in an age-dependent manner. In line with this hypothesis, the levels of Syn expression were markedly increased in NTera2 teratocarcinoma cells following retinoic acid–induced neuronal differentiation (a model of differentiated human neurons), suggesting that Syn expression in neurons may be upregulated during differentiation.[46] Indeed, rat Syn was highly and selectively upregulated at the mRNA and protein levels after 7 days of NGF (nerve growth factor) treatment, but was neither sufficient nor necessary for the neuritic sprouting that occurs within 1–2 days of NGF treatment.[47] These last results suggest that Syn upregulation may be a component of a late neuronal maturational response or plasticity.

The widely described upregulation of Syn expression by MPP^+ in various models of neurodegeneration has been recently linked to its neuroprotective action.[48,49] The highest increase in Syn expression after MPP^+ exposure of SH-SY5Y neuroblastoma cells was observed with the lowest, least toxic, concentrations of MPP[+] tested.[48] Parallel to the increase in Syn expression, MPP[+] induced in these cells an activation of the MEK1/2 and of the downstream ERK pathway, which is usually associated with cell proliferation or promoting cell survival, but not of the SAPK/JNK or p38MAPK kinase pathways, which are usually activated in conditions inducing cell death.[48]

The most compelling evidence of a possible role for Syn in neuroprotection was obtained in *in vivo* models of apoptotic death. Indeed, an upregulation of Syn was observed by mRNA differential display in a rodent model of apoptotic death of substantia nigra dopaminergic neurons induced by developmental injury to their target, the striatum.[50] Upregulation of Syn mRNA was associated with an increase in the number of neuronal profiles immunostained for Syn protein. At a cellular level, Syn was almost exclusively expressed in normal neurons rather than in apoptotic profiles, suggesting that upregulation of Syn expression may be a compensatory response in neurons destined to survive.[50] Moreover, Syn mRNA and protein expression were found to be reduced as substantia nigra dopaminergic neurons die after intrastriatal injection of 6-hydroxydopamine in rodents.[51] There was again a complete dissociation between apoptotic morphology and synuclein protein expression, suggesting that Syn may play a role in protection or restoration of the dopaminergic neurons which survive.[51] Similarly, no correlation between Syn expression and apoptotic death was observed in NGF-differentiated PC12 cells following trophic deprivation.[47] These observations are in accordance with the observation by ribonuclease protection assay that Syn mRNA was significantly decreased in the substantia nigra (but not in cortex) of PD patients compared to the control subjects.[52]

Inhibition of proteasome activity has been shown to induce cytoplasmic inclusions or aggresomes containing Syn, which have several morphologic and molecular similarities to LBs.[1,12] In HEK293T-transformed human embryonic kidney cells overexpressing both Syn and one of its interacting partner, synphilin-1, an inhibition of proteasome activity elicited the formation of juxtanuclear synphilin-1-containing aggresomes where the phosphorylated form of Syn colocalized. Interestingly, aggresomes were found in 60% of nonapoptotic cells but in only 10% of apoptotic cells, and inhibitors of apoptosis had no impact on the percentage of aggresome-positive cells, suggesting a disconnection between aggresome formation and apoptosis. These data suggested a neuroprotective role for these Syn inclusions from the toxicity associated with the combined overexpression of Syn and synphilin-1.[53]

α-Synuclein Effects on Synaptic Vesicles

As it is highly expressed in presynaptic terminals, a role for Syn in synaptic plasticity has been envisaged, given the strong modulation of Syn expression that has been observed in physiological situations of plastic remodeling of neuronal networks, such as song systems in birds or long-term potentiation in the mammalian hippocampus.[3,13,54] In particular, Syn knock-out mice exhibited significant impairments in synaptic response to tetanic stimulation, suggesting that Syn may regulate synaptic vesicle mobilization at nerve terminals.[55] Moreover, when Syn expression was knocked down with antisense oligonucleotides, cultured hippocampal neurons had fewer synaptic vesicles than were found in their control littermates, particularly in the reserve pool, and the replenishment of docked vesicles by reserve pool vesi-

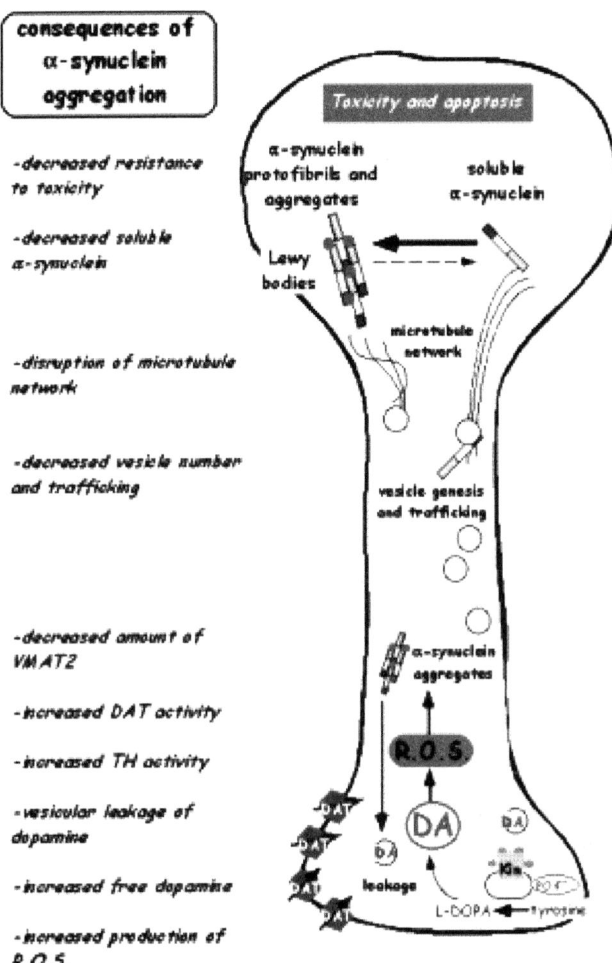

FIGURE 2. Overview of the consequences of α-synuclein aggregation that turn it from a neuroprotective to a toxic molecule. Formation of protofibrils or aggregates and LBs diminishes the availability of the physiological forms of soluble Syn. Consequences of this phenomenon are listed at left. Decreasing the availability of physiological Syn is favoring an increase in TH activity mediated by protein kinases and 14-3-3 proteins. It can also decrease the normal rate of synaptic vesicle formation, lowering thereby the amount of VMAT2 required to efficiently clear cytoplasmic dopamine. Then, lower amounts of physiological Syn at the nerve terminals promote the recruitment of the dopamine transporter (DAT) from a cytoplasmic compartment to the plasma membrane, increasing the load of extracellular dopamine into the neuronal cytoplasm. This contributes, overall, to increase free cytoplasmic dopamine and the formation of reactive oxygen species (ROS). This contrasts strikingly with the normal situation, where physiological Syn tends to decrease the amount of free dopamine inside neurons, and its possible bio-conversion into reactive and highly toxic species.

cles after depletion was slower in the mutant synapses.[56] Thus, Syn may be required for the genesis and/or maintenance of a reserve pool of presynaptic vesicles.[15,17,20] Syn-depleted neurons also exhibited decreased expression levels of synapsin,[56] an essential protein for synaptic vesicle recycling,[17] suggesting that a putative key function of Syn may be to regulate synaptic vesicle recycling (FIG. 2). This action of Syn may be partly mediated through the ability of its N-terminal repeat region (residues 7–87) to physically interact with, and inhibit, the activity of phospholipase D2 (PLD2) and, to a lesser, extent PLD1.[57,58] Activation of PLD2 in the plasma-lemmal endosomal membranes regulates the recycling of synaptic vesicles at or near the plasma membrane or endosomal compartments in response to external stimuli. It is also instrumental in vesicle formation through production of phosphatidic acid that recruits adaptor molecules, which, in turn, trigger the building of vesicles from donor membranes.[17,20] The modulation of vesicle recycling by Syn may also be partly mediated through its putative ability to transfer fatty acids, which are highly enriched in synaptic vesicles, to sites of synaptic vesicle formation (i.e., early endosomes) and/or regulate, as a lipid chaperone, the turnover or local organization of polyunsaturated fatty acid acyl groups, which have been implicated in clathrin-mediated endocytosis and, thus, in vesicle recycling.[17,20] These fatty acid-binding protein (FABP) properties of Syn rely on two observations: (1) Its N-terminal lipid (and vesicle) binding domain (residues 7–87) bears significant homology with the lipid-binding class A apolipoproteins, A2 and C1-3—proteins implicated in lipid transport[59] and which are major components of LBs.[1] (2) Short amino acyl stretches in Syn N- and C-termini share more than 55–67% identity with a cytosolic fatty acid–binding motif of FABPs.[59]

This regulatory effect of Syn on synaptic vesicle recycling may be tightly regulated by various seryl/threonyl or tyrosyl protein kinases.[15,17] Phosphorylation of Syn by G-protein–coupled receptor kinases, for example, lowers its ability to inhibit PLD2 activity and reduces its binding to phospholipids.[15,17] Thus, through reduction of its tonic inhibition of PLD2, phosphorylated Syn might promote vesicle recycling during periods of high neuronal activity and favor synaptic plasticity, whereas non-phosphorylated Syn may suppress synaptic vesicle formation during periods of low neuronal activity.[15] Moreover, the observed competition for Syn binding between calmodulin and artificial membranes suggests that the amount of membrane-bound Syn regulating PLD2 and therefore synaptic vesicle recycling may be regulated via an interaction between Syn and calmodulin, or via signalization pathways mobilizing calmodulin, as Syn and its familial PD-linked mutants bind to calmodulin in a Ca^{2+}-dependent manner.[15]

Finally, Syn has been suggested to interfere with axonal transport of synaptic vesicles by interacting with several proteins that either bind to or are part of the cytoskeleton, such as tubulin, *tau*, MAP1B, MAP2, synphilin-1, and torsin A.[15,60]

Nevertheless, these effects of Syn are very general and cannot account for a specific role in the neurodegeneration of dopaminergic neurons in PD. However, emerging studies suggest that the effects of Syn on synaptic vesicles may be responsible for affecting the vesicular content of dopamine in dopaminergic neurons, its storage, and its release into the synapse.[15,17,20] It is therefore likely that the physiological role of Syn in the regulation of synaptic vesicle formation and neuronal plasticity is probably impaired in dopaminergic neurons during the pathologic process of PD.

FUNCTIONS OF α-SYNUCLEIN IN DOPAMINERGIC NEURONS

α-Synuclein Regulates the Functional Activity of Tyrosine Hydroxylase, Modulating the Amount of Dopamine Synthesized

Dopamine synthesis depends on a rate-limiting step: the conversion of tyrosine into L-dopa by phosphorylated tyrosine hydroxylase [TH] before being converted into dopamine by the rather ubiquitous aromatic amino acid decarboxylase. Since only phosphorylated TH is active, the regulation of the phosphorylation/dephosphorylation of TH is primary in the regulation of dopamine biosynthesis.[15,19] In particular, there may be a reciprocal interplay between Syn and 14-3-3 proteins for the regulation of TH activity.[15,19,61] The binding of the chaperone protein, 14-3-3, to phospho-TH is necessary for maximal phosphorylation of the enzyme, protects TH from dephosphorylation, and increases the half-life of activated TH in neurons.[15,19] Syn colocalizes with TH and directly binds to the dephosphorylated form of TH; it tends to maintain TH in an inactive form in an opposite and symmetric manner to 14-3-3 proteins (FIG. 2), causing an overall net decrease in enzymatic activity and dopamine synthesis.[19,62] Since TH activity is dependent on the phosphorylation of the enzyme by several kinases, opposite actions of 14-3-3 protein and Syn on the activity of these kinases may also partly mediate their opposite action on TH activity.[15,19] Indeed, 14-3-3 proteins favor the activity of calcium-calmodulin-dependent kinases and of the mitogen-activated protein (MAP) kinase, ERK, by acting at different steps of the MAP kinase and protein kinase C pathways.[15,19,63] By contrast, Syn tends to inhibit the activity of ERK through its direct binding to the MAP kinase, an effect common with the A53T mutant.[34,35] This inhibitory effect of Syn can be extended to other kinases, such as calcium-calmodulin-dependent kinases and PKC, and contributes to dampening TH activity.[15] Another study also shows that *wt* Syn negatively modulates TH activity by decreasing its gene expression.[36]

Since the A30P and A53T mutants of Syn have the same inhibitory effects on TH activity as the *wt* protein,[19,62] some authors proposed that altered regulation of TH by the three Syn variants may not play a role in the pathogenesis of PD.[17] However, it is conceivable that aggregation of Syn during the pathological process of PD reduces the availability of the physiological form of the protein, leading to an increase in TH activity mediated by 14-3-3 protein as already hypothesized by our group[15] and others.[19] The resulting imbalance between the effects of Syn and 14-3-3 protein is highly deleterious since overproduction of cytosolic dopamine generates highly reactive oxidative species[15,19] Moreover, since certain isoforms of the 14-3-3 proteins are necessary to maintain, in an inactive form, pro-apoptotic proteins in the cytoplasm, such as Bad or the kinases Fkhrl1 and Ask1 (see ref. 61 and therein), the formation of complexes between 14-3-3 and Syn, when this latter tends to aggregate, lowers the ability of 14-3-3 proteins to inhibit several steps of the apoptotic process.[15,19] Trapping of 14-3-3 proteins by Syn during its aggregation certainly further contributes to render the dopamine-synthesizing neurons more sensitive to oxidative stress,[15,19,60] thereby initiating a vicious circle of cell injury and neurodegeneration.

wt Syn, but not its A30P and A53T mutants, also decreases the synthesis of dopamine by decreasing aromatic acid decarboxylase gene expression—and, therefore, the synthesis of its precursor L-dopa[36]—and by inhibiting the key enzymes involved in the production of tetrahydrobiopterin, a cofactor necessary for the catalytic activity of TH, including dihydropteridine reductase, GTP cyclohydrolase, and sepiapterin reductase.[36]

α-*Synuclein May Regulate the Storage of Catecholamines inside Synaptic Vesicles and Their Synaptic Release at Nerve Terminals*

In dopaminergic neurons, synthesized dopamine is immediately taken up into synaptic vesicles and stored through the activity of the vesicular monoamine transporter 2 (VMAT2), a transporter that uses the proton gradient across vesicular membranes as the driving force to sequester dopamine and other monoamines into vesicles.[64] The acidic pH environment of such storage vesicles hinders dopamine breakdown by spontaneous autoxidation and prevents its oxidative catabolism by monoamine oxidases.[64] Under normal conditions, efficient dopamine sequestration into storage vesicles is the major means by which dopamine neurons protect themselves from the deleterious effects of dopamine oxidation.[15,17,64] Moreover, the presence of VMAT2 in presynaptic vesicles attenuates the deleterious effect of MPTP (1-methyl-4-phenyl-1,2,3,6-tetrahydropyridine), a neurotoxin associated with the development of parkinsonian syndromes in human drug addicts. Indeed, in VMAT2-heterozygous knock-out mice, MPTP is twice as toxic as in wild-type mice, probably because VMAT2 is normally responsible for sequestrating MPP^+ (1-methyl-4-phenylpyridinium), the toxic metabolite of MPTP.[65,66]

Since Syn knock-out or knock-down mice show a decrease of paired-pulse depression in striatal terminals, Syn may act as a negative regulator of dopamine release into the synapse, probably via its inhibitory action on PLD2 activity.[15,17,20] The ability of nonphosphorylated Syn to suppress synaptic vesicle formation during periods of low neuronal activity may also be implicated in its negative modulatory effect on dopamine release (FIG. 2).[15] Indeed, PC12 pheochromocytoma cells expressing the A53T mutant, but not *wt* Syn, show a loss of both catecholamine-secreting dense core granules and of the capacity for depolarization-induced dopamine release.[67] These studies were later confirmed in human differentiated MESC2.10 mesencephalic cells, where the expression of the A53T mutant by lentiviral technology was found to decrease both potassium-induced dopamine release and vesicular dopamine storage through downregulation of the expression levels of VMAT2, but with an increase in amphetamine-mediated release of dopamine, indicating a depletion of vesicular dopamine and an accumulation of cytoplasmic dopamine.[68] A selective reduction in the number of dopamine storage vesicles or DA storage capacity may be a pathogenic feature of PD (FIG. 2) since *in vivo* positron emission tomography imaging studies of patients with idiopathic PD show a larger reduction of VMAT2 labeling than expected from measurement of neuronal loss marker by 18F-L-DOPA (18-fluoro-L-DOPA).[69] Moreover, Syn protofibrils with an annular shape, the most toxic species of Syn, may form integral pores in membranes,[70,71] including vesicular membranes, leading to dopamine leakage from the storage vesicles and increased levels of free cytoplasmic oxidizable dopamine in neurons, resulting in neuronal damage.[15,17]

α-*Synuclein Modulates the Functional Activity of the Dopamine Transporter*

As Syn, the dopamine transporter (DAT) is expressed in the presynaptic terminals of *SNpc* dopaminergic neurons where it mediates the re-uptake of dopamine back into the dopaminergic nerve terminals.[72] DAT is a member of a large gene family of Na^+- and Cl^--dependent transporters,[73,74] which share a common topology with 12 putative transmembrane domains, numerous consensus sequences for N-linked glycosylation, and putative phosphorylation sites for PKA, PKC, and calmodulin kinase II.[73,75] DAT is also the sole means by which the parkinsonian syndrome-inducing neurotoxin, MPP^+, the active metabolite of MPTP, is transported into nigral dopaminergic neurons, which preferentially degenerate in PD.[76] An enhanced DAT activity would increase intracellular levels of dopamine with a resulting increased oxidative stress within the dopaminergic neuron and neuronal death.[15,16] The regulation of DAT may thus be a crucial component in the maintenance of dopaminergic neurotransmission and the integrity of dopaminergic neurons (FIG. 2). The principal means by which DAT function is regulated is through the rapid and transient shuttling of the transporter molecule to and from the plasma membrane.[75] Reduced DAT activity may be directly correlated to a possible phosphorylation of DAT by kinases, causing its rapid redistribution and internalization away from the plasma membrane.[15,16,75] Participation of kinases, such as protein kinase C, which are dynamically activated by changes in intracellular (Ca^{2+}) levels, suggests rapid adaptations of the neuron to attenuate DAT function in response to signal transduction–induced changes in cellular calcium fluxes.[75] Interestingly, phosphorylation of the DAT by the MAP kinases, ERK1/2, upon signal transduction at the neuronal plasma membrane, was recently shown to increase the amount of DAT at the cell surface and dopamine re-uptake.[77] Since Syn binds to the MAP kinase ERK and tends to inhibit its activity,[34,35] it is very likely that the presence of Syn at the nerve terminals tends to blur the MAP kinase activity and decrease the amount of DAT at the cell surface of dopaminergic nerve terminals.

In agreement with these last results, our laboratories[15,16] have shown that upon transient co-expression in L*tk*$^-$ fibroblasts, or in basal conditions in mesencephalic neurons, wild-type (*wt*) human Syn tends to markedly decrease (by 30–50%) the activity of the human DAT by reducing the re-uptake of dopamine.[78,79] This *wt* Syn-mediated attenuation of DAT activity was because of a decrease in dopamine uptake velocity by the transporter without any changes in either its affinity for dopamine or its expression levels. As a consequence, there was diminished dopamine-induced oxidative stress and cytotoxicity upon exposure of transiently cotransfected cells to dopamine. In the presence of *wt* Syn, the transporter was dynamically trafficked away from the plasma membrane into the cytoplasm, as indexed by reduced DAT presence at the plasma membrane by biotinylation experiments (FIG. 2).[79] Co-immunoprecipitation studies showed that *wt* Syn can form a protein:protein heteromeric complex with the DAT via direct protein interactions between the NAC domain (residues 58–107) of Syn and the last 22 amino acids of the carboxy-terminal (CT) tail of DAT, both in cotransfected cell lines, rat substantia nigra, and rat primary mesencephalic neurons.[79] The A30P mutant also attenuated DAT function in a similar way to *wt* Syn by trafficking the DAT away from the plasma membrane, as indexed by biotinylation experiments, again via the formation of a DAT:A30P heteromeric protein:protein complex mediated through interactions between the NAC domain (residues 58–107) of A30P and the last 22 amino acids of the CT tail of DAT.[80,81] Interestingly, the A53T mutant was unable to modulate DAT function, and subsequent studies showed that this protein only very weakly interacted with the DAT.[80]

In an earlier study, *wt* Syn was found to have an opposite effect on DAT—that is, to increase the functional activity of the transporter.[82] This discrepancy is probably owing to the fact that the cells used in this study were batch-transfected and exposed to trypsin after transfection,[81] suggesting that cell adhesion may play a role in dictating the functional outcome of DAT:Syn interactions. Hence, mild trypsinization of cotransfected cells or neurons, under conditions that do not cause cell dissociation, reversed the attenuation of DAT function by *wt* Syn, increasing the presence of DAT at the cell surface.[79,81] Interestingly, our results showed that the parkinsonian syndrome–inducing agent, MPP^+, whose transport into cells occurs specifically through the DAT, reversed the inhibitory effects of Syn on the activity of the transporter—that is, induced a dysregulation of the Syn-mediated regulation of DAT activity.[79] Under all experimental conditions where the control of DAT activity by Syn was dysregulated, there was increased re-uptake of dopamine and dopamine-induced neurotoxicity,[79] suggesting that disruption of the ability of Syn to regulate DAT function may be an important determinant in the genesis of dopaminergic neurodegeneration (FIG. 2).

DOPAMINE-LINKED ABERRATIONS CONVERT α-SYNUCLEIN INTO A TOXIC MOLECULE

This overview of the putative physiological functions of Syn shows a tight link between the general roles of *wt* Syn in neurons and the regulation of dopaminergic tone in dopaminergic neurons while highlighting and reconciling the ubiquitous nature of Syn expression in the brain with the relative specificity of degeneration of the *SNpc* dopaminergic neurons in PD.[15,16] In the normal brain, *wt* Syn may have a neuroprotective effect by increasing the activity/expression of some anti-apoptotic molecules and decreasing the expression/activity of pro-apoptotic molecules.[39–45] In normal *SNpc* dopaminergic neurons, in addition to this neuroprotective effect, Syn tends to turn down the amount of cytoplasmic dopamine in dopaminergic nerve terminals, thereby limiting its conversion to highly reactive oxidative species and the resulting oxidative stress.[15,16] Indeed, the nonaggregated, physiological form of Syn is able to (1) decrease the activity of TH;[19,62] (2) regulate the availability of synaptic vesicles and the storage of dopamine mediated by VMAT2;[17,20,68] and (3) reduce the maximal DAT-mediated re-uptake of dopamine from the nigrostriatal synapse.[15,16,78,79]

However, as soon as Syn begins to form protofibrils and/or aggregates, the bioavailability of the physiological form of Syn is decreased and the toxic potential of dopamine at nerve terminals is increased since the protein can no longer participate in the intricate physiological processes necessary for the maintenance of healthy dopaminergic neurons.[15,16] These series of events will favor an accumulation of free dopamine in the neuronal cytosol—an intraneuronal production of highly toxic, dopamine-derived, oxidative species, and oxidative stress—through (1) relief of the inhibitory mechanism exerted by Syn on TH activity and/or its phosphorylation-dependent regulation;[15,19] (2) impaired storage of dopamine into synaptic vesicles via both alterations in synaptic vesicles formation/recycling and induction of dopamine leakage out of the vesicles through permeabilization of the vesicular membrane by protofibrils;[17,83] and (3) increase in the amount of extracellular dopamine taken up by the DAT.[15,16] The accumulated, free intracellular dopamine, in turn, favors the formation of more protofibrils since dopamine and L-DOPA were shown to disaggregate Syn amyloid fibrils.[84] Thus, a vicious circle of events is triggered, which may significantly contribute to the rather specific degeneration of the dopaminergic *SNpc* neurons in human PD (FIG. 3).

This hypothesis certainly does not recapitulate all the possible mechanisms envisaged to exist at the onset of PD, but it has the merit to include other well-demonstrated components of PD etiology, including genetic components and toxins, which may all enter, at multiple entry points, into the deleterious cycle of Syn aggregation and reactive oxygen species production (FIG. 3). Starting from the formation of Syn protofibrils, it is clear that free radicals, such as free iron or iron-centered radicals[85] and oxidized dopamine,[9,84] and catecholamines structurally related to dopamine,[9] accelerate and stabilize the formation of Syn protofibrils, the most toxic species of Syn,[18,83] by inhibiting the conversion of toxic soluble protofibrils into insoluble fibrils.[9,84] The formation of Syn protofibrils is also clearly facilitated by the A53T mutation in the Syn sequence or increased expression levels of Syn, as shown both *in vitro*[86] and in transgenic animals.[87,88] Interestingly, expression of human recombinant Syn carrying both substitution mutations (A30P and A53T) in nigrostriatal terminals, resulted in a slightly but nonsignificant increased density of the DAT and enhanced toxicity to the neurotoxin MPTP.[88] In transgenic *Drosophila*, the neuronal degeneration resulting from the formation of Syn aggregates is preferentially found in neurons that express TH and DAT.[89] These findings support the view of a close link between Syn and components of the dopaminergic neurons in the pathophysiological process of PD neurodegeneration.[15,16] Thus, it should be stressed again that Syn is by no means cytotoxic in itself, but that, on the contrary, significant levels of nonaggregated *wt* Syn tend to protect neurons against several neurotoxic events, including oxidative stress.[39–45]

The level of protofibrils and aggregated forms of Syn is also likely to be modulated through the ubiquitin-proteasome pathway.[90] Interestingly, the nonaggregated form of Syn cannot be ubiquitinated by the protein parkin, one of the genes which, when mutated, is linked to early-onset familial PD.[29] Parkin is an E3 ligase required to transfer ubiquitin onto proteins targeted for proteasome degradation and, in transgenic flies, overexpression of parkin can mitigate Syn-induced neuritic pathology and suppress its toxicity.[91] A causal link between a decrease in proteasomal degradation and high amounts of Syn aggregates has not yet been demonstrated. However, UCH-L1 (ubiquitin carboxy-terminal hydrolase L1), another gene linked to a familial form of PD, is also a component of the ubiquitination pathway, rendering even more probable the involvement of this degradation pathway in the pathological process linking Syn aggregation to neuronal degeneration.[12]

Still another well-demonstrated entry point into the parkinsonian neurodegeneration is exposure to toxins triggering oxidative stress in dopamine neurons. In this respect, studies linking MPP[+] and Syn effects highlight the central role of the determinants of dopaminergic systems in the induction of the processes leading to Syn toxicity (FIG. 3). Here, the expression of DAT confers the selectivity of MPP[+] towards *SNpc* dopaminergic neurons.[15,16] Once in the dopaminergic neurons, MPP[+]

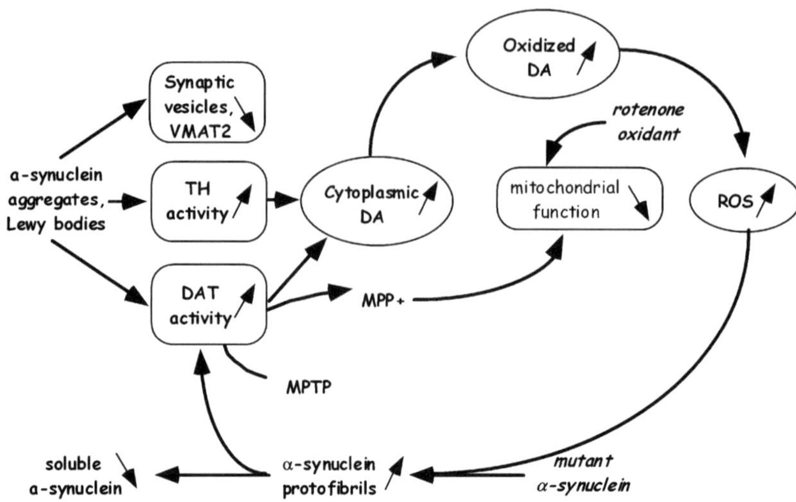

FIGURE 3. The cycle of deleterious interactions between α-synuclein and dopamine. The formation of protofibrils and aggregates by Syn and the oxidative stress triggered by free dopamine in neurons can be a self-maintained cycle, which ultimately may promote preferential degeneration of dopaminergic neurons of the substantia nigra in PD. Several well-known etiological factors of PD could enter the cycle at different point by either directly enhancing oxidative stress (rotenone, MPTP) or by altering the cellular milieu, thereby favoring the aggregation of Syn (Syn mutants and other mutants).

inhibits complex I of the mitochondrial respiratory chain, releasing cytochrome c, which accelerates aggregation of Syn[92]—ultimately affecting the properties of Syn. The presence of *wt* Syn and its A53T mutant has been shown to increase the vulnerability of cells to MPP[+] exposure.[93] Interestingly, Syn null mice are essentially resistant to MPTP-induced degeneration of dopaminergic neurons and dopamine release, and this resistance is because of an inability of the toxin to inhibit complex I of the mitochondria.[94] This further suggests that Syn has a facilitative role in enhancing, either directly or indirectly, the observed toxicity of MPP[+].[15,16]

Formation of protofibrils and aggregation of Syn may also dampen the "anti-apoptotic" and neuroprotective effects of the physiological concentrations of *wt* Syn, and the protein may become pro-apoptotic with an increased expression and/or activity of the neurotoxic JNKs, in particular. Some of the anti-apoptotic and neuroprotective effects of *wt* Syn may also be lost by the familial PD-linked mutants.[43] Exposure to certain neurotoxins, such as 6-OHDA,[39] has also been shown to block the neuroprotective function of *wt* Syn. Finally, an overexpression of the protein may block its neuroprotective properties. Indeed, supraphysiological concentrations of the *wt* protein have been shown to be pro-apoptotic in the study of Seo *et al.*,[42] secondary to increased expression levels and activity of numerous pro-apoptotic proteins, such as Bax, Bad, or caspase 3, among others. The intraneuronal expression levels of the protein can increase either as a result of its overexpression, which can be induced by some neurotoxins—in particular, dopaminergic neurotoxins, such as

MPP[+15,16]—or as a result of alterations in the degradation of the protein.[1,2,90] In line with a pro-apoptotic effect of high-expression levels of either *wt* Syn or its mutants, our group has recently shown[95] the following in dopamine-treated human SH-SY5Y neuroblastoma cells transiently co-expressing the human DAT, and either *wt*, A30P, or A53T variant of Syn: (1) Low expression levels of *wt* Syn, reminiscent of the expression levels found in normal rat substantia nigra,[14] reduced dopamine-induced oxidative stress and cell death compared to cells expressing human DAT alone by negatively regulating human DAT activity, as extensively shown by our group[15,16]—an effect that may be considered as neuroprotective. (2) In the presence of high-expression levels of A30P and, to a lesser extend, *wt* Syn, dopamine accelerated production of reactive oxygen species and cell death compared to cells expressing only DAT.[95] (3) High-expression levels of A53T only slightly increased dopamine-induced oxidative stress and cell death compared to cells expressing only DAT.[95] High-expression levels of both *wt* Syn and A30P and dopamine caused rapid decreases in levels of intracellular potassium, which is indicative of a possible inhibition of the plasmalemmal Na^+/K^+-ATPase. This is then followed by mitochondrial damage and cytochrome *c* leakage, and finally decreased cellular metabolism and depletion of metabolic energy assessed by high-resolution NMR, compared to cells expressing only human DAT; high levels of A53T, however, only slightly affected these parameters compared to cells expressing only DAT.[95] A similar pathologic staging of neurotoxicity was seen in dopamine-treated rat primary mesencephalic neuronal cultures, suggesting its pathophysiological relevance.[95] The lower amount of Syn immunoreactivity observed by us in the substantia nigra, compared to other brain areas, suggests that nigral dopaminergic neurons may be particularly vulnerable to a pathological increase in Syn protein levels (see ref. 14 and citations therein).

A striking aspect of our studies is the absence of any modulation by the A53T mutant of Syn on DAT function[15,16] and the observation of a differential cytotoxicity induced by the A53T compared to the two other variants of Syn.[80,95] These observations suggest a different mode of action, for the A53T, in inducing cell death. Interestingly, with increased levels of cytosolic dopamine, the A53T mutant decreased the protein expression levels of VMAT2 in a mesencephalic cell line and enhanced superoxide production and cytotoxicity.[68] Although the mechanisms of the A53T-induced depletion of VMAT2 is not known, it is probable that a decrease in the number of synaptic vesicles plays a role in this decreased amount of VMAT2 inside the synapses. These observations suggest that the effect of the A53T on the vesicular storage of dopamine and on the expression levels of VMAT2 may be particularly important in the pathomechanism of the neurodegeneration induced by this mutant form of Syn.

To conclude, there is ample evidence to propose that, overall, Syn in itself is not a toxic compound, but that it can be converted to a toxic compound in the presence of specific components of the dopaminergic systems, thereby conferring the selectivity for degeneration for the *SNpc* dopaminergic neurons characteristic of PD.[15–17,19] Through its peculiar biochemical properties, Syn is able to interact differently with numerous molecular systems, contributing in more than one way to the pathophysiology of PD. Considering Syn as a central regulator of the dopamine life cycle, and as an effector of dopamine-dependent oxidative stress, paves the way for a more accurate understanding of both the physiology and the pathology of dopamine neurotransmission.

ACKNOWLEDGMENTS

This work was supported in part by grants from the National Institutes of Health (NS-34914 and NS-45326).

REFERENCES

1. MARIES, E., B. DASS, T.J. COLLIER, *et al.* 2003. The role of alpha-synuclein in Parkinson's disease: insights from animal models. Nat. Rev. Neurosci. **4:** 727–738.
2. GOEDERT, M. 2001. Alpha-synuclein and neurodegenerative diseases. Nat. Rev. Neurosci. **2:** 492–501.
3. GEORGE, J.M. 2002. The synucleins. Genome Biol. **3:** 1–6.
4. GOEDERT, M. & M.G. SPILLANTINI. 1998. Lewy body diseases and multiple system atrophy as alpha-synucleinopathies. Mol. Psychiatry **3:** 462–465.
5. POLYMEROPOULOS, M.H., C. LAVEDAN, E. LEROY, *et al.* 1997. Mutation in the alpha-synuclein gene identified in families with Parkinson's disease. Science **276:** 2045–2047.
6. KRUGER, R., W. KUHN, T. MULLER, *et al.* 1998. Ala30Pro mutation in the gene encoding alpha-synuclein in Parkinson's disease. Nat. Genet. **18:** 106–108.
7. CHAN, P., X. JIANG, L.S. FORNO, *et al.* 1998. Absence of mutations in the coding region of the alpha-synuclein gene in pathologically proven Parkinson's disease. Neurology **50:** 1136–1137.
8. SCOTT, W.K., L.H. YAMAOKA & J.M. STAJICH. 1999. The alpha-synuclein gene is not a major risk factor in familial Parkinson disease. Neurogenetics **2:** 191–192.
9. CONWAY, K.A., J.C. ROCHET, R.M. BIEGANSKI, *et al.* 2001. Kinetic stabilization of the alpha-synuclein protofibril by a dopamine-alpha-synuclein adduct. Science **294:** 1346–1349.
10. GOEDERT, M., M.G. SPILLANTINI & S.W. DAVIES. 1998. Filamentous nerve cell inclusions in neurodegenerative diseases. Curr. Opin. Neurobiol. **8:** 619–632.
11. EL-AGNAF, O.M. & G.B. IRVINE. 2002. Aggregation and neurotoxicity of alpha-synuclein and related peptides. Biochem. Soc. Trans. **30:** 559–565.
12. DAWSON, T.M. & V.L. DAWSON. 2003. Molecular pathways of neurodegeneration in Parkinson's disease. Science **302:** 819–822.
13. CLAYTON, D.F. & J.M. GEORGE. 1998. The synucleins: a family of proteins involved in synaptic function, plasticity, neurodegeneration and disease. Trends Neurosci. **21:** 249–254.
14. WERSINGER, C., M. BANTA & A. SIDHU. 2004. Comparative analyses of alpha-synuclein expression levels in rat brain tissues and transfected cells. Neurosci. Lett. **358:** 95–98.
15. SIDHU, A., C. WERSINGER & P. VERNIER. 2004. Does alpha-synuclein modulate dopaminergic synaptic content and tone at the synapse? FASEB J. **18:** 637–647.
16. SIDHU, A., C. WERSINGER & P. VERNIER. 2004. Alpha-synuclein regulation of the dopaminergic transporter: a possible role in the pathogenesis of Parkinson's disease. FEBS Lett. **565:** 1–5.
17. LOTHARIUS, J. & P. BRUNDIN. 2002. Impaired dopamine storage resulting from alpha-synuclein mutations may contribute to the pathogenesis of Parkinson's disease. Hum. Mol. Genet. **11:** 2395–2407.
18. LEE, H.J. & S.J. LEE. 2002. Characterization of cytoplasmic alpha-synuclein aggregates: fibril formation is tightly linked to the inclusion-forming process in cells. J. Biol. Chem. **277:** 48976–48983.
19. PEREZ, R.G. & T.G. HASTINGS. 2004. Could a loss of α-synuclein function put dopaminergic neurons at risk? J. Neurochem. **89:** 1318–1324.
20. LOTHARIUS, J. & P. BRUNDIN. 2002. Pathogenesis of Parkinson's disease: dopamine, vesicles and α-synuclein. Nat. Rev. Neurosci. **3:** 932–942.
21. IWAI, A., E. MASLIAH, M. YOSHIMOTO, *et al.* 1995. The precursor protein of non-Aβ component of Alzheimer's disease amyloid is a presynaptic protein of the central nervous system. Neuron **14:** 467–475.
22. KAHLE, P.J., M. NEUMANN, L. OZMAN, *et al.* 2000. Subcellular localization of wild-type and Parkinson's disease-associated mutant α-synuclein in human and transgenic mouse brain. J. Neurosci. **20:** 6365–6373.

23. GALVIN, J.E., T.M. SCHUCK, V.M. LEE & J.Q. TROJANOWSKI. 2001. Differential expression and distribution of alpha-, beta-, and gamma-synuclein in the developing human substantia nigra. Exp. Neurol. **168:** 347–355.

24. UVERSKY, V.N. 2003. A protein-chameleon: conformational plasticity of alpha-synuclein, a disordered protein involved in neurodegenerative disorders. J. Biomol. Struct. Dyn. **21:** 211–234.

25. GIASSON, B.I., I.V. MURRAY, J.Q. TROJANOWSKI & V.M. LEE. 2001. A hydrophobic stretch of 12 amino acid residues in the middle of alpha-synuclein is essential for filament assembly. J. Biol. Chem. **276:** 2380–2386.

26. DU, H.N., L. TANG, X.Y. LUO, *et al.* 2003. A peptide motif consisting of glycine, alanine, and valine is required for the fibrillization and cytotoxicity of human alpha-synuclein. Biochemistry **42:** 8870–8878.

27. DAVIDSON, W.S., A. JONAS, D.F. CLAYTON & J.M. GEORGE. 1998. Stabilization of alpha-synuclein secondary structure upon binding to synthetic membranes. J. Biol. Chem. **273:** 9443–9449.

28. CHANDRA, S., X. CHEN, J. RIZO, *et al.* 2003. A broken alpha-helix in folded alpha-synuclein. J. Biol. Chem. **278:** 15313–15318.

29. SHIMURA, H., M.G. SCHLOSSMACHER, N. HATTORI, *et al.* 2001. Ubiquitination of a new form of alpha-synuclein by parkin from human brain: implications for Parkinson's disease. Science **293:** 263–269.

30. OSTREROVA, N., L. PETRUCELLI, M. FARRER, *et al.* 1999. Alpha-synuclein shares physical and functional homology with 14-3-3 proteins. J. Neurosci. **19:** 5782–5791.

31. EELLS, J.B. 2003. The control of dopamine neuron development, function and survival: insights from transgenic mice and the relevance to human disease. Curr. Med. Chem. **10:** 857–870.

32. QUILTY, M.C., W.P. GAI, D.L. POUNTNEY, *et al.* 2003. Localization of alpha-, beta-, and gamma-synuclein during neuronal development and alterations associated with the neuronal response to axonal trauma. Exp. Neurol. **182:** 195–207.

33. JENSEN, P.H. & W.P. GAI. 2001. Alpha-synuclein: axonal transport, ligand interaction and neurodegeneration. Adv. Exp. Med. Biol. **487:** 129–134.

34. IWATA, A., M. MARUYAMA, I. KANAZAWA & N. NUKINA. 2001. Alpha-synuclein affects the MAPK pathway and accelerates cell death. J. Biol. Chem. **276:** 45320–45329.

35. IWATA, A., S. MIURA, I. KANAZAWA, *et al.* 2001. Alpha-synuclein forms a complex with transcription factor Elk-1. J. Neurochem. **77:** 239–252.

36. BAPTISTA, M.J., C. O'FARRELL, S. DAYA, *et al.* 2003. Co-ordinate transcriptional regulation of dopamine synthesis genes by alpha-synuclein in human neuroblastoma cell lines. J. Neurochem. **85:** 957–968.

37. SATOH, J. & Y. KURODA. 2002. The constitutive and inducible expression of Nurr1, a key regulator of dopaminergic neuronal differentiaton, in human neural and non-neural cell lines. Neuropathology **22:** 219–232.

38. SCHERZER, C.R., R.V. JENSEN, S.R. GULLANS & M.B. FEANY. 2003. Gene expression changes presage neurodegeneration in a *Drosophila* model of Parkinson's disease. Hum. Mol. Genet. **12:** 2457–2466.

39. ALVES DA COSTA, C., K. ANCOLIO & F. CHECLER. 2000. Wild-type but not Parkinson's disease-related ala-53→Thr mutant alpha-synuclein protects neuronal cells from apoptotic stimuli. J. Biol. Chem. **275:** 24065–24069.

40. ALVES DA COSTA, C., E. PAITEL, B. VINCENT. & F. CHECLER. 2002. Alpha-synuclein lowers p53-dependent apoptotic response of neuronal cells: abolishment by 6-hydroxydopamine and implications for Parkinson's disease. J. Biol. Chem. **277:** 50980–50984.

41. LEE, M.H., D.H. HYUN, B. HALLIWELL & P. JENNER. 2001. Effect of the overexpression of wild-type or mutant alpha-synuclein on cell susceptibility to insult. J. Neurochem. **76:** 998–1009.

42. SEO, J.H., J.C. RAH, S.H. CHOI, *et al.* 2002. Alpha-synuclein regulates neuronal survival via Bcl-2 family expression and PI3/Akt kinase pathway. FASEB J. **16:** 1826–1828.

43. HASHIMOTO, M., L.J. HSU, E. ROCKENSTEIN, *et al.* 2002. Alpha-synuclein protects against oxidative stress via inactivation of the c-Jun N-terminal kinase stress-signaling pathway in neuronal cells. J. Biol. Chem. **277:** 11465–11472.

44. MANNING-BOG, A.B., A.L. MCCORMACK, M.G. PURISAI, *et al.* 2003. Alpha-synuclein overexpression protects against paraquat-induced neurodegeneration. J. Neurosci. **23:** 3095–3099.
45. JENSEN, P.J., B.J. ALTER & K.L. O'MALLEY. 2003. Alpha-synuclein protects naïve but not dbcAMP-treated dopaminergic cell types from 1-methyl-4-phenylpyridinium toxicity. J. Neurochem. **86:** 196–209.
46. SATOH, J.I. & Y. KURODA. 2001. Alpha-synuclein expression is up-regulated in NTera2 cells during neuronal differentiation but unaffected by exposure to cytokines and neurotrophic factors. Parkinsonism Relat. Disord. **8:** 7–17.
47. STEFANIS, L., N. KHOLODILOV, H.J. RIDEOUT, *et al.* 2001. Synuclein-1 is selectively up-regulated in response to nerve growth factor treatment in PC12 cells. J. Neurochem. **76:** 1165–1176.
48. GOMEZ-SANTOS, C., I. FERRER, J. REIRIZ, *et al.* 2002. MPP+ increases alpha-synuclein expression and ERK/MAP-kinase phosphorylation in human neuroblastoma SH-SY5Y cells. Brain Res. **935:** 32–39.
49. KALIVENDI, S.V., S. CUNNINGHAM, S. KOTAMRAJU, *et al.* Alpha-synuclein up-regulation and aggregation during MPP$^+$-induced apoptosis in neuroblastoma cells: intermediacy of transferring receptor iron and hydrogen peroxide. J. Biol. Chem. **279:** 15240–15247.
50. KHOLODILOV, N.G., T.F. OO & R.E. BURKE. 1999. Synuclein expression is decreased in rat substantia nigra following induction of apoptosis by intrastriatal 6-hydroxy-dopamine. Neurosci. Lett. **275:** 105–108.
51. KHOLODILOV, N.G., M. NEYSTAT, T.F. OO, *et al.* 1999. Increased expression of at synuclein in the substantia nigra pars ompacta identified by mRNA differential display in a model of developmental target injury. J. Neurochem. **73:** 2586–2599.
52. NEYSTAT, M., T. LYNCH, S. PRZEDBORSKI, *et al.* Alpha synuclein expression in substantia nigra and cortex in Parkinson's disease. Mov. Disord. **14:** 417–422.
53. TANAKA, M., Y.M. KIM, G. LEE, *et al.* 2004. Aggresomes formed by alpha-synuclein and synphilin-1 are cytoprotective. J. Biol. Chem. **279:** 4625–4631.
54. STEPHAN, A., S. DAVIS, H. SALIN, *et al.* 2002. Age-dependent differential regulation of genes encoding APP and alpha-synuclein in hippocampal synaptic plasticity. Hippocampus **12:** 55–62.
55. ABELIOVICH, A., Y. SCHMITZ, I. FARINAS, *et al.* 2000. Mice lacking alpha-synuclein display functional deficits in the nigrostriatal pathway. Neuron **25:** 239–252.
56. CABIN, D.E., K. SHIMAZU, D. MURPHY, *et al.* 2002. Synaptic vesicle depletion correlates with attenuated synaptic responses to prolonged repetitive stimulation in mice lacking alpha-synuclein. J. Neurosci. **22:** 8797–8807.
57. JENCO, J.M., A. RAWLINGSON, B. DANIELS & A.J. MORRIS. 1998. Regulation of phospholipase D2: selective inhibition of mammalian phospholipase D isoenzymes by α- and β-synucleins. Biochemistry **37:** 4901–4909.
58. AHN, B.H., H. RHIM, S.Y. KIM, *et al.* 2002. α-Synuclein interacts with phospholipase D isozymes and inhibits pervanadate induced phospholipase D activation in human embryonic kidney 293 cells. J. Biol. Chem. **277:** 12334–12342.
59. SHARON, R., M.S. GOLDBERG, I. BAR-JOSEF, *et al.* 2001. Alpha-synuclein occurs in lipid-rich high molecular weight complexes, binds fatty acids, and shows homology to the fatty acid-binding proteins. Proc. Natl. Acad. Sci. USA **98:** 9110–9115.
60. PAYTON, J.E., R.J. PERRIN, D.F. CLAYTON & J.M. GEORGE. 2001. Protein-protein interactions of alpha-synuclein in brain homogenates and transfected cells. Brain Res. Mol. Brain Res. **95:** 138–145.
61. XU, J., S.Y. KAO, F.J. LEE, *et al.* 2002. Dopamine-dependent neurotoxicity of alpha-synuclein: a mechanism for selective neurodegeneration in Parkinson's disease. Nat. Med. **8:** 600–606.
62. PEREZ, R.G., J.C. WAYMIRE, E. LIN, *et al.* 2002. A role for α-synuclein in the regulation of dopamine biosynthesis. J. Neurosci. **22:** 3090–3099.
63. TOSKA, K., R. KLEPPE, C.G. ARMSTRONG, *et al.* 2002. Regulation of tyrosine hydroxylase by stress-activated protein kinases. J. Neurochem. **83:** 775–783.
64. WEIHE, E. & L.E. EIDEN. 2000. Chemical neuroanatomy of the vesicular amine transporters. FASEB J. **14:** 2435–2449.

65. GAINETDINOV, R.R., F. FUMAGALLI, Y.M. WANG, *et al.* 1998. Increased MPTP neurotoxicity in vesicular monoamine transporter 2 heterozygote knockout mice. J. Neurochem. **70:** 1973–1978.

66. UHL, G.R., S. LI, N. TAKAHASHI, *et al.* 2000. The VMAT2 gene in mice and humans: amphetamine responses, locomotion, cardiac arrhythmias, aging, and vulnerability to dopaminergic toxins. FASEB J. **14:** 2459–2465.

67. STEFANIS, L., K.E. LARSEN, H.J. RIDEOUT, *et al.* 2001. Expression of A53T mutant but not wild-type alpha-synuclein in PC12 cells induces alterations of the ubiquitin-dependent degradation system, loss of dopamine release, and autophagic cell death. J. Neurosci. **21:** 9549–9560.

68. LOTHARIUS, J., S. BARG, P. WIEKOP, *et al.* 2002. Effect of mutant alpha-synuclein on dopamine homeostasis in a new human mesencephalic cell line. J. Biol. Chem. **277:** 38884–38894.

69. LEE, C.S., A. SAMII, V. SOSSI, *et al.* 2000. In vivo positron emission tomographic evidence for compensatory changes in presynaptic dopaminergic nerve terminals in Parkinson's disease. Ann. Neurol. **47:** 493–503.

70. VOLLES, M.J. & P.T.. LANSBURY, JR. 2002. Vesicle permeabilization by protofibrillar alpha-synuclein is sensitive to Parkinson's disease-linked mutations and occurs by a pore-like mechanism. Biochemistry **41:** 4595–4602.

71. LASHUEL, H.A., B.M. PETRE, J. WALL, *et al.* 2002. Alpha-synuclein, especially the Parkinson's disease-associated mutants, forms pore-like annular and tubular protofibrils. J. Mol. Biol. **322:** 1089–1092.

72. CHEN, N. & M.E. REITH. 2000. Structure and function of the dopamine transporter. Eur. J. Pharmacol. **405:** 329–339.

73. NELSON, N. 1998. The family of Na+/Cl- neurotransmitter transporters. J. Neurochem. **71:** 1785–1803.

74. TORRES, G.E., R.R. GAINETDINOV & M.G. CARON. 2003. Plasma membrane monoamine transporters: structure, regulation and function. Nat. Rev. Neurosci. **4:** 13–25.

75. ZAHNISER, N.R. & S. DOOLEN. 2001. Chronic and acute regulation of Na^+/Cl^--dependent neurotransmitter transporters: drugs, substrates, presynaptic receptors, and signaling systems. Pharmacol. Ther. **92:** 21–55.

76. GAINETDINOV, R.R., F. FUMAGALLI, S.R. JONES & M.G. CARON. 1997. Dopamine transporter is required for in vivo MPTP neurotoxicity: evidence from mice lacking the transporter. J. Neurochem. **69:** 1322–1325.

77. MORON, J.A., I. ZAKHAROVA, J.V. FERRER, *et al.* 2003. Mitogen-activated protein kinase regulates dopamine transporter surface expression and dopamine transport capacity. J. Neurosci. **23:** 8480–8488.

78. WERSINGER, C. & A. SIDHU. 2003. Attenuation of dopamine transporter activity by alpha-synuclein. Neurosci. Lett. **340:** 189-192.

79. WERSINGER, C., D. PROU, P. VERNIER & A. SIDHU. 2003. Modulation of dopamine transporter function by alpha-synuclein is altered by impairment of cell adhesion and by induction of oxidative stress. FASEB J. **17:** 2151–2153.

80. WERSINGER, C., D. PROU, P. VERNIER, *et al.* 2003. Mutations in the lipid-binding domain of α-synuclein confer overlapping, yet distinct, functional properties in the regulation of dopamine transporter activity. Mol. Cell. Neurosci. **24:** 91–105.

81. WERSINGER C., P. VERNIER & A. SIDHU. 2004. Trypsin disrupts the trafficking of the human dopamine transporter by alpha-synuclein and its A30P mutant. Biochemistry **43:** 1242–1253.

82. LEE, F.J., F. LIU, Z.B. PRISTUPA & H.B. NIZNIK. 2001. Direct binding and functional coupling of alpha-synuclein to the dopamine transporters accelerate dopamine-induced apoptosis. FASEB J. **15:** 916–926.

83. VOLLES, M.J. & P.T. LANSBURY, JR. 2003. Zeroing in on the pathogenic form of alpha-synuclein and its mechanism of neurotoxicity in Parkinson's disease. Biochemistry **42:** 7871–7878.

84. LI, J., M. ZHU, A.B. MANNING-BOG, *et al.* 2004. Dopamine and L-DOPA disaggregate amyloid fibrils: implications for Parkinson's and Alzheimer's disease. FASEB J. **18:** 962–964.

85. YOUDIM, M.B. 2003. What have we learnt from cDNA microarray gene expression studies about the role of iron in MPTP induced neurodegeneration and Parkinson's disease? J. Neural Transm. Suppl. **65:** 73–88.
86. CONWAY, K.A., S.J. LEE, J.C. ROCHET, *et al.* 2000. Acceleration of oligomerization, not fibrillization, is a shared property of both alpha-synuclein mutations linked to early-onset Parkinson's disease: implications for pathogenesis and therapy. Proc. Natl. Acad. Sci. USA **97:** 571–576.
87. GIASSON, B.I., J.E. DUDA, S.M. QUINN, *et al.* 2002. Neuronal alpha-synucleinopathy with severe movement disorder in mice expressing A53T human alpha-synuclein. Neuron **34:** 521–533.
88. RICHFIELD, E.K., M.J. THIRUCHELVAM, D.A. CORY-SLECHTA, *et al.* 2002. Behavioral and neurochemical effects of wild-type and mutated human alpha-synuclein in transgenic mice. Exp. Neurol. **175:** 35–48.
89. FEANY, M.B. & W.W. BENDER. 2000. A *Drosophila* model of Parkinson's disease. Nature **404:** 394–398.
90. GIASSON, B.I. & V.M. LEE. 2003. Are ubiquitination pathways central to Parkinson's disease? Cell **114:** 1–8.
91. YANG, Y., I. NISHIMURA, Y. IMAI, *et al.* 2003. Parkin suppresses dopaminergic neuron-selective neurotoxicity induced by Pael-R in *Drosophila*. Neuron **37:** 911–924.
92. KAKIMURA, J., Y. KITAMURA, K. TAKATA, *et al.* 2001. Release and aggregation of cyto-chrome c and alpha-synuclein are inhibited by the antiparkinsonian drugs, talipexole and pramipexole. Eur. J. Pharmacol. **417:** 59–67.
93. KANDA, S., J.F. BISHOP, M.A. EGLITIS, *et al.* 2000. Enhanced vulnerability to oxidative stress by alpha-synuclein mutations and C-terminal truncation. Neuroscience **97:** 279–284.
94. DAUER, W., N. KHOLODILOV, M. VILA, *et al.* 2002. Resistance of alpha-synuclein nul mice to the parkinsonian neurotoxin MPTP. Proc. Natl. Acad. Sci. USA **99:** 14524–14529.
95. MOUSSA, C., C. WERSINGER, Y. TOMITA & A. SIDHU. 2004. Differential cytotoxicity of human wild type and mutant alpha-synuclein in human neuroblastoma SH-SY5Y cells in the presence of dopamine. Biochemistry **43:** 5539–5550.

Blockade of PKCδ Proteolytic Activation by Loss of Function Mutants Rescues Mesencephalic Dopaminergic Neurons from Methylcyclopentadienyl Manganese Tricarbonyl (MMT)–Induced Apoptotic Cell Death

V. ANANTHARAM, M. KITAZAWA, C. LATCHOUMYCANDANE,
A. KANTHASAMY, AND A. G. KANTHASAMY

Parkinson's Disorder Research Laboratory, Department of Biomedical Sciences, Iowa State University, Ames, Iowa 50011-1250, USA

ABSTRACT: The use of methylcyclopentadienyl manganese tricarbonyl (MMT) as a gasoline additive has raised health concerns and increased interest in understanding the neurotoxic effects of manganese. Chronic exposure to inorganic manganese causes Manganism, a neurological disorder somewhat similar to Parkinson's disease. However, the cellular mechanism by which MMT, an organic manganese compound, induces neurotoxicity in dopaminergic neuronal cells remains unclear. Therefore, we systematically investigated apoptotic cell-signaling events following exposure to 3–200 μM MMT in mesencephalic dopaminergic neuronal (N27) cells. MMT treatment resulted in a time- and dose-dependent increase in reactive oxygen species generation and cell death in N27 cells. The cell death was preceded by sequential activation of mitochondrial-dependent proapoptotic events including cytochrome *c* release, caspase-3 activation, and DNA fragmentation, indicating that the mitochondrial-dependent apoptotic cascade primarily triggers MMT-induced apoptotic cell death. Importantly, MMT induced proteolytic cleavage of protein kinase Cδ (PKCδ), resulting in persistently increased kinase activity. The proteolytic activation of PKCδ was suppressed by treatment with 100 μM Z-VAD-FMK and 100 μM Z-DEVD-FMK, suggesting that caspase-3 mediates the proteolytic activation of PKCδ. Pretreatment with 100 μM Z-DEVD-FMK and 5 μM rottlerin (a PKCδ inhibitor) also significantly attenuated MMT-induced DNA fragmentation. Furthermore, overexpression of either the kinase inactive dominant negative PKCδ^{K376R} mutant or the caspase cleavage resistant PKCδ^{D327A} mutant rescued N27 cells from MMT-induced DNA fragmentation. Collectively, these results demonstrate that the mitochondrial-dependent apoptotic cascade mediates apoptosis via proteolytic activation of PKCδ in MMT-induced dopaminergic degeneration and suggest that PKCδ may serve as an attractive therapeutic target in Parkinson-related neurological diseases.

Address for correspondence: Dr. A. G. Kanthasamy, Professor, Parkinson's Disorder Research Laboratory, Department of Biomedical Sciences, 2062 Veterinary Medicine Building, Iowa State University, Ames, IA 50011. Voice: 515-294-2516; fax: 515-294-2315.
akanthas@iastate.edu

Ann. N.Y. Acad. Sci. 1035: 271–289 (2004). © 2004 New York Academy of Sciences.
doi: 10.1196/annals.1332.017

KEYWORDS: manganese; neurotoxicity; neuroprotection; PKCdelta; oxidative stress; kinase; caspases; Parkinson's disease (PD)

INTRODUCTION

Parkinson's disease (PD) is an idiopathic neurodegenerative disorder affecting 3% of the population over the age of 65.[1–9] PD is characterized by profound loss of dopaminergic neurons in the nigrostriatal tract and the presence of intraneuronal cytoplasmic inclusions called Lewy bodies, causing a disturbance in coordinated movement.[10–12] Several studies implicate aging, environmental factors, and genetic defects as potential risk factors in the development of PD.[13–17] Epidemiological evaluation of thousands of twins demonstrated that genetic factors do not play a role in the pathogenesis of geriatric onset of PD, supporting the view that environmental factors are dominant risk factors in the etiology of PD.[18] The role of environmental factors in the development of PD is further supported by several epidemiological studies that suggest that certain pesticides and manganese-containing compounds, such as inorganic manganese, manganese ethylene-bis-dithiocarbamate (MANEB, a fungicide), and Bazooka (a cocaine-based drug), are positively associated with increased incidences of PD.[19–21] Furthermore, occupational exposure to manganese has caused Manganism in miners.[19,22–24] Exposure to MANEB and Bazooka among farm workers and abusers, respectively, has been shown to result in adverse neurological defects similar to those observed in PD.[25–28] Recently, methylcyclopentadienyl manganese tricarbonyl (MMT), an anti-knock gasoline agent, replaced tetraethyl lead [$(CH_3CH_2)_4Pb$] in gasoline in the United States.[29–34] Since MMT is a manganese containing compound, possible adverse health risks associated with its exposure are of great concern.[1,29,33–36]

Administration or exposure to MMT causes pronounced accumulation of manganese in rat brain,[37] produces seizures in mice,[38] depletes dopamine in mouse striatum,[39,40] and effectively inhibits mitochondrial complex I.[41] We recently demonstrated that MMT is acutely cytotoxic to dopamine-producing (PC-12) cells, which are more susceptible to the cytotoxic effects of MMT than nondopaminergic cells (cerebellar granule cells). Subsequently, we demonstrated that MMT exposure induces reactive oxygen species (ROS) generation, dopamine depletion, and activation of a series of cellular factors including cytochrome c release, caspase-3 activation, proteolytic activation of PKCδ, and apoptotic cell death in dopamine-producing rat pheochromocytoma (PC12) cells.[42,43] Although PC12 cells are a commonly used dopaminergic cell model, we recently established that N27 cells are a superior cell culture model for studying dopaminergic neurodegeneration. N27 cells are derived from the mesencephalon, a brain region directly affected by PD, and represent a homogenous population of tyrosine hydroxylase positive cells with functional characteristics resembling dopaminergic neurons.[44] Using a combination of pharmacological inhibitors and overexpression of PKCδ dominant negative and caspase-resistant mutants, we demonstrate that suppression of proteolytic activation of PKCδ rescues N27 cells from MMT-induced dopaminergic cell death.

EXPERIMENTAL METHODS

Cell Culture

Immortalized rat mesencephalic cells (N27) were grown in RPMI medium supplemented with 10% fetal bovine serum, 1% L-glutamine, penicillin (100 units/mL), and streptomycin (100 units/mL), and maintained at 37°C in a humidified atmosphere of 5% CO_2 as described previously.[43,45]

Transient Transfections

Transient transfection assays were performed according to the manufacturer's protocol supplied with the Cell Line Nucleofector™ Kit V. Briefly, after 2–3 days in culture, N27 cells were harvested, washed with 1× PBS, and resuspended in transfection solution (supplied with the kit) at a cell density of 2×10^6 cells/100 µL. Plasmid DNA and pPKCδ^{K376R}-GFP, pPKCδ^{D327A}-GFP, and pEGFPN1 DNA were added separately to 100 µL of cell suspension, transferred into a Nucleofector cuvette, and electroporated using the Nucleofector device. Cells were immediately transferred from the cuvette to 24-well plates after dilution with growth media. After 24 h, GFP expressing cells were observed under a TE2000 Nikon fluorescence microscope, and the transfection efficiency was estimated to be between 70% and 75%. At this point, cells were harvested and used for apoptosis assays as described below.

Treatment Paradigm

After 1–2 days in culture, wild-type and transfected N27 cells were harvested and treated with varying concentrations of MMT (3–200 µM) over a period of 15 min to 3 h at 37°C in serum-free RPMI medium. In inhibitor studies, rottlerin (PKCδ inhibitor, 5 µM), Z-DEVD-FMK (caspase-3-specific inhibitor, 100 µM), or Z-VAD-FMK (a broad spectrum caspase inhibitor, 100 µM) was added 30 min prior to the addition of MMT. After treatment, cells were lysed and used for measurement of cytosolic cytochrome c, caspase-3 enzymatic activity, PKCδ cleavage, PKCδ activity, and DNA fragmentation. For measurement of ROS generation and apoptosis by flow cytometry, cells were harvested and cell suspensions were treated with MMT. DMSO (dimethyl sulfoxide, 0.5–1%) was used as a vehicle in control experiments.

Flow Cytometric Measurement of ROS Generation

ROS generation was detected in the cells using hydroethidine with a Becton Dickenson FACScan™ flow cytometer (Becton Dickinson, San Francisco, CA) as described previously.[43,45] Flow cytometric data were analyzed by Cellquest™ data analysis software. Briefly, N27 cells were resuspended with Hanks balanced salt solution (HBSS) with 2 mM calcium at a density of 0.5×10^6 cells/mL and then incubated with 10 µM hydroethidine for 15 min at 37°C in the dark. After removing the excess dye, cells were resuspended with HBSS and treated with MMT (3–100 µM), and ROS generation was measured at 0, 15, 30, 45, and 60 min after exposure in the fluorescence activated cell sorter in the flow cytometer.

Cytochrome c Release ELISA Assay

Cytochrome *c* release was quantified using an ELISA kit as described previous-ly.[43,45] Briefly, after 1–2 days in culture, N27 cells were exposed to 100 µM and 200 µM MMT for 15–30 min at 37°C in serum-free growth medium. After treatment, the cells were harvested, washed once with PBS, resuspended, and homogenized in buffer containing 10 mM Tris HCl (pH 7.5), 0.3 M sucrose, and protease inhibitors. After homogenization, the samples were centrifuged for 60 min at 12,000 rpm and the supernatants were collected as cytosolic fractions. These fractions were then used for ELISA assay. The optical density (O.D.) of each well was then measured at 450 nm using a microplate reader. The 620-nm reading was used as a reference blank and subtracted from the 450-nm reading.

Caspase-3 Enzymatic Assay

Caspase-3 activity was performed as previously described.[43,45] Briefly, after treatment, cells were directly lysed with assay buffer [50 mM Tris HCl (pH 7.4), 1 mM EDTA, and 10 mM EGTA] containing 10 µM digitonin for 20 min at 37°C. Lysates were centrifuged and the resulting supernatants were incubated with the fluorogenic caspase-3 substrate Ac-DEVD-AMC (50 µM) for 1 h at 37°C. Levels of cleaved (active) caspase substrate were monitored at excitation wavelength of 380 nm and emission wavelength of 460 nm using a microplate reader. The protein concentrations were determined using the Bio-Rad protein assay reagent.

Isolation of Cytoplasmic Fractions

Cytoplasmic fractions were prepared as described in our previous publications.[43,45] Briefly, after treatment, N27 cells were washed with 1× PBS, homogenized, sonicated, and centrifuged as described previously.[43,45] The supernatants were collected as cytosolic fractions, and protein concentrations were determined and used for SDS-gel electrophoresis.

Western Blotting

Cytoplasmic fractions containing equal amounts of protein were loaded in each lane and separated on a 10–12% SDS-PAGE gel as described previously.[43,45] Proteins were then transferred to nitrocellulose membrane, and nonspecific binding sites were blocked by treating with 5% nonfat dry milk powder. The membranes were then treated with primary antibody directed against PKCδ (1:2000 dilution), which was followed by treatment with secondary HRP-conjugated anti-rabbit. Secondary antibody-bound proteins were detected using Amersham's ECL chemiluminescence kit. To confirm equal protein loading, blots were reprobed with a β-actin antibody (1:5000 dilution). Western blot images were captured with a Kodak 2000 MM imaging system.

Immunoprecipitation Kinase Assays

PKCδ enzymatic activity was assayed using an immunoprecipitation kinase assay described previously.[43,45] Briefly, after treatment with 100 and 200 µM MMT for 2 h, N27 cells were washed with 1× PBS and resuspended in PKC lysis buffer [25 mM

HEPES (pH 7.5), 20 mM β-glycerophosphate, 0.1 mM sodium orthovanadate, 0.1% Triton X 100, 0.3 M NaCl, 1.5 mM $MgCl_2$, 0.2 mM EDTA, 0.5 mM DTT, 10 mM NaF, and protease inhibitors]. The cell lysates were centrifuged, and supernatants were collected as cell lysates. Samples of 400 μL of cell lysates containing 200 μg proteins were immunoprecipitated overnight at 4°C with anti-PKCδ antibody. The immunoprecipitates were then incubated with Protein-A–sepharose (Sigma) for 1 h and then washed three times with PKC lysis buffer and three times with 2× kinase buffer [40 mM Tris (pH 7.4), 20 mM $MgCl_2$, 20 μM ATP, and 2.5 mM $CaCl_2$]. Finally, the protein-A-bound PKCδ immunoprecipitates were resuspended in 100 μL of 2× kinase buffer. The kinase reaction was started by adding 25 μL of reaction buffer containing 0.4 mg histone H1 and 5 μCi of [γ-^{32}P]ATP (3000 Ci/mM) to 25 μL of immunoprecipitated samples and incubated for 10 min at 30°C. SDS gel loading buffer (2×) was added to terminate the reaction, the samples were boiled for 5 min, and the products were separated on a 12% SDS-PAGE gel. The H1 phosphorylated bands were detected using a Personal Molecular Imager (FX model, Bio-Rad) and quantified using Quantity One 4.2.0 software.

Assessment of Apoptosis by Annexin V/PI Double-Staining Assay

Externalization or flipping of phosphatidylserine in the plasma membrane occurs during apoptosis. This externalization is followed by the collapse of cytoskeletal elements, resulting in increased membrane permeability. Annexin V, a calcium-dependent antiphosphatidylserine antibody, recognizes the translocated phosphatidylserine and is used to detect cells in the early apoptotic stage. Propidium iodide (PI) stains the nucleus when the integrity of the cell membrane is compromised during the late apoptotic or necrotic stage. In this experiment, apoptotic cells were identified by double staining with recombinant FITC (fluorescein isothiocyanate)–conjugated annexin V and PI using the Annexin V–FITC Apoptosis Detection Kit (Molecular Probes). Flow cytometry analysis was performed on a FACScan™ flow cytometer (Becton Dickinson, San Francisco, CA). Briefly, after 1–2 days in culture, N27 cells were treated with 500 μM MMT for 1 h. After treatment, the cells were washed twice with 1× PBS and resuspended in a binding buffer supplied with the kit (10 mM HEPES, pH 7.4, 140 mM NaCl, and 2.5 mM $CaCl_2$) at a concentration of 0.5×10^6 cells/mL. Cell suspensions (100 μL) were incubated with annexin V–FITC (5 μL) and PI (2 μL) for 15 min at RT in the dark. An average of 5000 cells from each sample were counted. Viable, apoptotic, and necrotic cells in control and treated samples were then detected by a fluorescence-activated cell sorter in the flow cytometer. Annexin V–FITC and PI negative cells were designated as viable cells, annexin V positive and PI negative cells were designated as early apoptotic cells (EA), both annexin V and PI positive cells were designated as late apoptotic cells (LA), and annexin V negative and PI positive cells were designated as necrotic cells (N). Data acquisition and analysis were obtained using a CellQuest software.

DNA Fragmentation Assay

DNA fragmentation was measured using a Cell Death Detection ELISA Plus Assay Kit, as described previously.[43,45,46] N27 cells (0.1×10^6 cells) were subcultured in 24-well culture plates for 24 h and then exposed to 100 μM MMT with or without

100 μM Z-DEVD-FMK and 5 μM rottlerin for 3 h. N27 cells were pretreated with 5 μM rottlerin and 100 μM Z-DEVD-FMK for 30 min prior to the addition of MMT. In addition, 24 h after transfection, N27 cells transiently expressing PKCδ^{K376R}-GFP, PKCδ^{D327A}-GFP, and GFP alone were exposed to 100 μM MMT for 3 h and processed for DNA fragmentation. Quantitative determination of the amount of fragmented DNA retained by anti-DNA-HRP in the immunocomplex was determined spectrophotometrically with ABTS as an HRP substrate (supplied with the kit). Measurements were made at 405 nm against an ABTS solution as a blank (reference wavelength, 490 nm) using a Molecular Devices Spectramax Microplate Reader.

Data Analysis

Data analysis was performed using Prism 3.0 software (GraphPad Software, San Diego, CA). Data from caspase activity, cytochrome c release, and DNA fragmentation assays were first analyzed using one-way ANOVA. Dunnett's post-test or Bonferroni's multiple comparison test was then performed to compare treated samples, and $P < 0.05$ was considered significant.

RESULTS

MMT Treatment Induces ROS Production in N27 Cells

Recently, oxidative stress has been suggested to play an important role in the neurodegenerative process of PD.[47–51] Further, we previously showed that exposure of PC12 cells to MMT resulted in a dose- and time-dependent increase in ROS production. In this study, we examined whether MMT treatment induces ROS production

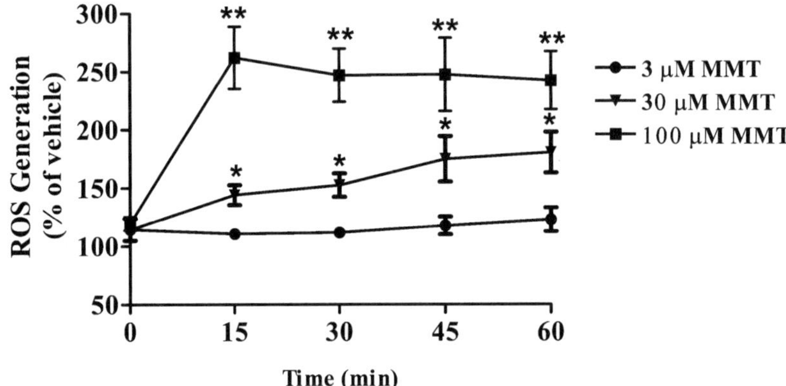

FIGURE 1. MMT induces dose- and time-dependent increases in ROS production in N27 cells. N27 cells were treated with 3, 30, and 100 μM MMT, and ROS generation was measured every 15 min for 1 h using hydroethidine fluorescence by flow cytometry as described in the EXPERIMENTAL METHODS section. Cells treated with 0.5% DMSO were used as the vehicle control. Data represent the mean ± SEM from 4–8 measurements. Asterisks (*$P < 0.5$; **$P < 0.01$) indicate significant differences compared with the time-matched vehicle-treated cells.

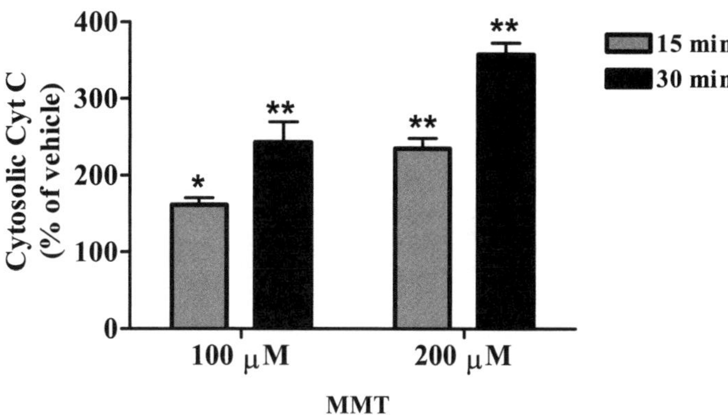

FIGURE 2. Effect of MMT on cytochrome *c* release. N27 cells were exposed to 100 and 200 μM MMT for 15 and 30 min; after treatment, cytosolic cytochrome *c* was detected using an ELISA kit as described in the EXPERIMENTAL METHODS section. Cells treated with 0.5% DMSO were used as the vehicle control. Data represent the mean ± SEM for 4 measurements. Asterisks (*$P < 0.05$; **$P < 0.01$) indicate a significant difference between vehicle- and MMT-treated cells.

in immortalized mesencephalic dopaminergic clonal cells (N27 cells). Exposure of N27 cells to MMT resulted in a time- and dose-dependent increase in ROS production, as revealed by flow cytometric analysis (FIG. 1). Exposure to 3, 30, and 100 μM MMT for 45 min resulted in increases of 118%, 174%, and 247% in ROS production compared to vehicle-treated N27 cells, respectively. Similarly, exposure to 100 μM MMT resulted in increases of 262%, 247%, 247%, and 242% in ROS production at 15, 30, 45, and 60 min, respectively, compared to time-matched vehicle treated N27 cells. The time course study of ROS production in 100 μM MMT-treated cells revealed a clear pattern of dramatic increase in ROS generation peaking within 15 min and remaining constant up to 1 h, whereas exposure to 30 μM MMT resulted in a linear increase in ROS production over time. ROS production was not statistically different in 3 μM MMT-treated cells from vehicle-treated N27 cells at all time points.

MMT Treatment Induces Mitochondrial Cytochrome c Release

Cellular ROS production is known to activate many cellular factors, including release of mitochondrial cytochrome *c* into the cytosol; then, the released cytochrome *c* activates the caspase cascade to trigger apoptotic cell death.[52–54] Therefore, we examined whether MMT induces mitochondrial release of cytochrome *c* in N27 mesencephalic clonal cells using a highly sensitive ELISA sandwich assay. FIGURE 2 shows a dose-dependent increase in cytosolic cytochrome *c* as early as 15 min following exposure. Exposure to 100 μM MMT for 15 and 30 min resulted in increases of 161% and 242% in cytosolic cytochrome *c* compared to the vehicle-treated group, respectively. Similarly, exposure to 200 μM MMT resulted in increases of 234% and 358% in cytosolic cytochrome *c* compared to the vehicle-treated group, respectively.

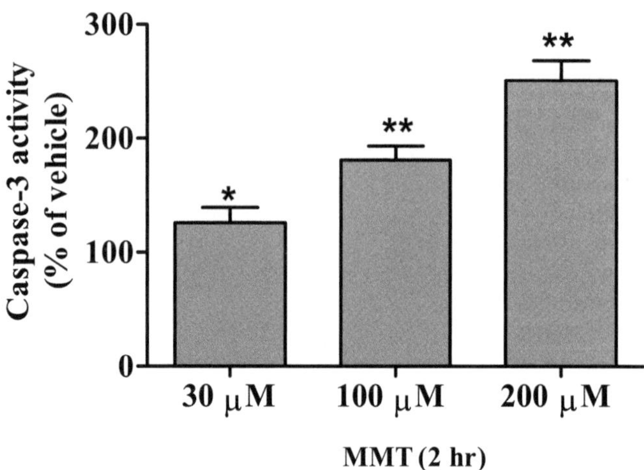

FIGURE 3. Effect of MMT on caspase-3 enzymatic activity. N27 cells were exposed to 30, 100, and 200 μM MMT for 1 h. Caspase-3 activity in cell lysates was measured by incubation with 50 μM Ac-DEVD-AMC for 1 h at 37°C. Cells were also treated with 0.5% DMSO for use as the vehicle control. Data are expressed as the percent vehicle control, and data points represent the mean ± SEM for 6–9 measurements. Asterisks (*$P < 0.05$; **$P < 0.01$) indicate significant differences compared with vehicle-treated cells.

MMT Treatment Induces Dose-Dependent Increase in Caspase-3 Activity

Release of cytochrome c activates a series of cysteine proteases, namely caspases including caspase-3.[55–59] Previously, we showed that exposure of PC12 cells to MMT resulted in caspase-3 and caspase-9 activation, but not caspase-8 activation.[42] In this study, we examined whether MMT treatment induces caspase-3 activation in N27 mesencephalic clonal cells. FIGURE 3 shows a dose-dependent increase in caspase-3 activation in N27 cells. Exposure to 30, 100, and 200 μM MMT for 2 h resulted in increases of 126%, 181%, and 251% in caspase-3 enzymatic activity when compared to vehicle-treated cells, respectively.

Caspase-3 Mediates Proteolytic Cleavage of PKCδ in MMT-Treated Cells

PKCδ can be activated by membrane translocation, tyrosine phosphorylation, or caspase-3-dependent proteolytic activation. Under normal circumstances, PKCδ is primarily activated by translocation to the cellular membrane during stimulation with lipid signaling molecules—phospholipid (PL), diacylglycerol (DAG), or phorbol ester (TPA).[42,45,60–63] Recently, we and others demonstrated that PKCδ is a prominent endogenous substrate for caspase-3 in many different cell types undergoing apoptotic cell death.[42,45,60–63] Caspase-3 cleaves PKCδ to yield a 41-kDa catalytically active subunit and a 38-kDa regulatory subunit. Proteolytic cleavage of PKCδ results in the permanent dissociation of the regulatory domain from the catalytic fragment, resulting in persistently active kinase. Previously, we demonstrated MMT-induced proteolytic cleavage of PKCδ, but not of PKCα, β, or γ; thus, MMT is

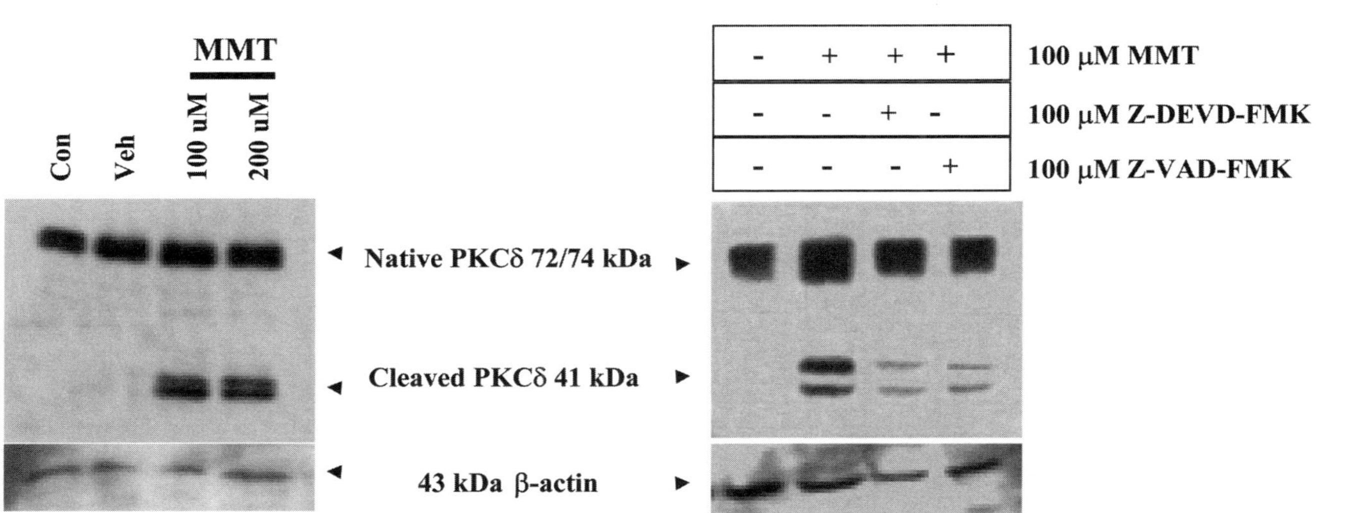

FIGURE 4. Caspase-3 mediates MMT-induced PKCδ cleavage in N27 cells. **(A)** Dose-dependent increase in PKCδ cleavage and **(B)** effect of Z-DEVD-FMK and Z-VAD-FMK on PKCδ cleavage. N27 cells were exposed to 100 and 200 μM MMT for 2 h. In the inhibitor study, cells were pretreated with 100 μM Z-DEVD-FMK and 100 μM Z-VAD-FMK for 30 min prior to the addition of 100 μM MMT. Cells treated with 0.5% DMSO were used as the vehicle control. After treatment, cytosolic fractions were collected and equal amounts of proteins were resolved on 10% SDS-PAGE followed by Western blotting with polyclonal PKCδ antibody. Native PKCδ appears at 72–74 kDa and catalytically active cleaved PKCδ appears at ~41 kDa. Equal protein loading was confirmed by reprobing with β-actin (43 kDa). Con: Untreated control cells; Veh: 0.5% DMSO-treated vehicle cells.

isoform-specific in PC12 cells. Since MMT exposure resulted in caspase-3 activation in N27 cells (FIG. 3), we examined the proteolytic cleavage of PKCδ in MMT-treated N27 cells. A 2-h MMT treatment induced PKCδ cleavage (FIG. 4A) and the extent of cleavage was similar following both 100 µM and 200 µM MMT treatments. However, no cleavage of PKCδ was observed in vehicle-treated cells. In subsequent experiments, we used cell-permeable caspase inhibitors, Z-VAD-FMK (a pan caspase inhibitor) and Z-DEVD-FMK (a caspase-3-specific inhibitor), to confirm that PKCδ cleavage is mediated by caspase-3. Although not completely, pretreatment with 100 µM Z-VAD-FMK and 100 µM Z-DEVD-FMK significantly attenuated 100 µM MMT-induced PKCδ cleavage (FIG. 4B), suggesting that the cleavage is indeed mediated by caspase-3. Nitrocellulose membranes were reprobed with β-actin antibody to confirm equal protein loading. On the other hand, we did not observe translocation of PKCδ to the membrane in MMT-treated cells (data not shown). Overall, these data suggest that activation of PKCδ occurs primarily via caspase-3 cleavage rather than translocation to the membrane.

Increased PKCδ Kinase Activity in MMT-Treated N27 Cells

To determine if the MMT-induced PKCδ cleavage also leads to an increase in PKCδ enzyme activity, we performed immunoprecipitation kinase assays by examining the ability of immunoprecipitated PKCδ to phosphorylate histone H1 using [^{32}P]ATP. MMT exposure resulted in a dose-dependent increase in PKCδ kinase activity (FIG. 5A). Exposure to 100 µM and 200 µM MMT for 2 h resulted in

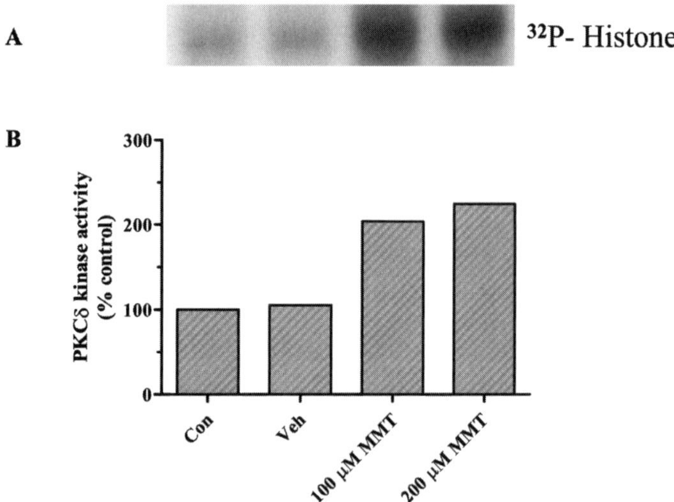

FIGURE 5. Dose-dependent increases in PKCδ kinase activity in MMT-treated cells: (**A**) ^{32}P phosphorylation of histones and (**B**) densitometric analysis. N27 cells were exposed to 100 and 200 µM MMT for 2 h. Cells treated with 0.5% DMSO were used as the vehicle control. The immunoprecipitation kinase assay was performed as described in the EXPERIMENTAL METHODS section. After scanning the dried gel, the histone phosphorylated bands were detected by a PhosphoImager. The histone bands were then quantified using Quantity One software. Data are expressed as the percent of control.

increases of 204% and 225% in PKCδ kinase activity when compared to untreated control cells, as revealed by densitometric analysis of phosphorylated histone H1 bands (FIG. 5B). The increase in PKCδ kinase activity coincided with generation of PKCδ cleavage. Since the kinase assay was performed in the absence of lipids, we attribute this increased kinase activity to the persistently active PKCδ catalytic fragment, but not the native full-length PKCδ.

Caspase-3 and PKCδ Mediate MMT-Induced Apoptotic Cell Death in N27 Cells

To understand the functional consequence of activation of ROS production, cytochrome *c* release, and caspase-3 and PKCδ activation, we tested whether MMT induces apoptosis. We used the annexin V/PI double-staining assay to identify apoptotic and necrotic cells using a flow cytometer. Flow cytometric analysis revealed that MMT treatment induces apoptotic cell death in N27 cells (FIG. 6). Exposure to 500 µM MMT for 1 h resulted in 48% EA cells and 44% LA cells compared to 9% and 13% in vehicle-treated cells, respectively. On the other hand, the percentage of viable cells decreased from 75% in vehicle-treated cells to 7% in MMT-treated cells.

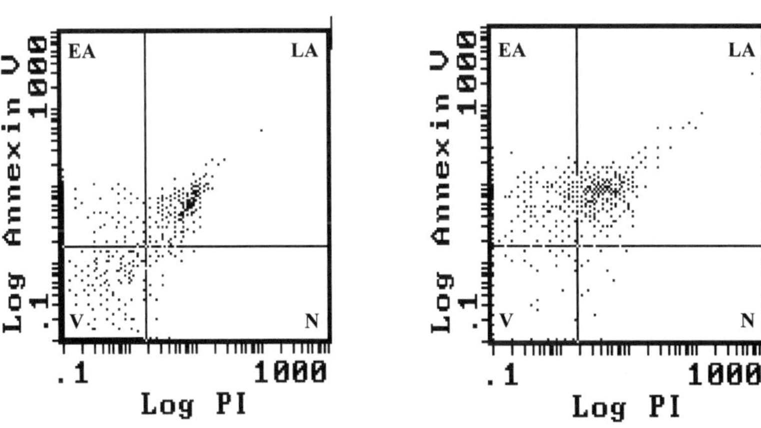

Cell population	Viable (V) Annexin V & PI -ve	Early Apoptotic (EA) Annexin V +ve	Late Apoptotic (LA) Annexin V & PI + ve	Necrotic (N) PI +ve
Vehicle	75%	9 %	13 %	3 %
500 µM MMT	7 %	48 %	44 %	1 %

FIGURE 6. Fluorescence-activated cell sorter analysis for annexin V and PI staining. After treatment with 500 µM MMT for 1 h, N27 cells were double-stained with annexin V–FITC and PI as described in the EXPERIMENTAL METHODS section. Cells treated with 0.5% DMSO were used as the vehicle control. Sorter analysis revealed the presence of viable cells (V), early apoptotic cells (EA), late apoptotic cells (LA), and necrotic cells (N). The table represents the percentage of data obtained from the log plot.

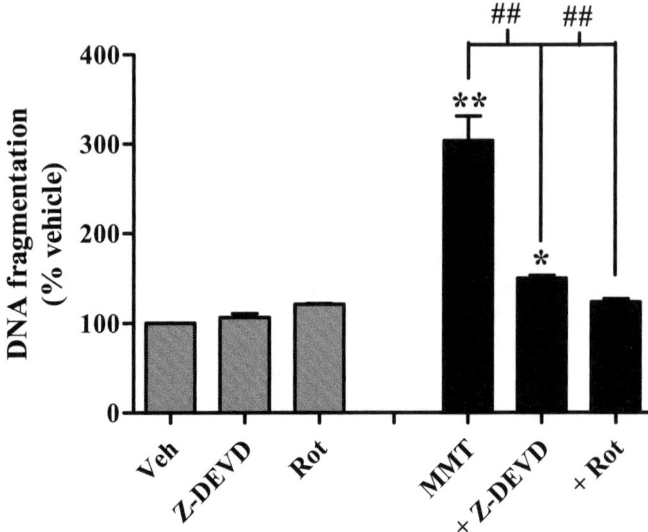

FIGURE 7. Caspase-3 and PKCδ mediate MMT-induced DNA fragmentation. Cells were treated with 100 μM MMT for 3 h, and the level of DNA fragmentation was quantified using a DNA ELISA kit. For the inhibitor study, N27 cells were treated with 100 μM Z-DEVD-FMK and 5 μM rottlerin for 30 min prior to treatment with 100 μM MMT. Cells treated with 0.5% DMSO were used as the vehicle control. Data are expressed as the percent vehicle control, and data points represent the mean ± SEM for 6–9 measurements. Asterisks (*$P < 0.05$; **$P < 0.01$) indicate significant differences compared with vehicle-treated cells; "pound" signs (##$P < 0.01$) indicate a significant difference between MMT-treated cells and inhibitor-treated cells. Terms—Z-DEVD: Z-DEVD-FMK; Rot: rottlerin.

To further confirm the results obtained by flow cytometry and to determine the involvement of caspases and PKCδ in mediation of apoptosis, we performed a quantitative DNA ELISA fragmentation assay. FIGURE 7 shows that the MMT-induced DNA fragmentation in N27 cells is significantly attenuated in cells pretreated with caspase-3 and PKCδ inhibitors. Exposure to 100 μM MMT for 3 h caused a 303% increase in DNA fragmentation compared to vehicle-treated cells, while pretreatment with 100 μM Z-DEVD-FMK and 5 μM rottlerin (a PKCδ inhibitor) resulted in increases of only 150% and 124% in DNA fragmentation in comparison to vehicle-treated cells (FIG. 7). DNA fragmentation in cells treated independently with 100 μM Z-DEVD-FMK or 5 μM rottlerin was not significantly different from vehicle-treated groups. Together, these data suggest that both caspase-3 and PKCδ contribute to MMT-induced DNA fragmentation.

Overexpression of PKCδ^{D327A}-CRM and PKCδ^{K376R}-DNM Rescues N27 Cells from MMT-Induced Apoptotic Cell Death

To support the data obtained with pharmacological inhibitors, we used loss of function approaches to demonstrate that caspase-3-dependent proteolytic activation of PKCδ mediates apoptotic cell death in dopaminergic neuronal cells. We used two

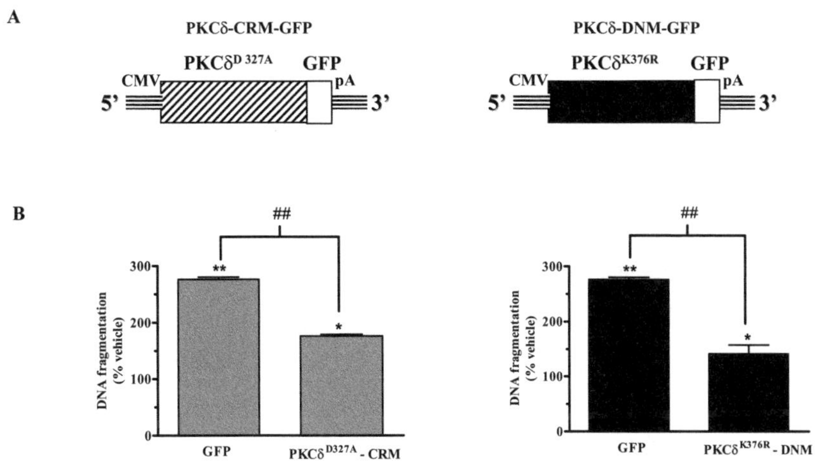

FIGURE 8. Overexpression of PKCδ^{D327A}-CRM and PKCδ^{K376R}-DNM mutant proteins rescues N27 cells from MMT-induced apoptotic cell death: **(A)** plasmid description and **(B)** DNA fragmentation. Briefly, N27 cells transiently expressing caspase cleavage resistant PKCδ^{D327A}-CRM, dominant negative PKCδ^{K376R}-DNM, and GFP alone were exposed to 100 µM MMT for 3 h. DNA fragmentation was quantified using an ELISA assay as described in the EXPERIMENTAL METHODS section. Cells treated with 0.5% DMSO were used as the vehicle control. Data are expressed as a percentage of DNA fragmentation observed in vehicle-treated cells. Data points represent the mean ± SEM for 6–9 measurements. Asterisks (*P < 0.05; **P < 0.01) indicate significant differences compared with vehicle-treated cells; "pound" signs ($^{##}P$ < 0.01) indicate significant differences between MMT-treated GFP expressing cells and MMT-treated PKCδ^{D327A}-CRM or PKCδ^{K376R}-DNM expressing N27 cells.

PKCδ mutants to evaluate the loss of function approach: the PKCδ^{D327A}-CRM mutant in which the cleavage site is mutated to render PKCδ resistant to cleavage by caspase-3 with the catalytic site intact; and the PKCδ^{K376R}-DNM mutant in which the caspase-3 cleavage site is intact, but the catalytic site is mutated to render the kinase inactive. We examined whether MMT-induced apoptotic cell death is suppressed in PKCδ^{D327A}-CRM and PKCδ^{K376R}-DNM overexpressing N27 cells (FIG. 8A). N27 cells expressing GFP alone were used as controls. FIGURE 8B shows that MMT-induced DNA fragmentation is significantly reduced in N27 cells overexpressing PKCδ^{K376R} and PKCδ^{D327A} mutant protein as compared to GFP vector expressing cells. Exposure to 100 µM MMT for 3 h resulted in increased DNA fragmentation by 276%, 176%, and 142% in GFP, PKCδ^{K376R}, and PKCδ^{D327A} overexpressing cells, respectively, compared to vehicle-treated cells. Overall, these data suggest overexpression of PKCδ^{K376R} and PKCδ^{D327A} mutant proteins can partially rescue N27 cells from MMT-induced dopaminergic cell death.

DISCUSSION

We recently reported that exposure of PC12 cells to MMT induces dopamine depletion, caspase-3 and PKCδ activation, and subsequently apoptotic cell death.[42,43] The present study extends the apoptotic action of MMT to N27 mesencephalic dopaminergic neuronal cells. Exposure to MMT resulted in a sequential activation of ROS production, cytochrome c release into the cytosol, activation of caspase-3, proteolytic activation of PKCδ, and nuclear DNA breakdown. Furthermore, blockade of proteolytic cleavage or activation of PKCδ using caspase cleavage resistant PKCδ[D327A] or dominant negative kinase inactive PKCδ[K376R] mutant proteins can partially rescue N27 cells from MMT-induced apoptotic cell death. Our data strongly suggest that proteolytic activation of PKCδ mediates oxidative stress–induced apoptotic cell death in mesencephalic clonal cells following MMT exposure.

In this study, MMT exposure elevated intracellular ROS levels in a time- and dose-dependent manner as early as 15 min after exposure. Although the source of ROS generation during MMT exposure is unclear, mitochondria may contribute to the oxidative stress because previous studies have shown that MMT impairs oxidative phosphorylation.[41–43,64] Alternatively, cytotoxic radicals may be generated because of autooxidation of dopamine in dopaminergic cells since manganese-containing compounds are known to cause autooxidation of dopamine.[43,65–67] ROS has been shown to activate mitochondrial transition pore opening to induce cytochrome c release.[55,68–72] We observed an accumulation of cytosolic cytochrome c in N27 cells within 15 min following MMT treatment, suggesting that ROS may be an initial signal for the release of cytochrome c. Our data are consistent with other dopaminergic toxin activity, including MPP$^+$ (1-methyl-4-phenylpyridinium), 6-OHDA (6-hydroxydopamine), manganese, and dieldrin, which induce ROS-mediated cytochrome c release.[45,53,54,73–75] Once in the cytosol, cytochrome c forms a complex with apoptotic protease activating factor (Apaf-1) to initiate the caspase cascade.[55]

Activation of caspases is an early and essential step in the apoptotic signaling pathway.[55,56,58,59,62,76] It is well established that caspase-3 mediates the execution phase of programmed cell death.[55,56,58,59,62,76] In this study, MMT treatment of N27 cells results in activation of caspase-3, consistent with effects of dieldrin, MMT, MPP$^+$, and 6-OHDA in cell culture models.[42,45,73,75] A recent study emphasizes the importance of caspase-3 activation as an indicator of apoptosis in dopaminergic neurons in both an MPTP mouse model and human patients with PD.[77,78]

Recently, we and others established PKCδ as an emerging putative substrate for caspase-3.[61–63] MMT exposure induces both PKCδ cleavage and kinase activity in N27 dopaminergic cells, which can be effectively blocked by caspase-3 inhibitors, indicating that the cleavage is mediated by caspase-3. Proteolytic cleavage of PKCδ by caspase-3 results in the persistent activation of PKCδ in cytosol, which might initiate a myriad of vital signaling cascades.[61–63] However, in these cells, MMT did not induce translocation of full-length PKCδ to the membrane. Recently, we showed that the proteolytic cleavage of PARP, a key DNA repair enzyme, is dependent on PKCδ activation.[79] Furthermore, we and others have demonstrated the existence of a positive feedback regulation of caspase-3 by PKCδ.[42,45,46,80,81] Studies have also implicated the proteolytically activated PKCδ in apoptotic cell death in nonneuronal cell systems.[61–63] We recently demonstrated that MMT is acutely cytotoxic, and dopamine-producing cells (PC12 and N27 cells in this study) appear to be more susceptible to cytotoxic effects than nondopaminergic cells (cerebellar granule cells).[43]

DNA fragmentation and chromatin condensation are terminal events in the apoptotic process and are considered biochemical hallmarks of apoptosis.[56,82–90] Flow cytometric analysis using annexin V and PI staining revealed that both flipping of phosphatidylserine and increased membrane permeability due to collapse of cytoskeletal elements occurred during MMT treatment, suggesting that the cells were undergoing apoptosis. Quantitative ELISA assays also revealed that MMT induced chromatin condensation and DNA fragmentation in N27 cells. MMT induced a dose-dependent increase in DNA fragmentation and apoptotic cell death in N27 cells. Furthermore, pretreatment with caspase-3 and PKCδ inhibitors significantly suppressed MMT-induced DNA fragmentation, indicating that caspase-3 and PKCδ activities mediate the cell death event. Further confirmation of the role of proteolytically activated PKCδ fragments in MMT-induced apoptosis is supported by dominant negative experiments performed in N27 cells overexpressing caspase cleavage resistant PKCδ^{D327A} and kinase dead PKCδ^{K376R} mutant proteins. MMT treatment produced a significant increase in DNA fragmentation in GFP expressing control cells, whereas MMT failed to induce DNA fragmentation in PKCδ^{D327A} or PKCδ^{K376R} overexpressing cells, thus confirming the key functional role of proteolytically activated PKCδ in MMT-induced apoptotic cell death.

In conclusion, the present study demonstrates that MMT induces a sequential activation of cell signaling events beginning with ROS production, followed by cytochrome *c* release, caspase-3 activation, proteolytic activation of PKCδ, and DNA fragmentation, which eventually results in apoptotic cell death. More importantly, MMT induces dopaminergic degeneration by a novel apoptotic pathway mediated by caspase-3-dependent proteolytic activation of PKCδ. This study emphasizes that PKCδ is a key critical downstream target of MMT-induced apoptotic dopaminergic cell death. Furthermore, blockade of proteolytic cleavage and activation of PKCδ rescue mesencephalic neurons from MMT-induced dopaminergic degeneration and, therefore, may have therapeutic implications in Parkinson-like diseases.

ACKNOWLEDGMENTS

This study was supported by National Institutes of Health (NIH) Grant Nos. ES10586, NS38644, and NS45133.

REFERENCES

1. DOBSON, A.W., K.M. ERIKSON & M. ASCHNER. 2004. Manganese neurotoxicity. Ann. N.Y. Acad. Sci. **1012:** 115–128.
2. LANG, A.E. & J.A. OBESO. 2004. Time to move beyond nigrostriatal dopamine deficiency in Parkinson's disease. Ann. Neurol. **55:** 761–765.
3. LANG, A.E. & J.A. OBESO. 2004. Challenges in Parkinson's disease: restoration of the nigrostriatal dopamine system is not enough. Lancet Neurol. **3:** 309–316.
4. LANGSTON, J.W. 2002. Parkinson's disease: current and future challenges. Neurotoxicology **23:** 443–450.
5. LANGSTON, J.W. 1989. Mechanisms underlying neuronal degeneration in Parkinson's disease: an experimental and theoretical treatise. Mov. Disord. **4**(suppl. 1)**:** S15–25.

6. GIASSON, B.I. & V.M. LEE. 2001. Parkin and the molecular pathways of Parkinson's disease. Neuron **31**: 885–888.
7. BALDI, I. *et al.* 2003. Neurodegenerative diseases and exposure to pesticides in the elderly. Am. J. Epidemiol. **157**: 409–414.
8. DI MONTE, D.A. 2003. The environment and Parkinson's disease: is the nigrostriatal system preferentially targeted by neurotoxins? Lancet Neurol. **2**: 531–538.
9. DI MONTE, D.A., M. LAVASANI & A.B. MANNING-BOG. 2002. Environmental factors in Parkinson's disease. Neurotoxicology **23**: 487–502.
10. DIETZ, V., J. QUINTERN & W. BERGER. 1981. Electrophysiological studies of gait in spasticity and rigidity. Evidence that altered mechanical properties of muscle contribute to hypertonia. Brain **104**: 431–449.
11. MASLIAH, E. & M. HASHIMOTO. 2002. Development of new treatments for Parkinson's disease in transgenic animal models: a role for beta-synuclein. Neurotoxicology **23**: 461–468.
12. SHASTRY, B.S. 2003. Neurodegenerative disorders of protein aggregation. Neurochem. Int. **43**: 1–7.
13. OERTEL, W.H. & A. KUPSCH. 1993. Pathogenesis and animal studies of Parkinson's disease. Curr. Opin. Neurol. Neurosurg. **6**: 323–332.
14. LANGSTON, J.W. 1998. Epidemiology versus genetics in Parkinson's disease: progress in resolving an age-old debate. Ann. Neurol. **44**: S45–52.
15. ASCHNER, M. 2000. Manganese: brain transport and emerging research needs. Environ. Health Perspect. **108**(suppl. 3): 429–432.
16. ASCHNER, M. 2000. Interactions between pesticides and glia: an unexplored experimental field. Neurotoxicology **21**: 175–180.
17. SIMON, D.K. *et al.* 2000. Mitochondrial DNA mutations in complex I and tRNA genes in Parkinson's disease. Neurology **54**: 703–709.
18. TANNER, C.M. *et al.* 1999. Parkinson disease in twins: an etiologic study. JAMA **281**: 341–346.
19. GORELL, J.M. *et al.* 1999. Occupational exposure to manganese, copper, lead, iron, mercury and zinc and the risk of Parkinson's disease. Neurotoxicology **20**: 239–247.
20. LIOU, H.H. *et al.* 1997. Environmental risk factors and Parkinson's disease: a case-control study in Taiwan. Neurology **48**: 1583–1588.
21. SEIDLER, A. *et al.* 1996. Possible environmental, occupational, and other etiologic factors for Parkinson's disease: a case-control study in Germany. Neurology **46**: 1275–1284.
22. MENA, I. *et al.* 1967. Chronic manganese poisoning: clinical picture and manganese turnover. Neurology **17**: 128–136.
23. BARBEAU, A. 1984. Manganese and extrapyramidal disorders (a critical review and tribute to Dr. George C. Cotzias). Neurotoxicology **5**: 13–35.
24. DONALDSON, J. 1987. The physiopathologic significance of manganese in brain: its relation to schizophrenia and neurodegenerative disorders. Neurotoxicology **8**: 451–462.
25. ROELS, H. *et al.* 1987. Epidemiological survey among workers exposed to manganese: effects on lung, central nervous system, and some biological indices. Am. J. Ind. Med. **11**: 307–327. [Published erratum: Am. J. Ind. Med. **12**: 119–120.]
26. ROELS, H. *et al.* 1987. Relationship between external and internal parameters of exposure to manganese in workers from a manganese oxide and salt producing plant. Am. J. Ind. Med. **11**: 297–305.
27. FERRAZ, H.B. *et al.* 1988. Chronic exposure to the fungicide maneb may produce symptoms and signs of CNS manganese intoxication. Neurology **38**: 550–553.
28. THIRUCHELVAM, M. *et al.* 2000. Potentiated and preferential effects of combined paraquat and maneb on nigrostriatal dopamine systems: environmental risk factors for Parkinson's disease? Brain Res. **873**: 225–234.
29. LYNAM, D.R. *et al.* 1999. Environmental effects and exposures to manganese from use of methylcyclopentadienyl manganese tricarbonyl (MMT) in gasoline. Neurotoxicology **20**: 145–150.
30. ZAYED, J. *et al.* 1999. Airborne manganese particulates and methylcyclopentadienyl manganese tricarbonyl (MMT) at selected outdoor sites in Montreal. Neurotoxicology **20**: 151–157.

31. ZAYED, J. 2001. Use of MMT in Canadian gasoline: health and environment issues. Am. J. Ind. Med. **39:** 426–433.

32. ZAYED, J. *et al.* 2003. Estimation of annual Mn emissions from MMT source in the Canadian environment and the Mn pollution index in each province. Sci. Total Environ. **312:** 147–154.

33. ZAYED, J., A. VYSKOCIL & G. KENNEDY. 1999. Environmental contamination and human exposure to manganese-contribution of methylcyclopentadienyl manganese tricarbonyl in unleaded gasoline. Int. Arch. Occup. Environ. Health **72:** 7–13.

34. KAISER, J. 2003. Manganese: a high-octane dispute. Science **300:** 926–8.

35. FRUMKIN, H. & G. SOLOMON. 1997. Manganese in the U.S. gasoline supply. Am. J. Ind. Med. **31:** 107–115.

36. DAVIS, J.M. 1998. Methylcyclopentadienyl manganese tricarbonyl: health risk uncertainties and research directions. Environ. Health Perspect. **106**(suppl. 1): 191–201.

37. ZHENG, W., H. KIM & Q. ZHAO. 2000. Comparative toxicokinetics of manganese chloride and methylcyclopentadienyl manganese tricarbonyl (MMT) in Sprague-Dawley rats. Toxicol. Sci. **54:** 295–301.

38. FISHMAN, B.E., P.A. MCGINLEY & G. GIANUTSOS. 1987. Neurotoxic effects of methylcyclopentadienyl manganese tricarbonyl (MMT) in the mouse: basis of MMT-induced seizure activity. Toxicology **45:** 193–201.

39. GIANUTSOS, G. & M.T. MURRAY. 1982. Alterations in brain dopamine and GABA following inorganic or organic manganese administration. Neurotoxicology **3:** 75–81.

40. GIANUTSOS, G. *et al.* 1985. Brain manganese accumulation following systemic administration of different forms. Arch. Toxicol. **57:** 272–275.

41. AUTISSIER, N. *et al.* 1977. Effects of methylcyclopentadienyl manganese tricarbonyl (MMT) on rat liver mitochondria. II. Activity-structure relation. Toxicology **8:** 125–133.

42. ANANTHARAM, V. *et al.* 2002. Caspase-3-dependent proteolytic cleavage of protein kinase Cδ is essential for oxidative stress-mediated dopaminergic cell death after exposure to methylcyclopentadienyl manganese tricarbonyl. J. Neurosci. **22:** 1738-1751.

43. KITAZAWA, M. *et al.* 2002. Oxidative stress and mitochondrial-mediated apoptosis in dopaminergic cells exposed to methylcyclopentadienyl manganese tricarbonyl. J. Pharmacol. Exp. Ther. **302:** 26–35.

44. PRASAD, K.N. *et al.* 1998. Efficacy of grafted immortalized dopamine neurons in an animal model of parkinsonism: a review. Mol. Genet. Metab. **65:** 1–9.

45. KAUL, S. *et al.* 2003. Caspase-3 dependent proteolytic activation of protein kinase Cδ mediates and regulates 1-methyl-4-phenylpyridinium (MPP+)-induced apoptotic cell death in dopaminergic cells: relevance to oxidative stress in dopaminergic degeneration. Eur. J. Neurosci. **18:** 1387–1401.

46. REYLAND, M.E. *et al.* 1999. Protein kinase Cδ is essential for etoposide-induced apoptosis in salivary gland acinar cells. J. Biol. Chem. **274:** 19115–19123.

47. CAAP-AHLGREN, M. & O. DEHLIN. 2002. Factors of importance to the caregiver burden experienced by family caregivers of Parkinson's disease patients. Aging Clin. Exp. Res. **14:** 371–377.

48. CASSARINO, D.S. *et al.* 1997. Elevated reactive oxygen species and antioxidant enzyme activities in animal and cellular models of Parkinson's disease. Biochim. Biophys. Acta **1362:** 77–86.

49. HOYT, K.R. *et al.* 1997. Characterization of hydrogen peroxide toxicity in cultured rat forebrain neurons. Neurochem. Res. **22:** 333–340.

50. LEE, H.S., C.W. PARK & Y.S. KIM. 2000. MPP(+) increases the vulnerability to oxidative stress rather than directly mediating oxidative damage in human neuroblastoma cells. Exp. Neurol. **165:** 164–171.

51. WONG, S.S., R.H. LI & A. STADLIN. 1999. Oxidative stress induced by MPTP and MPP(+): selective vulnerability of cultured mouse astrocytes. Brain Res. **836:** 237–244.

52. TAN, S., M. WOOD & P. MAHER. 1998. Oxidative stress induces a form of programmed cell death with characteristics of both apoptosis and necrosis in neuronal cells. J. Neurochem. **71:** 95–105.

53. CASSARINO, D.S. *et al.* 1999. The parkinsonian neurotoxin MPP+ opens the mitochondrial permeability transition pore and releases cytochrome c in isolated mitochondria via an oxidative mechanism. Biochim. Biophys. Acta **1453:** 49–62.

54. CASSARINO, D.S. & J.P. BENNETT, JR. 1999. An evaluation of the role of mitochondria in neurodegenerative diseases: mitochondrial mutations and oxidative pathology, protective nuclear responses, and cell death in neurodegeneration. Brain Res. Brain Res. Rev. **29:** 1–25.
55. JIANG, X. & X. WANG. 2004. Cytochrome c-mediated apoptosis. Annu. Rev. Biochem. **73:** 87–106.
56. COHEN, G.M. 1997. Caspases: the executioners of apoptosis. Biochem. J. **326:** 1–16.
57. EARNSHAW, W.C., L.M. MARTINS & S.H. KAUFMANN. 1999. Mammalian caspases: structure, activation, substrates, and functions during apoptosis. Annu. Rev. Biochem. **68:** 383–424.
58. JELLINGER, K.A. 2001. Cell death mechanisms in neurodegeneration. J. Cell. Mol. Med. **5:** 1–17.
59. SCHULZ, J.B. *et al.* 2000. Glutathione, oxidative stress and neurodegeneration. Eur. J. Biochem. **267:** 4904–4911.
60. GHAYUR, T. *et al.* 1996. Proteolytic activation of protein kinase Cδ by an ICE/CED3-like protease induces characteristics of apoptosis. J. Exp. Med. **184:** 2399–2404.
61. BRODIE, C. & P.M. BLUMBERG. 2003. Regulation of cell apoptosis by protein kinase Cδ. Apoptosis **8:** 19–27.
62. KANTHASAMY, A.G. *et al.* 2003. Role of proteolytic activation of protein kinase Cδ in oxidative stress-induced apoptosis. Antioxid. Redox Signal. **5:** 609–620.
63. KIKKAWA, U., H. MATSUZAKI & T. YAMAMOTO. 2002. Protein kinase Cδ: activation mechanisms and functions. J. Biochem. (Tokyo) **132:** 831–839.
64. AUTISSIER, N. *et al.* 1977. Effects of methylcyclopentadienyl manganese tricarbonyl (MMT) of rat liver mitochondria. I. Effects, in vitro, on the oxidative phosphorylation. Toxicology **7:** 115–22.
65. GRAHAM, D.G. 1984. Catecholamine toxicity: a proposal for the molecular pathogenesis of manganese neurotoxicity and Parkinson's disease. Neurotoxicology **5:** 83–95.
66. KANTHASAMY, A.G. & J.R. WAGNER. 2000. Enviromental Factors-Induced Oxidative Stress in Dopaminergic Degeneration: Relevance to the Etiopathogenesis of Parkinson's Disease. Prominent Press. Phoenix, AZ.
67. KITAZAWA, M., V. ANANTHARAM & A.G. KANTHASAMY. 2001. Dieldrin-induced oxidative stress and neurochemical changes contribute to apoptopic cell death in dopaminergic cells. Free Radical Biol. Med. **31:** 1473–1485.
68. JIANG, X. & X. WANG. 2000. Cytochrome *c* promotes caspase-9 activation by inducing nucleotide binding to Apaf-1. J. Biol. Chem. **275:** 31199–31203.
69. LIU, X. *et al.* 1996. Induction of apoptotic program in cell-free extracts: requirement for dATP and cytochrome *c*. Cell **86:** 147–157.
70. PETIT, P.X. *et al.* 1996. Mitochondria and programmed cell death: back to the future. FEBS Lett. **396:** 7–13.
71. BLACKSTONE, N.W. & D.R. GREEN. 1999. The evolution of a mechanism of cell suicide. Bioessays **21:** 84–88.
72. LEE, H.C. & Y.H. WEI. 2000. Mitochondrial role in life and death of the cell. J. Biomed. Sci. **7:** 2–15.
73. KITAZAWA, M., V. ANANTHARAM & A.G. KANTHASAMY. 2002. Dieldrin induces apoptosis by promoting caspase-3 dependent proteolytic cleavage of protein kinase Cδ in dopaminergic cells: relevance to pathogenesis of Parkinson's disease. Neuroscience. Submitted.
74. LEIST, M. *et al.* 1998. 1-Methyl-4-phenylpyridinium induces autocrine excitotoxicity, protease activation, and neuronal apoptosis. Mol. Pharmacol. **54:** 789–801.
75. DODEL, R.C. *et al.* 1999. Caspase-3-like proteases and 6-hydroxydopamine induced neuronal cell death. Brain Res. Mol. Brain Res. **64:** 141–148.
76. SHI, Y. 2004. Caspase activation: revisiting the induced proximity model. Cell **117:** 855–858.
77. HARTMANN, A. *et al.* 2000. Caspase-3: a vulnerability factor and final effector in apoptotic death of dopaminergic neurons in Parkinson's disease. Proc. Natl. Acad. Sci. USA **97:** 2875–2880.
78. HARTMANN, A. & E.C. HIRSCH. 2001. Parkinson's disease: the apoptosis hypothesis revisited. Adv. Neurol. **86:** 143–153.

79. KITAZAWA, M. *et al.* 2004. Dieldrin promotes proteolytic cleavage of poly(ADP-ribose) polymerase and apoptosis in dopaminergic cells: protective effect of mitochondrial anti-apoptotic protein Bcl-2. Neurotoxicology **25:** 589–598.

80. KITAZAWA, M., V. ANANTHARAM & A.G. KANTHASAMY. 2003. Dieldrin induces apoptosis by promoting caspase-3-dependent proteolytic cleavage of protein kinase Cδ in dopaminergic cells: relevance to oxidative stress and dopaminergic degeneration. Neuroscience **119:** 945–964.

81. KANTHASAMY, A.G. *et al.* 2003. Proteolytic activation of proapoptotic kinase PKCδ is regulated by overexpression of Bcl-2: implications for oxidative stress and environmental factors in Parkinson's disease. Ann. N.Y. Acad. Sci. **1010:** 683–686.

82. PRZEDBORSKI, S. 2004. Programmed cell death in amyotrophic lateral sclerosis: a mechanism of pathogenic and therapeutic importance. Neurologist **10:** 1–7.

83. ZHIVOTOVSKY, B. 2004. Apoptosis, necrosis and between. Cell Cycle **3:** 64–66.

84. SAELENS, X. *et al.* 2004. Toxic proteins released from mitochondria in cell death. Oncogene **23:** 2861–2874.

85. HONG, S.J., T.M. DAWSON & V.L. DAWSON. 2004. Nuclear and mitochondrial conversations in cell death: PARP-1 and AIF signaling. Trends Pharmacol. Sci. **25:** 259–264.

86. LU, C.X. *et al.* 2003. Apoptosis-inducing factor and apoptosis. Sheng Wu Hua Xue Yu Sheng Wu Wu Li Xue Bao (Shanghai) **35:** 881–885.

87. BOHM, I. & H. SCHILD. 2003. Apoptosis: the complex scenario for a silent cell death. Mol. Imaging Biol. **5:** 2–14.

88. REGO, A.C. & C.R. OLIVEIRA. 2003. Mitochondrial dysfunction and reactive oxygen species in excitotoxicity and apoptosis: implications for the pathogenesis of neurodegenerative diseases. Neurochem. Res. **28:** 1563–1574.

89. HIGUCHI, Y. 2003. Chromosomal DNA fragmentation in apoptosis and necrosis induced by oxidative stress. Biochem. Pharmacol. **66:** 1527–1535.

90. NAGATA, S. *et al.* 2003. Degradation of chromosomal DNA during apoptosis. Cell Death Differ. **10:** 108–116.

New Therapeutic Strategies and Drug Candidates for Neurodegenerative Diseases

p53 and TNF-α Inhibitors, and GLP-1 Receptor Agonists

NIGEL H. GREIG,[a] MARK P. MATTSON,[a] TRACYANN PERRY,[a] SIC L. CHAN,[a] TONY GIORDANO,[b] KUMAR SAMBAMURTI,[c] JACK T. ROGERS,[d] HAIM OVADIA,[e] AND DEBOMOY K. LAHIRI[f]

[a]*Laboratory of Neurosciences, Intramural Research Program, National Institute on Aging, National Institutes of Health, Baltimore, Maryland 21224, USA*

[b]*Department of Molecular Biology and Biochemistry, Louisiana State University, Shreveport, Louisiana 71130, USA*

[c]*Department of Physiology and Neuroscience, Medical University South Carolina, Charleston, South Carolina 29425, USA*

[d]*Genetics and Aging Unit, Massachusetts General Hospital, Harvard Medical School, Charlestown, Massachusetts 02129, USA*

[e]*Department of Neurology, The Agnes Ginges Center for Human Neurogenetics, Hadassah Hebrew University Hospital, Jerusalem, Israel*

[f]*Department of Psychiatry, Institute of Psychiatric Research, Indiana University School of Medicine, Indianapolis, Indiana 46202, USA*

ABSTRACT: Owing to improving preventative, diagnostic, and therapeutic measures for cardiovascular disease and a variety of cancers, the average ages of North Americans and Europeans continue to rise. Regrettably, accompanying this increase in life span, there has been an increase in the number of individuals afflicted with age-related neurodegenerative disorders, such as Alzheimer's disease, Parkinson's disease, and stroke. Although different cell types and brain areas are vulnerable among these, each disorder likely develops from activation of a common final cascade of biochemical and cellular events that eventually lead to neuronal dysfunction and death. In this regard, different triggers, including oxidative damage to DNA, the overactivation of glutamate receptors, and disruption of cellular calcium homeostasis, albeit initiated by different genetic and/or environmental factors, can instigate a cascade of intracellular events that induce apoptosis. To forestall the neurodegenerative process, we have chosen specific targets to inhibit that are at pivotal rate-limiting steps within the pathological cascade. Such targets include TNF-α, p53, and GLP-1 receptor. The cytokine TNF-α is elevated in Alzheimer's disease, Parkinson's disease, stroke, and amyotrophic lateral sclerosis. Its synthesis can be reduced via posttranscriptional mechanisms with novel analogues of the classic drug,

Address for correspondence: Nigel H. Greig, Drug Design and Development Section, Laboratory of Neurosciences, Gerontology Research Center, 5600 Nathan Shock Drive, Baltimore, MD 21224.
greign@grc.nia.nih.gov

Ann. N.Y. Acad. Sci. 1035: 290–315 (2004). © 2004 New York Academy of Sciences.
doi: 10.1196/annals.1332.018

thalidomide. The intracellular protein and transcription factor, p53, is activated by the Alzheimer's disease toxic peptide, Aβ, as well as by excess glutamate and hypoxia to trigger neural cell death. It is inactivated by novel tetrahydrobenzothiazole and -oxazole analogues to rescue cells from lethal insults. Stimulation of the glucagon-like peptide-1 receptor (GLP-1R) in brain is associated with neurotrophic functions that, additionally, can protect cells against excess glutamate and other toxic insults.

KEYWORDS: TNF-α; p53; GLP-1 receptor (GLP-1R)

INTRODUCTION

Gaining from our expanding understanding of the medical sciences and from the discovery and introduction of new drug classes, human life span increased by more than 50% in most industrialized nations during the 20th century. Longer life is associated with both merits and costs. Hence, the continuing increase in longevity has major implications on both the societies and economies of these countries. Although hardly uncommon at the turn of the 20th century, neurodegenerative diseases were not a major cause of morbidity. In contrast, with an effective armamentarium of drugs for common infectious diseases—killers of yesteryear—together with improved preventative, diagnostic, and therapeutic measures for cardiovascular disease and a variety of cancers, degenerative disorders of the nervous system, including stroke, Alzheimer's disease (AD), Parkinson's disease (PD), and Huntington's disease, motor neuron diseases, and prion diseases are among the most common causes of death. They are also currently among the most debilitating illnesses and force an enormous strain on both social and healthcare budgets throughout the world.

Different brain areas are primarily affected in each of these diseases: for example cortical and striatal neurons in stroke, hippocampal and cortical neurons in AD, and substantia nigral and midbrain dopaminergic neurons in PD. However, each disorder likely develops from the activation of common final cascades of biochemical and cellular events that eventually lead to neuronal cell dysfunction and death.[1] This may involve genetic or different external triggers, such as oxidative damage to DNA, the overactivation of glutamate receptors, or the disruption of cellular calcium homeostasis, to initiate the shared cascade of intracellular events causing either acute or chronic perturbations of physiological function, cell death, and clinical manifestations (TABLE 1).[2–4] Within this shared cascade, competing biochemical pathways can steer a cell towards survival or death, even at a late stage after a potentially lethal insult. Two targets that will be discussed further and that can alter this cell survival/death balance are the GLP-1 receptor and the transcription factor p53. Very often, inflammatory reaction accompanies the pathological processes that underpin neurodegeneration and it can be initiated in numerous ways.[5–8] For example, glial activation occurs as part of a defense mechanism to facilitate tissue repair by removing unwanted cell debris. Unfortunately, such valuable actions can go awry. Activated microglial cells can produce and secrete proinflammatory cytokines, in particular TNF-α, as well as cytotoxic elements like reactive oxygen species (ROS), nitric oxide (NO), and excitatory amino acids (e.g., glutamate), and induce a self-propagating cycle of events.

Characterization of the shared biochemical cascades has provided prospective targets to intervene and potentially slow or halt the disease process. Which, if any,

TABLE 1. Examples of genetic and environmental triggers in neurodegenerative disorders

Disorder	Gene	Environmental factor
Stroke	NOTCH3, KRIT1, CST3, BRI	Smoking, lipids, calories
Alzheimer's disease	APP, presenilin-1 and -2, ApoE	Head trauma, education, physical and mental activity, calories
Parkinson's disease	α-Synuclein, parkin, DJ-1, UCHL-1, PINK1	Head trauma, toxins, calories
Amyotrophic lateral sclerosis	Cu/Zn-SOD	Autoimmune response, toxins
Huntington's disease	Huntingtin	

NOTE: PINK1, PTEN-induced putative kinase 1; UCHL-1, ubiquitin C-terminal hydrolase gene; KRIT1 encodes for Krev-1/rap1 interaction trapped 1 protein.

are pivotal and rate-limiting is a focus of ongoing research and, in part, will rely on the design, synthesis, and development of pharmacological tools to selectively bind and inhibit the function of the individual protein members within the biochemical cascade. The application of medicinal chemistry to cell biology and molecular and *in vivo* pharmacology is providing us the means of testing new therapeutic strategies to both validated and unvalidated disease targets. Our overarching focus has been to incorporate features into our initial drug design and medicinal chemistry that optimize *in vivo* targeting and provide appropriate druglike properties (pharmaco-kinetic and pharmacodynamic parameters) to our pharmacological tools to facilitate their rapid utility as drug candidates in proof-of-concept studies.

HALTING NEURONAL APOPTOSIS BY INACTIVATION OF p53

All differentiated cells are able to trigger their own death via activation of a genetically encoded suicide program, termed apoptosis. This biological phenomenon was originally described by Kerr and colleagues,[9] and is characterized by the presence of chromatin condensation, nuclear fragmentation, cell contraction, and dissolution into small fragments, termed apoptotic bodies, that are surrounded by plasma membrane. Phagocytosis, thereafter, removes apoptotic cells without accompanying inflammation as the integrity of the plasma membrane and organelles is maintained during the cell death process and there is no spillage of the intracellular contents. In contrast, in necrotic cell death rapid swelling and cell rupture occur and cause substantial secondary damage in surrounding tissues due to inflammation. Whereas apoptosis and necrosis differ both structurally and biochemically and hence were classified as two separate forms of cell death, both can occur side by side as a consequence of a traumatic injury with the affected cells showing a continuum of features of apoptosis and necrosis.[10,11]

From a physiological perspective, apoptosis plays a crucial role in morphogenesis during embryogenic development of the central and peripheral nervous systems,[12] where it is pronounced when the genesis of synapses occurs. In the adult, it is also a critical mechanism for maintaining the cell number within and size of an organ or tissue that has proliferative capacity, such as the immune system or intestinal mucosa. For cells that have sustained an irreversible level of DNA damage, it represents a means of removing them from the organism and allowing their replacement by a new viable cell. While valuable in tissues with proliferative capacity by ultimately protecting the genome from accumulating excess mutations, for nervous tissue the value of this same process in the adult is questionable. Neurons that are terminally differentiated have no capacity to divide; hence, apoptosis may not be beneficial to survival, as a functioning but damaged neuron may be more useful than a dead one.

Apoptosis is a tightly regulated process that can be initiated by a variety of factors that then trigger specific biochemical pathways (FIG. 1). These have been categorized as extrinsic and intrinsic, with various interlinks. Whereas the external pathway is initiated by cell surface activation, for example, TNF-α receptor signaling through cytokine binding and activation of TNF-related apoptosis-inducing ligand (TRAIL) receptors, the intrinsic pathway is often triggered by DNA or mitochondria damage. The principal molecular components of the apoptosis program in neurons have been reviewed,[8,10,13] and broadly include Apaf-1 (apoptotic protease-activating factor 1) and proteins in the Bcl-2 and caspase families (FIG. 1).

The caspases, with 15 members in mammalian cells that can be divided into initiators (caspases 2, 8, 9, and 10) that activate effectors (caspases 3, 6, and 7), are the proteolytic enzymes responsible for mitochondrial damage, nuclear membrane breakdown, DNA fragmentation, chromatin condensation, and eventual cell death.[14] The initiator caspases possess long amino-terminal domains that contain specialized motifs that promote specific protein-protein interactions. Via these domains, as exemplified by initiator caspases 8 and 9, activation occurs by interaction with the adapter molecules, Apaf1 and FADD (Fas-associating protein with death domain). The activated initiator caspases thereafter cleave the effector ones into their active forms. Caspases, hence, provide a potential target for therapeutic intervention and significant medicinal chemistry has focused on this area.[15–17] Selective caspase inhibition has proved promising in the laboratory,[18] although some consider that they act too late in cell death pathways to have a substantial effect on long-term survival.[19] In addition, the value of this approach in brain has been limited by the poor blood-brain barrier penetration of current inhibitors[20] as these primarily are peptide-based compounds.

Another strategy would be to interrupt the apoptotic cascade upstream of caspase activation. In this regard, an important regulatory step in apoptosis occurs at mitochondrial membranes where members of the Bcl-2 family of proteins either promote (Bax and Bad) or prevent (Bcl-2 and Bcl-XL) membrane permeability transition. The ratio of specific Bcl-2 family members is hence critical as to whether cell death or protection occurs. Although signaling events acting upstream of mitochondrial changes in apoptosis are yet to be fully elucidated, the tumor suppressor protein p53, a transcription factor, clearly plays a key role[21,22] by stimulating production or mitochondrial translocation of the pro-apoptotic protein Bax and release of cytochrome c[23,24] among numerous other pro-apoptotic actions.[8] Whether intrinsically or extrinsically initiated, it is clear that p53 protein levels are greatly increased and the ability of p53 to bind specific DNA sequences is activated in response to cellular damage. p53 protein levels are primarily regulated posttranscriptionally, and hence

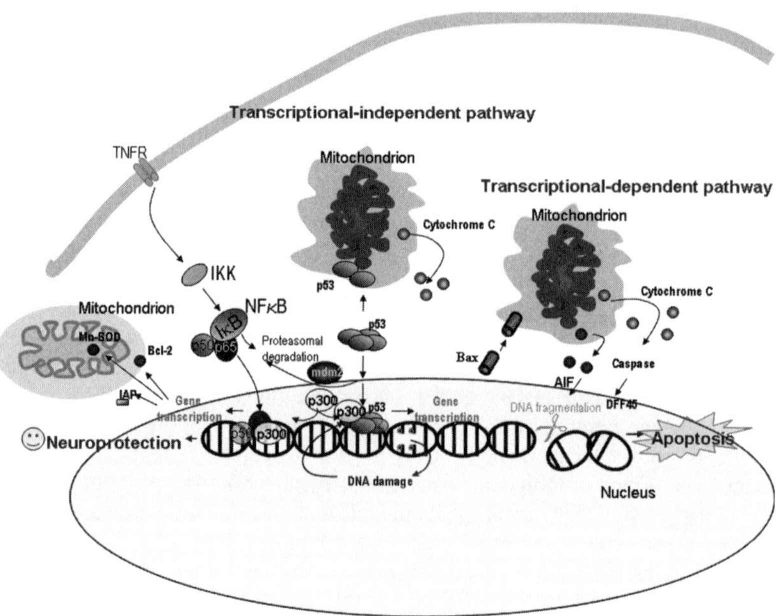

FIGURE 1. Various apoptotic stimuli, including DNA damage, induce p53 activation. This involves posttranslational modification of the p53 protein resulting in reduced proteasomal targeting by Mdm2 and, hence, increased stability and elevated p53 levels. The proapoptotic action of p53 involves its function as transcription factor inducing the synthesis and mitochondrial translocation of Bax and other p53-inducible genes, such as PUMA and Noxa. Bax induces release of apoptosis-inducing factor (AIF) and cytochrome *c* from the mitochondria. Cytochrome *c* activates caspases that cleave a series of substrates including DNA fragmentation factor (DFF45). Both AIF and DFF45 induce DNA fragmentation. Recently, mechanisms independent of p53 transcriptional activity may also be involved in p53-mediated apoptosis. p53 can translocate to the mitochondria wherein it induces release of cytochrome *c*. p53 can also block the activity of other transcription factors such as nuclear factor-κB (NFκB). NFκB is activated by downstream signaling cascades induced by tumor necrosis factor receptor (TNFR). In neurons, NFκB supports survival signaling by inducing the expression of anti-apoptotic factors, for example anti-apoptotic Bcl-2 family members, manganese superoxide dismutase (MnSOD), and inhibitors of apoptosis (IAP). p53 binds to and sequesters p300, a co-activator for various transcription factors including NFκB.

damage-induced accumulation of p53 results largely from increased stability. Phosphorylation, too, likely plays an important role in regulating its stability (such as by reducing the ability of the p53 binding protein, Mdm2, to complex and increase p53 degradation) and regulating its DNA binding activity.[25] As illustrated in FIGURE 1, the p53-dependent cascades leading to programmed cell death invoke transcription-dependent and -independent pathways with numerous regulatory feedback mechanisms to culminate eventually in cellular protection or apoptosis.

Our studies have focused on the antihelminthic (antiparasitic) compound, pifithrin-α (PFTα), as a pharmacophore for drug design (FIG. 2) because the agent

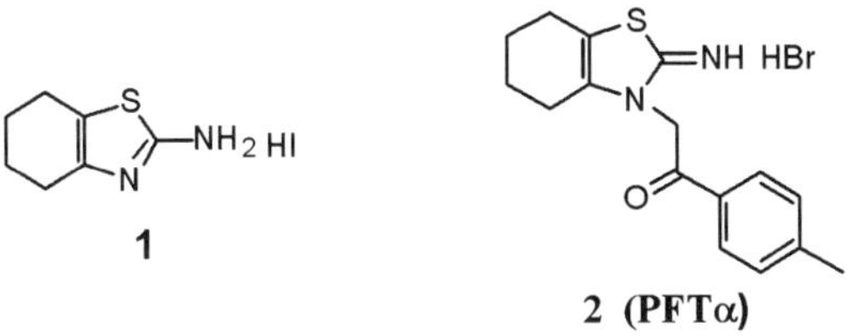

FIGURE 2. Chemical structures of the p53 inactivators, PFTα and precursor (compounds 2 and 1, respectively).

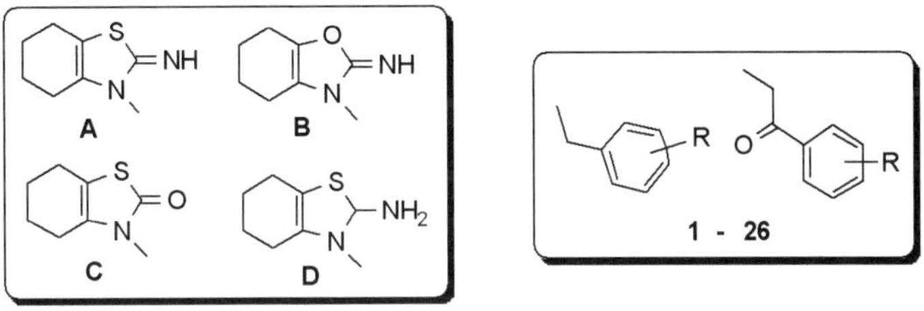

FIGURE 3. Heterocycle and *N*-substituent modifications to create PFTα analogues.

was recently reported to inhibit p53-mediated transcription.[26] Our initial studies demonstrated that compound 2, but not its precursor (compound 1) (FIG. 2), was effective in protecting cultured primary hippocampal neurons against death induced by the DNA-damaging topoisomerase I and II inhibitors, camptothecin and etoposide, respectively.[27] These agents induce neuronal apoptosis via a mechanism that involves p53 induction and caspase activation,[28,29] which parenthetically were suppressed in the presence of compound 2. Compound 2, additionally, protected neuronal cells against fatality induced by glutamate and Aβ,[27] which similarly induce p53-mediated neuronal death.[1,30] However, it was ineffective in preventing cell death caused by trophic factor withdrawal,[27] which is known to kill cells in a p53-independent manner.[31,32] These studies confirmed the activity of compound 2 as a p53 inactivator and hence provided a lead compound for medicinal chemistry.

The inactivity of the PFTα precursor, compound 1, indicates that the *N*-substituent group of compound 2 is critical for p53 inactivation. Modifications were therefore initially made to this moiety to elucidate structure-activity relationships for neuroprotective activity. Analogues were synthesized to assess the importance of the carbonyl and aryl groups, together with substitution of electron-donating and electron-withdrawing moieties on the latter.[33] In addition, heterocyclic modifications also were undertaken to optimize the pharmacophore for greatest neuroprotective activity (FIG. 3). Numerous novel analogues were synthesized, possessing calculated log D values (clog D: octanol/water partition coefficient at physiological pH) that primarily ranged between 0 to 2.5, in line with the Lipinski "Rule of 5"[34] to optimize absorption and brain delivery.[35] The log D value provides an indication of blood-brain barrier penetrability and the upper value is in line with that of the classic CNS active drug valium. Illustrated in FIGURE 4 are examples, among many modifications, which result in altered activity. Interestingly, and as depicted by B5 vs. A5 (FIG. 4), replacement of the heterocycle S by an O (resulting in tetrahydrobenzoxazoles rather than -thiazoles) resulted in greater potency (as determined by a lower EC_{50} value for protecting PC12 cells from camptothecin-induced apoptosis). Modifications in the *N*-substituent group of the parent compound, such as removal of the carbonyl function (depicted by A19 vs. A5, FIG. 4) resulted in loss of activity. However, incorporation of a halogen within aryl function (depicted by A15 and A17 vs. A5) reinstated biological activity and, indeed, improved it depending on the position of substitution. Likewise, as depicted by A7, A8, and A9 vs. A5 (FIG. 4), replacement of an aryl methyl group by an electron-donating methoxy dramatically altered biological activity depending on the position of substitution.[33] In this manner, a wide variety of compounds of varying p53 inhibitory potency were synthesized with physicochemical characteristics to either augment or restrict brain uptake for neurodegenerative and systemic diseases, respectively, together with modifications to protect against plasma lability.[33]

The mechanisms underpinning p53 inactivation remain to be fully elucidated. PFTα and active analogues lowered the basal level of p53 DNA-binding activity in resting, unchallenged neuronal cells in culture, without affecting basal levels of p53-responsive genes, as exemplified by Bax.[27] Consequent to an insult with Aβ or camptothecin, however, PFTα markedly suppressed p53 induction, phosphorylation, the induction of Bax, and downstream events associated with apoptosis, such as stabilizing mitochondrial function and suppressing caspase activation.[27,36]

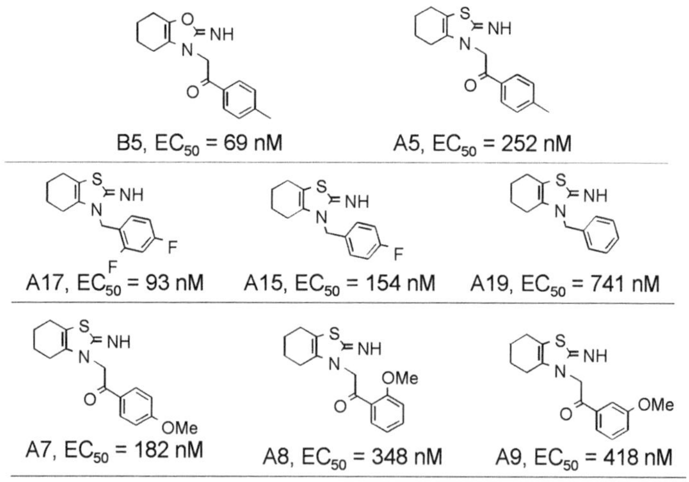

FIGURE 4. PFTα analogues: examples of structure-activity relations. EC_{50} values were determined in PC12 cells challenged with a lethal dose of camptothecin, which induces cell death via a p53-dependent mechanism (EC_{50} represents the concentration of compound required to protect 50% of cells from death).[33,117]

Preclinical studies have focused on the selection of analogues as candidates for potential clinical development. In this regard, "proof of concept" preclinical efficacy studies have been undertaken in a variety of models, exemplified by stroke and PD, to assess the potential of transient p53 inactivation.[27,33,36,37] Such studies, together with classic pharmacokinetic and pharmacodynamic studies in rodent models, aid in compound selection to determine which of the numerous agents available should be developed as experimental drug candidates. A potentially serious adverse action of this class of compounds is the risk that they may induce or increase the risk of tumors. p53 knockout mice have an increased incidence of cancer. In contrast, its overactivation induces premature aging-associated phenotypes in mice.[38,39] Consequently, transient and relatively short-term inhibition of p53 in the treatment of acute catastrophic insults, exemplified by stroke or head trauma, could prove efficacious, as could long-term inhibition of induced p53 rather than constitutive, basal levels during a devastating, longer term disorder, such as PD and AD. Only classical toxicological studies can define whether risk/benefit ratios are appropriate to support the strategy in specific indications.

Most research has focused on stroke, utilizing the classical middle cerebral artery occlusion (MCAO) model in the mouse, wherein focal ischemia is induced by either transient or permanent occlusion. An ischemic infarct results in damage to the ipsilateral cerebral cortex and striatum, whose size can be measured at a fixed time thereafter (e.g., 24 or 48 h) by staining brain sections with a dye taken up by functioning mitochondrion.[27,33,36] In both stroke models, p53 inhibition lowered infarct volume[33] (as achieved with PFTα, FIG. 5), with reductions occurring in the ischemic penumbra as opposed to the central core.[36] A concentration-dependent effect was

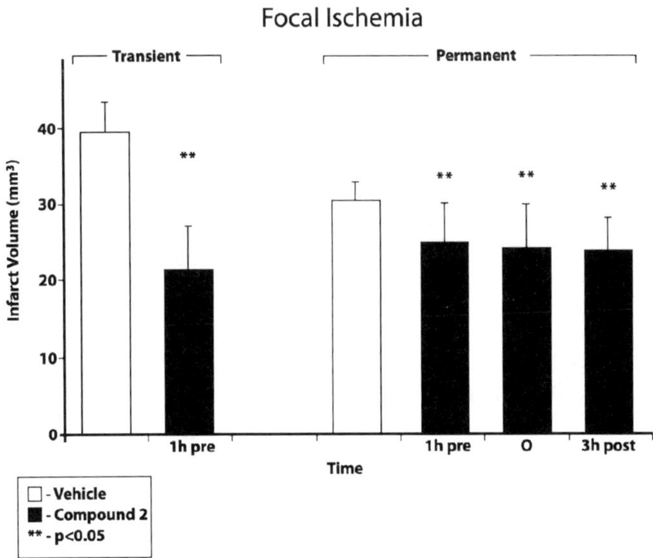

FIGURE 5. Protective effect of PFTα (compound 2) (2 mg/kg i.p.) in mice before and after focal ischemia. Infarct volume was assessed at 24 h.[33]

evident, which demonstrated a classical inverted U-shaped curve, with a loss of protective activity occurring at high doses.[36] Reduced infarct size was associated with lower disability scores and could be achieved within a therapeutic window of some 4 h after MCAO. Administration of p53 inactivators in stroke, similar to cell culture studies assessing other apoptotic insults, was associated with lowered levels of both induced and phosphorylated p53, a reduced expression of its targeted genes p21[WAF] and Bax, and less activation of caspases in the infarct tissue, compared to untreated animals after MCAO.[36] Of particular interest, immunohistochemical staining for p53 and p21[WAF] within the ischemic penumbra of PFTα treated and untreated mice demonstrated a similar number of p53-positive cells in each, p53 localization in the cytoplasm in the former as opposed to the nucleus for the latter, and a lack of p21[WAF] staining in the former.[36] This is indicative of PFTα and analogues acting at the level of p53 translocation into the nucleus and the prevention of its binding to specific DNA sites. Likewise, studies in cortical synaptosomes have demonstrated that p53 has a role in synaptic dysfunction and loss that occurs during the early stages of the neuronal death process, which can be protected by PFTα that blocks the translocation of p53 to mitochondria.[40]

Similarly, p53 inactivators have been employed in a mouse model of seizure-induced brain damage, in which intrahippocampal administration of the excitotoxic kainate induces seizures and selective degeneration of pyramidal neurons in regions CA1 and CA3 of the hippocampus. Here too, PFTα provided neuroprotection,[27] as well as in a classic mouse model of PD, wherein selective dopaminergic cell death was induced by the mitochondrial poison, MPTP.[37] Whereas the mechanisms whereby PFTα and analogues inhibit p53 transcriptional-dependent and -independent activities remains largely unknown, they reliably inhibit activation of p53-responsive genes in neuronal cells in both cell culture and *in vivo*.[27,33,36,37,40] The specificity of these agents is confirmed by their inability to protect cells lacking p53 or tumor cells with p53 mutations against apoptosis.[26,40] The factors that cause p53-mediated apoptosis in neurodegenerative diseases, such as PD and AD, are not fully understood, but likely involve common cascades, albeit initiated by different environmental as well as genetic factors, leading to mitochondrial impairment and increased oxidative stress. Thus, our data, which show that chemical inhibitors of p53 can prevent apoptosis of different vulnerable neurons in a host of insults in cell culture as well as in animal models, and yet preserve motor function, suggest that their use, if sufficiently well tolerated, might delay or halt the neurodegenerative processes associated with a variety of acute and chronic insults.

INHIBITING THE INFLAMMATORY PROCESS ASSOCIATED WITH NEURODEGENERATION

Inflammatory processes play a critical role in promoting the degenerative processes in a wide variety of neurodegenerative disorders, including AD, PD, ALS, and MS.[5,41–43] Although inflammation represents a first line of defense against injury and infection, a disproportionate inflammatory response can cause additional injury to neural cells. Indeed, many neurodegenerative disorders are associated with the accumulation of abnormal protein assemblies, exemplified by Aβ in AD and α-synuclein in PD. There is increasing support to suggest that such assemblies can instigate cellular stress and neuro-inflammation, to which neurons have a relatively low tolerance, thus potentially initiating a self-propagating cycle of autodestructive immune and inflammatory processes that hamper the recovery of neurological function at sites of inflammation or that even intensify neuronal injury.[44]

The characteristic markers of chronic inflammation are associated with most neurodegenerative disorders,[5,6] amongst which there is upregulation of the pro-inflammatory cytokines interleukin-1β (IL-1β), interleukin-6 (IL-6), and TNF-α, as well as the prostaglandin generating cyclooxygenases, COX-1 and COX-2.[7,44–46] In AD, the impact of these inflammatory processes is now well accepted. In PD, however, although inflammatory markers in the substantia nigra were reported long ago[5] and the high number of microglia associated with this area may underpin its vulnerability,[47] the impact of these processes remains a matter of debate. Nevertheless, anti-inflammatory therapy may represent a promising therapeutic intervention.[43,48] The question remains as to the choice of target.

The potential that COX-1 and COX-2 inhibitors have demonstrated in cell culture and animal models has, unfortunately, not yet been realized in clinical AD trials focused on disease progression. Although the results have been disappointing,[49] the use of non-steroidal anti-inflammatory agents has been associated with a lower risk of the disease.[6,50] This has stimulated interest in the potential value of inhibiting other specific cytokines. In this regard, the role of IL-1β in neuroinflammation and AD has recently been examined,[51] as has TNF-α.[52] Both IL-1β and TNF-α are expressed in microglia around developing amyloid plaques in brain cells[53,54] and have been shown to stimulate APP turnover into its pathological Aβ form.[55–57] Indeed, these cytokines are potent stimulators of γ-secretase, resulting in the increased production of Aβ through a pathway involving the c-Jun N-terminal kinase (JNK)–dependent MAPK pathway[58] and, additionally, upregulate the APP expression of cells.[59–61] Furthermore, astrocytes and microglia, both representing key components of the cellular environment surrounding neurons, are non-neuronal sources of APP that are activated in the presence of amyloid plaques[62,63] as well as by fibrillar Aβ, through a cell surface receptor complex, to further increase their production of TNF-α and IL-1β.[64,65]

These same cytokines represent a useful target in PD, where there is evidence of the upregulation of TNF-α, in particular, in both brain and CSF.[66–68] In addition, an earlier onset of sporadic PD has been reported in Japanese patients with a polymorphism in the promotor region of the TNF-α gene.[69] The genetic ablation of TNF-α in mice provides them resistance to MPTP toxicity[70] as well as to EAE.[71] Finally, overexpression of TNF-α is found in brain trauma and cerebral ischemia,[46,72] multiple sclerosis,[73] as well as ALS.[74] Clearly, cytokines have a beneficial role, as evidenced in their reported neuroprotective actions in β-amyloid toxicity,[75] focal cerebral ischemia, and epileptic seizures.[76] Their actions are concentration- and time-dependent, and a reduction of their levels towards basal ones could prove to be efficacious in several neurodegenerative conditions.

In our continuing effort to design and develop agents of potential clinical value, we focused on the pharmacophore of thalidomide to synthesize novel and pharmacologically useful agents. Thalidomide (*N*-α-phthalimidoglutarimide) (FIG. 6) is a glutamic acid derivative that was introduced onto the market as a sedative hypnotic in 1956. It was withdrawn from the market in 1961 due to the development of severe congenital abnormalities in babies born to mothers using it for morning sickness.[77,78] Interest in the agent was rekindled after thalidomide was found clinically effective in the treatment of erythema nodosum leprosum (ENL)[79] and in the treatment of HIV wasting syndrome and various cancers.[80] Mechanistic studies of its ENL activity demonstrated an anti–TNF-α action. Specifically, thalidomide enhances the degradation of TNF-α RNA and thereby lowers TNF-α synthesis and secretion.[81,82] Further studies have defined it as a co-stimulator of both CD8+ and CD4+ T cells,[83] an inhibitor of angiogenesis[84] via its inhibitory actions on basic fibroblast growth factor (bFGF) and vascular endothelial growth factor (VEGF), and an inhibitor of NFκB. However, it is the action of thalidomide on TNF-α that has provided our

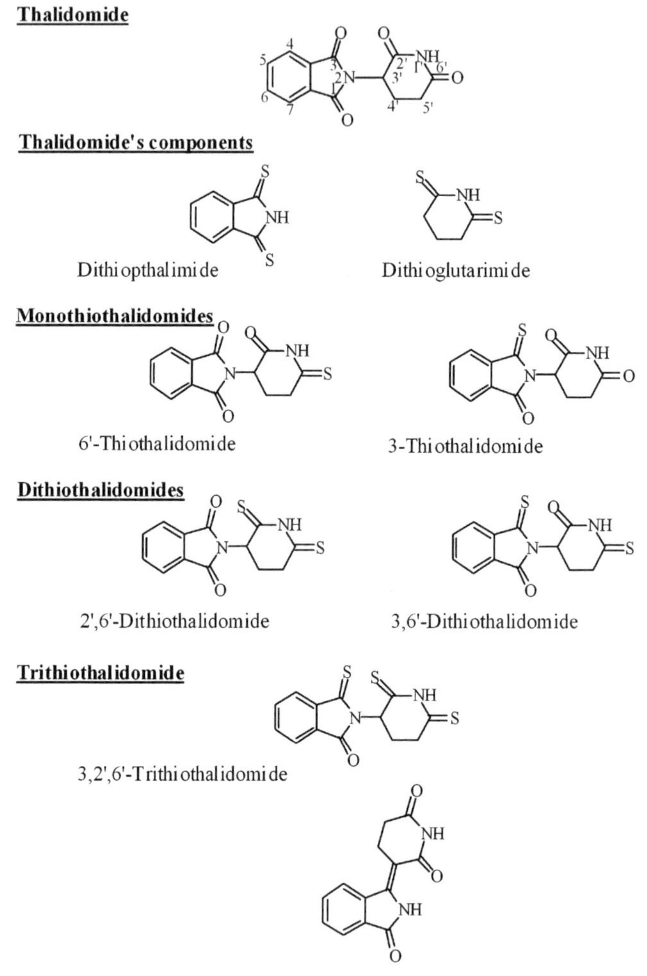

FIGURE 6. Chemical structures of analogues of 3-phthalimidoglutarimide: thalidomide.

initial focus. Clearly, this critical cytokine has numerous fundamental roles beyond neurodegeneration, as its overproduction exacerbates inflammatory and autoimmune responses in a wide number of systemic diseases, including rheumatoid arthritis, ENL, septic shock, graft-versus-host disease, Crohn's disease, and AIDS.

The mechanisms underlying thalidomide's diverse actions, together with identification of the active species (since it generates numerous metabolites) remain an area of intense research. Seldom has such a simple molecule had such a controversial history and held so much therapeutic promise. Our focus was the design of agents with improved TNF-α inhibitory potency plus a balanced lipohilicity to combine a reasonable solubility in the aqueous phase of plasma with the ability to penetrate biological membranes readily, such as the gastrointestinal tract and blood-brain barrier. Prior research had primarily focused on exploring the structural modification of the phthaloyl ring or glutarimide ring of thalidomide, including *N*-phthaloyl 3-amino-3-arylpropionic acid derivatives, amino-phthaloyl substituted and tetra-fluorophthaloyl substituted analogues of thalidomide, and *N*-substituted phthalimides with a simplified glutarimide moiety.[82,85–88] In addition, as the anti-angiogenic property of thalidomide has been attributed to its hydroxylated metabolites,[89,90] the open-ring metabolites have also been synthesized.[89,91]

To discover novel isosteric analogues of thalidomide, we focused on the carbonyl moiety and synthesized a novel series of thiothalidomides and analogues (exemplified by compounds in FIG. 6). Their TNF-α inhibitory activity was thereafter assessed in human peripheral blood mononuclear cells (PBMCs) that were stimulated with lipopolysaccharide (LPS) to elevate levels of constitutively expressed TNF-α. As shown in TABLE 2 and FIGURE 7, thalidomide was essentially devoid of activity at 30 μM, requiring a concentration of ~200 μM to induce a 50% inhibition (IC_{50}) of TNF-α secretion. By comparison, the monothiothalidomides, 3-thiothalidomide and 6′-thiothalidomide demonstrated albeit minor but nevertheless significant activity

TABLE 2. Thalidomide and analogue-induced inhibition of LPS-stimulated TNF-α production in PBMCs and cell viability

Compound	IC_{50} (μM)	Percent inhibition at 30 μM	Percent cell viability at 30 μM	Clog D value (lipophilicity)
Thalidomide	~200	None	100	−0.83
6′-Thiothalidomide	>30	31	100	−0.57
3-Thiothalidomide	>30	23	94	−0.57
2′,6′-Dithiothalidomide	20	52	69	−0.56
3,6′-Dithiothalidomide	11	61	100	−0.56
3,2′,6′-Trithiothalidomide	6	79	94	−0.30
Dithioglutarimide	8	75	100	−0.48
Dithiophthalimide	3	95	54	+0.27
ODYPD	>30	37	100	+0.29

NOTE: Clog D value: measure of solubility in aqueous/lipophilic environment, with minus value representing aqueous solubility and plus value representing lipophilic solubility.[35]

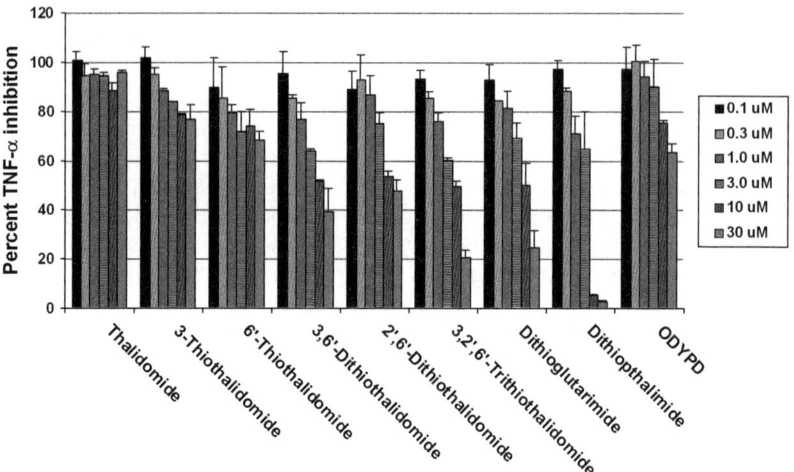

FIGURE 7. Concentration-dependent activity of thalidomide and analogues to lower LPS-stimulated TNF-α levels in human PBMCs (Mean±SEM, $N \geq 3$).

at 30 μM, inducing a 23% and a 31% inhibition of TNF-α secretion, respectively, without a loss of cell viability.

In contrast, the dithiothalidomides, 3,6'-dithiothalidomide and 2',6'-dithiothalidomide, proved to be yet more potent (FIG. 7). They induced a 61% and 53% TNF-α inhibition at 30 μM, albeit with a slight loss of cell viability for only the latter compound, and possessed IC$_{50}$ values of 19.5 μM and 11.5 μM, respectively. In line with the illustrated augmented TNF-α inhibitory action with successive isoteric carbonyl to thiocarbonyl replacement, the trithiothalidomide, 3,2',6'-trithiothalidomide, inhibited TNF-α production with an IC$_{50}$ of 6.2 μM without any accompanying toxicity. As shown in FIGURE 7, an increasing concentration-dependent inhibition was achieved that induced a 79% reduction in secreted TNF-α levels at 30 μM. Hence, replacement of successive carbonyl groups with a thiocarbonyl group led to an increased inhibitory activity compared to thalidomide, of up to 30-fold for 3,2',6'-trithiothalidomide, that was unassociated with toxicity, but coupled to an elevated lipid solubility, as assessed by clog D values (TABLE 2), to aid in driving the compound into the brain.

As thalidomide comprises of two distinct chemical moieties, specifically adjoining glutarimide and phthalimide rings, dithioglutarimide and dithiophthalimide were therefore synthesized and evaluated for biological activity against TNF-α. Interestingly, both proved to be substantially more potent than thalidomide; inducing a dramatic inhibition of 75% and 95% at a 30 μM concentration, respectively, albeit with some toxicity for the latter. However, such toxicity was not found at the IC$_{50}$ concentrations, which were 8 and 3 μM for dithioglutarimide and dithiophthalimide, respectively. Furthermore, as the pthalimide and glutarimide rings are conjoined at the 2- and 3'-positions, modification of this was undertaken by the synthesis of ODYPD, whose TNF-α inhibition was more potent than thalidomide (37% vs. no inhibition at 30 μM, respectively), indicating that thionation of this as well as other thalidomide-like backbones could provide increased TNF-α activity.

Additional studies were undertaken to elucidate the mechanism underpinning the activity of the thalidomide analogues on TNF-α. TNF-α and other cytokines and protooncogenes are known to be regulated at the posttranscriptional level.[92,93] Seeing that thalidomide has been reported to act via the 3′-UTR of TNF-α mRNA that contains an AU-rich area,[81] specific studies were undertaken to assess this with dithioglutarimide and 3,2′,6′-trithiothalidomide. In this regard, a cell-based assay consisting of two stably transfected cell lines derived from the mouse macrophage line (RAW264.7) was used. One line expressed a luciferase reporter construct without any UTR sequences, whereas the other expressed a luciferase reporter construct with the entire 3′-UTR of human TNF-α inserted directly downstream of the luciferase coding region. As illustrated in FIGURE 8, concentration-dependent reductions in the ratio of the luciferase plus 3′-UTR versus the luciferase minus 3′-UTR were found that paralleled reductions in PBMC TNF-α levels. This suggests translational regulation as an underlying mechanism, whereby TNF-α mRNA is destabilized in the presence of the compounds to lower newly synthesized TNF-α protein levels. Current studies are assessing whether or not the described reductions translate into *in vivo* models and are efficacious in specific neurodegenerative diseases.

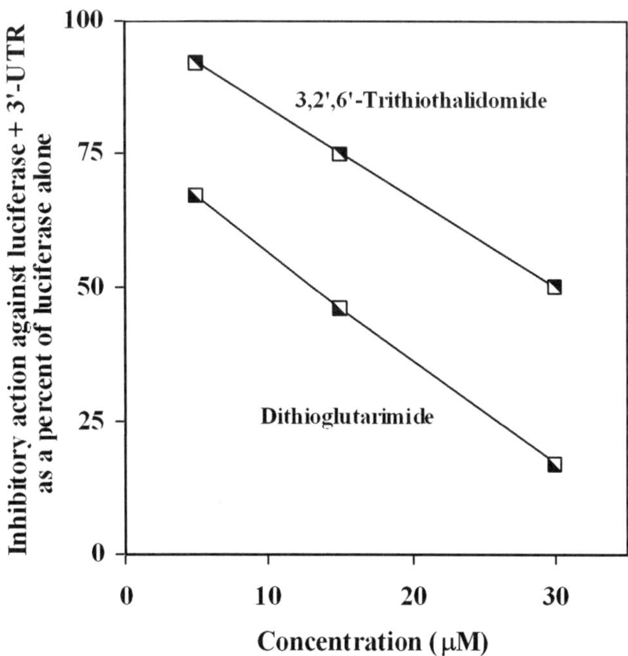

FIGURE 8. The inhibitory actions of dithioglutarimide and 3,2′,6′-trithiothalidomide in mouse macrophage cells (RAW264.7) expressing a luciferase reporter element together with the 3′-UTR of human TNF-α compared to cells lacking the 3′-UTR.

Interestingly, TNF-α inhibition is a validated therapeutic strategy for the treatment of adult and juvenile rheumatoid arthritis and other systemic indications involving inflammatory processes, with the approval of the prescription medications, Enbrel (Etanercept, Amgen/Wyeth) and Remicade (infliximab, Centocor/Schering-Plough). These medications, however, are large macromolecules that minimally traverse biological barriers, require subcutaneous and intravenous injection, respectively, for administration and have negligible brain penetration—thereby precluding their utility in neurodegenerative disorders. In contrast, thalidomide analogues are orally bioavailable and, if well tolerated in toxicological studies and not administered during pregnancy, may be of potential in a wide spectrum of diseases.

GLP-1 RECEPTOR ANALOGUES AS NEUROPROTECTIVE AGENTS

GLP-1 is an endogenous insulinotropic peptide that controls plasma glucose levels via its action on the pancreas; specifically, via the G-protein coupled GLP-1 receptor (GLP-1R) (FIG. 9). The peptide derives from the posttranslational modification of proglucagon and is released from intestinal L cells in response to the presence of food in the gastrointestinal tract.[94] It has an array of reported physiological actions that include glucose-dependent stimulation of insulin secretion and inhibition of glucagon secretion,[95] the inhibition of small bowel motility as well as gastric emptying, and a reduction of hunger.[94–96] GLP-1 additionally acts as a trophic agent, inducing pancreatic β-cell proliferation and neogenesis as well as an inhibition of β-cell apoptosis.[97,98] As a consequence, GLP-1 is an important regulator of β-cell mass, which, together with its other physiological actions, has spurred the development of GLP-1R agonists as a treatment strategy for type 2 diabetes. An advantage of this approach is that many of its effects are glucose-dependent and hence its use is associated with a low risk of hypoglycemia. A disadvantage is that, like most endogenous peptides, GLP-1 is short-lived. It is rapidly degraded by the enzyme, dipeptidyl peptidase IV (DPPIV), and then cleared by the kidney. Hence, its biological activity is short-lived in humans and rodents.[99,100] This, however, has been overcome by both peptide modification, to provide DPPIV-resistant analogues such as exendin-4 (FIG. 9), as well as by the use of DPPIV inhibitors.[94,97,100]

Although predominantly localized to pancreatic islets, numerous reports have documented GLP-1R expression in both the rodent[101,102] and human brain.[103,104] Whether or not GLP-1 is produced by neural cells, though, remains to be determined. It is clear, however, that GLP-1 present in the bloodstream can enter brain.[105]

GLP-1 (7-36 amide) **HAEGTFTSDVSSYLEGQAAKEFIAWLVKGR.**
Exendin-4 (1-39)   **HGEGTFTSDLSKQMEEEAVRLFIEWLKNGGPSSGAPPPS**

FIGURE 9. Amino acid sequences of GLP-1 and its long-acting analogues, exendin-4. GLP-1 is cleaved at the amino terminal by DPPIV (*light gray* amino acids) to end its biological action. The replacement of HA by HG dramatically reduces this. *Underlined* amino acids differentiate GLP-1 and exendin-4, and the 9 amino acid carboxy terminal tail associated with the latter provides it higher potency at the GLP-1R.[100,118,119]

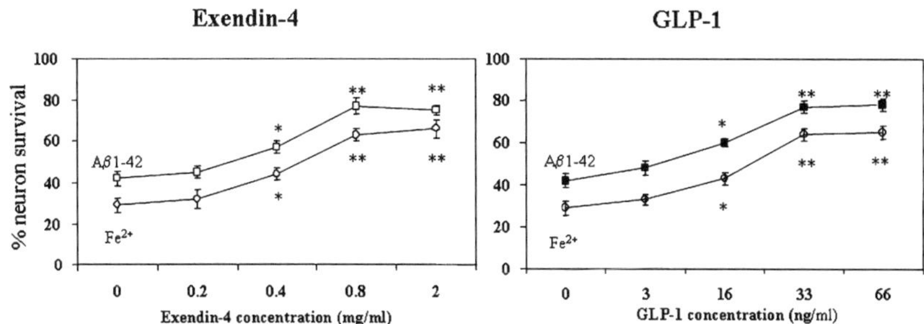

FIGURE 10. GLP-1R stimulation by either GLP-1 or its long-acting analogue, exendin-4, dose-dependently protected cultured rat primary hippocampal cells against apoptosis induced by $A\beta_{1-42}$ (2 mM) or iron (1 mM) (*$P<.05$, **$P<.01$).[108]

In light of the described trophic action of GLP-1R stimulation on β cells, together with its coupling to the cyclic AMP (cAMP) second messenger pathway, increases in which are well documented to be associated with neuroprotection, we characterized the action of GLP-1 analogues on neuronal cells both in cell culture and animal studies.[106–108]

Cell culture studies with both rat pheochromocytoma (PC12) and rat primary hippocampal cells established that the cells express GLP-1 receptors and that GLP-1R activation stimulated adenylyl cyclase, leading to an increase in intracellular cAMP in a manner similar to pancreatic β cells.[106] In addition, GLP-1 together with long-acting analogues induced differentiation in PC12 cells in a manner similar to nerve growth factor (NGF), which was reversed by co-incubation with a selective GLP-1R antagonist. Furthermore, GLP-1 analogues enhanced NGF-initiated differentiation and partly rescued degenerating cells from NGF-mediated withdrawal, in the absence of cellular dysfunction or toxicity.[106] Competitive binding studies demonstrated that the binding affinity of GLP-1 for receptors on hippocampal neurons (IC$_{50}$ of 14 nM) was similar to pancreatic β cells. In addition, GLP-1 analogues provided complete protection against apoptotic cell death induced by glutamate neurotoxicity in cultured hippocampal neurons,[107] as has been shown with other neurotrophic factors.[109,110] Likewise, and as illustrated in FIGURE 10, hippocampal cells were protected against cell death induced by $A\beta_{1-42}$ as well as from oxidative stress and membrane lipid peroxidation caused by iron.[108] Together, these data suggest that GLP-1 agonists may play a significant role in protecting neurons against several types of brain injury, including excitotoxic and oxidative damage.

Whereas much is known about the cellular signaling pathways that occur following GLP-1R stimulation in pancreatic β cells,[97,98] as yet, less has been elucidated in neuronal cells. Our findings implicate participation of phosphatidylinositol-3 kinase (PI3-kinase) and extracellular signal–regulated mitogen-activated protein kinase (ERK MAPK)–dependent pathways in GLP-1–mediated neurite outgrowth and neuroprotection, with additional involvement of protein kinase-A (PKA) signaling.[106,108,111,112] As illustrated in FIGURE 11, stimulation of these and related pathways can divert signaling away from apoptosis towards cell survival.

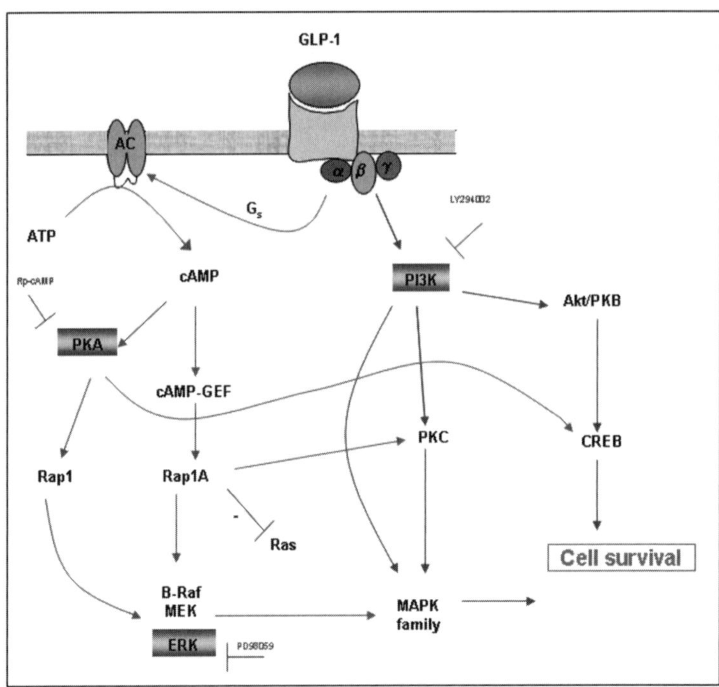

FIGURE 11. Putative signaling pathways stimulated by GLP1-R binding and activation supporting cell survival.GLP-1 action is mediated following binding to a specific G-protein coupled GLP-1R that is coupled positively to the adenylate cyclase (AC) system. Ligand activation of the Gα subunit of the GLP-1R stimulates AC, which leads to an increase in intracellular cAMP and activation of PKA. cAMP activates a GTPase of the Ras superfamily, Rap1, following PKA-dependent phosphorylation. However, cAMP also activates multiple intracellular signaling pathways independently of its activation of PKA. One such pathway has been postulated in β cells, which involves two types of cAMP-GEFs (which are activated by binding cAMP and result in activation of Rap1A). Rap1A subsequently inhibits Ras, but activates PKC and B-Raf, both of which result in activation of MAPKs. The Gβγ dimer activates PI3K, which subsequently activates MAPKs by a PKC-dependent (*dark gray arrows*) or independent (*light gray arrows*) mechanism. Inhibition of PI3K (with LY294002) or ERK/MAPK (with PD98059) results in limited GLP-1 stimulated neurite outgrowth,[106] whereas simultaneous inhibition of both pathways blocks differentiation. GLP-1R activation has been shown to protect against apoptotic insult in a number of different cell types, which can be abolished by Rp-cAMP (a cAMP-dependent inhibitor of PKA), which indicates cAMP is a positive mediator in the prevention of apoptosis. Likewise, the PI3K inhibitor with LY294002 inhibits the anti-apoptotic activity of GLP-1, which indicates this effect is at least in part, regulated in a PI3K-dependent manner.[106] Interestingly, inhibition of MAPK/ERK with PD98059 does not inhibit the protective properties of GLP-1, suggesting that MAP/ERK signaling is not critically involved in cell survival in insulinoma cells. Such studies have not yet been addressed in neuronal cells and there is insufficient evidence to rule out a role for all MAPK pathways in the anti-apoptotic action of GLP-1. It seems likely that the protective properties of GLP-1 are mediated through PI3K-induced phosphorylation and activation of Akt, with subsequent CREB-stimulated gene expression of nuclear targets.

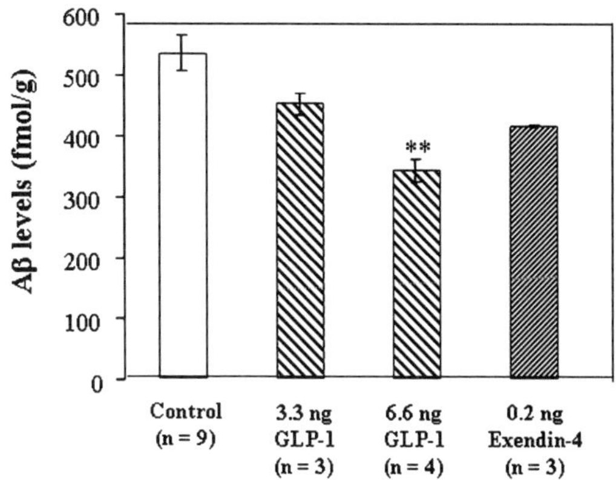

FIGURE 12. GLP-1R stimulation lowered brain levels of Aβ in mice following a single administration of either GLP1 or its long-acting analogue, exendin-4 (Aβ levels were assayed by sandwich ELISA of whole brain homogenates 48 h after administration, using a mouse-specific antibody, **P<.01).[108]

In light of the protective action of GLP-1R stimulation against toxic insults in neuronal cells, the physiological relevance of GLP-1 analogues was assessed in rodents. Specifically, the ability of GLP-1 to modify the synthesis/processing of APP and Aβ was evaluated, together with its potential to protect neurons against apoptosis in a classic model involving the ablation of presynaptic cholinergic neurons that mimics the cholinergic deficit associated with early AD. As shown in FIGURE 12, GLP-1 analogues lower Aβ in normal mouse brain by some 20%. The mechanism(s) underpinning this activity remains to be elucidated, as Aβ levels can be altered via numerous processes.[57,113] In cell culture studies, GLP-1 analogues lowered both secreted and cellular APP levels,[108] suggesting a reduction in APP synthesis, in a manner analogous to that reported for the AD experimental drug, phenserine,[114] which acts posttranscriptionally to destabilize APP mRNA at the level of its 5′-untranslated region and, consequently, lower APP protein synthesis. This, in turn, can lower Aβ levels. Alternatively, reductions in APP and Aβ could be mediated via cAMP, which, as discussed, is dramatically elevated by GLP-1R activation, or by direct action on α-, β-, or γ-secretases, which has not yet been assessed.

In a well-established rodent model of cholinergic neurodegeneration,[115] we have shown complete amelioration of an ibotenic acid–induced cholinergic marker deficit following infusion of GLP-1. As illustrated in FIGURE 13, a partial unilateral ibotenic acid basal nucleus lesion was followed by infusion of GLP-1 agonists or vehicle (artificial CSF) into the right lateral ventricle for 14 days. Choline acetyltransferase (ChAT)–positive immunoreactivity as the marker for cholinergic cell bodies within the basal forebrain, showed that GLP-1R stimulation significantly decreased the loss of ChAT-positive cell bodies in the lesion area compared to the vehicle-treated lesion group,[107] to an extent that there was no difference between rats with a lesion that

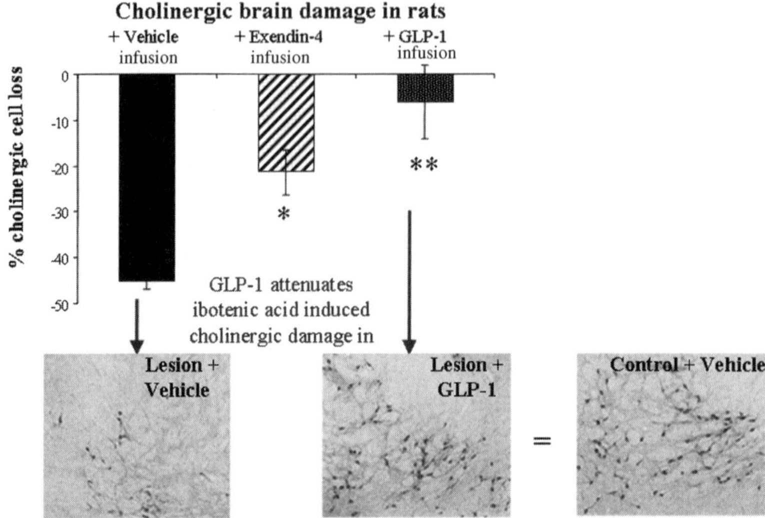

FIGURE 13. Percent difference in the Abercrombie-corrected number of ChAT-immuno-reactive cell bodies in the lesioned basal nucleus relative to the intact contralateral basal nucleus in sham and ibotenic acid animals receiving i.c.v. infusion of vehicle, GLP-1 (0.8 nM/kg/min) or its long-acting analogue, exendin-4 (0.08 nM/kg/min), for 14 days. Vertical error bars represent the standard error of the difference between the means. Significant difference from ibotenic acid vehicle group: *$P<.05$ and **$P<.01$. Representative areas of ChAT-positive stained cells in the nucleus basalis are shown for control + vehicle (i.e., no lesion) and animals with a lesion that were either administered vehicle or GLP-1. There is no discernible difference between animals without a lesion and those with +GLP-1, in relation to ChAT-positive neurons.[107]

were administered GLP-1 and control rats without a lesion administered vehicle (FIG. 13).

Based on our combined studies, we hypothesize that GLP-1 and analogues possess neurotrophic capabilities that are not specific for excitotoxic or, indeed, cholinergic neuronal death, but may represent a trophic property for all neuronal GLP-1R expressing cells.[95] Ongoing studies are currently testing this hypothesis in a wide variety of degenerative models of clinical relevance. This is particularly interesting as the receptors for NGF and related neurotrophins (tyrosine kinase family members) and for GLP-1 (G protein–coupled receptor family member) have been characterized and are vastly different. Furthermore, there is minimal structural similarity between GLP-1 (30 amino acids) and the far larger NGF (118 amino acids). Nevertheless, there are numerous cross-overs in the biochemical pathways that are initiated by activation of their respective receptors that lead towards cell survival. This suggests that GLP-1R activation may prove a useful therapeutic strategy in neurodegenerative disorders, particularly as a loss of the TrkA receptor for NGF, together with the large size of the protein, may negatively impact its value in some disorders, such as AD. In contrast, the brain uptake of GLP-1 is surprisingly high.[116]

The abundance and localization of the GLP-1R in brain and the peripheral nervous system in health, aging, and disease remain to be fully elucidated, but have not been reported to be lost.

SUMMARY

Many advances have been made during the last decade to progress our understanding of the key mechanisms that regulate cell survival and death in response to a wide number of physiological insults, via programmed cell death. A critical process in sculpting the developing brain, the very same biochemical cascades, albeit activated by different stimuli, appear to be consistently involved in a wide variety of neurodegenerative disorders. Certainly programmed cell death is not the sole mediator of cell loss seen in these disorders but, as assessed with a number of experimental mouse models, it represents a key mechanism. As illustrated in FIGURES 1 and 11, the molecular complexity of the cascades associated with programmed cell death or survival offers numerous potential targets for modulation. Few, however, are classical or validated, which has forced groups associated with drug design to think "outside the box" and collaborate more broadly with experts in molecular and cellular biology to characterize un-validated targets. We have reviewed three novel and different therapeutic strategies with potential for a wide variety of neurodegenerative disorders and described small compounds and peptides that already possess interesting pharmacological profiles in cellular and *in vivo* models. It is important to define the molecular point-of-no-return associated with specific acute (e.g., stroke and head trauma) and chronic (e.g., AD, PD, and ALS) disorders, to determine the point when neurons become irreversibly committed to die, and the window of therapeutic opportunity that this provides. In addition, it remains to be determined whether or not the toxicological profile associated with such strategies will allow their use for intervention in humans. It could well be that a synergistic combination of rational therapeutic approaches may prove optimal and, for chronic disorders, likely will require the initiation of intervention well before a cellular "suicide" decision has been made. This could potentially slow or halt processes that gradually render neurons dysfunctional well before their loss of function leaves them all but worthless.

ACKNOWLEDGMENTS

This paper is dedicated to our collaborator and close friend, Arnold Brossi, University of North Carolina (Chapel Hill, NC), on the occasion of his 81st birthday. We are grateful to Harold W. Holloway, Laboratory of Neurosciences, Intramural Research Program, National Institute on Aging, National Institutes of Health, for his critical input into this article.

REFERENCES

1. MATTSON, M.P. 2000. Apoptosis in neurodegenerative disorders. Nat. Rev. **1:** 120–129.
2. MATTSON, M.P, S.L. CHAN & W. DUAN. 2002. Modification of brain aging and neurodegenerative disorders by genes, diet, and behavior. Physiol. Rev. **82:** 637–672.

3. MATTSON, M.P. 2003. Excitotoxic and excitoprotective mechanisms: abundant targets for the prevention and treatment of neurodegenerative disorders. Neuromol. Med. **3:** 65–94.

4. MATTSON, M.P. 2004. Pathways towards and away from Alzheimer's disease. Nature **430:** 631–639.

5. MCGEER, P.L., S. ITAGAKI, B.E. BOYES & E.G. MCGEER. 1988. Reactive microglia are positive for HLA-DR in the substantia nigra of Parkinson's and Alzheimer's disease brains. Neurology **38:** 1285–1291.

6. MCGEER, P.L., M. SCHULZER & E.G. MCGEER. 1996. Arthritis and anti-inflammatory agents as possible protective factors for Alzheimer's disease: a review of 17 epidemiologic studies. Neurology **47:** 425–432.

7. MCGEER, P.L. & E.G. MCGEER. 2001. Inflammation, autotoxicity and Alzheimer disease. Neurobiol. Aging **22:** 799–809.

8. VILA, M. & S. PRZEDBORSKI. 2003. Targeting programmed cell death in neurodegenerative diseases. Nat. Rev. Neurosci. **4:** 365–375.

9. KERR, J.F., A.H. WYLLIE & A.R. CURRIE. 1972. Apoptosis: a basic biological phenomenon with wide-ranging implications in tissue kinetics. Br. J. Cancer **26:** 239–257.

10. JESENBERGER, V. & S. JENTSCH. 2002. Deadly encounter: ubiquitin meets apoptosis. Nat. Rev. Mol. Cell Biol. **3:** 112–121.

11. KERMER, P., J. LIMAN, J.H. WEISHAUPT & M. BÄHR. 2003. Neuronal apoptosis in neurodegenerative diseases: from basic research to clinical application. Neurodegenerative Disease **1:** 9–19.

12. MEIER, P., A. FINCH & G. EVAN. 2000. Apoptosis in development. Nature **407:** 796–801.

13. YUAN, J. & B.A. YANKNER. 2000. Apoptosis in the nervous system. Nature **407:** 802–809.

14. MATTSON, M.P. & G. KROEMER. 2003. Mitochondria in cell death: novel targets for neuroprotection and cardioprotection. Trends Mol. Med. **9:** 196–205.

15. RUDEL, T. 1999. Caspase inhibitors in prevention of apoptosis. Herz **24:** 236–241.

16. CHARRIAUT-MARLANGUE, C. 2004. Apoptosis: a target for neuroprotection. Therapie **59:** 185–190.

17. SUN, H., Z. NIKOLOSKA-COLESKA, C.Y. YANG, et al. 2004. Structure-based design, synthesis, and evaluation of conformationally constrained mimetics of the second mitochondria-derived activator of caspase that target the X-linked inhibitor of apoptosis protein/caspase-9 interaction site. J. Med. Chem. **47:** 4147–4150.

18. RAY, A.M., D.E. OWEN, M.L. EVANS, et al. 2000. Caspase inhibitors are functionally neuroprotective against oxygen glucose deprivation induced CA1 death in rat organotypic hippocampal slices. Brain Res. **867:** 62–69.

19. MCCARTHY, N.J., M.K.B. WHYTE, S.C. GILBERT & G.I. EVAN. 1997. Inhibition of Ced-3/ICE-related proteases does not prevent cell death induced by oncogenes, DNA damage, or the Bcl-2 homologue Bak. J. Cell Biol. **136:** 215–227.

20. SCHULZ, J.B., M. WELLER & M.A. MOSKOWITZ. 1999. Caspases as treatment targets in stroke and neurodegenerative diseases. Ann. Neurol. **45:** 421–429.

21. HUGHES, P.E., T. ALEXI & S.S. SCHREIBER. 1997. A role for the tumour suppressor gene p53 in regulating neuronal apoptosis. Neuroreport **8:** 5–12.

22. CREGAN, S.P., J.G. MACLAURIN, C.G. CRAIG, et al. 1999. Bax-dependent caspase-3 activation is a key determinant in p53-induced apoptosis in neurons. J. Neurosci. **19:** 7860–7869.

23. CHEN, R.W., P.A. SAUNDERS, H. WEI, et al. 1999. Involvement of glyceraldehyde-3-phosphate dehydrogenase (GAPDH) and p53 in neuronal apoptosis: evidence that GAPDH is upregulated by p53. J. Neurosci. **19:** 9654–9662.

24. SHEIKH, M.S., M.C. HOLLANDER & A.J. FORNANCE, JR. 2000. Role of Gadd45 in apoptosis. Biochem. Pharmacol. **59:** 43–45.

25. CHAO, C., S. SAITO, J. KANG, et al. 2000. p53 transcriptional activity is essential for p53-dependent apoptosis following DNA damage. EMBO J. **19:** 4967–4975.

26. KOMAROV, P.G., E.A. KOMAROVA, R.V. KONDRATOV, et al. 1999. A chemical inhibitor of p53 that protects mice from the side effects of cancer therapy. Science **285:** 1733–1737.

27. CULMSEE, C., X. ZHU, Q.S. YU, et al. 2001. A synthetic inhibitor of p53 protects neurons against death induced by ischemic and excitotoxic insults, and amyloid beta-peptide. J. Neurochem. **77:** 220–228.

28. CRUMRINE, R.C., A.L. THOMAS & P.F. MORGAN. 1994. Attenuation of p53 expression protects against focal ischemic damage in transgenic mice. J. Cereb. Blood Flow Metab. **14:** 887–891.

29. TAKIMOTO, C.H., L.V. KIEFFER, M.E. KIEFFER, *et al.* 1999. DNA topoisomerase I poisons. Cancer Chemother. Biol. Response Modif. **18:** 81–124.

30. MORRISON, R.S., H.J. WENZEL, Y. KINOSHITA, *et al.* 1996. Loss of the p53 tumor suppressor gene protects neurons from kainate-induced cell death. J. Neurosci. **16:** 1337–1345.

31. FREEMAN, R.S., S. ESTUS & E.M. JOHNSON, JR. 1994. Analysis of cell cycle-related gene expression in postmitotic neurons: selective induction of cyclin D1 during programmed cell death. Neuron **12:** 343–355.

32. SADOUL, R., A.L. QUIQUEREZ, I. MARTINOU, *et al.* 1996. p53 protein in sympathetic neurons: cytoplasmic localization and no apparent function in apoptosis. J. Neurosci. Res. **43:** 594–601.

33. ZHU, X., T. GIORDANO, Q.S. YU, *et al.* 2003. Thiothalidomides: novel isosteric analogues of thalidomide with enhanced TNF-α inhibitory activity. J. Med. Chem. **46:** 5222–5229.

34. LIPINSKI, C.A. 2000. Drug-like properties and the causes of poor solubility and poor permeability. J. Pharmacol. Toxicol. Methods **44:** 235–249.

35. GREIG, N.H. 1992. Drug entry to the brain and its pharmacologic manipulation. Handb. Exp. Pharmacol. **103:** 487–523.

36. LEKER, R.R, M. AHARONOWIZ, N.H. GREIG & H. OVADIA. 2004. The role of p53-induced apoptosis in cerebral ischemia: effects of the p53 inhibitor pifithrin alpha. Exp. Neurol. **187:** 478–486.

37. DUAN, W., X. ZHU, B. LADENHEIM, *et al.* 2002. p53 inhibitors preserve dopamine neurons and motor function in experimental parkinsonism. Ann. Neurol. **52:** 597–606.

38. TYNER, S.D., S. VENKATACHALAM, J. CHOI, *et al.* 2002. p53 mutant mice that display early ageing-associated phenotypes. Nature **415:** 45–53.

39. DUMBLE, M., C. GATZA, S. TYNER, *et al.* 2004. Insights into aging obtained from p53 mutant mouse models. Ann. N.Y. Acad. Sci. **1019:** 171–177.

40. GILMAN, C.P., S.L. CHAN, Z. GUO, *et al.* 2003. p53 is present in synapses where it mediates mitochondrial dysfunction and synaptic degeneration in response to DNA damage, and oxidative and excitotoxic insults. Neuromol. Med. **3:** 159–172.

41. HIRSCH, E.C., S. HUNOT, P. DAMIER & B. FAUCHEUX. 1998. Glial cells and inflammation in Parkinson's disease: a role in neurodegeneration? Ann. Neurol. **44:** S115–S120.

42. NAGATSU, T., M. MOGI, H. ICHINOSE & A. TOGARI. 2000. Cytokines in Parkinson's disease. J. Neural. Transm. Suppl. **58:** 143–151.

43. LIU, B. & J.-S. HONG. 2003. Role of microglia in inflammation-mediated neurodegenerative diseases: mechanisms and strategies for therapeutic intervention. J. Pharmacol. Exp. Ther. **304:** 1–7.

44. WYSS-CORAY, T. & L. MUCKE. 2002. Inflammation in neurodegenerative disease—a double-edged sword. Neuron **35:** 419–432.

45. CAMPBELL, I.L., A.K. STALDER, Y. AKWA, *et al.* 1998. Transgenic models to study the actions of cytokines in the central nervous system. Neuroimmunomodulation **5:** 126–135.

46. SHOHAMI, E., I. GINIS & J.M. HALLENBECK. 1999. Dual role of tumor necrosis factor alpha in brain injury. Cytokine Growth Factor Rev. **10:** 119-130.

47. LAWSON, L.J., V.H. PERRY, P. DRI & S. GORDON. 1990. Heterogeneity in the distribution and morphology of microglia in the normal adult mouse brain. Neuroscience **39:** 151–170.

48. GAO, H.-M., B. LIU, W. ZHANG & J.-S. HONG. 2003. Novel anti-inflammatory therapy for Parkinson's disease. Trends Pharmacol. Sci. **24:** 395–401.

49. AISEN, P.S. 2000. Anti-inflammatory therapy for Alzheimer's disease: implications of the prednisone trial. Acta Neurol. Scand. **176:** 85–89.

50. STEWART, W.F., C. KAWAS, M. CORRADA & E.J. METTER. 1997. Risk of Alzheimer's disease and duration of NSAID use. Neurology **48:** 626–632.

51. MRAK, R.E. & W.S. GRIFFIN. 2001. Interleukin-1, neuroinflammation, and Alzheimer's disease. Neurobiol. Aging **22:** 903–908.

52. CACQUEVEL, M., N. LEBEURRIER, S. CHEENNE & D. VIVIEN. 2004. Cytokines in neuro-inflammation and Alzheimer's disease. Curr. Drug Targets **5:** 529–534.
53. DAS, S. & H. POTTER. 1995. Expression of the Alzheimer amyloid-promoting factor antichymotrypsin is induced in human astrocytes by IL-1. Neuron **4:** 447–456.
54. GRIFFIN, W.S., L.C. STANLEY, C. LING, *et al.* 1989. Brain interleukin 1 and S-100 immunoreactivity are elevated in Down syndrome and Alzheimer disease. Proc. Natl. Acad. Sci. USA **86:** 7611–7615.
55. SELKOE, D.J. 2001. Alzheimer's disease: genes, proteins, and therapy. Physiol. Rev. **81:** 741–766.
56. AVRAMOVICH, Y., T. AMIT & M.B.H. YOUDIM. 2002. Non-steroidal anti-inflammatory drugs stimulate secretion of non-amyloidogenic precursor protein. J. Biol. Chem. **277:** 31466–31473.
57. LAHIRI, D.K., M.R. FARLOW, K. SAMBAMURTI, *et al.* 2003. A critical analysis of new molecular targets and strategies for drug developments in Alzheimer's disease. Curr. Drug Targets **4:** 97–112.
58. LIAO, Y.F., B.J. WANG, H.T. CHENG, *et al.* 2004. Tumor necrosis factor-alpha, inter-leukin-1beta, and interferon-gamma stimulate gamma-secretase-mediated cleavage of amyloid precursor protein through a JNK-dependent MAPK pathway. J. Biol. Chem. [Epub ahead of print].
59. ROGERS, J.T., L.M. LEITER, J. MCPHEE, *et al.* 1999. Translation of the Alzheimer amyloid precursor protein mRNA is up-regulated by interleukin-1 through 5′-untranslated region sequences. J. Biol. Chem. **274:** 6421–6431.
60. ROGERS, J.T., J.D. RANDALL, C.M. CAHILL, *et al.* 2002. An iron-responsive element type II in the 5′-untranslated region of the Alzheimer's amyloid precursor protein transcript. J. Biol. Chem. **277:** 45518–45528.
61. LAHIRI, D.K., D. CHEN, D. VIVIEN, *et al.* 2003. Role of cytokines in the gene expression of amyloid β-protein precursor: identification of a 5′-UTR-binding nuclear factor and its implications in Alzheimer's disease. J. Alz. Dis. **5:** 81–90.
62. FUNATO, H., M. YOSHIMURA, T. YAMAZAKI, *et al.* 1998. Astrocytes containing amyloid beta-protein (Abeta)-positive granules are associated with Abeta40-positive diffuse plaques in the aged human brain. Am. J. Pathol. **152:** 983–992.
63. AKIYAMA, H., S. BARGER, S. BARNUM, *et al.* 2002. Inflammation and Alzheimer's disease. Neurobiol. Aging **21:** 383–421.
64. BAMBERGER, M.E., M.E. HARRIS, D.R. MCDONALD, *et al.* 2003. A cell surface receptor complex for fibrillar beta-amyloid mediates microglial activation. J. Neurosci. **23:** 2665–2674.
65. COMBS, C.K., J.C. KARLO, S.C. KAO & G.E. LANDRETH. 2001. Beta-amyloid stimula-tion of microglia and monocytes results in TNF alpha-dependent expression of inducible nitric oxide synthase and neuronal apoptosis. J. Neurosci. **21:** 1179–1188.
66. MOGI, M., M. HARADA, P. RIEDERER, *et al.* 1994. Tumor necrosis factor-alpha (TNF-alpha) increases both in the brain and in the cerebrospinal fluid from Parkinsonian patients. Neurosci. Lett. **165:** 208–210.
67. HUNOT, S., N. DUGAS, B. FAUCHEUX, *et al.* 1999. FcepsilonRII/CD23 is expressed in Parkinson's disease and induces, in vitro, production of nitric oxide and tumor necrosis factor-alpha in glial cells. J. Neurosci. **19:** 3440–3447.
68. KRUGER, R., C. HARDT, F. TSCHENTSCHER, *et al.* 2000. Genetic analysis of immuno-modulating factors in sporadic Parkinson's disease. J. Neural Transm. **107:** 553–562.
69. NISHIMURA, M., I. MIZUTA, E. MIZUTA, *et al.* 2001. Tumor necrosis factor gene poly-morphisms in patients with sporadic Parkinson's disease. Neurosci. Lett. **311:** 1–4.
70. FERGER, B., B. LENG, A. MURA, *et al.* 2004. Genetic ablation of tumor necrosis factor-alpha (TNF-α) and pharmacological inhibition of TNF-synthesis attenuates MPTP toxicity in mouse striatum. J. Neurochem. **89:** 822–833.
71. GHEZZI, P. & T. MENNINI. 2004. Tumor necrosis factor and motoneuronal degeneration: an open problem. Neuroimmunomodulation **9:** 178–182.
72. HAYES, R.L., K. YANG, R. RAGHUPATHI & T.K. MCINTOSH. 1995. Changes in gene-expression following traumatic brain injury in the rat. J. Neurotrauma **12:** 779–790.
73. HOFMAN, F.M., D.R. HINTON, K. JOHNSON & J.E. MERRILL. 1989. Tumor necrosis factor identified in multiple-sclerosis brain. J. Exp. Med. **170:** 607–612.

74. HENSLEY, K., J. FEDYNYSHYN, S. FERRELL, *et al.* 2003. Message and protein-level elevation of tumor necrosis factor alpha (TNF alpha) and TNF alpha-modulating cytokines in spinal cords of the G93A-SOD1 mouse model for amyotrophic lateral sclerosis. Neurobiol. Dis. **14:** 74–80.

75. BARGER, S.W., D. HÖRSTER, K. FURUKAWA, *et al.* 1995. Tumor necrosis factors alpha and beta protect neurons against amyloid beta-peptide toxicity: evidence for involvement of a kappa B-binding factor and attenuation of peroxide and Ca^{2+} accumulation. Proc. Natl. Acad. Sci. USA **92:** 9328–9332.

76. BRUCE, A.J., W. BOLING, M.S. KINDY, *et al.* 1996. Altered neuronal and microglial responses to excitotoxic and ischemic brain injury in mice lacking TNF receptors. Nat. Med. **2:** 788–794.

77. EGER, K., M. JALALIAN, E.J. VERSPOHL & N.P. LUPKE. 1990. Synthesis, central nervous system activity and teratogenicity of a homothalidomide. Arzneim. Forsch. **40:** 1073–1075.

78. KLING, J. 2000. Redeeming thalidomide. Modern Drug Discovery **3:** 35–36.

79. SHESKIN, J. 1965. Thalidomide in the treatment of lepra reaction. Clin. Pharmacol. Ther. **6:** 303–310.

80. KUMAR, S., T.E. WITZIG & S.V. RAJKUMAR. 2002. Thalidomide as an anti-cancer agent. J. Cell Mol. Med. **6:** 160–174.

81. MOREIRA, A.L., E.P. SAMPAIO, A. ZMUIDZINAS, *et al.* 1993. Thalidomide exerts its inhibitory action on tumor necrosis factor α by enhancing mRNA degradation. J. Exp. Med. **177:** 1675–1680.

82. NIWAYAMA, S., B.E. TURK & J.O. LIU. 1996. Potent inhibition of tumor necrosis factor α production by tetrafluorothalidomide and tetrafluorophthalimides. J. Med. Chem. **39:** 3044–3045.

83. HASLETT, P.A., W.A. HANEKOM, G. MULLER & G. KAPLAN. 2003. Thalidomide and a thalidomide analogue drug costimulate virus-specific CD8+ T cells in vitro. J. Infect. Dis. **187:** 946–955.

84. D'AMATO, R.J., M.S. LOUGHNAN, E. FLYNN & J. FOLKMAN. 1994. Thalidomide is an inhibitor of angiogenesis. Proc. Natl. Acad. Sci. USA **91:** 4082–4085.

85. MULLER, G.W., L.G. CORRAL, M.G. SHIRE, *et al.* 1996. Structural modifications of thalidomide produce analogs with enhanced tumor necrosis factor inhibitory activity. J. Med. Chem. **39:** 3238–3240.

86. MULLER, G.W., R. CHEN, S-Y. HUANG, *et al.* 1999. Amino-substitutes thalidomide analogs: potent inhibitors of TNF-α production. Bioorg. Med. Chem. Lett. **9:** 1625–1630.

87. TEUBERT, U., K. ZWINGENBERGER, W. STEPHAN & K. EGER. 1998. 5'-Substituted thalidomide analogs as modulators of TNF-α. Arch. Pharm. Med. Chem. **331:** 7–12.

88. HASHIMOTO, Y. 2002. Structural development of biological response modifiers based on thalidomide. Bioorg. Med. Chem. **10:** 461–479.

89. BAUER, K.S., S.C. DIXON & W.D. FIGG. 1998. Inhibition of angiogenesis by thalidomide requires metabolic activation, which is species-dependent. Biochem. Pharmacol. **55:** 1827–1834.

90. LUZZIO, F.A., A.V. MAYOROV, S.S. NG, *et al.* 2003. Thalidomide metabolites and analogues: 3. Synthesis and antiangiogenic activity of the teratogenic and TNFalpha-modulatory thalidomide analogue 2-(2,6-dioxopiperidine-3-yl)phthalimidine. J. Med. Chem. **46:** 3793–3799.

91. PRICE, D.K., Y. ANDO, E.A. KRUGER, *et al.* 2002. 5'-OH-Thalidomide, a metabolite of thalidomide, inhibits angiogenesis. Ther. Drug Monit. **24:** 104–110.

92. KRUYS, V., O. MARINX, G. SHAW, *et al.* 1989. Translational blockade imposed by cytokine-derived UA-rich sequences. Science **245:** 852–855.

93. KRUYS, V. & G. HUEZ. 1994. Translational control of cytokine expression by 3′ AU-rich sequences. Biochimie **76:** 862–866.

94. KNUDSEN, L.B. 2004. Glucagon-like peptide-1: the basis of a new class of treatment for type 2 diabetes. J. Med. Chem. **47:** 4128–4134.

95. GROMADA, J., J.J. HOLST & P. RORSMAN. 1998. Cellular regulation of islet hormone secretion by the incretin hormone GLP-1. Pflug. Arch. Eur. J. Phys. **435:** 583–594.

96. PERRY, T. & N.H. GREIG. 2003. The glucagon-like peptides: a double-edged therapeutic sword? Trends Pharmacol. Sci. **24:** 377–383.

97. DRUCKER, D.J. 2003. Glucagon-like peptide-1 and the islet beta-cell: augmentation of cell proliferation and inhibition of apoptosis. Endocrinology **144:** 5145–5148.

98. BRUBAKER, P.L. & D.J. DRUCKER. 2004. Minireview: Glucagon-like peptides regulate cell proliferation and apoptosis in the pancreas, gut, and central nervous system. Endocrinology **145:** 2653–2659.

99. DEACON, C.F., M.A. NAUCK, X. TOFT-NIELSEN, *et al.* 1995. Both subcutaneously and intravenously administered glucagon-like peptide-1 are rapidly degraded from the NH_2-terminus in type II diabetic patients and in healthy subjects. Diabetes **44:** 1126–1131.

100. GREIG, N.H., H.W. HOLLOWAY, K.A. DE ORE, *et al.* 1999. Once daily injection of exendin-4 to diabetic mice achieves long-term beneficial effects on blood glucose concentrations. Diabetologia **42:** 45–50.

101. GOKE, R., P.J. LARSEN, J.D. MIKKELSEN & S.P. SHEIKH. 1995. Distribution of GLP-1 binding sites in the rat brain: evidence that exendin-4 is a ligand of brain GLP-1 binding sites. Eur. J. Neurosci. **7:** 2294–2300.

102. SHUGHRUE, P.J., M.V. LANE & I. MERCHENTHALER. 1996. Glucagon-like peptide-1 receptor (GLP1-R) mRNA in the rat hypothalamus. Endocrinology **137:** 5159–5162.

103. WEI, Y. & S. MOJSOV. 1995. Tissue-specific expression of the human receptor for glucagon-like peptide-I: brain, heart and pancreatic forms have the same deduced amino acid sequences. FEBS Lett. **358:** 219–224.

104. SATOH, F., S.A. BEAK, C.J. SMALL, *et al.* 2000. Characterization of human and rat glucagon-like peptide-1 receptors in the neurointermediate lobe: lack of coupling to either stimulation or inhibition of adenylyl cyclase. Endocrinology **141:** 1301–1309.

105. ORSKOV, C., S.S. POULSEN, M. MOLLER & J.J. HOLST. 1996. Glucagon-like peptide I receptors in the subfornical organ and the area postrema are accessible to circulating glucagon-like peptide I. Diabetes **45:** 832–835.

106. PERRY, T., D.K. LAHIRI, D. CHEN, *et al.* 2002. A novel neurotrophic property of glucagon-like peptide 1: a promoter of nerve growth factor-mediated differentiation in PC12 cells. J. Pharmacol. Exp. Ther. **300:** 958–966.

107. PERRY, T., N.J. HAUGHEY, M.P. MATTSON, *et al.* 2002. Protection and reversal of excitotoxic neuronal damage by glucagon-like peptide-1 and exendin-4. J. Pharmacol. Exp. Ther. **302:** 881–888.

108. PERRY, T., D.K. LAHIRI, K. SAMBAMURTI, *et al.* 2003. Glucagon-like peptide-1 decreases endogenous amyloid-beta peptide (Abeta) levels and protects hippocampal neurons from death induced by Abeta and iron. J. Neurosci. Res. **72:** 603–612.

109. CHENG, B. & M.P. MATTSON. 1994. NT-3 and BDNF protect CNS neurons against metabolic/excitotoxic insults. Brain Res. **640:** 56–67.

110. MATTSON, M.P., M.A. LOVELL, K. FURUKAWA & W.R. MARKESBERY. 1995. Neurotrophic factors attenuate glutamate-induced accumulation of peroxides, elevation of intracellular Ca^{2+} concentration, and neurotoxity and increase antioxidant enzyme activities in hippocampal neurons. J. Neurochem. **65:** 1740–1751.

111. PERRY, T. & N.H. GREIG. 2002. The glucagon-like peptides: a new genre in therapeutic targets for intervention in Alzheimer's disease. J. Alzheimers Dis. **4:** 487–496.

112. PERRY, T. & N.H. GREIG. 2004. A new Alzheimer's disease interventive strategy: GLP-1. Curr. Drug Targets **5:** 565-571.

113. SAMBAMURTI, K., N.H. GREIG & D.K. LAHIRI. 2002. Advances in the cellular and molecular biology of the beta-amyloid protein in Alzheimer's disease. Neuromol. Med. **1:** 1–31.

114. SHAW, K.T.Y., T. UTSUKI, J. ROGERS, *et al.* 2001. Phenserine regulates translation of β-amyloid precursor mRNA by a putative interleukin-1 responsive element, a target for drug development. Proc. Natl. Acad. Sci. USA **98:** 7605–7610.

115. HAROUTUNIAN, V., P.D. KANOF, G.K. TSUBOYAMA, *et al.* 1986. Animal models of Alzheimer's disease: behavior, pharmacology, transplants. Can. J. Neurol. Sci. **13:** 385–393.

116. KASTIN, A.J., V. AKERSTROM & W. PAN. 2002. Interactions of glucagon-like peptide-1 (GLP-1) with the blood-brain barrier. J. Mol. Neurosci. **18:** 7–14.

117. GREIG, N.H., T. GIORDANO, X. ZHU, *et al.* 2004. Thalidomide-based TNF-alpha inhibitors for neurodegenerative diseases. Acta Neurobiol. Exp. **64:** 1–9.

118. DOYLE, M.E., N.H. GREIG, H.W. HOLLOWAY, *et al.* 2001. Insertion of an N-terminal 6-aminohexanoic acid after the 7 amino acid position of glucagon-like peptide-1 produces a long-acting hypoglycemic agent. Endocrinology **142:** 4462–4468.
119. DOYLE, M.E., M.J. THEODORAKIS, H.W. HOLLOWAY, *et al.* 2003. The importance of the nine-amino acid C-terminal sequence of exendin-4 for binding to the GLP-1 receptor and for biological activity. Regul. Pept. **114:** 153–158.

Nicotinic Receptor Modulation for Neuroprotection and Enhancement of Functional Recovery Following Brain Injury or Disease

J. R. PAULY,[a,b] C. M. CHARRIEZ,[a] M. V. GUSEVA,[a] AND S. W. SCHEFF[b,c]

[a]*Department of Pharmaceutical Sciences, College of Pharmacy,*
[b]*Spinal Cord and Brain Injury Research Center,* [c]*Sanders Brown Center on Aging,*
University of Kentucky, Lexington, Kentucky, USA

ABSTRACT: Despite the well-known adverse health effects of tobacco smoking, numerous studies have shown that nicotine, the principal pharmacologically active alkaloid in tobacco smoke, exerts neuroprotective properties in several animal models of neurodegeneration. Furthermore, cigarette smoking appears to significantly reduce the risk of developing Parkinson's disease in human subjects. We review the animal and human studies that investigated possible neuroprotective actions of nicotine and other nicotinic receptor agonists and antagonists. We demonstrate that nicotine is not neuroprotective in all animal models of neurodegenerative disease. In fact, C57Bl/6 mice pretreated with nicotine have an increased sensitivity to 3-nitropropionic acid, a neurotoxin used in mice to mimic some aspects of Huntington's disease. The actions of nicotine on dopamine release may explain the variable effects of nicotine in animal models of Parkinson's and Huntington's diseases. Finally, we focus on some future directions for studies that evaluate neuroprotective properties of nicotinic agonists and antagonists.

KEYWORDS: nicotine; neurodegeneration; neuroprotection

INTRODUCTION

Nicotine is thought to be the principal component of tobacco smoke that underlies the addictive properties of cigarette smoking. However, in spite of the well-recognized adverse effects of cigarette smoking, some studies suggest that nicotine may have "beneficial" actions that might be useful for therapeutic purposes. Numerous recent studies have suggested that drugs that modify the activity of CNS nicotinic cholinergic receptors (nAChRs) may be useful for the treatment of human neurological disorders. Significant deficits in nAChR expression have been shown to occur in several neurological disorders including Alzheimer's disease (AD), Parkinson's disease (PD), and Down syndrome. The loss of nicotinic receptors in these conditions may be a major contributor to cognitive deficits associated with these disorders. In addition,

Address for correspondence: James R. Pauly, Department of Pharmaceutical Sciences, College of Pharmacy, University of Kentucky, Lexington, KY 40536-0082. Voice: 859-323-8164.
jpauly@uky.edu

Ann. N.Y. Acad. Sci. 1035: 316–334 (2004). © 2004 New York Academy of Sciences.
doi: 10.1196/annals.1332.019

nicotinic receptor agonists and antagonists have been shown to be neuroprotective in a variety of *in vivo* and *in vitro* experimental models.[1,2] Unfortunately the neuro-biological mechanisms that underlie nicotine-induced cellular preservation and/or increased cognitive function are not well established. The purpose of this review article is to summarize information regarding the various models that have been employed to demonstrate neuroprotective actions of nicotine or nicotinic receptor–mediated facilitation of functional recovery from brain injury. Some potential mechanisms involved with nicotinic receptor–mediated neuroprotection will also be discussed.

OVERVIEW OF NICOTINIC RECEPTOR NEUROBIOLOGY

Nicotinic acetylcholine receptors are members of the ligand-gated ion channel receptor superfamily. Activation of nAChRs causes a rapid increase in cellular per-meability to cations, including Na^+ and Ca^{2+}. Although many different nAChR phenotypes are expressed in the mammalian CNS, the functional significance of this diversity remains to be elucidated. Nicotinic receptors are pentamers comprising alpha and beta subunits. To date, five different alpha subunits (alpha 2–6) have been shown to combine with four possible beta subunits (beta 2–5) to form heteromeric nicotinic receptors. The brain alpha-bungarotoxin (BTX) receptor is a homomeric receptor consisting of only alpha 7 nAChR subunits.[3] The two most prominent nAChRs expressed in the mammalian CNS are those consisting of either alpha 4/beta 2 subunits or homomeric alpha 7 receptors. The alpha 7 receptor is unique because of its high permeability to calcium. Numerous studies have shown that alpha 7 receptors are involved with cognition, synaptic plasticity, and presynaptic neurotransmitter release and regulation of immune function.[4]

MODELS USED TO EVALUATE NEUROPROTECTIVE EFFECTS OF NICOTINIC RECEPTOR AGONISTS

Excitotoxins

Numerous studies have shown that nicotinic receptor agonists have neuroprotec-tive properties against excitotoxins related to glutamatergic neurotransmission. The original studies by Akiake[5] and Marin[6] used cortical or striatal primary cultures that were pretreated for 1–24 h with different concentrations of nicotine, prior to appli-cation of N-methyl-D-aspartate (NMDA) to the cultured neurons. Nicotine pretreat-ment significantly attenuated toxicity mediated by NMDA receptor. Acetylcholine, carbachol (a mixed muscarinic/nicotinic agonist) and nornicotine (a nicotine metab-olite with agonist properties) also had neuroprotective properties in striatal cultures.[6] The neuroprotective action of nicotine was blocked by pre-exposure to the ganglionic blocker, hexamethonium, but not by pretreatment with the muscarinic receptor blocker, atropine. Since these initial reports, other research has supported and extended these results using other nicotinic receptor agonists, such as ABT-418[7] and the low affinity but selective alpha 7 agonist choline.[8] In addition, Takada[9] reported that the acetylcholinesterase inhibitor, donepezil, was neuroprotective in cultured cortical neurons exposed to excitotoxins. The neuroprotective actions of donepezil were blocked with nicotinic antagonists (mecamylamine, dihydro-beta-erythroidine [DHBE] and methyllycaconatine [MLA]) but not muscarinic antagonists. The vast majority of the studies evaluating nicotine protection against cytotoxicity mediated by NMDA receptor have used pretreatment times ranging from 30 minutes to 7 days. In spite of the various models used, variations in the timing of pretreatment have not greatly influenced the outcome of the experiments. In many cases, 30–120 min of nicotine pretreatment afforded the same neuroprotection as more prolonged pretreatment intervals. This finding may suggest that changes in nAChR functional status (i.e., activated, desensitized, etc.) may be more important than nicotine-induced receptor upregulation following chronic nicotine administration. Nicotinic stimulation following excitotoxic insult has not been widely reported as neuroprotective, but one study showed that it was as effective as pretreatment.[10]

The nAChR subtype(s) responsible for mediation of nicotine's neuroprotective effects against glutamate toxicity is not known and there is evidence to support involvement of both alpha 4/beta 2 and alpha 7 receptor subtypes. Pharmacologically, the cytoprotective effects of nicotine are commonly blocked by pretreatment with alpha 7 antagonists, such as BTX and MLA.[7,11–13] Gahring[14] showed that nicotine-induced protection against NMDA toxicity was lost in transgenic mice that have mutations in the alpha 7 receptor. However, Stevens and colleagues[15] demonstrated that neuroprotective actions of nicotine are lost in cortical cultures obtained from animals that have a genotypic deletion of beta 2–containing neuronal nAChRs. Thus, pharmacological and genetic perspectives each support the involvement of multiple receptor subtypes in nicotine-mediated neuroprotection against excessive NMDA receptor stimulation.

Nicotine's neuroprotective actions are calcium dependent and generally restricted to cytotoxicity caused by glutamate or NMDA. Several studies have shown that nicotine is not neuroprotective against cell death mediated by AMPA (DL-amino-3-hydroxy-5-methyl-isoxazole-4-propionic acid) in cortical and hippocampal cell cultures.[5,16] However, in one study, nicotine (and choline) blocked AMPA-induced dark cell degeneration in cerebellar Purkinje neurons in a MLA-sensitive fashion.[8] The cellular mechanisms involved with nicotine-induced neuroprotection against excitotoxins are not well established, but previous studies have pointed to upregulation of intracellular calcium binding proteins,[15,17] changes in nitric oxide mediated signaling,[16] and other signaling events downstream from nicotinic receptor activation.[1,2]

In vivo experiments, although less common than *in vitro* approaches, also have shown some evidence of nicotine mediated neuroprotection against excitotoxicity. Rats pretreated with nicotine had less kainic acid–induced neurotoxicity based on the number of "wet dog shakes" that were observed. Nicotine pretreated animals also had less hippocampal damage based on preservation of AChE staining, which was significantly decreased in animals not pretreated with nicotine.[18] Similar results have been reported in a neonatal model of glutamate mediated excitotoxicity.[19] O'Neill and colleagues[20] used bilateral injections of quinolinic acid into the dorsal hippocampus to produce cognitive impairment associated with a loss of pyramidal and granule cells in the hippocampus. Chronic nicotine pretreatment via osmotic minipumps prevented the histological and behavioral deficits produced by quinolinic acid infusions. The spastic Han-Wistar rat is known to demonstrate overactivity of glutamatergic signaling, which causes significant damage to the hippocampus and cerebellum. Chronic nicotine administration via the drinking solution caused significant improvement in motor function in these animals and also increased longevity.[21] Finally, Kim and colleagues[22] exposed rats to cigarette smoke for 10 minutes per day, 6 days per week, for 4 weeks, followed by intraperitoneal injections of kainic acid. Cigarette exposure reduced kainic acid–induced convulsions, mortality, and cell loss in the hippocampus. While the protective effects of tobacco smoke cannot be directly ascribed to nicotine, daily treatment with the nicotinic antagonist mecamylamine, blocked the apparent protective actions of smoke exposure.[22]

Beta-Amyloid-Mediated Cell Death

The chief histopathological markers associated with Alzheimer's disease are neurofibrillary tangles and neuritic plaques containing beta-amyloid, while the main clinical feature of AD is a loss of cognitive function. In spite of years of research, the relationship between cognitive dysfunction in AD and pathological markers found at autopsy remains elusive. One consistent finding in many studies of the postmortem AD brain is degeneration of basal forebrain cholinergic neurons that innervate the hippocampus.[23] The loss of cholinergic input into the hippocampus may contribute significantly to cognitive impairment seen in AD patients. Acetylcholinesterase inhibitors, which increase synaptic levels of acetylcholine remain a mainstay for the clinical treatment of the disease. The factors that impart selective vulnerability to the cholinergic system in AD are not known, but numerous studies have shown that nicotinic receptor stimulation reduces the neurotoxic actions of beta-amyloid. Early studies by Shimohama[24] and Kihara[25,26] pretreated cultured rat cortical neurons with nicotine and observed a dose-dependant neuroprotection against beta-amyloid–induced cytotoxicity. The effects of nicotine were antagonized by hexamethonium, mecamylamine, DHBE, and BTX, indicating the involvement of multiple nicotinic receptor subtypes. More recent studies have attempted to unravel some aspects of the downstream signaling events that mediate the protective effects of nicotine. Shaw[27] showed that nicotinic stimulation of alpha 7 nAChRs in PC12 cells causes neuroprotection through transduction of phosphatidylinositol mediated cell signaling. Alpha 7–mediated calcium entry activated PI-3 kinase and Akt, leading to activation of Janus kinase 2 (JAK2). Inhibitors of JAK2 blocked the effects of nicotine. Other studies with PC12 cells suggest that nicotine attenuation of beta-amyloid–induced lipid peroxidation may account for some of the neuroprotection afforded by nicotine.[28] Some of nicotine's protective actions could be through anti-apoptotic actions. Studies using cultured hippocampal neurons exposed to beta-amyloid have shown that nicotine reduces caspase activation, attenuates increases in cytoplasmic calcium levels, and reduces free radical generation.[29] Other nicotinic agonists[30] and galantamine (a weak acetylcholinesterase inhibitor and nicotinic allosteric potentiating ligand) also are neuroprotective against beta-amyloid.[31]

The search for a mechanistic link between AD neuropathology and degradation of the cholinergic system has been further stimulated by the finding that soluble beta-amyloid interacts directly with alpha 7 nAChRs. Wang and colleagues[32] first demonstrated that beta-amyloid 1-42 binds with high affinity and selectivity to alpha 7 nAChRs, with a K_i in the low picomolar range. However controversy still exists as to the nature of the interaction between beta-amyloid and alpha 7 nAChRs, as some studies indicate that beta-amyloid may be an agonist at alpha 7 receptors,[33,34] while others report that it may be an antagonist.[35–37] Additional studies report that beta-amyloid acts as an agonist[39] or an antagonist[39] at non-alpha 7 nicotinic receptor subtypes. Thus, there is an intriguing but as of yet unresolved relationship between beta-amyloid and direct interactions with nicotinic receptors in the brain. Future studies in this area are required for a greater understanding of this interaction and the clinical significance in AD patients.

Dopaminergic Neurotoxins

Epidemiological studies have consistently shown a protective effect of tobacco use on the incidence and development of PD. More than 35 such studies have been published and virtually all have indicated a lower incidence of PD in cigarette smokers (see Quik and Kulak[40] for a recent review). These studies have estimated that cigarette smokers have approximately one-half the risk of age-matched nonsmokers for developing PD. This appears to be a global effect since retrospective and prospective studies performed on different populations of individuals from North America, Europe, Asia, and Australia have all demonstrated an inverse correlation between cigarette smoking and PD. Furthermore, some studies have shown a gradient for risk of developing PD with current smokers being the least probable to have PD, former smokers having an intermediate chance, and the highest incidence of PD in never smokers. Thus the preponderance of evidence from epidemiological studies suggests that cigarette smoking is protective against unknown neurochemical changes that lead to the development of PD. Study biases or other confounding variables are unlikely to explain the consistency of the findings that show an inverse relationship between cigarette smoking and PD. While the protective agent(s) in tobacco smoke is (are) difficult to define, many studies support the notion that nicotine's effects on dopaminergic neurons could be the source of the protection.[40] However, tobacco smoke also contains monoamine oxidase inhibitors that could also alter brain dopaminergic function.[41]

In vitro and *in vivo* studies using neurotoxins or mechanical lesions to produce experimental parkinsonism have been employed to investigate the interaction between nicotine and dopaminergic neurotoxins. Early studies by Janson and colleagues[42,43] used a unilateral nigrostriatal hemitransection to cause a significant decrease in the level of dopamine in the striatum. Alzet minipumps primed with nicotine were implanted at the time of lesioning. Nicotine administration attenuated the loss of striatal dopamine caused by the lesions. Similar results have been shown in animals that have 6-hydroxydopamine (6OHDA) lesions in the substantia nigra.[44] However, in the 6OHDA experiment, nicotine treatment before, as well as after lesioning was required for significant neuroprotection. The long-lasting nicotinic receptor antagonist chlorasondamine blocked the neuroprotective action of nicotine.[44] Ryan and colleagues[45] showed that nicotine infusions delivered for one week prior to lesioning reduced 6OHDA-induced cellular damage, as assessed by ^{3}H-mazindol binding to dopamine transporters in the striatum. In addition, nicotine pretreatment attenuated methamphetamine-induced neurodegeneration in wild-type mice, but not alpha 4 nAChR knockout mice, indicating that alpha 4 stimulation may be crucial for nicotine-mediated neuroprotection. Studies with the dopaminergic neurotoxin, 1-methyl-4-phenyl 1,2,3,6-tetrahydropyridine (MPTP), have been more variable with some studies indicating that nicotine administration reduces the toxicity of MPTP,[46–48] some studies reporting increases in MPTP toxicity,[49] and others reporting no change.[50] *In vitro*, nicotine pretreatment of mesencephalic dopamine cell cultures reduced toxicity of 1-methyl-4-phenylpyridinium (MPP+).[51] Variability in the outcome of MPTP studies is likely to be due to fundamental differences between the studies in terms of nicotine and MPTP dosing regimens (dose, frequency, pre- or post-treatment administration, etc.) and the outcome measures that were employed. In general, the results of these studies suggest that chronic nicotine treatment by osmotic minipumps may have a greater chance to enhance MPTP toxicity compared to other dosing strategies.

Experimental Neurotrauma

Although studies using this approach are limited, there is good evidence that nicotine administration could be neuroprotective and/or enhance functional recovery in animal models of neurotrauma. Our lab has used rats subjected to controlled cortical contusion injuries to evaluate the effects of nicotine on cognitive recovery and tissue preservation following injury. In one study, osmotic minipumps containing nicotine were implanted in animals immediately following brain injury. Increased tissue sparing was seen in animals that received a low dose of nicotine, but a higher dose was associated with post-operative convulsions, impaired upregulation of non-alpha 7 nAChRs, and no tissue-sparing effect. Nevertheless, tissue sparing induced by low dose nicotine treatment following the injury was promising.[52] In a second study, intermittent nicotine injections initiated 24 h after injury resulted in significant improvement in cognitive performance following brain injury.[53] Importantly, nicotine pretreatment was not necessary in this study, as treatment was initiated 24 h after injury. Ravikumar[54] evaluated the effects of nicotine on recovery from spinal cord contusion injury. Rats were subjected to spinal cord trauma and nicotine was delivered as a single injection 2 h after injury. Nicotine administration caused a reduction in indices of oxidative stress and inflammation, possibly reflective of a neuroprotective action.

Other Models

Hypoxia/Ischemia

Employing a gerbil model of global ischemia, Nanri[55] demonstrated that nicotine or 2,4-dimethoxybenzilidene (DMXB, an alpha 7 partial agonist, also called GTS-21) pretreatment attenuated cognitive impairment and cell death that followed the insult. Nicotine has also been shown to be neuroprotective *in vitro*, against oxygen and glucose deprivation. Four hours of hypoxia induced apoptotic cell death in rat cortical culture. Nicotine pretreatment (sustained during the hypoxia) was neuroprotective as evidenced by a significant reduction in DNA fragmentation and caspase activation. The effects of nicotine were blocked by both DHBE and BTX in this study.[56] Sobrado and colleagues[57] reported that the acetylcholinesterase inhibitor galantamine was neuroprotective in hippocampal slices exposed to oxygen and glucose deprivation but specific receptor mechanisms involved were not elaborated in this study.

Removal of Trophic Support from Cultured Neurons

Growth, differentiation, and survival of cultured neurons is dependent on trophic support by growth factors such as nerve growth factor (NGF). Removal of the neurotrophins causes cells to enter an apoptotic death cascade. Li and colleagues[58] showed that DMXB was neuroprotective against NGF withdrawal in cultured PC12 cells. MLA pretreatment blocked the effect of DMXB, indicating possible mediation by alpha 7 nAChRs. Protein kinase C (PKC) inhibitors attenuated some of the actions of nicotine, suggesting involvement of downstream signaling events. Choline and structurally modified analogs of choline have also been shown to be neuroprotective in this model.[59]

Ethanol-Induced Neurotoxicity

The rate of cigarette smoking in alcoholic individuals is much higher than in non-drinkers.[60] While the neuropsychological mechanisms underlying this interaction are likely to involve numerous factors, nicotine may offset some of the detrimental effects of ethanol exposure.[60] *In vitro* models of alcohol-induced neurodegeneration have been employed to demonstrate neuroprotective actions of nicotinic agonists. Li and colleagues[61] used cultured hippocampal neurons to show that DMXB decreased cell loss caused by high dose ethanol exposure in a MLA-sensitive manner. The authors suggest that nicotine might act by stabilizing mitochondrial function, attenuating cytochrome *c* release, and reducing apoptotic cell death. Similar findings in studies using cerebellar granule cell cultures were reported by Tizabi.[62]

NICOTINIC RECEPTOR AGONISTS AND FUNCTIONAL RECOVERY FOLLOWING BRAIN DAMAGE

Collectively, the studies outlined above clearly indicate that agonist stimulation of neuronal nAChRs produces significant neuroprotection in a variety of models used to mimic some aspects of human neurological disorders. One limitation to these studies is that pretreatment with nicotine was routinely employed. While such studies may be useful for establishing feasibility and developing hypotheses, therapeutic aspects of nicotine pretreatments are not realistic in most cases (except possibly in cigarette smokers). Since it is still impossible to predict which individuals will eventually develop neurological disorders or have an injury, prophylactic pretreatments are not likely to be of great utility. However, drugs that enhance functional recovery following trauma or disease may be more clinically useful. Several studies have shown that nicotine treatment can attenuate cognitive deficits produced by medial septal lesions, lesions of the nucleus basalis, and traumatic brain injury.[53,63–68]

NEUROPROTECTIVE EFFECTS OF NICOTINIC RECEPTOR ANTAGONISTS

Compared to nicotinic receptor agonists, possible neuroprotective effects of nicotinic receptor antagonists have received little attention. Numerous studies have shown that NMDA receptor blockers such as MK-801, are neuroprotective against a wide variety of neurotoxic insults, including those outlined in this review article. Alpha 7 nAChRs have a calcium permeability that is equivalent to NMDA receptors and are prominently located in the hippocampus.[69] Thus, it is somewhat surprising that more studies have not evaluated possible neuroprotective properties of nicotinic receptor antagonists. Laudenbach and colleagues[19] demonstrated neuroprotective properties of the alpha 7 antagonist MLA in a neonatal model of neurotoxicity. Peptides isolated from cone snails may be specific antagonists for various nAChR subtypes and could exert neuroprotective properties in some models.[70] Our lab has shown preliminary data that suggest that post head injury administration of MLA could have significant neuroprotective effects and also may increase cognitive function following trauma.[71]

STUDIES THAT DO NOT SUPPORT NEUROPROTECTIVE ACTIONS OF NICOTINIC AGONISTS

Despite the volume of data in support of neuroprotective actions of nicotinic receptor agonists, nicotine is certainly not a "magic bullet." In human non-smokers that have used nicotine patches for various indications, autonomic side effects (nausea, vomiting, dizziness) often limit the usefulness of the patch. There is great need for development of nicotinic agonists that activate CNS nAChRs (most prominently alpha 4/beta 2 and/or alpha 7 receptors), while providing no stimulation of autonomic receptors containing an alpha 3 subunit. Also there is some evidence in animal models suggesting that nicotine might increase neurodegenerative processes. Fuxe[72] evaluated the effects of chronic nicotine infusions following unilateral transection of the fimbria fornix. Chronic nicotine treatment exacerbated the loss of choline acetyltransferase activity in the septohippocampal system. Berger and colleagues[73] showed an increase in apoptosis of hippocampal progenitor cells following nicotine exposure. However, following differentiation of these neurons, nicotine was found to reduce apoptosis. The major calcium buffer in these cells, calbindin D28K, is expressed only after differentiation and may mediate the delayed protective action of nicotine in this model.[73] In addition, Freir[74] showed that nicotine exposure increases long-term depression in the CA1 caused by beta-amyloid application, possibly indicative of a process that would impair cognitive function.

Our lab evaluated the effects of chronic oral nicotine exposure in a mouse model related to Huntington's disease (HD). HD is caused by a mutation of chromosome 4, which results in a specific trinucleotide expansion. An excess number of CAG repeats is thought to encode for an aberrant protein known as huntingtin, which causes cell death in the striatum. The loss of specific striatal neurons (especially GABA interneurons) leads to an involuntary, choreiform movement disorder and progressive dementia. Currently there are no pharmacological treatments that have been shown to cure HD or alter its progression.[75] 3-Nitropropionic acid (3-NP) is a naturally occurring neurotoxin that is produced by various fungi. Ingestion of fungal contaminated sugarcane has been known to cause outbreaks of motor dysfunction that resemble the choreiform movements seen in HD patients. Systemic administration of 3-NP to rodents produces a movement disorder that has been correlated with selective damage to the striatum. 3-NP is an irreversible inhibitor of succinate dehydrogenase in complex II of respiration and induces metabolic impairment/mitochondrial dysfunction that resembles that seen in animals treated with MPTP.[76,77]

Adult male C57Bl/6 mice (Harlan, Indianapolis, IN) were treated for four weeks with either nicotine (200 µg/mL) in 2% saccharin solution ($N = 22$) or 2% saccharin alone ($N = 14$) as a drinking solution. Previous studies from our lab have shown that oral nicotine exposure in mice causes nicotinic receptor upregulation and behavioral tolerance to acute nicotine challenge.[78] Mice were randomized to two treatment groups that received either repeated injections of saline or 3-NP (100 mg/kg body weight) on five consecutive days. Mice were euthanatized on the morning of the sixth day by rapid cervical dislocation and the brains were quickly removed and frozen in isopentane (–30°C) and stored at –80°C until sectioned. The effects of 3-NP on the striatum were evaluated through the use of three different markers: (1) Nissl staining, (2) dopamine transporter autoradiography, and (3) nicotinic receptor autoradiography. The presynaptic dopamine transporter was labeled using ^{125}I-RTI121, and ^{125}I-Epibatidine was used to identify non-alpha 7 nAChRs. Following completion of the receptor binding studies, tissue sections were stained with cresyl violet and the volume of the striatal lesion was determined using the Caverieri method. Six equally spaced sections were evaluated using a video-based image analysis system (NIH Image). The system was calibrated to measure the size of the striatal infarct in square millimeters. Analysis of variance was used for all data analysis.

Chronic nicotine treatment increased the toxicological actions of 3-NP as evidenced by increased weight loss (FIG. 1) and increased mortality (FIG. 2) compared to saccharin-treated mice. Striatal damage was also exacerbated in chronic nicotine-treated mice; there was a greater incidence of 3-NP–induced striatal lesions (FIG. 3), and the sizes of the lesions were larger in 3-NP–treated animals (FIGS. 4 and 5). Non-

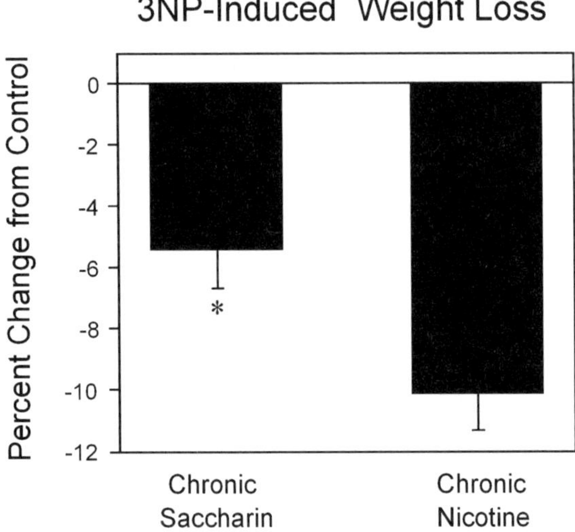

FIGURE 1. 3-NP-induced weight loss in animals pretreated with saccharin or nicotine. Mice that were exposed to the nicotine drinking solution were significantly more sensitive to the toxicological actions of 3-NP as assessed by changes in body mass that occurred during the ensuing week (F=6.8944, P<.0129).

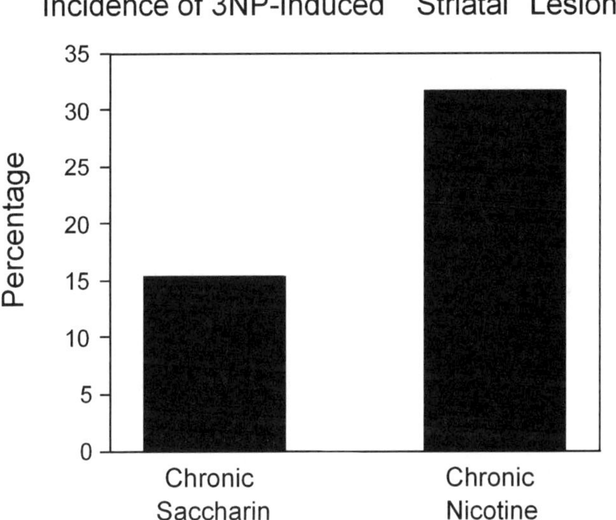

FIGURE 2. The incidence of 3-NP–induced striatal lesions in animals that were exposed to a saccharin or nicotine drinking solution. Nicotine-treated animals (7/22) has a greater percentage of striatal lesions compared to saccharin-treated mice (2/14).

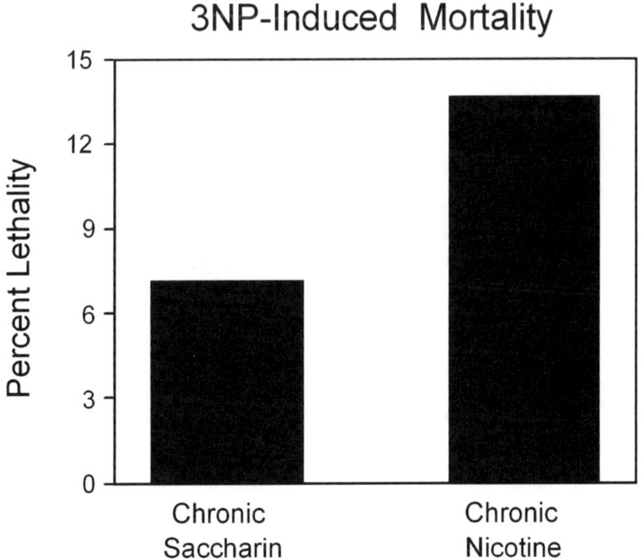

FIGURE 3. The percentage of 3-NP–induced mortality was higher in nicotine-exposed animals (3/22) compared with saccharin (1/14).

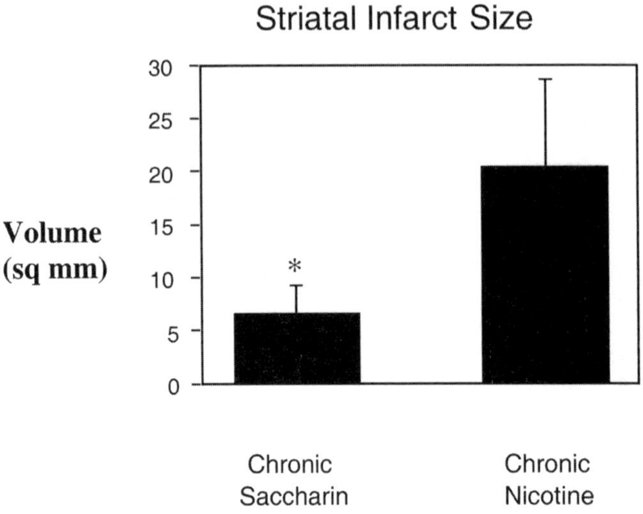

FIGURE 4. Lesion volume calculation in mice treated with saccharin (*N*=2) and with nicotine (*N*=7). Nicotine pretreatment caused a significant increase in the size of the striatal infarct.

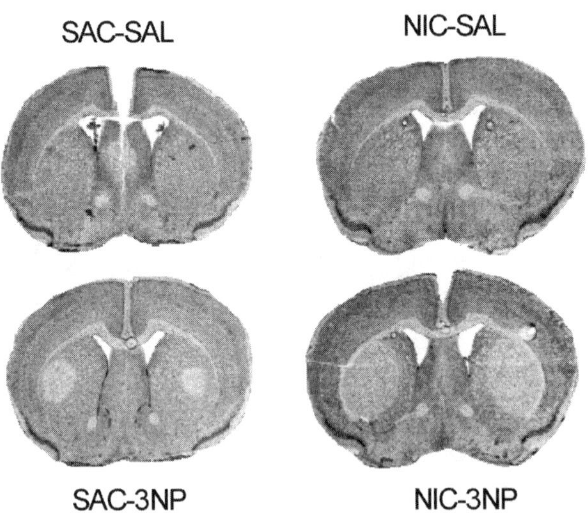

FIGURE 5. Nissl-stained sections taken from animals that were pre-exposed to nicotine or saccharin and then treated with saline or 3-NP. Striatal lesion size was larger in nicotine pretreated animals, indicating an greater sensitivity to the toxic actions of 3-NP.

alpha 7 nAChR binding receptor and dopamine transporter expression were not altered by 3-NP pretreatment (data not shown), indicating relative preservation of presynaptic nerve terminals that express these proteins. The cause for nicotine-mediated exacerbation of 3-NP mediated striatal damage remains to be determined. Gabrielson and colleagues[79] showed that, in addition to striatal toxicity, 3-NP administration to C57Bl/6 mice also results in significant cardiac toxicity. It may be that some of the effects of nicotine seen in the present study (e.g., weight loss and mortality) may be related to a peripheral mechanism of toxicity. However, we hypothesize that chronic nicotine may increase CNS toxicity of 3-NP (striatal lesion incidence and size) due to enhancement of dopaminergic function, since previous studies have shown that dopamine increases the toxicity of 3-NP in rodents.[80,81] We are not aware of any studies that have evaluated cigarette smoking in Huntington's disease patients, but these results suggest that nicotine derived from cigarette smoke could negatively impact the course of the disease and its treatment.

FUTURE DIRECTIONS FOR NICOTINIC MECHANISMS AND NEUROPROTECTION

Although there is a convincing body of literature to support the notion that nicotinic agonists and antagonists could be used for neuroprotection and/or enhancement of behavioral recovery following brain injury or disease, the underlying causative mechanisms are far from understood. In future studies, it will be important to consider some of the ten issues outlined below:

(1) In nicotine pretreatment studies, more attention should be paid to compensatory mechanisms that might occur following acute or prolonged nicotine pretreatment. One simple question to answer is: What is the relationship between changes in nicotinic receptor density and neuroprotective properties of the drug? In PC12 cells, Jonnala and Buccafusco concluded that nicotine-induced increases in the density of alpha 7 receptors correlated with the efficacy of ligands to exert neuroprotective actions.[82]

(2) The use of more sophisticated models (including whole animal studies) to evaluate nicotine-mediated neuroprotection would be useful. While cell culture approaches are valuable for ligand development and proof-of-concept experiments, the predominant presynaptic location of nAChRs makes data from culture models somewhat difficult to interpret. The use of other models including synaptoneurosomes or organotypic slice cultures would be welcomed.

(3) Future studies in this area should employ nicotinic exposure regimens that move beyond the common chronic pretreatment strategies that have been used in most previous studies. Pretreatment studies have limitations in clinical utility and interpretation. In cultured neurons, long-term, continuous nicotine treatment could cause adaptive changes in expression (or function) of other neurotransmitter receptors, transporters, intracellular enzymes, and drug metabolism pathways could all be involved with nicotine-mediated neuroprotection. Even short term nicotine treatment can cause significant

changes in dopamine transporter function.[83] Thus, long-term preincubation with nicotine may be neuroprotective due to a number of direct and indirect actions of nicotine exposure.

(4) The downstream signaling events involved with nicotine-induced neuroprotection require more scrutiny. While some limited information is provided by some studies, much greater detail, and a more systematic approach is required in these studies.

(5) The nicotinic receptor subtypes involved with the various neuroprotective actions of nicotine need to be clearly established. Unfortunately the development of subtype-selective agonists has been disappointing to date. The recent discovery of choline as a selective alpha 7 agonist[84] provides one possible tool for future studies. There is solid evidence for involvement of both alpha 4/beta 2 and alpha 7 nAChRs in nicotine-mediated neuroprotection.[1,2,85] In addition to the direct pharmacological studies that have been performed, studies using aged beta 2 knockout mice also support a role for this receptor in neurodegeneration. Aged beta 2 knockout mice display cognitive impairment as well as a loss of hippocampal pyramidal neurons, reactive gliosis and a significant elevation in plasma corticosterone levels.[86]

(6) Nicotinic receptors appear to have a predominant presynaptic location and facilitate the release of a number of different neurotransmitters and hormones including acetylcholine, GABA, glutamate, dopamine, serotonin, and norepinephrine.[2] When tissue slices or *in vivo* models are employed in neuroprotection studies, the possibility of nicotine induced neurotransmitter release factoring into the effect should be considered.

(7) The effects of nicotinic receptor stimulation or blockade on the expression of neuroprotective gene products need more attention. Several studies have shown that nicotine increases the expression of neurotrophic factor mRNA and/or protein.[87–89] One study also showed that nicotine increases the expression of NGF receptors in PC12 cells.[90] Prendergast and colleagues[17] showed that the neuroprotective effects of nicotine were mirrored by an increase in calbindin-D28K expression in the hippocampus. Increased expression of calcium binding proteins by nicotine could protect the cells from a number of insults that cause cellular damage secondary to increases in cytoplasmic calcium overload.[17,73]

(8) Studies evaluating interactions between nicotine and beta-amyloid peptide should consider studies that indicate that nicotine may play a role in alterations in beta-amyloid processing. Dickerson and Janda[91] showed that nornicotine, a nicotine metabolite that sequesters and accumulates in the CNS,[92] was shown to covalently bind to beta-amyloid, reducing its ability to aggregate. This would be expected to reduce plaque formation and/or possibly modify the clearance of preformed amyloid plaques. Interestingly, nicotine administered chronically through the drinking solution reduces amyloidosis in transgenic mice expressing the Swedish mutation of the amyloid precursor protein.[93] Nicotine treatment may also alter the neurobiology of APP processing, producing less toxic forms of beta-amyloid.[94] Hellstrom-Lindahl[95] found that amyloid load (beta-amyloid 1-40 and 1-42) was significantly less in AD patients that smoked cigarettes as compared with age-matched non-smoking AD patients.

(9) Nicotine has been shown to reduce apoptotic cell death in a wide variety of model systems including neurons, lung cancer cell lines, and the cardiovascular system.[96–99] In small cell lung cancer cultures, nicotine prevents apoptosis by increasing the phosphorylation of the anti-apoptotic cell protein Bcl2, possibly through a phospholipase C–mediated signaling mechanism.[100] Jin and colleagues[101] demonstrated that nicotine increased phosphorylation of Bad, which would also lead to a reduction in apoptotic cell death. Thus in cigarette smokers who develop lung cancer, tobacco smoke–derived nicotine could be a tumor promoter, leading to enhanced development of lung cancer and/or resistance to cancer chemotherapeutics. In the immature nervous system, apoptotic cell death is required for normal brain development. Perinatal cigarette smoke exposure has been correlated with a number of behavioral and neuropsychological impairments in children,[102] possibly as a direct effect of nicotine on apoptosis. It is interesting to consider that the effects of nicotine on apoptosis represent a plausible mechanism by which nicotine could provide benefit to the aged, diseased, or damaged nervous system but have significant deleterious actions during times of development when apoptosis must occur unchecked for normal brain development.

(10) While most studies have focused on neuroprotective actions of nicotinic agonists, it is also plausible that nicotinic antagonists may be useful for conditions involving cholinergically mediated excitotoxicity. However this possibility presents somewhat of a conundrum since in many previous studies nicotinic antagonists have been used to block the protective actions of agonists. However, there is still much to learn regarding the neurobiology of neuronal nicotinic cholinergic receptors. Because of rapid desensitization (and possibly permanent inactivation) of nicotinic receptors following agonist stimulation, it is possible that the long-term protective actions of nicotine agonists may be due to receptor inactivation, which in some respects may resemble the actions of a pharmacological antagonist.

ACKNOWLEDGMENTS

This work was supported by grants from the National Institutes of Health (NS42196 to J.R.P. and NS39828 to S.W.S.) and the Kentucky Tobacco Research and Development Center. We acknowledge the technical assistance of Melissa Yingling and Khaled Tanwir.

REFERENCES

1. DAJAS-BAILADOR, F. & S. WONNACOTT. 2004. Nicotinic acetylcholine receptors and the regulation of neuronal signalling. Trends Pharmacol Sci. **25:** 317–324.
2. O'NEILL, M.J., T.K. MURRAY, V. LAKICS, *et al.* 2002. The role of neuronal nicotinic acetylcholine receptors in acute and chronic neurodegeneration. Curr. Drug Targets CNS Neurol. Disord. **1:** 399–411.
3. HOGG, R.C., M. RAGGENBASS & D. BERTRAND. 2003. Nicotinic acetylcholine receptors: from structure to brain function. Rev. Physiol. Biochem. Pharmacol. **147:** 1–46.

4. KEM, W.R. 2000. The brain alpha7 nicotinic receptor may be an important therapeutic target for the treatment of Alzheimer's disease: studies with DMXBA (GTS-21). Behav. Brain Res. **113:** 169–181.
5. AKAIKE, A., Y. TAMURA, T. YOKOTA, *et al.* 1994. Nicotine-induced protection of cultured cortical neurons against N-methyl-D-aspartate receptor-mediated glutamate cytotoxicity. Brain Res. **644:** 181–187.
6. MARIN, P., M. MAUS, S. DESAGHER, *et al.* 1994. Nicotine protects cultured striatal neurons against N-methyl-D-aspartate receptor-mediated neurotoxicity. Neuroreport **5:** 1977–1980.
7. DONNELLY-ROBERTS, D.L., I.C. XUE, S. P. ARNERIC & J. P. SULLIVAN. 1996. In vitro neuroprotective properties of the novel cholinergic channel activator (ChCA), ABT-418. Brain Res. **719:** 36–44.
8. STRAHLENDORF, J.C., S. ACOSTA, R. MILES & H.K. STRAHLENDORF. 2001. Choline blocks AMPA-induced dark cell degeneration of Purkinje neurons: potential role of the alpha7 nicotinic receptor. Brain Res. **901:** 71–78.
9. TAKADA, Y., A. YONEZAWA, T. KUME, *et al.* 2003. Nicotinic acetylcholine receptor-mediated neuroprotection by donepezil against glutamate neurotoxicity in rat cortical neurons. J. Pharmacol. Exp. Ther. **306:** 772–777.
10. DAJAS-BAILADOR, F.A., P.A. LIMA & S. WONNACOTT. 2000. The alpha7 nicotinic acetylcholine receptor subtype mediates nicotine protection against NMDA excitotoxicity in primary hippocampal cultures through a Ca(2+) dependent mechanism. Neuropharmacology **39:** 2799–2807.
11. CARLSON, N.G., A. BACCHI, S.W. ROGERS & L.C. GAHRING. 1998. Nicotine blocks TNF-alpha-mediated neuroprotection to NMDA by an alpha-bungarotoxin-sensitive pathway. J. Neurobiol. **35:** 29–36.
12. KANEKO, S., T. MAEDA, T. KUME, *et al.* 1997. Nicotine protects cultured cortical neurons against glutamate-induced cytotoxicity via alpha7-neuronal receptors and neuronal CNS receptors. Brain Res. **765:** 135–140.
13. FERCHMIN, P.A., D. PEREZ, V.A. ETEROVIC & J. DE VELLIS. 2003. Nicotinic receptors differentially regulate N-methyl-D-aspartate damage in acute hippocampal slices. J. Pharmacol. Exp. Ther. **305:** 1071–1078.
14. GAHRING, L.C., E.L. MEYER & S.W. ROGERS. 2003. Nicotine-induced neuroprotection against N-methyl-D-aspartic acid or beta-amyloid peptide occurs through independent mechanisms distinguished by pro-inflammatory cytokines. J. Neurochem. **87:** 1125–1136.
15. STEVENS, T.R., S.R. KRUEGER, R.M. FITZSIMONDS & M.R. PICCIOTTO. 2003. Neuroprotection by nicotine in mouse primary cortical cultures involves activation of calcineurin and L-type calcium channel inactivation. J. Neurosci. **23:** 10093-10099.
16. SHIMOHAMA, S., A. AKAIKE & J. KIMURA. 1996. Nicotine-induced protection against glutamate cytotoxicity. Ann. NY Acad. Sci. **777:** 356–361.
17. PRENDERGAST, M.A., B.R. HARRIS, S. MAYER, *et al.* 2001. Chronic nicotine exposure reduces N-methyl-D-aspartate receptor-mediated damage in the hippocampus without altering calcium accumulation or extrusion: evidence of calbindin-D28K overexpression. Neuroscience **102:** 75–85.
18. BORLONGAN, C.V., R.D. SHYTLE, S.D. ROSS, *et al.* 1995. (−)-Nicotine protects against systemic kainic acid-induced excitotoxic effects. Exp. Neurol. **136:** 261–265.
19. LAUDENBACH, V., F. MEDJA, M. ZOLI, *et al.* 2002. Selective activation of central subtypes of the nicotinic acetylcholine receptor has opposite effects on neonatal excitotoxic brain injuries. FASEB J. **16:** 423–425.
20. O'NEILL, A.B., S.J. MORGAN & J.D. BRIONI. 1998. Histological and behavioral protection by (−)-nicotine against quinolinic acid-induced neurodegeneration in the hippocampus. Neurobiol. Learn. Mem. **69:** 46–64.
21. HILDEBRANDT, I.J., J.L. TERMEER, D. TOLEDO & R.W. COHEN. 2003. Characterization of chronic nicotine exposure on the survival of the spastic Han-Wistar rat. Nicotine Tob. Res. **5:** 827–836.
22. KIM, H.C., W.K. JHOO, K.H. KO, *et al.* 2000. Prolonged exposure to cigarette smoke blocks the neurotoxicity induced by kainic acid in rats. Life Sci. **66:** 317–326.

23. TERRY, A.V., JR. & J.J. BUCCAFUSCO. 2003. The cholinergic hypothesis of age and Alzheimer's disease-related cognitive deficits: recent challenges and their implications for novel drug development. J. Pharmacol. Exp. Ther. **306:** 821–827.

24. SHIMOHAMA, S. & T. KIHARA. 2001. Nicotinic receptor-mediated protection against beta-amyloid neurotoxicity. Biol. Psychiatry **49:** 233–239.

25. KIHARA, T., S. SHIMOHAMA, H. SAWADA, *et al.* 1997. Nicotinic receptor stimulation protects neurons against beta-amyloid toxicity. Ann. Neurol. **42:** 159–163.

26. KIHARA, T., S. SHIMOHAMA, M. URUSHITANI, *et al.* 1998. Stimulation of alpha4beta2 nicotinic acetylcholine receptors inhibits beta-amyloid toxicity. Brain Res. **792:** 331–334.

27. SHAW, S., M. BENCHERIF & M.B. MARRERO. 2002. Janus kinase 2, an early target of alpha 7 nicotinic acetylcholine receptor-mediated neuroprotection against Abeta-(1-42) amyloid. J. Biol. Chem. **277:** 44920–44924.

28. GUAN, Z.Z., H. MIAO, J.Y. TIAN, *et al.* 2001. Suppressed expression of nicotinic acetylcholine receptors by nanomolar beta-amyloid peptides in PC12 cells. J. Neural Transm. **108:** 1417–1433.

29. LIU, Q. & B. ZHAO. 2004. Nicotine attenuates beta-amyloid peptide-induced neurotoxicity, free radical and calcium accumulation in hippocampal neuronal cultures. Br. J. Pharmacol. **141:** 746–754.

30. MARRERO, M.B., R.L. PAPKE, B.S. BHATTI, *et al.* 2004. The neuroprotective effect of 2-(3-pyridyl)-1-azabicyclo[3.2.2]nonane (TC-1698), a novel alpha7 ligand, is prevented through angiotensin II activation of a tyrosine phosphatase. J. Pharmacol. Exp. Ther. **309:** 16–27.

31. ARIAS, E., E. ALES, N.H. GABILAN, *et al.* 2004. Galantamine prevents apoptosis induced by beta-amyloid and thapsigargin: involvement of nicotinic acetylcholine receptors. Neuropharmacology **46:** 103–114.

32. WANG, H.Y., D.H. LEE, C.B. DAVIS & R.P. SHANK. 2000. Amyloid peptide Abeta(1-42) binds selectively and with picomolar affinity to alpha7 nicotinic acetylcholine receptors. J. Neurochem. **75:** 1155–11561.

33. DINELEY, K.T., K.A. BELL, D. BUI & J.D. SWEATT. 2002. Beta-amyloid peptide activates alpha 7 nicotinic acetylcholine receptors expressed in Xenopus oocytes. J. Biol. Chem. **277:** 25056–25061.

34. DOUGHERTY, J.J., J. WU & R.A. NICHOLS. 2003. Beta-amyloid regulation of presynaptic nicotinic receptors in rat hippocampus and neocortex. J. Neurosci. **23:** 6740–6747.

35. LIU, Q., H. KAWAI & D.K. BERG. 2001. Beta-amyloid peptide blocks the response of alpha 7-containing nicotinic receptors on hippocampal neurons. Proc. Natl. Acad. Sci. USA **98:** 4734–4739.

36. GRASSI, F., E. PALMA, R. TONINI, *et al.* 2003. Amyloid beta(1-42) peptide alters the gating of human and mouse alpha-bungarotoxin-sensitive nicotinic receptors. J. Physiol. **547:** 147–157.

37. LI, X.D. & J.J. BUCCAFUSCO. 2003. Effect of beta-amyloid peptide 1-42 on the cytoprotective action mediated by alpha7 nicotinic acetylcholine receptors in growth factor-deprived differentiated PC-12 cells. J. Pharmacol. Exp. Ther. **307:** 670–675.

38. FU, W. & J.H. JHAMANDAS. 2003. Beta-amyloid peptide activates non-alpha7 nicotinic acetylcholine receptors in rat basal forebrain neurons. J. Neurophysiol. **90:** 3130–3136.

39. WU, J., Y.P. KUO, A.A. GEORGE, *et al.* 2004. Beta-amyloid directly inhibits human alpha 4 beta 2-nicotinic acetylcholine receptors heterologously expressed in human SH-EP1 cells. J. Biol. Chem. In press. [Epub ahead of print.]

40. QUIK, M. & J.M. KULAK. 2002. Nicotine and nicotinic receptors; relevance to Parkinson's disease. Neurotoxicology **23:** 581–594.

41. CASTAGNOLI, K., J.B. PETZER, S.J. STEYN, *et al.* 2003. Inhibition of human MAO-A and MAO-B by a compound isolated from flue-cured tobacco leaves and its neuroprotective properties in the MPTP mouse model of neurodegeneration. Inflammopharmacology **11:** 183–188.

42. JANSON, A.M., K. FUXE, L.F. AGNATI, *et al.* 1988. Chronic nicotine treatment counteracts the disappearance of tyrosine-hydroxylase-immunoreactive nerve cell bodies, dendrites and terminals in the mesostriatal dopamine system of the male rat after partial hemitransection. Brain Res. **455:** 332–345.

43. JANSON, A.M., J.J. MEANA, M. GOINY, *et al.* 1991. Chronic nicotine treatment counteracts the decrease in extracellular neostriatal dopamine induced by a unilateral transection at the mesodiencephalic junction in rats: a microdialysis study. Neurosci. Lett. **134:** 88–92.

44. COSTA, G., J.A. ABIN-CARRIQUIRY & F. DAJAS. 2001. Nicotine prevents striatal dopamine loss produced by 6-hydroxydopamine lesion in the substantia nigra. Brain Res. **888:** 336–342.

45. RYAN, R.E., S.A. ROSS, J. DRAGO & R.E. LOIACONO. 2001. Dose-related neuroprotective effects of chronic nicotine in 6-hydroxydopamine treated rats, and loss of neuroprotection in alpha4 nicotinic receptor subunit knockout mice. Br. J. Pharmacol. **132:** 1650–1656.

46. JANSON, A.M., K. FUXE, E. SUNDSTROM, *et al.* 1988. Chronic nicotine treatment partly protects against the 1-methyl-4-phenyl-2,3,6-tetrahydropyridine-induced degeneration of nigrostriatal dopamine neurons in the black mouse. Acta Physiol. Scand. **132:** 589–591.

47. PARAIN, K., V. MARCHAND, B. DUMERY & E. HIRSCH. 2001. Nicotine, but not cotinine, partially protects dopaminergic neurons against MPTP-induced degeneration in mice. Brain Res. **890:** 347–350.

48. PARAIN, K., C. HAPDEY, E. ROUSSELET, *et al.* 2003. Cigarette smoke and nicotine protect dopaminergic neurons against the 1-methyl-4-phenyl-1,2,3,6-tetrahydropyridine Parkinsonian toxin. Brain Res. **984:** 224–232.

49. HADJICONSTANTINOU, M., J.P. HUBBLE, T.A. WEMLINGER & N.H. NEFF. 1994. Enhanced MPTP neurotoxicity after treatment with isoflurophate or cholinergic agonists. J. Pharmacol. Exp. Ther. **270:** 639–644.

50. FUNG, Y.K., L.A. FISKE & Y.S. LAU. 1991. Chronic administration of nicotine fails to alter the MPTP-induced neurotoxicity in mice. Gen. Pharmacol. **22:** 669–672.

51. QUIK, M. & D.A. DI MONTE. 2001. Nicotine administration reduces striatal MPP+ levels in mice. Brain Res. **917:** 219–224.

52. VERBOIS, S.L., S.W. SCHEFF & J.R. PAULY. 2003. Chronic nicotine treatment attenuates alpha 7 nicotinic receptor deficits following traumatic brain injury. Neuropharmacology **44:** 224–233.

53. VERBOIS, S.L., D.M. HOPKINS, S.W. SCHEFF & J.R. PAULY. 2003. Chronic intermittent nicotine administration attenuates traumatic brain injury-induced cognitive dysfunction. Neuroscience **119:** 1199–1208.

54. RAVIKUMAR, R., G. FLORA, J.W. GEDDES, *et al.* 2004. Nicotine attenuates oxidative stress, activation of redox-regulated transcription factors and induction of proinflammatory genes in compressive spinal cord trauma. Brain Res. Mol. Brain Res. **124:** 188–198.

55. NANRI, M., J. YAMAMOTO, H. MIYAKE & H. WATANABE. 1998. Protective effect of GTS-21, a novel nicotinic receptor agonist, on delayed neuronal death induced by ischemia in gerbils. Jpn. J. Pharmacol. **76:** 23–29.

56. HEJMADI, M.V., F. DAJAS-BAILADOR, S.M. BARNS, *et al.* 2003. Neuroprotection by nicotine against hypoxia-induced apoptosis in cortical cultures involves activation of multiple nicotinic acetylcholine receptor subtypes. Mol. Cell Neurosci. **24:** 779–786.

57. SOBRADO, M., J.M. RODA, M.G. LOPEZ, *et al.* 2004. Galantamine and memantine produce different degrees of neuroprotection in rat hippocampal slices subjected to oxygen-glucose deprivation. Neurosci. Lett. **365:**132–136.

58. LI, Y., R.L. PAPKE, Y.J. HE, *et al.* 1999. Characterization of the neuroprotective and toxic effects of alpha7 nicotinic receptor activation in PC12 cells. Brain Res. **830:** 218–225.

59. JONNALA, R.R., J.H. GRAHAM, 3RD, A.V. TERRY, JR, *et al.* 2003. Relative levels of cytoprotection produced by analogs of choline and the role of alpha7-nicotinic acetylcholine receptors. Synapse **47:** 262–269.

60. LITTLETON, J. & H. LITTLE. 2002. Interactions between alcohol and nicotine dependence: a summary of potential mechanisms and implications for treatment. Alcohol Clin. Exp. Res. **26:** 1922–V1924.

61. LI, Y., E.M. MEYER, D.W. WALKER, *et al.* 2002. Alpha7 nicotinic receptor activation inhibits ethanol-induced mitochondrial dysfunction, cytochrome c release and neurotoxicity in primary rat hippocampal neuronal cultures. J. Neurochem. **81:** 853–858.

62. TIZABI, Y., M. AL-NAMAEH, K.F. MANAYE & R.E. TAYLOR. 2003. Protective effects of nicotine on ethanol-induced toxicity in cultured cerebellar granule cells. Neurotox. Res. **5**: 315–321.
63. ABDULLA, F.A., M.R. CALAMINICI, J.D. STEPHENSON & J.D. SINDEN. 1993. Chronic treatments with cholinoceptor drugs influence spatial learning in rats. Psychopharmacology (Berl.) **111**: 508–511.
64. BROWN, R.W., C.L. GONZALEZ & B. KOLB. 2000. Nicotine improves Morris water task performance in rats given medial frontal cortex lesions. Pharmacol. Biochem. Behav. **67**: 473–478.
65. DECKER, M.W., A.W. BANNON, P. CURZON, *et al.* 1997. ABT-089 [2-methyl-3-(2-(S)-pyrrolidinylmethoxy)pyridine dihydrochloride]: II. A novel cholinergic channel modulator with effects on cognitive performance in rats and monkeys. J. Pharmacol. Exp. Ther. **283**: 247–258.
66. DECKER, M.W., P. CURZON, J.D. BRIONI & S.P. ARNERIC. 1994. Effects of ABT-418, a novel cholinergic channel ligand, on place learning in septal-lesioned rats. Eur. J. Pharmacol. **261**: 217–222.
67. HODGES, H., P. SOWINSKI, J.D. SINDEN, *et al.* 1995. The selective 5-HT3 receptor antagonist, WAY100289, enhances spatial memory in rats with ibotenate lesions of the forebrain cholinergic projection system. Psychopharmacology (Berl.) **117**: 318–332.
68. RIEKKINEN, M. & P. RIEKKINEN, JR. 1997. Nicotine and D-cycloserine enhance acquisition of water maze spatial navigation in aged rats. Neuroreport **8**: 699–703.
69. BERG, D.K. & W.G. CONROY. 2002. Nicotinic alpha 7 receptors: synaptic options and downstream signaling in neurons. J. Neurobiol. **53**: 512–523.
70. HEADING, C.E. 2002. Conus peptides and neuroprotection. Curr. Opin. Invest. Drugs **3**: 915–920.
71. SRINIVASAN, D.M., L.A. PASS, D.A. HOPKINS, *et al.* 2003. Neuroprotective actions of the nicotinic receptor antagonist methyllycaconatine following experimental injury. Soc. Neurosci. Poster 683.6.
72. FUXE, K., L. ROSEN, A. LIPPOLDT, *et al.* 1994. Chronic continuous infusion of nicotine increases the disappearance of choline acetyltransferase immunoreactivity in the cholinergic cell bodies of the medial septal nucleus following a partial unilateral transection of the fimbria fornix. Clin. Invest. **72**: 262–268.
73. BERGER, F., F.H. GAGE & S. VIJAYARAGHAVAN. 1998. Nicotinic receptor-induced apoptotic cell death of hippocampal progenitor cells. J. Neurosci. **18**: 6871–6881.
74. FREIR, D.B. & C.E. HERRON. 2003. Nicotine enhances the depressive actions of A beta 1-40 on long-term potentiation in the rat hippocampal CA1 region in vivo. J. Neurophysiol. **89**: 2917–2922.
75. BONELLI, R.M. & P. HOFMANN. 2004. A review of the treatment options for Huntington's disease. Exp. Opin. Pharmacother. **5**: 767–776.
76. BROWNELL, A.L., Y.I. CHEN, M. YU, *et al.* 2004. 3-Nitropropionic acid-induced neurotoxicity—assessed by ultra high resolution positron emission tomography with comparison to magnetic resonance spectroscopy. J. Neurochem. **89**: 1206–1214.
77. FERNAGUT, P.O., E. DIGUET, N. STEFANOVA, *et al.* 2002. Subacute systemic 3-nitropropionic acid intoxication induces a distinct motor disorder in adult C57Bl/6 mice: behavioural and histopathological characterisation. Neuroscience **114**: 1005–1017.
78. SPARKS, J.A. & J.R. PAULY. 1999. Effects of continuous oral nicotine administration on brain nicotinic receptors and responsiveness to nicotine in C57Bl/6 mice. Psychopharmacology (Berl.) **141**:145–153.
79. GABRIELSON, K.L., B.A. HOGUE, V.A. BOHR, *et al.* 2001. Mitochondrial toxin 3-nitropropionic acid induces cardiac and neurotoxicity differentially in mice. Am. J. Pathol. **159**: 1507–1520.
80. FERNAGUT, P.O., E. DIGUET, M. JABER, *et al.* 2002. Dopamine transporter knock-out mice are hypersensitive to 3-nitropropionic acid-induced striatal damage. Eur. J. Neurosci. **15**: 2053–2056.
81. REYNOLDS, D.S., R.J. CARTER & A.J. MORTON. 1998. Dopamine modulates the susceptibility of striatal neurons to 3-nitropropionic acid in the rat model of Huntington's disease. J. Neurosci. **18**: 10116–10127.

82. JONNALA, R.R. & J.J. BUCCAFUSCO. 2001. Relationship between the increased cell surface alpha7 nicotinic receptor expression and neuroprotection induced by several nicotinic receptor agonists. J. Neurosci. Res. **66:** 565–572.

83. MIDDLETON, L.S., W.A. CASS & L.P. DWOSKIN. 2004. Nicotinic receptor modulation of dopamine transporter function in rat striatum and medial prefrontal cortex. J. Pharmacol. Exp. Ther. **308:** 367–377.

84. ALBUQUERQUE, E.X., E.F. PEREIRA, M.F. BRAGA & M. ALKONDON. 1998. Contribution of nicotinic receptors to the function of synapses in the central nervous system: the action of choline as a selective agonist of alpha 7 receptors. J. Physiol. (Paris) **92:** 309–316.

85. PRENDERGAST, M.A., B.R. HARRIS, S. MAYER, et al. 2001. Nicotine exposure reduces N-methyl-D-aspartate toxicity in the hippocampus: relation to distribution of the alpha7 nicotinic acetylcholine receptor subunit. Med. Sci. Monit. **7:** 1153–1160.

86. ZOLI, M., M.R. PICCIOTTO, R. FERRARI, et al. 1999. Increased neurodegeneration during ageing in mice lacking high-affinity nicotine receptors. EMBO J. **18:** 1235–1244.

87. BELLUARDO, N., G. MUDO, M. BLUM & K. FUXE. 2000. Central nicotinic receptors, neurotrophic factors and neuroprotection. Behav. Brain Res. **113:** 21–34.

88. GARRIDO, R., K. KING-POSPISIL, K.W. SON, et al. 2003. Nicotine upregulates nerve growth factor expression and prevents apoptosis of cultured spinal cord neurons. Neurosci. Res. **47:** 349–355.

89. GARRIDO, R., J.E. SPRINGER, B. HENNIG & M. TOBOREK. 2003. Apoptosis of spinal cord neurons by preventing depletion nicotine attenuates arachidonic acid-induced of neurotrophic factors. J. Neurotrauma **20:** 1201–1213.

90. TERRY, A.V., JR. & M.S. CLARKE. 1994. Nicotine stimulation of nerve growth factor receptor expression. Life Sci. **55:** PL91– PL98.

91. DICKERSON, T.J. & K.D. JANDA. 2003. Glycation of the amyloid beta-protein by a nicotine metabolite: a fortuitous chemical dynamic between smoking and Alzheimer's disease. Proc. Natl. Acad. Sci. USA **100:** 8182–8187.

92. GHOSHEH, O.A., L.P. DWOSKIN, D.K. MILLER & P.A. CROOKS. 2001. Accumulation of nicotine and its metabolites in rat brain after intermittent or continuous peripheral administration of [2′-(14)C]nicotine. Drug Metab. Dispos. **29:** 645–651.

93. NORDBERG, A., E. HELLSTROM-LINDAHL, M. LEE, et al. 2002. Chronic nicotine treatment reduces beta-amyloidosis in the brain of a mouse model of Alzheimer's disease (APPsw). J. Neurochem. **81:** 655–658.

94. UTSUKI, T., M. SHOAIB, H.W. HOLLOWAY, et al. 2002. Nicotine lowers the secretion of the Alzheimer's amyloid beta-protein precursor that contains amyloid beta-peptide in rat. J. Alzheimers Dis. **4:** 405–415.

95. HELLSTROM-LINDAHL, E., M. MOUSAVI, R. RAVID & A. NORDBERG. 2004. Reduced levels of Abeta 40 and Abeta 42 in brains of smoking controls and Alzheimer's patients. Neurobiol. Dis. **15:** 351–360.

96. GARRIDO, R., M.P. MATTSON, B. HENNIG & M. TOBOREK. 2001. Nicotine protects against arachidonic-acid-induced caspase activation, cytochrome c release and apoptosis of cultured spinal cord neurons. J. Neurochem. **76:** 1395–1403.

97. SUZUKI, J., E. BAYNA, E. DALLE MOLLE & W.Y. LEW. 2003. Nicotine inhibits cardiac apoptosis induced by lipopolysaccharide in rats. J. Am. Coll. Cardiol. **41:** 482–488.

98. OPANASHUK, L.A., J.R. PAULY & K.F. HAUSER. 2001. Effect of nicotine on cerebellar granule neuron development. Eur. J. Neurosci. **13:** 48–56.

99. WIELGUS, J.J., L. CORBIN DOWNEY, K.W. EWALD, et al. 2004. Exposure to low concentrations of nicotine during cranial nerve development inhibits apoptosis and causes cellular hypertrophy in the ventral oculomotor nuclei of the chick embryo. Brain Res. **1000:** 123–133.

100. MAI, H., W.S. MAY, F. GAO, et al. 2003. A functional role for nicotine in Bcl2 phosphorylation and suppression of apoptosis. J. Biol. Chem. **278:**1886–1891.

101. JIN, Z., F. GAO, T. FLAGG & X. DENG. 2004. Nicotine induces multi-site phosphorylation of Bad in association with suppression of apoptosis. J. Biol. Chem. **279:** 23837–23844.

102. SLOTKIN, T.A. 2002. Nicotine and the adolescent brain: insights from an animal model. Neurotoxicol. Teratol. **24:** 369–384.

Pharmacological Manipulation of Brain Kynurenine Metabolism

JOHN F. REINHARD, JR.

Brain Insights Incorporated and The California Brain Disorders Institute, Irvine, California 92614, USA

ABSTRACT: The amino acid tryptophan is a precursor for the neurotransmitter serotonin as well as for kynurenic and quinolinic acids. These latter molecules are antagonists and agonists, respectively, of the excitatory amino acid glutamate and arise through the kynurenine pathway of tryptophan metabolism. Significant differences exist in the sites and physiological control of serotonin versus kynurenine. While serotonin is formed within serotonin neurons (in the brain and intestine) and neuroendocrine cells of the intestine, kynurenine is formed by liver cells (as a precursor to nicotinic acid) and in macrophages, activated by inflammatory cytokines. Our studies are based on the hypothesis that inhibition of kynurenine metabolism (at the kynurenine hydroxylase [KH] step) allows the amino acid to be converted to kynurenic acid, a neuroprotective antagonist of excitatory amino acid receptors. Inhibition of KH also prevents formation of the neurotoxic species 3-hydroxykynurenine and quinolinic acid. To accomplish this end, inhibitors were identified and are described.

KEYWORDS: kynurenine; kynurenic acid (KynA); kynurenine hydroxylase (KH); metabolism; neuroprotection

INTRODUCTION

Strategies for neural protection are logically evolving with advances in the understanding of mechanisms through which neurons are damaged. In some cases, a physiologically important process can become pathologically relevant. One good example is glutamate. Acting through a variety of excitatory amino acid receptors,[1] synaptic glutamate influences a host of physiologically relevant processes. However, excessive stimulation of certain glutamate receptors, specifically the NMDA (for the prototypic agonist, N-methyl-D-aspartic acid), can lead to cell death.[2] In animal models, the neuronal damage resulting from cerebral ischemia can be reduced by antagonists of the NMDA receptor.[3]

Over the last 30 years, many antagonists of the NMDA have been identified. One of the best studied has been kynurenic acid (KynA). Medicinal chemists have used KynA as a starting point for the design of more potent inhibitors of the NMDA receptor.[4] Unfortunately, most of these molecules (like KynA) are carboxylic acids and appear to have poor brain bioavailability.[5]

Address for correspondence: John F. Reinhard, Ph.D., Brain Insights Inc., 17801 Sky Park Circle, Suite K, Irvine, CA 92614.

jfr02092003@yahoo.com

Ann. N.Y. Acad. Sci. 1035: 335–349 (2004). © 2004 New York Academy of Sciences.
doi: 10.1196/annals.1332.020

Among the endogenous agonists for the NMDA receptor, quinolinic acid (QUIN) has special attributes that distinguish it from the other amino acids. QUIN is a ubiquitous intermediate in the biosynthesis of nicotinic acid from which the redox cofactors NAD and NADP are formed. This formation appears highly conserved.[6] In mammals, QUIN is formed in liver as an NAD intermediate and is also formed in macrophages, which do not further metabolize the molecule but release it into the extracellular space.[7] In both liver and macrophage, the initial step involves cleavage of tryptophan's pyrrole ring through addition of O_2 to yield kynurenine.[8] The term "kynurenine pathway" is often used to distinguish this use of tryptophan from the formation of the neurotransmitter serotonin and the related hormone melatonin. For the kynurenine pathway, significant differences exist in the regulation within liver and macrophage. One significant similarity is that both cell types are "leaky", releasing the kynurenine intermediate. This intermediate can appear in the blood and is transported into the brain by the large, neutral amino acid transport protein (which also transports tryptophan).[9] In brain, kynurenine is a substrate for α-amino adipate transaminase (AAT, previously known as kynurenine amino transferase), which deaminates the amino acid to form KynA.[10] Thus, hepatic tryptophan metabolism can influence NMDA-receptor responsive neurons. In both liver and macrophage, kynurenine can also be hydroxylated by kynurenine-3-monooxygenase (a neurotoxic molecule[11]) that can be rapidly converted to the neurotoxic glutamate receptor agonist quinolinic acid.[12] The metabolism of tryptophan via these two pathways is depicted in FIGURE 1.

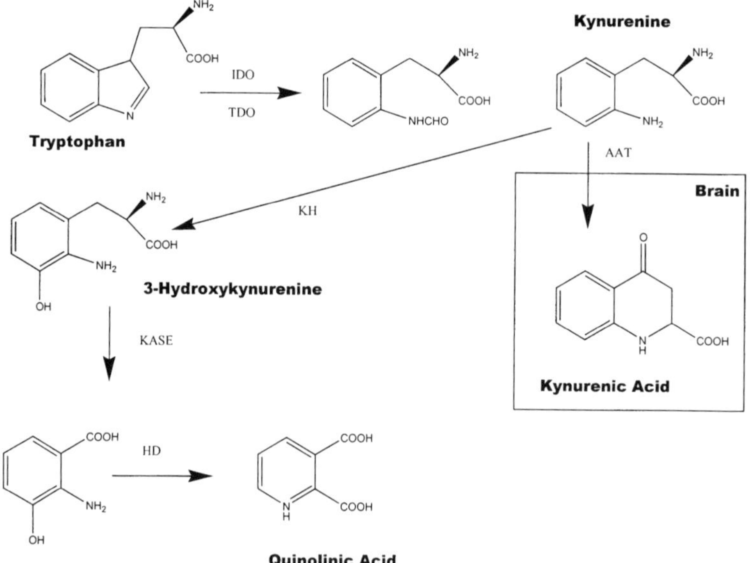

FIGURE 1. The metabolism of tryptophan by these two pathways. Enzyme abbreviations: IDO, indoleamine 2,3-dioxygenase (macrophage); TDO, tryptophan pyrrolase (liver); KH, kynurenine hydroxylase; AAT, α-aminoadipate aminotransferase (also known as kynurenine amino transferase); KASE, kynureninase; HD, 3-hydroxyanthranilate dioxygenase.

Kynurenine in the blood, irrespective of where it was formed, is transported into brain by the large neutral amino acid transporter.[13] In brain, extracellular kynurenine can be metabolized by glial AAT to yield kynurenic acid or by activated macrophages to the neurotoxins quinolinic acid and 3-hydroxykynurenine.

The neurotoxic potential of QUIN was first revealed by Lapin, who observed seizures in mice following the intracerebral injection of this molecule.[14] Stone and colleagues later reported QUIN to be an agonist of the NMDA receptor.[15] At high concentrations (5 mM), the toxicity of the molecule is apparent within minutes.[16] By contrast, in cultures of neuronal tissue QUIN toxicity was apparent at lower concentrations with significantly longer exposure times.[17] More recently, Brew and associates observed that media from activated macrophages (known to contain significant concentrations of QUIN) were toxic to neuronal cultures, and this toxicity was inhibited by inhibition of QUIN formation.[18]

Heyes and colleagues made the seminal discovery that QUIN was elevated in the cerebrospinal fluid of patients with HIV and the greatest concentrations were observed in those patients with HIV dementia.[19] These investigators later reported that QUIN could be formed from activated macrophages in response to the proinflammatory cytokine, interferon-γ.[20] Analysis of QUIN in cerebrospinal fluid from a variety of neurological disorders revealed an association between QUIN and diseases in which cerebral inflammation was a component.[21] Consistent with this hypothesis, our laboratory observed that brain microglia synthesized QUIN.[22]

As the working hypothesis, QUIN formed in brain by activated macrophages might damage neurons through activation of NMDA receptors. Inhibition of kynurenine hydroxylase, in brain macrophages and in liver, would attenuate QUIN formation while increasing serum and brain kynurenine that could preferentially form the neuroprotective NMDA antagonist KynA. Based on this rationale, inhibitors of kynurenine hydroxylase were prepared and evaluated.

METHODS

Stable isotope-labeled tryptophan and QUIN, $[^2H]$ and $[^{13}C]$, respectively, were obtained from Cambridge isotope labs (Andover, MA) and Li Laboratories (Milwaukee, WI). The $[^{13}C]$KynA was synthesized by Dr. William Pendergast (Burroughs Wellcome Co). Hexafluoroisopropanol, trifluoroacetylimidazole, and pentafluorobenzylbromide were purchased from Pierce. Inhibitors of kynurenine hydroxylase were prepared by M. Drysdale and W. Pendergast (Burroughs Wellcome). All other reagents were obtained commercially at analytical reagent grade purity.

Quinolinic and kynurenic acids were analyzed using gas chromatography with mass spectrometry (GS/MS) following conversion to their perfluoroacyl derivatives as described previously.[17]

Kynurenine hydroxylase activity was measured by the release of ^{3}HOH from 3-^{3}H-kynurenine (Amersham) as described[1] using crude, rat liver mitochondrial preparations as the enzyme source. Inhibition studies were conducted using a substrate concentration that yielded half-maximal velocity (K_m). Inhibitors were dissolved in dimethylsulfoxide and added in a volume (10 μL) corresponding to 10% of the total reaction volume. To assess the mechanism of inhibition, some inhibitors were tested at multiple concentrations of both substrate and inhibitor, as indicated in the text.

The inhibitor constant (K_i) was taken as the $(-)x$ intercept on secondary plots of K_m versus (I).

Macrophages were prepared from human monocyte preparations,[2] in 24-well plates (Costar, Waltham, MA) using Dulbecco's Modified Essential Medium (DMEM) containing gentamycin (3 µg/mL), fungizone (15 µg/mL) and human AB+ serum (6% vol/vol). Plates were maintained in a humid atmosphere under 95% O_2/ 5% CO_2 for 5 days in the presence of granulocyte-macrophage colony stimulating factor (GMCSF) (10 ng/mL) to promote differentiation into macrophages. Inhibition of quinolinate formation was studied by adding human interferon-γ (100 U/mL), followed 24 h later by the joint addition of the inhibitor and (^{2}H)-tryptophan (50 µM final concentration). Media was sampled 24–48 h thereafter and analyzed for nascent QUIN by GC/MS, monitoring the m/z fragment at 470.

Mice (male CD-1, Charles River, 20–25 g) were housed in an AAALAC-approved facility on a 12-h light-dark cycle with *ad libitum* access to food and water. Animals were housed in the facility for 7 days before use. Quinolinate formation was initiated by intraperitoneal injection with either bacterial lipopolysaccharide (*S. abortus equii*) or L-kynurenine, as indicated in the figure legends. Brain and blood were removed at necropsy and frozen on dry ice until analyzed for QUIN,[23] using [^{13}C]QUIN as the internal standard.

RESULTS

The regulation of QUIN formation in the CNS is different than for many other brain-derived toxins in that the primary cell of origin is not of neural crest origin. Rather, cells of the monocyte lineage (microglia and macrophages) appear to be the

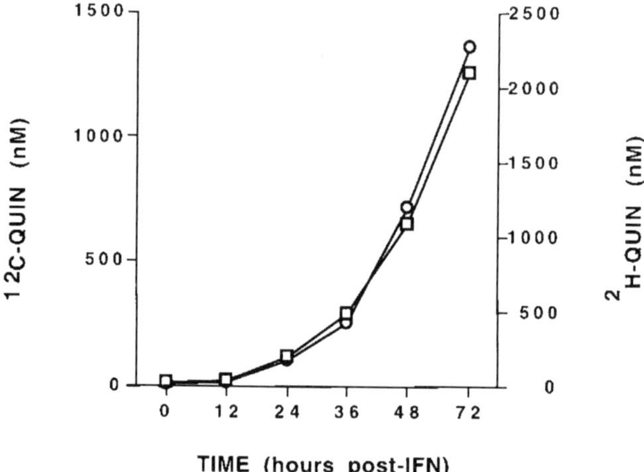

FIGURE 2. Effect of IFN-γ on nascent and endogenous QUIN. Data are the means ± SEM of four sister cultures per data point and represent the levels of endogenous and nascent QUIN, as determined by GC/MS, monitoring the fragments at 467 and 470 (m/z), respectively, in culture media of human monocyte-derived macrophages.

TABLE 1. Effect of cytokines on macrophage QUIN synthesis

Cytokine	Concentration	[^{2}H]QUIN
None		91 ± 12
IL-1	40 pg/mL	213 ± 47
IL-2	1000 U/mL	42 ± 1
IL-3	10 ng/mL	24 ± 4
IL-4	40 ng/mL	38 ± 8
IL-6	50 ng/mL	30 ± 10
IL-10	20 ng/mL	77 ± 25
TNF-α	300 ng/mL	106 ± 47
IFN-γ	1000 U/mL	1599 ± 30*

NOTE: Results are expressed as the means ± SEM (N=4) of (^{2}H)-QUIN (nM) following 48-h exposure to the cytokine and 50 μM [^{2}H]tryptophan macrophage culture media. *Significant difference from the control media (P<.05) as determined by one-way analysis of variance and posteriori analysis with the Neuman-Keuls test.

primary source of brain QUIN. We evaluated the suitability of human macrophage cultures as a test system in which candidate inhibitors could be tested against the relevant human enzymes. To accomplish this end, human peripheral blood-derived monocyte cultures were differentiated in culture for 5 days in the presence of GMCSF. Nascent QUIN formation was evaluated by adding [^{2}H]tryptophan (50 μM) and monitoring the formation of [^{2}H]QUIN. Media was sampled at different times after the addition of IFN-γ (FIG. 2). Induction of QUIN biosynthesis appeared to be restricted to IFN-γ, as suggested by comparison to maximally effective concentrations of other cytokines (TABLE 1).

Activation of indoleamine-2,3-dioxygenase, a key control step for the flux through the kynurenine pathway, has also been reported for other stimuli, including bacterial lipopolysaccharide, pokeweed mitogen, and poly I-C RNA.[24] Comparison of the lipopolysaccharide from different bacterial strains revealed marked differences in the ability to induce QUIN formation in macrophage cultures (FIG. 3). The data suggest that the macrophage response to pathogens differs in the apparent affinity of the lipopolysaccharide with no difference in the maximal induction of QUIN formed. Among the LPS tested, macrophages appeared to have greatest affinity for *S. typhenurium* and lowest for *P. aerugenosa*, with *S. abortus equii* being intermediate.

Based on early reports with *m*-nitrobenzoylalanine,[25] a series of related molecules were prepared and tested for their ability to inhibit rat liver kynurenine hydroxylase (KH), *in vitro*. The racemate and its (S)(+) enantiomer were prepared and tested. Data are presented in TABLE 2.

In addition to the *in vitro* and cell culture inhibition studies, (+/−) NBA was also evaluated for its ability to alter kynurenine metabolism in mice injected with tryptophan (FIG. 4). The data revealed that high doses of NBA could decrease QUIN formation from tryptophan. Further, this inhibition promoted flux of kynurenine to

TABLE 2. Benzoylalanine inhibitors of kynurenine hydroxylase

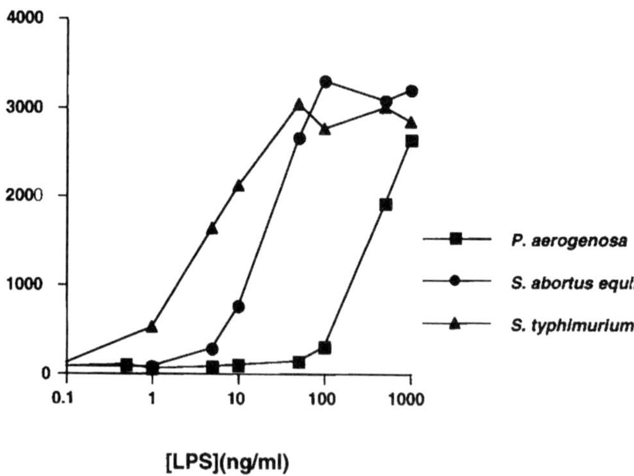

Compound	R	Chirality	IC$_{50}$ KH	IC$_{50}$ cells
(S)-NBA	3-NO$_2$	(S)(+)	4 μM	100 μM
NBA	3-NO$_2$	(R,S)(+/−)	8 μM	ND
I	3,4-Cl$_2$	(S)(+)	0.1 μM	0.7 μM
II	3,4-Cl$_2$	(R)(−)	85%*	2.5 μM

NOTE: Compounds were tested *in vitro* for inhibition of KH using rat liver preparations or for inhibition of QUIN formation in cultures of human monocyte-derived macrophages. ND: Experiment was not performed. *Maximum inhibition attained at a 10 μM concentration.

FIGURE 3. Bacterial lipopolysaccharides and macrophage QUIN. Monocyte-derived macrophage cultures were exposed to the lipopolysaccharides for 48 h in the presence of [²H]tryptophan. Results are the means ± SEM of three sister cultures as [²H]QUIN (nM). The *y*-axis represents the concentration of QUIN as nmol/L.

KynA, whose levels rose dramatically at doses of inhibitor that diminished QUIN formation.

In addition, enantiomers of the dichloro analog (DCBA) was also tested. The mode of inhibition was evaluated *in vitro*, assessing enzyme inhibition at multiple concentrations of substrate and inhibitor (FIG. 5). Secondary plots of K_m as a function of inhibitor concentration afforded an estimate of the K_i at 100 nM (not shown).

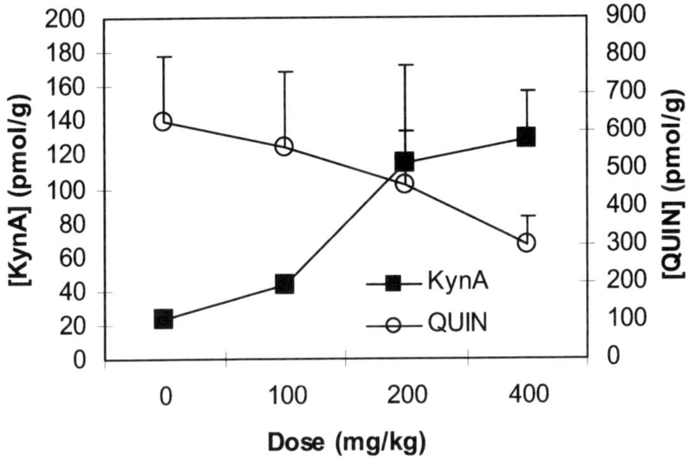

FIGURE 4. Effect of NBA dose effect on brain QUIN and KynA in mice. Data are the means ± SEM of groups of 4–5 mice injected intraperitoneally with kynurenine (30 mg/kg), 30 min before receiving NBA at the doses indicated, by the oral route. Brains were removed at necropsy 30 min thereafter and analyzed for QUIN and KynA as described.

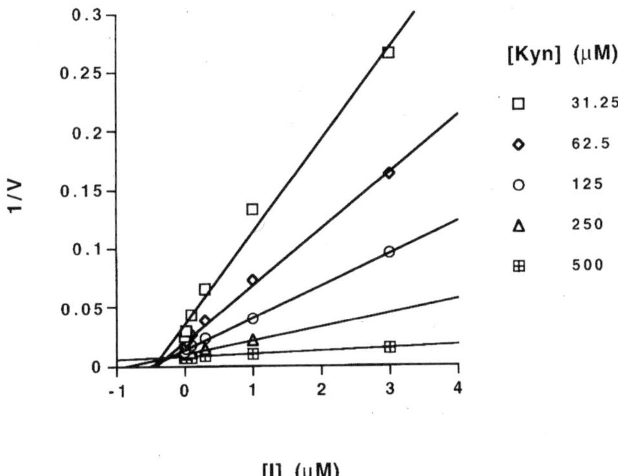

FIGURE 5. Inhibition of KH by L-3,4-dichlorobenzoylalanine. Data are the means of triplicate determinations at the concentrations of substrate and inhibitor.

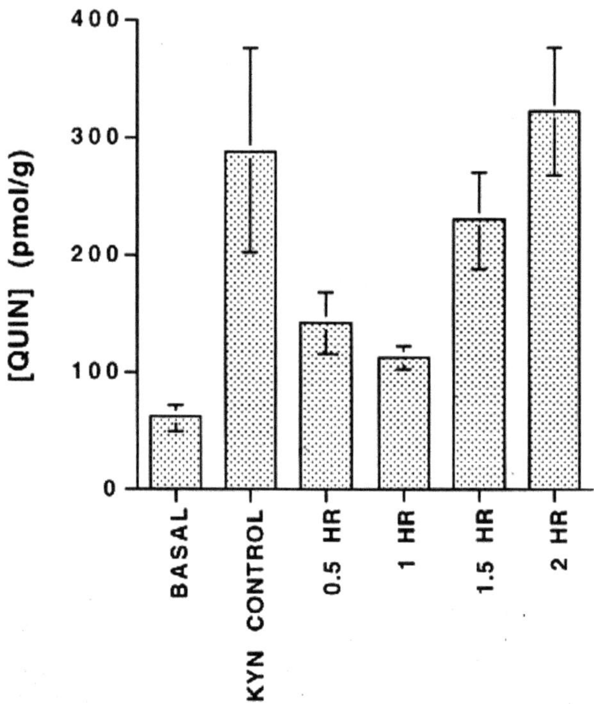

FIGURE 6. Time course inhibition of QUIN formation by (S)-3,4-dichlorobenzoyl-alanine. Data are the means of 4–5 animals per group, injected with kynurenine (30 mg/kg intraperitoneally), 30 min before receiving diluent (pH 8.0 Tris buffer, 50 mM) or the drug (10 mg/kg) by oral gavage. Animals were killed and brains removed for analysis at the times indicated.

In vivo testing in mice was performed at a single dose of 10 mg/kg to determine the effect on kynurenine-induced increases in brain QUIN at different times after dosing (FIG. 6). The *in vitro* and cell culture data further suggested a chiral preference for inhibition. KH inhibition by both nitrobenzoyllalanine and 3,4-dichloro-benzoyllalanine was greater for the (S) isomer than either the racemate (NBA) or the (R)-enantiomer (TABLE 1).

In an attempt to simplify the structural requirements for inhibition, a series of phenyl-oxo-butanoic acids lacking a chiral nitrogen was prepared. Surprisingly, the potency for inhibiting KH was greater than the benzoylalanines. Representative examples are presented in TABLE 3.

These data dissociated inhibitor affinity from the requirement of both the side-chain nitrogen and a chiral center. When tested on macrophage cultures, these aryloxobutanoates were among the most potent molecules tested for inhibiting the formation of QUIN. Random searching of related aryl olefinic acids identified several phenylcinnamic acids, some of which are presented as TABLE 4.

TABLE 3. Inhibition of kynurenine-3-hydroxylase by 4-aryl-2-hydroxy-4-oxobut-2-enoic acids and esters

Compound	R_1	R_2	IC_{50} KH	IC_{50} cells
III	3-Cl	CH_3	1.9 μM	0.006 μM
IV	3-Cl	H	0.32 μM	0.025 μM
V	3-F	CH_3	1.6 μM	5.6 μM
VI	3-F	F	0.58 μM	0.04 μM

NOTE: Compounds were tested *in vitro* for inhibition of KH using rat liver preparations or for inhibition of QUIN formation in cultures of human monocyte-derived macrophages.

TABLE 4. Inhibition of kynurenine-3-hydroxylase by phenylcinnamic acids

Compound	R_1	R_2	IC_{50} KH	IC_{50} cells
VII	$2\text{-}NO_2$	$2,4\text{-}Cl_2$	0.9 μM	75 μM
VIII	$2\text{-}NO_2$	$3\text{-}N_3$	10 μM (0.2 μM)*	ND
IX	$2,4\text{-}Cl_2$	2-Cl, $4\text{-}OCH_3$	0.5 μM	50 μM
X	$2,4\text{-}Cl_2$	$4\text{-}N(CH_3)_2$	2.9 μM	40 μM

NOTE: Compounds were tested *in vitro* for inhibition of KH using rat liver preparations or for inhibition of QUIN formation in cultures of human monocyte-derived macrophages. ND: Experiment was not performed. *Inhibition in the absence of light for an apparent photoaffinity ligand, while the value in parentheses is the inhibition after exposure to 302 nm light.

Although the potency of this series was less than that of the others, the latter series included an aryl azide (Compound VIII) that was evaluated for its ability to function as a photoaffinity ligand for KH. When exposed to 302 nm UV light, the effects were rapid (2 min, data not shown) and altered the pattern of inhibition (FIG. 7).

In the absence of light, VIII appeared as a competitive inhibitor of KH that increased the apparent K_m (126 vs. 70 μM) but not the V_{max} (310 vs. 344 pmol/

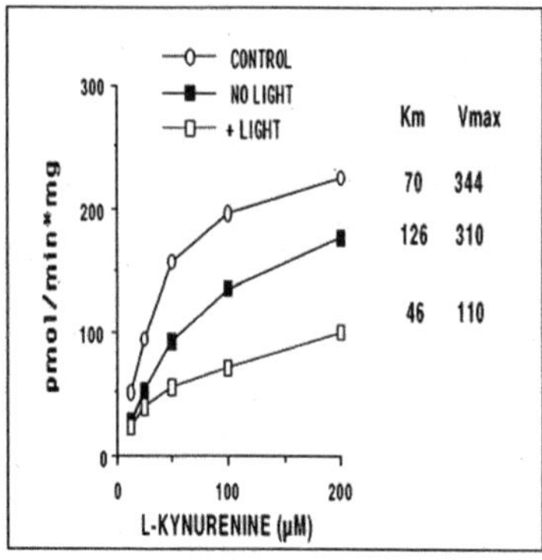

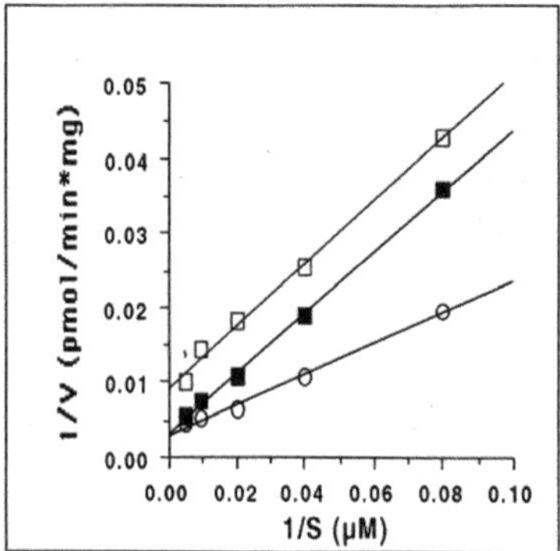

FIGURE 7. Effect of light on KH inhibition by Compound VIII. Data are the means of three estimates per data point of rat liver KH following exposure to light at 302 nm. Data are depicted as both direct linear (*left*) and double reciprocal (*right*) plots.

min·mg protein). By contrast, light exposure reduced the V_{max} by approximately 3-fold (110 vs. 344 pmol/min·mg protein) with only negligible alteration in the apparent affinity of the enzyme for its kynurenine substrate (46 vs. 70 µM).

DISCUSSION

The present work was undertaken based on a hypothetical relationship of kynurenine pathway metabolites to inflammatory CNS pathology. According to the hypothesis, in CNS inflammatory diseases, monocyte-derived macrophages and microglia appear at sites of injury. These cells become activated, principally by the proinflammatory cytokine IFN-γ (TABLE 1).[26] These data reveal that the neurotoxin QUIN is secreted from human macrophage cultures stimulated with either IFN-γ or bacterial LPS. It is hypothesized that the presence of QUIN at excitatory amino acid receptors in the CNS may either kill neurons or disrupt the otherwise regulated neuronal signaling at glutamatergic synapses. Assuming that this hypothesis is correct, inhibiting the flux of kynurenine to QUIN, via inhibition of KH, should divert the amino acid intermediate to the formation of KynA, a neuroprotective NMDA antagonist.

The origin of brain QUIN has variously ascribed to different cell types. Synthesis of QUIN by glial cells was initially suggested based on the ability of these cultures to convert 3-hydroxyanthranilic acid to QUIN[12] and six glioma cell lines to make the neurotoxin.[27] Isolation of [³H]QUIN, following intracerebroventricular infusion of [3,5-³H]kynurenine, argued for an intact kynurenine pathway in rat brain.[11] However, the levels of QUIN reported in rat brain were relatively low in comparison to mice, gerbils, and other species.[28] By comparison, synthesis of QUIN by macrophages and microglia was found to be robust, as demonstrated by mass spectrometry[14] (FIG. 2). Immunohistochemical localization of brain QUIN was further localized to immune cells, rather than neurons or astrocytes.[29] Using RT-PCR, Brew and coworkers demonstrated that human astrocytes can express IDO, kynureninase, KAT, and the quinolinate phosphoribosyl transferase (QPRT) but not KH.[30] The investigators further observed production of kynurenine and KynA that was increased by IFN-γ. Consistent with the lack of KH expression, the cultures did not form QUIN but did appear to express functional QPRT since the cultures actively degraded the neurotoxin. Given the preponderance of astrocytes (as compared to invading macrophages or microglia), their ability to degrade QUIN may be an important protective mechanism against QUIN neurotoxicity.

In addition to IFN-γ, bacterial LPS have been known to induce IDO[31] and to increase QUIN production.[29] The present data confirm and extend this observation. Surprisingly, the comparison of LPS from different bacterial strains revealed differences in the apparent affinity of these agents for inducing QUIN. The reason for this difference is unknown but could reflect differences in the affinities of the LPS to the Toll-like receptor 4.[16] However, induction of QUIN formation is not restricted to infectious agents.

In Alzheimer's disease, lesions include depositions of the amyloid-β peptide (1–42), which may be of functional importance in the disease. Inflammatory processes may be a component of Alzheimer pathogenesis.[32] It is also possible that QUIN may be a factor in lesions arising from inflammatory foci in the brain. It was recently reported that exposure of human macrophage cultures to aggregates of the amyloid-β peptide (1–42) elicited the production of QUIN. In contrast, a shorter form of the same peptide (1–40) and the prion peptide (106–126) did not promote QUIN formation.[33]

The KH inhibitor NBA was reported to be anticonvulsant,[12] suggesting a novel mechanistic approach to the control of seizure disorders. Based on the work of these investigators, other groups sought to identify KH inhibitors with better potency that might be amenable to pharmaceutical development. Investigators at Roche prepared and reported a promising lead with low nanomolar potency for inhibiting KH. The molecule, 3,4-dimethoxy-[N-4-(nitrophenyl)thiazol-2yl]-benzenesulfonamide (Ro 61-8048), was found to increase the KynA content of gerbil brain dialysates following oral administration of the compound.[14] The molecule has also proven effective in an animal model of dystonia,[34] suggesting a potential role for neuroactive kynurenines in this disorder.

In our hands, NBA was found to inhibit cell-free extracts of rat liver KH with an IC_{50} of 4 µM for the (S)-isomer and 8 µM for the racemate. By comparison, the potency in human macrophage cultures was only 100 µM. Such a difference in potency could result from poor cellular entry, rapid degradation or decreased affinity for the human enzyme. Regardless of the reason, low cellular potency is inconsistent with therapeutic utility.

As a tool, however, NBA inhibited QUIN formation in mice and, at these inhibitory doses, produced marked increases in the brain content of KynA. Both effects, however, were observed at relatively high, oral doses of the compound. The high doses required for these alterations in kynurenine pathway metabolism are consistent with the low cellular potency but may also result from poor oral bioavailability or other reasons. However, the data effectively confirm that KH inhibition can promote accumulation of KynA and identified benzoylalanines as a useful starting point for the discovery of other more potent inhibitors.

One such example was the discovery of 3,4-dichlorobenzoylalanine (DCBA) by investigators at Pharmacia. Reports on this molecule demonstrated effectiveness *in vitro* and *in vivo*, including ischemic damage in the gerbil.[35] We prepared this molecule for comparison to potentially more effective KH inhibitors. Tested against rat liver KH, a competitive pattern of inhibition with an apparent K_i of 100 nM was observed. Similar to NBA, DCBA is also chiral and the (S) isomer was found to be a more potent inhibitor of KH than the (R) isomer. In marked contrast to NBA, DCBA appeared quite potent on cultures of human macrophages, inhibiting QUIN formation with an apparent IC_{50} of 0.7 μM.

Administered to mice, DCBA was found to interfere with the kynurenine-induced elevations in brain QUIN. The effects, while significant, were short lived. The conditions used in this study, giving 30 mg/kg of kynurenine, are a difficult hurdle for a competitive inhibitor and may underestimate the actual biological duration that might be realized under conditions of human disease. While the short duration of action in mice was less than ideal, the chiral attributes of DCBA create an additional obstacle in the requirement for an efficient asymmetric synthetic method. We focused attention on simpler molecules.

The structural requirements for inhibition were further probed and resulted in the synthesis of 4-aryl-oxobutanoates and their esters[36] (TABLE 3). Among these molecules, unexpected differences were found in the relative potencies for cellular versus cell-free KH inhibition. Compound III, a methyl ester, was the most potent molecule tested for inhibition of QUIN formation in macrophage cultures with markedly lower affinity for the rat enzyme. Compound IV (the acid homolog of III) was slightly less effective on cells and more potent on the cell-free rat enzyme. Compound V, a methyl ester and fluoro analog of III, was equipotent for cell-free rat liver KH, but was much less potent on cellular QUIN formation. Surprisingly, compound VI (the acid of V) was comparable to IV on both cellular and cell-free measures of KH activity. The basis for these differences is not known. However, the rapid hydrolysis of esters (by intestinal and hepatic carboxylesterase) suggests that, administered to humans, the acid will be the predominant species available to inhibit QUIN formation. The historically poor brain bioavailability of acids makes this series less attractive for pharmaceutical development of CNS disorders.

The aryloxobutanoates were known to be capable of keto-enol tautomerism. Proton NMR showed that the intermediate methyl 4-aryl-2-hydroxy-4-oxobut-2-enoates III existed exclusively, and the corresponding acids IV existed mainly in their enol tautomeric form. These compounds may also be considered asymmetric olefins and are related to the cinnamic acids. Investigation of phenylcinnamic acids identified the phenylazide VIIII. In the absence of light, VIII and a non-azide, halogen-substituted analog (VII) appeared as simple competitive inhibitors of KH. However, following 2-min illumination at 302 nm, the pattern of inhibition changed for VIII to noncompetitive. Such a change is consistent with alkylation of the active site by the reactive species produced from the phenylazide by exposure to light. Compound VIII, while not a drug development candidate, is a useful tool for studies on the mechanism of KH.

Since the identification of seizures, resulting from intracerebral injection of QUIN,[37] our understanding of the kynurenine pathway has grown to a potential target for therapeutic intervention. It is possible that new therapies can be developed in which alterations in the balance between QUIN and KynA may find therapeutic benefit in wide-ranging neurological diseases.[38–51] Towards this end, the present work is a small step in a novel direction.

ACKNOWLEDGMENTS

The author thanks the skilled and dedicated efforts of Martin Drysdale and William Pendergast for their design and synthesis of the compounds described. The collaborative efforts of Ellen Flanagan, Mark Salter, Richard Knowles, and Chris Pogson are also gratefully acknowledged.

REFERENCES

1. LAPIN, I.P. 1978. Stimulant and convulsive effects of kynurenines injected into brain ventricles in mice. J. Neural Transm. **42:** 37–43.
2. STONE, T.W. & M.N. PERKINS. 1981. Quinolinic acid: a potent endogenous excitant at amino acid receptors in CNS. Eur. J. Pharmacol. **72:** 411–4412.
3. MELDRUM, B.S. *et al.* 1987. Protection against hypoxic/ischaemic brain damage with excitatory amino acid antagonists. Med. Biol. **65:** 153–157.
4. OZYURT, E. *et al.* 1988. Protective effect of the glutamate antagonist, MK-801 in focal cerebral ischemia in the cat. J. Cereb. Blood Flow Metab. **8:** 138–143.
5. SWAN, J.H., M.C. EVANS & B.S. MELDRUM. 1988. Long-term development of selective neuronal loss and the mechanism of protection by 2-amino-7-phosphonoheptanoate in a rat model of incomplete forebrain ischaemia. J. Cereb. Blood Flow Metab. **8:** 64–78.
6. BALSAMINI, C. *et al.* 1998. (E)-3-(2-(N-Phenylcarbamoyl)vinyl)pyrrole-2-carboxylic acid derivatives: a novel class of glycine site antagonists. J. Med. Chem. **41:** 808–820.
7. DI FABIO, R. *et al.* 1997. Substituted indole-2-carboxylates as in vivo potent antagonists acting as the strychnine-insensitive glycine binding site. J. Med. Chem. **40:** 841–850.
8. MUGNAINI, M. *et al.* 1998. [^{3}H]5,7-Dichlorokynurenic acid recognizes two binding sites in rat cerebral cortex membranes. J. Recept. Signal Transduct. Res. **18:** 91–112.
9. DANYSZ, W. *et al.* 1998. GlycineB antagonists as potential therapeutic agents: previous hopes and present reality. Amino Acids **14:** 235–239.
10. GHOLSON, R.K. 1966. The pyridine nucleotide cycle. Nature **212:** 933–935.
11. ISQUITH, A.J. & A.G. MOAT. 1966. Biosynthesis of NAD and nicotinic acid by *Clostridium butylicum*. Biochem. Biophys. Res. Commun. **22:** 565–571.
12. HEYES, M.P., K. SAITO & S.P. MARKEY. 1992. Human macrophages convert L-tryptophan into the neurotoxin quinolinic acid. Biochem. J. **283:** 633–635.
13. HEYES, M.P. *et al.* 1996. Human microglia convert l-tryptophan into the neurotoxin quinolinic acid. Biochem. J. **320:** 595–597.
14. ESPEY, M.G. *et al.* 1997. Activated human microglia produce the excitotoxin quinolinic acid. Neuroreport **8:** 431–434.
15. SALTER, M. & C.I. POGSON. 1985. The role of tryptophan 2,3-dioxygenase in the hormonal control of tryptophan metabolism in isolated rat liver cells: effects of glucocorticoids and experimental diabetes. Biochem. J. **229:** 499–504.
16. TAKIKAWA, O. *et al.* 1986. Tryptophan degradation in mice initiated by indoleamine 2,3-dioxygenase. J. Biol. Chem. **261:** 3648–3653.
17. FUKUI, S. *et al.* 1991. Blood-brain barrier transport of kynurenines: implications for brain synthesis and metabolism. J. Neurochem. **56:** 2007–2017.
18. GOH, D.L. *et al.* 2002. Characterization of the human gene encoding alpha-aminoadipate aminotransferase (AADAT). Mol. Genet. Metab. **76:** 172–180.
19. BUCHLI, R. *et al.* 1995. Cloning and functional expression of a soluble form of kynurenine/alpha-aminoadipate aminotransferase from rat kidney. J. Biol. Chem. **270:** 29330–29335.
20. OKUDA, S. *et al.* 1996. Hydrogen peroxide-mediated neuronal cell death induced by an endogenous neurotoxin, 3-hydroxykynurenine. Proc. Natl. Acad. Sci. USA **93:** 12553–12558.
21. WEI, H. *et al.* 2000. Neuronal apoptosis induced by pharmacological concentrations of 3-hydroxykynurenine: characterization and protection by dantrolene and Bcl-2 over-expression. J. Neurochem. **75:** 81–90.

22. REINHARD, J.F., JR., J.B. ERICKSON & E.M. FLANAGAN. 1994. Quinolinic acid in neurological disease: opportunities for novel drug discovery. Adv. Pharmacol. **30:** 85–127.

23. GARTHWAITE, G. & J. GARTHWAITE. 1984. Differential sensitivity of rat cerebellar cells in vitro to the neurotoxic effects of excitatory amino acid analogues. Neurosci. Lett. **48:** 361–367.

24. WHETSELL, W.O. & R. SCHWARCZ. 1989. Prolonged exposure to submicromolar concentrations of quinolinic acid causes excitotoxic damage in organotypic cultures of rat corticostriatal system. Neurosci. Lett. **97:** 271–275.

25. KERR, S.J. et al. 1997. Kynurenine pathway inhibition reduces neurotoxicity of HIV-1-infected macrophages. Neurology **49:** 1671–1681.

26. HEYES, M.P. et al. 1989. Cerebrospinal fluid quinolinic acid concentrations are increased in acquired immune deficiency syndrome. Ann. Neurol. **26:** 275–277.

27. HEYES, M.P. et al. 1993. A mechanism of quinolinic acid formation by brain in inflammatory neurological disease. Attenuation of synthesis from L-tryptophan by 6-chlorotryptophan and 4-chloro-3-hydroxyanthranilate. Brain **116:** 1425–1450.

28. HEYES, M.P. et al. 1992. Quinolinic acid and kynurenine pathway metabolism in inflammatory and non-inflammatory neurological disease. Brain **115:** 1249–1273.

29. HEYES, M.P. & S.P. MARKEY. 1988. Quantification of quinolinic acid in rat brain, whole blood, and plasma by gas chromatography and negative chemical ionization mass spectrometry: effects of systemic L-tryptophan administration on brain and blood quinolinic acid concentrations. Anal. Biochem. **174:** 349–359.

30. ERICKSON, J.B. et al. 1992. A radiometric assay for kynurenine 3-hydroxylase based on the release of ^3H_2O during hydroxylation of L-[3,5-^{3}H]kynurenine. Anal. Biochem. **205:** 257–262.

31. NOTTET, H.S. et al. 1996. The regulation of quinolinic acid in human immunodeficiency virus-infected monocytes. J. Neurovirol. **2:** 111–117.

32. CARPENEDO, R. et al. 1994. Inhibitors of kynurenine hydroxylase and kynureninase increase cerebral formation of kynurenate and have sedative and anticonvulsant activities. Neuroscience **61:** 237–243.

33. SMITH, D.G. et al. 2001. Quinolinic acid is produced by macrophages stimulated by platelet activating factor, Nef and Tat. J. Neurovirol. **7:** 56–60.

34. FOSTER, A.C., R.J. WHITE & R. SCHWARCZ. 1986. Synthesis of quinolinic acid by 3-hydroxyanthranilic acid oxygenase in rat brain tissue in vitro. J. Neurochem. **47:** 23–30.

35. VEZZANI, A. et al. 1991. Production of quinolinic acid and kynurenic acid by human glioma. Adv. Exp. Biol. Med. **294:** 691–695.

36. GUIDETTI, P., C.L. EASTMAN & R. SCHWARCZ. 1995. Metabolism of [5-^{3}H]kynurenine in the rat brain in vivo: evidence for the existence of a functional kynurenine pathway. J. Neurochem. **65:** 2621–2632.

37. SAITO, K. & M.P. HEYES. 1996. Kynurenine pathway enzymes in brain: properties of enzymes and regulation of quinolinic acid synthesis. Adv. Exp. Med. Biol. **398:** 485–492.

38. SAITO, K., S.P. MARKEY & M.P. HEYES. 1992. Effects of immune activation on quinolinic acid and neuroactive kynurenines in the mouse. Neuroscience **51:** 25–39.

39. HEYES, M.P. et al. 1997. Species heterogeneity between gerbils and rats: quinolinate production by microglia and astrocytes and accumulations in response to ischemic brain injury and systemic immune activation. J. Neurochem. **69:** 1519–1529.

40. MOFFETT, J.R. et al. 1993. Antibodies to quinolinic acid reveal localization in select immune cells rather than neurons or astroglia. Brain Res. **623:** 337–340.

41. GUILLEMIN, G.J. et al. 2001. Kynurenine pathway metabolism in human astrocytes: a paradox for neuronal protection. J. Neurochem. **78:** 842–853.

42. SAITO, K. et al. 1996. Cytokine and drug modulation of kynurenine pathway metabolism by blood mononuclear cells. Adv. Exp. Med. Biol. **398:** 161–165.

43. HAJJAR, A.M. et al. 2002. Human Toll-like receptor 4 recognizes host-specific LPS modifications. Nat. Immunol. **3:** 354–359.

44. EIKELENBOOM, P. & W.A. VAN GOOL. 2004. Neuroinflammatory perspectives on the two faces of Alzheimer's disease. J. Neural Transm. **111:** 281–294.

45. GUILLEMIN, G.J. et al. 2003. A beta 1-42 induces production of quinolinic acid by human macrophages and microglia. Neuroreport **14:** 2311–2315.

46. PELLICCIARI, R. *et al.* 1994. Modulation of the kynurenine pathway in search for new neuroprotective agents: synthesis and preliminary evaluation of (m-nitrobenzoyl)alanine, a potent inhibitor of kynurenine-3-hydroxylase. J. Med. Chem. **37:** 647–655.
47. ROVER, S. *et al.* 1997. Synthesis and biochemical evaluation of N-(4-phenylthiazol-2-yl)-benzenesulfonamides as high-affinity inhibitors of kynurenine 3-hydroxylase. J. Med. Chem. **40:** 4378–4385.
48. RICHTER, A. & M. HAMANN. 2003. The kynurenine 3-hydroxylase inhibitor Ro 61-8048 improves dystonia in a genetic model of paroxysmal dyskinesia. Eur. J. Pharmacol. **478:** 47–52.
49. SPECIALE, C. *et al.* 1996. (R,S)-3,4-Dichlorobenzoylalanine (FCE 28833A) causes a large and persistent increase in brain kynurenic acid levels in rats. Eur. J. Pharmacol. **315:** 263–267.
50. SPECIALE, C. *et al.* 1996. Kynurenic acid-enhancing and anti-ischemic effects of the potent kynurenine 3-hydroxylase inhibitor FCE 28833 in rodents. Adv. Exp. Med. Biol. **398:** 221–227.
51. DRYSDALE, M.J. *et al.* 2000. Synthesis and SAR of 4-aryl-2-hydroxy-4-oxobut-2-enoic acids and esters and 2-amino-4-aryl-4-oxobut-2-enoic acids and esters: potent inhibitors of kynurenine-3-hydroxylase as potential neuroprotective agents. J. Med. Chem. **43:** 123–127.

Cooperative Ideas about Cooperative Strategies

STEVEN W. BARGER

Departments of Geriatrics and Neurobiology and Developmental Sciences, University of Arkansas for Medical Sciences, and Geriatric Research Education and Clinical Center, Central Arkansas Veterans Healthcare System, Little Rock, Arkansas 72205, USA

ABSTRACT: There is little precedence for rational design of pharmacological strategies that utilize multiple sites of action. However, such pharmaceutical and nutraceutical multitasking may be just the ticket to combat the multifactorial nature of neurodegeneration. This paper summarizes the discussion on several cooperative ideas, particularly on intellectual property issue, current research funding status, and limitations of public and private funding.

KEYWORDS: cooperative; medicine; pharmacology; science; strategy

The nature of biomedical research in general, and neuroscience especially, has always included movement toward higher levels of complexity. The multidisciplinary lines of investigation intersecting from the fields of nutrition, phytopharmacology, nutraceuticals, and alternative medicine have certainly perpetuated that trend. Traditional pharmacology depends on the rigor of molecular reductionism, yet emerging data indicate that the benefits derived from a healthful diet will be realized only through the cooperative actions of multiple compounds. As fortunate as these synergistic actions may be for the beneficiaries of cooperative pharmaceuticals, their interdependence is equally unfortunate for scientists. There is little precedence for rational design of pharmacological strategies that utilize multiple sites of action. However, according to the participants at the *VIIth International Conference on Protective Strategies for Neurodegenerative Diseases*, such pharmaceutical and nutraceutical multitasking may be just the ticket to combat the multifactorial nature of neurodegeneration.

In discussions to conclude the conference and to derive a consensus from its presentations, three main topics arose: First, several participants remarked on the lack of financial incentive for pharmaceutical companies to invest in research on public-domain agents such as natural products. While a unique formula combining agents that work cooperatively can be patented, few companies would pursue this strategy because of the ability of competitors to alter the composition slightly and thereby subvert intellectual property protections, according to Greg Cole. In order to lay claim to the novelty and utility required of patents, a company would need to show that its concoction was significantly more effective than a competitor's mixture that included or lacked even a trivial component.

Address for correspondence: Dr. Steven W. Barger, Reynolds Center on Aging, 629 Jack Stephens Drive, #807, Little Rock, AR 72205. Voice: 501-526-5811; fax: 501-526-5830.
sbarger@uams.edu

Ann. N.Y. Acad. Sci. 1035: 350–353 (2004). © 2004 New York Academy of Sciences.
doi: 10.1196/annals.1332.021

The obvious solution for nonpatentable therapeutic opportunities is research sponsored by the National Institutes of Health. While a great deal of this research is being performed extramurally and through unprecedented levels of cooperation between public and private endeavors, intramural NIH programs are also committed to therapeutic discovery. Nigel Greig, for instance, has identified promising neuroprotective molecules among an array of compounds released from proprietary protection by commercial interests. However, provided that therapeutic drugs are identified in the public domain, there remains the problem of production and distribution. It is not clear that private industry could always be convinced that such an undertaking would be profitable without a proprietary claim.

One business model has been provided by Joe Marwah and colleagues (Biotechnology Discovery, Inc.). They have developed an innovative method for single-step purification of lycopene. While this neuroprotective tomato-derived compound cannot be claimed itself as intellectual property, such a novel production strategy can provide a competitive incentive.

The second significant issue tackled by the attendees was the inadequacy of methods historically utilized in pharmacology. As Jim Pauly emphasized, pharmacologists have always sought to whittle down a lead molecule to its active moieties; and specificity, restriction of the drug's target, has traditionally been considered insurance against undesirable side effects. However, some of the most successful compounds may derive their power from the breadth of their effects. As an example, curcumin and other polyphenols would appear to have utility in Alzheimer's disease not only because of their dual function as antiinflammatory/antioxidant agents, but also because several of them can structurally interfere with the fibrillization of amyloid β-peptide.[1] Curcumin and melatonin may also provide superior antioxidant protection because their various metabolites parse to both hydrophilic and hydrophobic compartments within a biological tissue. A concoction of several discretely acting drugs can provide a similar multitarget synergy. However, systematic approaches to discovering and optimizing such synergies are not supported by tradition within pharmacological sciences or, indeed, within science at all.

The rise of combinatorial chemistry has ushered in the simultaneous synthesis and coordinate testing of entire libraries of compounds. Patents (and thus financial incentive) can be applied to the libraries themselves or even to the methodology that creates them. However, the general practice has been to test combinatorial libraries by performing rounds of subdivision, splitting the library into smaller and smaller mixtures that retain bioactivity—usually, a very discrete and easily assayed bioactivity—with the goal of eventually isolating a single compound. This process might divorce two or more molecules that have cooperative effects. Worse yet, the simplicity of the assay may overlook such cooperative effects altogether if they impact a biological system rather than a single enzyme or receptor. The first problem could be alleviated through decision trees that include assays of overlapping groups, for example, testing mixes of sublibraries obtained by distinct purification techniques. The second problem is exacerbated by the fact that a given combinatorial library will usually be generated by a single set of reaction conditions with a single "scaffold" molecule, so its constituents are likely to be structurally similar and thus impact a single target. Therefore, it might also be helpful to assay "combinatorial combinations", or mixtures of multiple libraries, and to do so in more complex test models. In such a strategy, greater attention would need to be focused on the library subdivision steps at which bioactivity was lost rather than on the ultimate isolation of a single molecule.

These strategies, like the entire intersection between nutraceuticals and alternative medicine, run the risk of appearing phenomenological. However, science and medicine always stand to gain when mechanisms can be understood, and discussions took this turn as conference participants considered the possible intersection of nutraceutical effects with the transcriptional control highlighted by several presentations in the program. Considerable evidence now indicates that dietary manipulations can have a dramatic effect on epigenetic mechanisms that influence gene expression. Among the mechanisms for mediating epigenetic effects are methylation of DNA and modification of histones, including acetylation, methylation, and phosphorylation. Resveratrol, a polyphenol in red wine that has been touted for its antioxidant effects, also stimulates a member of the sirtuin family of NAD^+-dependent histone deacetylases.[2] Sirtuin deacetylases are necessary for the life span–enhancing effects of caloric restriction in some models; and while they may have additional protein substrates, histones at specific gene loci can be influenced by their activity. DNA methylation, as well, has been connected to both age-related inflammation and dietary manipulation. Folate or B_{12} insufficiency can hamper the one-carbon system necessary for maintaining the DNA methylation patterns,[3] and methylation is critical for suppressing transcription of tumor necrosis factor, interferon-γ, and a host of other genes that can contribute to inflammatory neurodegeneration.[4] One indicator of such an attenuation of one-carbon anabolism is an increase in homocysteine, a phenomenon already documented in Alzheimer's disease, Parkinson's disease, and stroke.[5] Among other things, such epigenetic mechanisms provide a perfect explanation for cases in which an infection or injury provokes a prolonged inflammation or primes the CNS for a more robust subsequent inflammatory response.[6–9] Specific or acquired immunity has long been recognized for a type of a "memory", mediated in that case by chromatin rearrangement. The innate immune system (which contributes critically to neurodegenerative conditions) would be unlikely to undergo such a genetic alteration, but epigenetic events are quite probable.

In essence, none of the individual opinions ventured forth by this particular event focusing on protective strategies for neurodegeneration may have been entirely novel. The precise mix of concepts discussed, however, may have been entirely unique. Perhaps, by analogy, such a productive mix of ideas serves as a fitting justification for the development of neuroprotective therapies from innovative combinations of nutraceutical and pharmaceutical compounds.

REFERENCES

1. ONO, K., K. HASEGAWA, H. NAIKI & M. YAMADA. 2004. Curcumin has potent anti-amyloidogenic effects for Alzheimer's β-amyloid fibrils in vitro. J. Neurosci. Res. **75:** 742–750.
2. HOWITZ, K.T. *et al.* 2003. Small molecule activators of sirtuins extend *Saccharomyces cerevisiae* lifespan. Nature **425:** 191–196.
3. FRISO, S. & S.W. CHOI. 2002. Gene-nutrient interactions and DNA methylation. J. Nutr. **132:** 2382S–2387S.
4. GOLDBERG, B., H.B. URNOVITZ & R.B. STRICKER. 2000. Beyond danger: unmethylated CpG dinucleotides and the immunopathogenesis of disease. Immunol. Lett. **73:** 13–18.

5. MATTSON, M.P. 2003. Gene-diet interactions in brain aging and neurodegenerative disorders. Ann. Intern. Med. **139:** 441–444.
6. KURTZ, J. & K. FRANZ. 2003. Innate defence: evidence for memory in invertebrate immunity. Nature **425:** 37–38.
7. SCHWAB, J.M., K. SEID & H.J. SCHLUESENER. 2001. Traumatic brain injury induces prolonged accumulation of cyclooxygenase-1 expressing microglia/brain macrophages in rats. J. Neurotrauma **18:** 881–890.
8. LING, Z.D. *et al.* 2004. Combined toxicity of prenatal bacterial endotoxin exposure and postnatal 6-hydroxydopamine in the adult rat midbrain. Neuroscience **124:** 619–628.
9. LUE, L.F. *et al.* 2001. Inflammatory repertoire of Alzheimer's disease and nondemented elderly microglia in vitro. Glia **35:** 72–79.

Index of Contributors

Anantharam, V., 271–289

Babusikova, E., 21–33
Barger, S.W., 133–146, 350–353
Begum, A., 68–84
Bondy, S.C., 197–215, 216–230
Bush, A.I., 34–48

Callier, S., 231–249
Campbell, A., 117–132, 197–215
Chan, S.L., 290–315
Charriez, C.M., 316–334
Chen, D., 216–230
Cole, G.M., 68–84

Dobrota, D., 21–33

Eder, P., 34–48

Fisk, L., 1–20, 21–33
Frautschy, S.A., 68–84

Giordano, T., 34–48, 290–315
Greig, N.H., 34–48, 216–230, 290–315
Guseva, M.V., 316–334

Kanthasamy, A., 271–289
Kanthasamy, A.G., 271–289
Kellaway, L.A., 147–164
Kitazawa, M., 85–103, 271–289
Kochkina, E.G., 21–33
Kotwal, G.J., 147–164, 165–178
Kulkarni, A.P., 147–164

LaFerla, F.M., 85–103
Lahiri, D.K., ix–xiii, 34–48, 147–164,
    165–178, 197–215, 216–230, 290–
    315
Lahiri, P., 216–230
Latchoumycandane, C., 271–289

Lim, G.P., 68–84

Mattson, M.P., 290–315
McGeer, E.G., 104–116
McGeer, P.L., 104–116
Mengsheng, Q., 165–178
Morassutti, D.J., 165–178
Moret, F., 231–249
Morihara, T., 68–84
Moussa, C.E-H., 250–270

Nalivaeva, N.N., 1–20, 21–33

Ovadia, H., 290–315

Pappolla, M.A., 179–196
Pauly, J.R., 316–334
Perreau, V.M., 197–215
Perry, T.A., 290–315
Plesneva, S.A., 21–33

Qing, H., 49–67

Reinhard, J.F., Jr., 335–349
Reiter, R.J., 179–196
Reynolds, D.N., 165–178
Rogers, J.T., 34–48, 216–230, 290–315

Sambamurti, K., 290–315
Scheff, S.W., 316–334
Sharman, E.H., 197–215
Sharman, K.Z., 197–215
Shields, C.B., 165–178
Sidhu, A., 231–249, 250–270
Smith, S.A., 165–178
Snapyan, M., 231–249
Song, W., 49–67

Tan, D.-X., 179–196
Tong, Y., 49–67

Turner, A.J., 1–20, 21–33

Venti, A., 34–48
Vernier, P., 231–249, 250–270

Wersinger, C., 231–249, 250–270
Wu, S., 133–146

Yamasaki, T.R., 85–103
Yang, F., 68–84

Zhang, Y.P., 165–178
Zhou, J., 197–215
Zhou, W., 49–67
Zhuravin, I.A., 21–33